# COMBAT CASUALTY CARE
## *Lessons Learned from OEF and OIF*

**Edited by**
Eric Savitsky, MD
Colonel Brian Eastridge, MD

Pelagique, LLC
Los Angeles, California

University of California at Los Angeles
Los Angeles, California

Office of The Surgeon General
United States Army, Falls Church, Virginia

AMEDD Center & School
Fort Sam Houston, Texas

Borden Institute
Fort Detrick, Maryland

# COMBAT CASUALTY CARE
## *Lessons Learned from OEF and OIF*

**Published by the**
Office of the Surgeon General
Department of the Army, United States of America

*Editor in Chief*
Martha K. Lenhart, MD, PhD
Colonel, MC, US Army
Director, Borden Institute
Assistant Professor of Surgery
F. Edward Hébert School of Medicine
Uniformed Services University of the Health Sciences

*Medical Content Editor*
Eric Savitsky, MD
UCLA Professor of Emergency Medicine/Pediatric Emergency Medicine
Executive Director, UCLA Center for International Medicine
Director, UCLA EMC Trauma Services and Education

*Military Editor*
Brian Eastridge, MD, FACS
Colonel, MC, US Army
Trauma and Surgical Critical Care
Director, Joint Trauma System Program
Trauma Consultant, US Army Surgeon General

For sale by the Superintendent of Documents, U.S. Government Printing Office
Internet: bookstore.gpo.gov   Phone: toll free (866) 512-1800;   DC area (202) 512-1800
Fax: (202) 512-2104 Mail: Stop IDCC, Washington, DC 20402-0001

ISBN 978-0-16-091390-7

# COMBAT CASUALTY CARE
## *Lessons Learned from OEF and OIF*

**Editors**
Eric Savitsky, MD
Colonel Brian Eastridge, MD

**Associate Editors**
Dan Katz, MD
Richelle Cooper, MD

Office of The Surgeon General
United States Army
Falls Church, Virginia

AMEDD Center & School
Fort Sam Houston, Texas

Borden Institute
Fort Detrick, Maryland

2012

**Editorial Staff:**

**BORDEN INSTITUTE**
Vivian Mason
*Technical Editor*

Douglas Wise
*Senior Layout Editor*

Bruce Maston
*Visual Information Specialist*

**PELAGIQUE, LLC**
Dan Katz, MD
*Associate Medical Editor*

**UCLA**
Richelle Cooper, MD
*Research Methodology Editor*

**PELAGIQUE, LLC**
Nicole Durden, MPP
*Digital Media Editor*

**PELAGIQUE, LLC**
Koren Bertolli, MIA
*Copy Editor*

This volume was prepared for military medical educational use. The focus of the information is to foster discussion that may form the basis of doctrine and policy. The opinions or assertions contained herein are the private views of the authors and are not to be construed as official or as reflecting the views of the Department of the Army or the Department of Defense.

**Dosage Selection:**
The authors and publisher have made every effort to ensure the accuracy of dosages cited herein.
However, it is the responsibility of every practitioner to consult appropriate information sources to ascertain correct dosages for each clinical situation, especially for new or unfamiliar drugs and procedures. The authors, editors, publisher, and the Department of Defense cannot be held responsible for any errors found in this book.

**Use of Trade or Brand Names:**
Use of trade or brand names in this publication is for illustrative purposes only and does not imply endorsement by the Department of Defense.

**Neutral Language:**
Unless this publication states otherwise, masculine nouns and pronouns do not refer exclusively to men.

Published by the Office of The Surgeon General
Borden Institute
Fort Detrick, MD 21702-5000

**Library of Congress Cataloging-in-Publication Data**

Combat casualty care : lessons learned from OEF and OIF / editor-in-chief, Martha K. Lenhart; medical editor, Eric Savitsky; military editor, Brian Eastridge.
    p. ; cm.
    Includes bibliographical references and index.
    I. Lenhart, Martha K. II. Savitsky, Eric. III. Eastridge, Brian. IV. United States. Dept. of the Army. Office of the Surgeon General. V. Borden Institute (U.S.)
    [DNLM: 1. Military Medicine--methods. 2. Wounds and Injuries--surgery. 3. Afghan Campaign 2001-. 4. Iraq War, 2003-2011. 5. War. WO 800]

    616.9'8023--dc23

                2011032530

PRINTED IN THE UNITED STATES OF AMERICA
19, 18, 17, 16, 15, 14        5 4 3 2

# Contents

# Contributors

Rocco A. Armonda, MD, LTC, MC, US Army
Kenneth S. Azarow, MD, FACS, FAAP, COL (Ret), MC, US Army
Alec C. Beekley, MD, FACS, LTC, MC, US Army
Randy Bell, MD
John Belperio, MD
Lorne H. Blackbourne, MD, COL, MC, US Army
Harold Bohman, MD, CAPT, MC, US Navy
Sidney B. Brevard, MD, MPH, FACS, COL, US Air Force
Frank K. Butler, MD, FACS, CAPT (Ret), US Navy
Leopoldo C. Cancio, MD, FACS, COL, MC, US Army
Howard Champion, MD, FRCS, FACS
Raymond I. Cho, MD, LTC, MC, US Army
William P. Cranston, PA, CPT, SP, US Army
Henry Cryer, MD
Robert A. De Lorenzo, MD, MSM, FACEP, COL, US Army
Brian J. Eastridge, MD, COL, MC, US Army
James R. Ficke, MD, COL, MC, US Army
Gelareh Gabayan, MD
Robert T. Gerhardt, MD, MPH, FACEP, FAAEM, LTC, US Army
Robert G. Hale, DDS, COL, US Army
David K. Hayes, MD, COL, US Army
John Hiatt, MD
Jay Johannigman, MD, COL, US Air Force Reserve
Dan Katz, MD
Jess M. Kirby, MD, MAJ, MC, US Army
John F. Kragh, Jr., MD, COL, MC, US Army
Geoffrey S. F. Ling, MD, PhD, COL, US Army
Robert L. Mabry, MD, FACEP, MAJ(P), US Army
Swaminatha Mahadevan, MD
Scott A. Marshall, MD
Jonathan Martin, MD
Phillip Mason, MD, MAJ, US Air Force
Alan Murdock, MD, LTC, US Air Force
David Norton, MD, LTC, MC, US Air Force
George Orloff, MD
Jeremy G. Perkins, MD, FACP, LTC, MC, US Army
Kyle Peterson, DO, CDR, US Navy
David B. Powers, DMD, MD, COL, US Air Force
Todd Rasmussen, MD, LTC, US Air Force
Evan M. Renz, MD, FACS, LTC(P), MC, US Army
Eric Savitsky, MD
Danielle Schindler, MD
Philip C. Spinella, MD
Areti Tillou, MD, MsED, FACS
Raymond F. Topp, MD, LTC, MC, US Army
Lee Ann Young, BSME, MA

# Photo Contributors

We thank the following individuals and organizations for providing some of the images used in this book.

American Academy of Neurology Practice Parameter on
  Management of Concussions
Applied Research Associates, Inc.
Harold Bohman, MD, CAPT, MC, US Navy
Borden Institute, Office of The Surgeon General,
  Washington, DC
David Burris, MD, COL, MC, US Army
Leopoldo C. Cancio, MD, FACS, COL, MC, US Army
David Carmack, MD
Center for Sustainment of Trauma and Readiness Skills
  (C-STARS)
Combat Medical Systems™
Composite Resources, Inc.
Subrato Deb, MD, CDR
Defense Imagery Management Operations Center (DIMOC)
Defense-Update.com
Delfi Medical Innovations, Inc.
Robert H. Demling, MD, Harvard Medical School
DJO, LLC
Brian J. Eastridge, MD, FACS, COL, US Army
Elsevier
James R. Ficke, MD, COL, MC, US Army
J. Christian Fox, MD, University of California–Irvine
Aletta Frazier, MD, Illustrator
GlobalSecurity.org
Mitchell Goff, MD
Tamer Goksel, DDS, MD, COL, US Army
Chris Gralapp, Illustrator
Robert R. Granville, MD, COL, MC, US Army
Kurt W. Grathwohl, MD, COL, MC, US Army
Timothy Hain, MD, Northwestern University
Robert G. Hale, DDS, COL, US Army
John B. Holcomb, MD, COL (Ret), MC, US Army
iCasualties.org
Joint Combat Trauma Management Course, 2007
Joint Theater Trauma Registry
Joint Theater Trauma Systems Program, US Army Institute
  of Surgical Research
Dan Katz, MD
Glenn J. Kerr, MD, MAJ, MC, US Army
John F. Kragh, Jr., MD, COL, MC, US Army
Donald C. Kowalewski, LTC, MC, US Air Force
LearningRadiology.com
Gene Liu, MD, Cedars-Sinai Medical Center
Michael Shaun Machen, MD, COL, MC, US Army
Swaminatha V. Mahadevan, MD, Stanford University
Jonathan Martin, MD, Connecticut Children's Medical
  Center
Massachusetts Medical Society
Bruce Maston, Illustrator
Alan Murdock, MD, LTC, US Air Force
Juan D. Nava, Medical Illustrator, Brooke Army Medical
  Center

Joel Nichols, MD
North American Rescue, LLC
David Norton, MD, LTC, MC, US Air Force
Pelagique, LLC
Pelvic Binder, Inc.
David B. Powers, DMD, MD, COL, US Air Force
Rady Rahban, MD
Todd Rasmussen, MD, LTC, US Air Force
Reichert Technologies
Evan M. Renz, MD, FACS, LTC(P), MC, US Army
Jessica Shull, Illustrator
Philip C. Spinella, MD
Stryker Instruments
Raymond F. Topp, MD, LTC, MC, US Army
Trauma.org
UCLA Center for International Medicine
United Nations Mine Action Service
University of Michigan Kellogg Eye Center
Eric D. Weichel, MD
Wikimedia Commons

# Acknowledgments

We extend our gratitude to Robert (Bob) Foster, Director of Biosystems (Ret), Office of the Director, Defense Research and Engineering; and Colonel (Ret) John Holcomb for their vision and guidance in support of this project.

This educational effort was made possible through the Defense Health Program Small Business Innovation Research (SBIR) Program and Telemedicine and Advanced Technology and Research Center (TATRC).

A special thanks to Colonel Lorne Blackbourne (USAISR), Colonel Karl Friedl (TATRC), and Jessica Kenyon (TATRC) for their support and guidance throughout this effort.

# Preface

To enhance combat casualty care (CCC) pre-deployment education for all healthcare providers, this contemporary educational program was developed through the Small Business Innovative Research Program in partnership with civilian industry and the Office of the Secretary of Defense for Health Affairs. This military medicine textbook is designed to deliver CCC information that will facilitate transition from a continental United States (CONUS) or civilian practice to the combat care environment. Establishment of the Joint Theater Trauma System (JTTS) and the Joint Theater Trauma Registry (JTTR), coupled with the efforts of the authors, has resulted in the creation of the most comprehensive, evidence-based depiction of the latest advances in CCC.

Lessons learned in Operation Enduring Freedom (OEF) and Operation Iraqi Freedom (OIF) have been fortified with evidence-based recommendations with the intent of improving casualty care. The chapters specifically discuss differences between CCC and civilian sector care, particularly in the scheme of "echelonized" care. Overall, the educational curriculum was designed to address the leading causes of preventable death and disability in OEF and OIF. Specifically, the generalist CCC provider is presented requisite information for optimal care of US combat casualties in the first 72 to 96 hours after injury. The specialist CCC provider is afforded similar information, which is supplemented by lessons learned for definitive care of host nation patients.

These thirteen peer-reviewed and well-referenced chapters were authored by military subject matter experts with extensive hands-on experience providing CCC during the course of OEF and OIF, and were edited by an experienced team of physicians and research methodologists. Together they will provide readers with a solid understanding of the latest advances in OEF and OIF CCC. This information provides an excellent supplement to pre-deployment CCC training and education. Ideally, readers will aptly apply the newly acquired knowledge toward improving CCC.

Eric Savitsky, MD
UCLA Professor of Emergency Medicine/Pediatric Emergency Medicine
Executive Director, UCLA Center for International Medicine
Director, UCLA EMC Trauma Services and Education

Los Angeles, CA
June 2011

# Prologue

*"War is Hell."* — William Tecumseh Sherman

The battlefield will challenge your medical skills, knowledge, personal courage, and perseverance. However, in the end, you and the Wounded Warrior will be better for it.

It is 0200. You are on a forward operating base in the high desert somewhere in southwest Asia. The radio in the TOC (Tactical Operations Center) crackles to life, breaking the silence of the night:

> This is Whiskey … Foxtrot … Tango … Niner. Inbound in six mikes with two urgent surgicals from an IED. Requesting a hot offload … TIC in progress … more casualties to pick up. … Over.

Outside of the resuscitation area, over the whisper of the cold wind, you hear the whir of the rotor blades of the approaching MEDEVAC Blackhawks. Setting down on the landing zone with a deafening roar, all you can see is the static electrical discharge from the spinning rotors. Appearing from the darkness are wheeled litter carriers bearing casualties and teams of attendants racing alongside. Now, it's your turn. This is our calling, the reason we are here … for the Warrior. The content of this book was composed for you by those who have "been in your boots."

Similar situations have played out over 47,000 times for US military combat casualties. Survival from injury on the modern battlefield is unprecedented; the current case fatality rate is 11%. This is even more astonishing, considering the complexity of injury and evacuation of casualties through multiple levels of care across the globe. Throughout history, armed conflict has shaped advances in medicine and surgery. These conflicts are no different. However, with the progress of technology and communication, we are better able to potentiate and disseminate recent lessons learned.

The paradigm of tactical combat casualty care has dramatically altered pre-hospital management of the combat casualty. Tourniquets have saved countless lives. The novel concept of damage control resuscitation was born on these battlefields and has reduced the mortality rate of casualties requiring massive transfusion from 40% to less than 20%. The Joint Theater Trauma System (JTTS) was implemented to enhance injury care performance and to improve provider communication and dissemination of lessons learned across the vast continuum of care. Efforts of the trauma system have lead to the development of more than 30 evidence-based battlefield relevant clinical practice guidelines, and decreased morbidity and mortality from combat injury.

The legacy of this conflict will not only be what we have learned, but also how rapidly we were able to disseminate, educate, and change practice on the battlefield in nearly "real-time," and to translate many combat lessons learned into trauma care in the civilian environment. This text is a natural complement of our efforts contributing to evolution of casualty care on the battlefield.

Brian Eastridge, MD, FACS
Colonel, MC, US Army
Trauma Consultant, US Army Surgeon General

San Antonio, TX
June 2011

# MODERN WARFARE

## *Chapter 1*

**Contributing Authors**
Alec C. Beekley, MD, FACS, LTC, MC, US Army
Harold Bohman, MD, CAPT, MC, US Navy
Danielle Schindler, MD

# Table of Contents

# Introduction

War has historically provided an opportunity for medical advancement and innovation. Military medical personnel face the challenge of managing a high volume of severe multisystem injuries, relative to what is encountered in civilian practice. Combat casualty care (CCC) providers face injury and illness in the context of an austere wartime environment, in which transport times may be unpredictable and supplies and staff limited. The frequency of multiple or mass casualties may overwhelm available resources. In addition, CCC providers not only care for injured members of the military, but for injuries and illnesses suffered by the local population and enemy combatants (Fig. 1).

Such challenges have fostered innovation in all aspects of CCC. Since 2001, significant changes including the organization of medical teams, new resuscitation practices, new technologies, and changes in evacuation strategies have been implemented. The creation of a database of all military casualties from the current conflicts in Iraq and Afghanistan, known as the Joint Theater Trauma Registry (JTTR), has allowed for an unprecedented level of analysis of wartime injuries

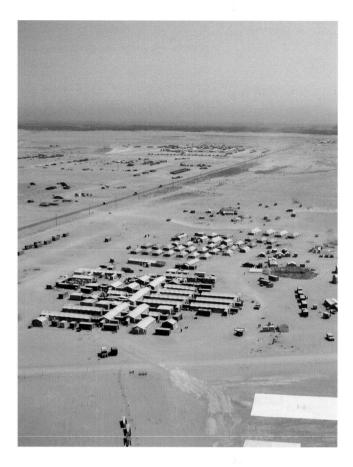

Figure 1. *Level III Combat Support Hospital. Image courtesy of the Borden Institute, Office of The Surgeon General, Washington, DC.*

and deaths. Such analysis has been used to identify potentially preventable causes of death and paved the way for implementation of new technologies and practices targeted towards reduction of morbidity and mortality from combat.[1,2]

> Combat casualty care providers face multiple challenges in wartime including an austere environment, limited supplies or staff, multiple-casualty-incidents, and caring for the local population or enemy combatants.

Comparing Operation Enduring Freedom (OEF) and Operation Iraqi Freedom (OIF) to Vietnam, the mortality rate of combat-sustained injury has decreased by nearly half.[1] The survival rate in these conflicts exceeds 90 percent, which is higher than prior conflicts.[3,4] Wounding patterns in OEF/OIF differ from that of previous conflicts (World War II, Korea, Vietnam, and the Persian Gulf War), which had a higher proportion of thoracic injuries and fewer head and neck injuries.[5,6,7,8,9] There has been a decreased incidence of wounds to the abdomen since the Persian Gulf War.[10] The percentage of blast-related injuries is now higher.[9]

The resources and evacuation systems used to treat casualties have seen substantial improvements since the prior conflicts. A special emphasis has been placed upon identifying wounding patterns, adverse outcomes, and preventable deaths.[9,11,12,13,14] Improvements in body armor, military tactics, and the ability to respond quickly and effectively to trauma in a combat environment has led to dramatic improvements in morbidity and mortality.[1,13]

## Lessons Learned - Know Your Environment

The following is an experience of a general surgeon during an early deployment:

*I was assigned to a Forward Surgical Team (FST) that took us two hours driving south of Baghdad to reach by ground vehicle. It was my first time there; I was nervous about convoys, because we were driving through a heavily attacked route; and my intern classmate (a general surgeon) had been killed on an FST three weeks before I left for Iraq. Needless to say, my mind really wasn't on how far we were from the nearest Combat Support Hospital (CSH), what the evacuation times were, or even how far we were actually driving (we were going very slowly, stopping and starting a lot). So when we arrived at our FST site, it felt like we had come a long way to get there. On my prior FST experience in Afghanistan, our FST was two and one-half hours by fixed-wing aircraft to the nearest CSH.*

*It turns out that we were only about 15 minutes by helicopter from the CSH. I assumed that we were much farther away. The proximity to more robust hospital support clearly makes a difference regarding how you triage multiple patients and what kind of operations you undertake. Nobody had oriented me to this, and at the time I didn't think to ask. I was at the FST 17 days before our first casualties arrived. There were four wounded casualties from an improvised explosive device (IED) attack. So here I am, three years out of residency, used to taking calls two to four times a month at a relatively slow Level II trauma center. I had performed maybe four or five blunt trauma-related operations in that period, and only a few penetrating trauma cases from Afghanistan. Now I had to simultaneously care for four wounded, multisystem trauma patients with one other surgeon, who was less than a year out of residency.*

*We actually thought we did okay. One guy had an abdominal fragment wound but was stable and had a negative focused assessment with sonography in trauma (FAST). Two of the guys had extremity wounds and fractures, but were able to be splinted and were not hemorrhaging. One guy, however, had a systolic blood pressure (SBP) of 70 mm Hg, an inadequate improvised tourniquet on his leg, and open femur, tibial, and fibular fractures. He also had an injury to his distal superficial femoral artery. We spent some time getting proximal control in the groin, then dissecting out his artery through his huge, hematoma-laden, torn and distorted thigh, and putting in a temporary vascular shunt. We transfused him most of our blood bank of 20 units of red blood cells (RBCs). He was hemodynamically stabilized. He was cold, slightly acidemic, and coagulopathic when he left, but we had restored flow to his foot.*

*Sorting out all these casualties took us maybe one and one-half hours. We finally got them on a helicopter and on their way about two hours after they arrived to us. When they arrived to the CSH, the patient with the vascular injury had clotted off his shunt. He went back to the operating room (OR) at the CSH and was revascularized, but had too much ischemia time and ended up losing his leg.*

*When the trauma consultant to the Surgeon General came to visit us at the FST a few weeks later, he noted that it took him 17 minutes by slow-flying helicopter to get there from the CSH. As I reviewed the case with him, we realized that rather than a vascular shunt, which ended up being harder than it sounded and cost us a lot of blood products and time, we could have simply applied secure tourniquets to this guy, resuscitated him, and sent him on his way to the CSH. He would have reached a facility with vascular surgery support, robust blood bank and critical care services, and everything else he needed within an hour.*

*Dr. Alec Beekley, LTC*
*United States Army Medical Corps*

Upon arriving at your area of deployment, get to know your CCC environment and resources. Rapid evacuation to a higher level of care may be the best contribution you provide to a casualty (Fig. 2). In some Combat Support Hospitals, specialists from trauma surgery, orthopedics, vascular surgery, ophthalmology, and critical care are available. Knowing the approximate evacuation time to a higher level of care may change critical decisions of whether to operate on a critically injured patient who will ultimately need transfer, or whether to transport immediately. What is the nearest Combat Support Hospital? How can transport be arranged? What is the fastest method of transport and expected transport time? How many critically-injured patients is your unit prepared to handle? If this number is exceeded, casualties who would otherwise stay for operative intervention may instead need to be transferred.

Know your CCC environment and recognize your resources and limitations.

The nature of war is that it is unpredictable. In civilian surgical practice, although the number and acuity of patients ebbs and flows, rarely is full capacity exceeded. In civilian urban settings, most injured patients are only 15 to 20 minutes from a Level I or II trauma center, and mass casualties are uncommon. In a combat environment, multiple-casualty-incidents are quite common (Fig. 3). The most common causes of injuries, explosions or exchanges of gunfire, are likely to create several casualties at once. Time to reach medical care may vary drastically not only by location, but by the tactical situation (i.e., ability to safely evacuate a casualty from a combat area without excessive endangerment of others).

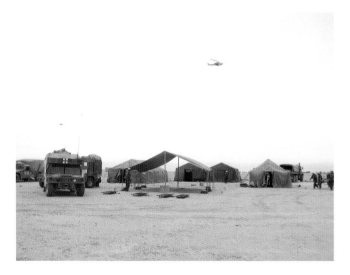

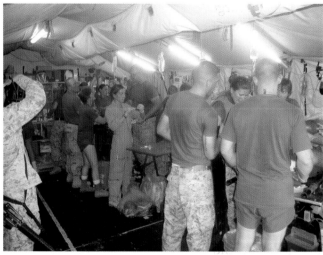

Figure 2. *Level II FRSS-6/STP-7 in Southern Iraq in March, 2003.*

Figure 3. *Initial evaluation and resuscitation during a multiple-casualty-incident occurring at the Surgical Shock Trauma Platoon (SSTP) at Camp Taqaddum, Iraq 2006.*

Although Level III Combat Support Hospitals are well equipped with trauma specialists, blood banks, and multiple operating tables, many casualties first present to smaller, mobile medical and surgical units, such as Army Forward Surgical Teams (FSTs) or Marine Corps Forward Resuscitative Surgical System (FRSS) teams. Critical decisions on whether and when to intervene and when to transport critically ill casualties are made in these smaller mobile facilities (Table 1). These decisions will change with every new location, and even hour-by-hour with the availability of personnel, equipment, and transport. It is critical to know, to the best extent possible, what is occurring on the battlefield to prepare for the arrival of casualties. The chief surgeon or surgeon-of-the-day is usually the ultimate clinical decision maker and manages the clinical function of the unit and its resources. Attention to details, situational awareness of both internal and external conditions and good communication with the team are essential.

| Service | Level II Facilities |
|---------|---------------------|
| Air Force | Mobile Field Surgical Team (MFST)<br>Expeditionary Medical Support (EMEDS) |
| Army | Level II Medical Treatment Facility (MTF)<br>Forward Surgical Team (FST) |
| Marine Corps | Forward Resuscitative Surgical System (FRSS) |
| Navy | Casualty Receiving and Treatment Ships (CRTS) |

Table 1. *Level II treatment facilities with surgical capabilities according to military service branch. Adapted from Rasmussen, 2006.*[76]

All surgeons at forward surgical facilities need to have situational awareness that extends beyond taking care of patients in the operating room. The factors outlined in Table 2 are critical to optimal decision making.

Physicians in wartime are rarely fully prepared to treat combat-related injuries on their initial deployment. Explosive injuries comprise the majority of severe combat-related injuries (Fig. 4).[9,13] In peacetime, even experienced surgeons rarely encounter injuries from explosions. Explosions combine primary blast, blunt, and penetrating mechanisms to create multisystem, high-energy injuries with extensive soft-tissue damage, wound contamination, and hemorrhage from multiple sites. In addition to encountering unfamiliar injury patterns, newly deployed physicians must also learn a new medical system, with policies and logistics far different from the civilian sector. While standards of medical care remain the same, physicians are challenged to meet these standards in a new and often stressful environment.

> Physicians in wartime are rarely fully prepared to treat combat-related injuries on their initial deployment. Unfamiliar injury patterns, such as explosive injuries, and a new medical system with policies and logistics differing from the civilian sector contribute to a unique and often stressful environment. Rehearsing scenarios of care may prove beneficial to newly deployed careproviders.

Because time and circumstance may not afford a thorough orientation, it is critical to ask questions, learn from those with experience, and become familiar with available resources before the arrival of your first critically-injured patient. Care of the severely-injured combat casualty requires a team effort, and with

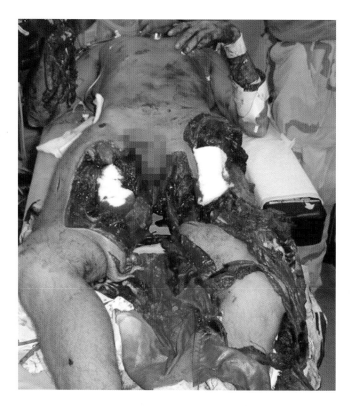

Figure 4. (Left) *US serviceman injured by a large mortar round explosion, with traumatic amputation of the right hand, near amputation of the left leg, and extensive soft-tissue wounds to the right leg. Image courtesy of the Borden Institute, Office of The Surgeon General, Washington, DC.*

Figure 5. (Below) *FRSS patient care team at Forward Operating Base St. Michael outside Mahmudiyah, Iraq in March 2004.*

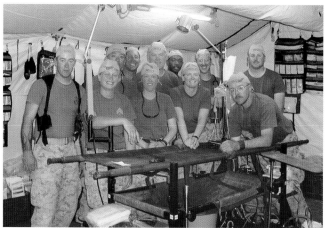

## FORWARD SURGERY - LESSONS LEARNED

| Triage Issues | Situational Awareness |
|---|---|
| • Triage Officer responsible for: <br>   • Clinical function of facility <br>     -Ultimate clinical decision maker <br>     -Status of all casualties <br>     -Consider tactical situation <br>   • Management of available resources <br>     -Personnel, supplies, ORs, blood bank <br>     -Control of walking blood bank <br>   • Initial triage of arriving casualty groups <br>   • Evacuation priorities | • Internal <br>   • Status personnel/supplies <br>   • Number and physiologic status of casualties <br>   • OR availability <br>   • Blood products <br>   • En-route-care capability <br> • External <br>   • Evacuation assets <br>   • Time/distance to facility with resources to provide appropriate care <br>   • Weather conditions <br>   • Tactical situation |

Table 2. *Forward Surgery - Lessons Learned.*

every team there is a learning curve. An important lesson learned from Forward Surgical Teams has been that teams need to rehearse scenarios of caring for multiple casualties before the first true casualties arrive (Fig. 5). This is extremely critical to improving the skills of corpsman, medics, and nurses unfamiliar with the care of critically-injured patients, and in improving the efficiency of physicians and the team. An open, critical, and nonjudgmental review after every major casualty incident, a "hot wash," has been found to improve the performance of Forward Surgical Teams.[15]

# Joint Theater Trauma Registry (JTTR)

The civilian trauma systems and practice patterns in place today have emerged largely from the lessons learned during wartime. Military medicine has been the driving force behind many of the major advancements in trauma care. In the Civil War, the concept of a field hospital emerged, as did the link between treatment time and survival rates. In World War I, blood banks and the use of blood transfusions were developed. In World War II, antibiotics were put into widespread use, and the triage system was used to prioritize casualty evacuations.[16] The Korean War brought the development of Mobile Army Surgical Hospital (MASH) units, and with Vietnam, improvements were made in rapid evacuation systems with helicopters.[16,17]

Combat casualty care providers must use the lessons learned from wartime to improve subsequent patient care. The military medical system is capable of adopting new changes more quickly and efficiently than is the civilian sector, and the large number of severe injuries seen in a relatively short span of time allows for rapid evaluation of new innovations.

With the aim of improving CCC, the US Army established the Joint Theater Trauma System (JTTS) in 2004 to oversee the organization of medical facilities and resources as well as aeromedical evacuation systems.[18] Among its many roles, the JTTS has established the Joint Theater Trauma Registry (JTTR), an extensive database of every United States (US) combat casualty.[1] This comprehensive clinical database now contains over 40,000 entries.[19] The JTTR allows for retrospective analysis of the type and severity of combat injuries and the identification of potentially survivable injuries. It is the cornerstone by which performance improvement measures can be developed, implemented, and analyzed.

> With over 40,000 entries, the JTTR has allowed retrospective analysis and actionable research of combat injuries.

Data from medical charts, hospital records, transport records, and elsewhere are gathered, reviewed, and coded by a team of nurses and coders (Figs. 6 and 7). This allows for an unprecedented amount of medical data to be collected on US casualties. Important epidemiological questions, such as what is the rate of primary amputation or what is the percentage of thoracic injury with and without body armor, can now be answered. Moreover, the JTTR allows for analysis of changes that have been implemented, such as: are decreased transport times from the battlefield to medical aid associated with an improvement in survival, or does the rate of uncontrolled hemorrhage upon arrival to the hospital decrease with an increase in tourniquet use?

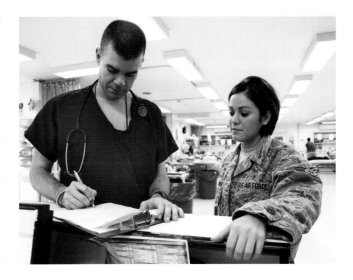

Figure 6. *An unprecedented amount of information is collected on US casualties allowing retrospective analysis and actionable research. Image courtesy of Defense Imagery Management Operations Center (DIMOC).*

## PHYSICIAN TRAUMA ADMITTING RECORD (Theater Hospitalization Capability) - Previously Level 3

**(All shaded areas mandatory for Joint Theater Trauma Registry data collection)**

DATE: _____

**VITAL SIGNS**

TIME OF INJURY: _____

TIME OF ARRIVAL: _____ T____ P____ R___ BP __/__ O2 Sat ___

LOCATION OF PRE-HOSP. CARE: _____

**TRIAGE CATEGORY**
- ☐ Immediate
- ☐ Minimal
- ☐ Delayed
- ☐ Expectant

### HISTORY & PHYSICAL

**INJURY DESCRIPTION**

(AB)rasion
(AMP)utation
(AV)ulsion
(BL)eeding
(B)urn %TBSA_____
(C)repitus
(D)eformity
(DG)Degloving
(E)cchymosis
(FX)Fracture
(F)oreign Body
(GSW)Gun Shot Wound
(H)ematoma
(LAC)eration
(PW)Puncture Wound
(SS)Seatbelt Sign

R          L          L          R

ANTERIOR          POSTERIOR

**Pulses Present:**
S= Strong
W= Weak
D= Doppler
A=Absent

**HISTORY AND PRESENTING ILLNESS:** _____

### MECHANISM OF INJURY

- ☐ Assault/Fight
- ☐ Biological
- ☐ Blast/Explosion
- ☐ Blunt Trauma
- ☐ Bomb
- ☐ Building Collapse
- ☐ Burn
- ☐ Chemical
- ☐ Crush
- ☐ Drowning
- ☐ Fall
- ☐ Flying Debris
- ☐ Grenade
- ☐ GSW/Bullet
- ☐ Helo Crash
- ☐ Hot Obj/Liquid
- ☐ IED
- ☐ Knife/Edge
- ☐ Landmine
- ☐ Machinery
- ☐ Mortar
- ☐ Multi-frag
- ☐ MVC
- ☐ Plane Crash
- ☐ Rad/Nuclear
- ☐ Single Frag
- ☐ UXO
- ☐ Other _____

### CARE DONE PRIOR TO ARRIVAL

Pre-hospital Airway: ☐ no ☐ yes

Pre-hosp. Tourniquet : ☐ no ☐ yes Type: ____ TIME On:____ Off:____

Pre-hosp. Chest Tube: ☐ no ☐ yes R L (circle as applicable)

Temp Control Measure: ☐ no ☐ yes Type: ☐ body bag ☐ other

Intraosseous Access: ☐ no ☐ yes

### HISTORY & PHYSICAL

**Head & Neck:**

**Tymp Membranes**
Clear R ☐ L ☐
Blood R ☐ L ☐

**Chest:**

**Abdomen:**

**Pelvis:** ☐ Stable ☐ Unstable

**Upper Extremities:**

**Lower extremities:**

**Neuro:** GCS:_____
E __/4 M __/6 V __/5
C-Spine Tender
☐ Yes ☐ No

**Motor Deficit:**
None
R UE/LE
L UE/LE

**Skin:** Burn: 1st 2nd 3rd %TBSA

**Vision: Pupils** R L
Brisk ☐ ☐
Sluggish ☐ ☐
NR ☐ ☐
Hand Motion ☐ ☐
Light Perception ☐ ☐
No Light Perception ☐ ☐
Size ___ mm ___ mm

### INITIAL PROCEDURES / DIAGNOSTICS

- ☐ C-Collar
- ☐ Airway (oral/ nasal)
- ☐ Chest tube R ☐ L ☐ Output
- ☐ Needle decompression R ☐ L ☐ Output:
- ☐ Pericardiocentesis
- ☐ Intubate
- ☐ CRIC
- ☐ Thoracotomy
- Canthotomy (circle L/R)
- Cantholysis (circle L/R)
- Blood: mls ____ ☐ Air
- ☐ Blood: mls _____ ☐ Air

Rectal Exam
Tone_____
Gross Blood +/-
Prostate_____
GYN_____
- ☐ FAST
- ☐ DPL
- ☐ NG/OG
- ☐ Pelvic Binder
- ☐ Foley

- ☐ Closed Reduction ☐ EXT Fixation
- ☐ Splint ☐ Wound Washout
- ☐ Tourniquet Type CAT / SOFTT / Oth Time On:____ Time Off:____

- ☐ Closed reduction ☐ EXT Fixation
- ☐ Splint ☐ Wound washout
- ☐ Tourniquet Type CAT / SOFTT / Oth Time on:____ Time off:____

- ☐ Sedated
- ☐ Chemically Paralyzed
- ☐ Seizure Protocol
- ☐ Mannitol
- ☐ Intraosseus
- ☐ Central Line
- ☐ A-Line

### HYPO / HYPERTHERMIA CONTROL MEASURES

Beginning Temp _____ Time/date
Ending Temp _____ Time/date
Temperature Control Procedure
- ☐ Bair Hugger
- ☐ Chill Buster
- ☐ Cooling Blanket
- ☐ Fwd Resus Fluid Warmer
- ☐ Body Bag
- ☐ Other _____

### LABORATORY

**CBC**

**CHEMISTRY 7**

**LFT**
Amylase: _____
Alk Phos: _____
LDH: _____
Bili: _____
SGOT: _____
SGPT: _____
Other: _____

**URINALYSIS**
SpGr: _____
pH: _____
Chem: _____
Micro: _____
RBC: _____
WBC: _____
Bact: _____
HCG: _____

**ALLERGIES**
- ☐ NKDA
- ☐ ASA
- ☐ PCN
- ☐ Sulfa
- ☐ Morphine
- ☐ Codeine
- ☐ Latex
- ☐ Other

**PT/ INR/ PTT**
____/____/____

**ABG**
FiO2: _____ VENT:
pH: _____ YES NO
pCO2: _____ ETT Size: ____
pO2: _____
HCO3: _____
Sat: _____
BE: _____

**MEDICATIONS**
- ☐ DT
- ☐ Abx _____
- ☐ Versed
- ☐ Morphine
- ☐ Fentanyl
- ☐ Other:

**IV FLUIDS/BLOOD PRODUCTS**
- ☐ Crystalloids _____ cc's NS LR
- ☐ Colloids _____ cc's
- ☐ PRBC's _____
- ☐ FFP _____ units
- ☐ Whole Bld _____ units
- ☐ Cryo _____ _____ units
- ☐ PLT's _____ packs

**PMH**
- ☐ Unknown ☐ HTN
- ☐ None ☐ DM
- ☐ Cardiac ☐ Ulcer
- ☐ Respiratory ☐ Other
- ☐ Seizure

**Patient NAME/ID:**

Last:                First                MI

SSN/ID                DOB/AGE

**DATE: (dd,mm,yy)**

**MTF transferred from:**

ASD(HA) September 2005 (March 2010 Interim Update)          This Form is Subject to the Privacy Act of 1974          Page 1 of 2

Figure 7. *Joint Theater Trauma Registry Treatment Record (front). Image courtesy of Joint Theater Trauma Systems Program, US Army Institute of Surgical Research.*

By understanding how deaths and injuries occur, investigators are best able to identify potential areas in which survival and other outcomes can be improved. Research by the JTTS and military healthcare providers remains ongoing, resulting in continued improvements in products, techniques, and systems-level aspects of medical care.

## Combat Injury Patterns

Analysis of injury patterns and deaths during OEF and OIF indicates that most combat-related injuries occur as a result of injury from explosions, followed by gunshot wounds.[9,11] Only a small percentage of injuries are related to motor vehicle accidents and other causes. Injury patterns demonstrate that the highest rate of injury is to the extremities, followed by the abdomen, face, and head.[9,11] There is a low rate of thoracic injury, likely due to improvements in body armor.[9, 10,12]

---

Published data from the JTTR database from 2001 to 2005 demonstrated the following casualty data:[9]
- Mechanism of Injury – explosions (78 percent), gunshot wounds (18 percent)
- Injury Distribution –  extremity (54 percent)
  abdomen (11 percent)
  face (10 percent)
  head (8 percent)
  thorax (6 percent)
  eyes (6 percent)
  neck (3 percent)
  ears (3 percent)

---

With extremity injury, there is a high frequency of penetrating soft-tissue injury and associated fractures due to explosive fragments and gunshots (Fig. 8). Accordingly, there is a much higher proportion of open fractures in combat casualties compared to civilian practice.[11,20]

## Causes of Preventable Death

Analysis of JTTR statistics and data from prior conflicts has demonstrated that hemorrhage is by far the leading cause of potentially preventable combat-related death.[13,21] The case fatality rate has decreased significantly since Vietnam, from 16.5 percent to 8.8 percent.[1] The improvements in mortality are due not only to advancements in CCC, but improvements in body armor and rapid evacuation. A large part of the JTTS's mission is to analyze casualties, both wounded and killed, for the purpose of identifying, implementing, and evaluating potential improvements at any point in the medical system from first response to long-term care and rehabilitation.

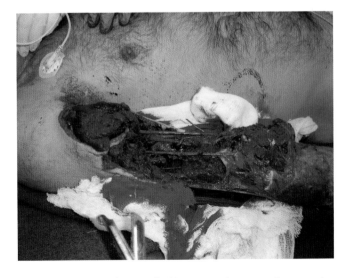

Figure 8. *Fragmentation wound with near complete traumatic amputation of the right arm. The injury was nonsalvageable and required a completion amputation. Image courtesy of CDR Subrato Deb.*

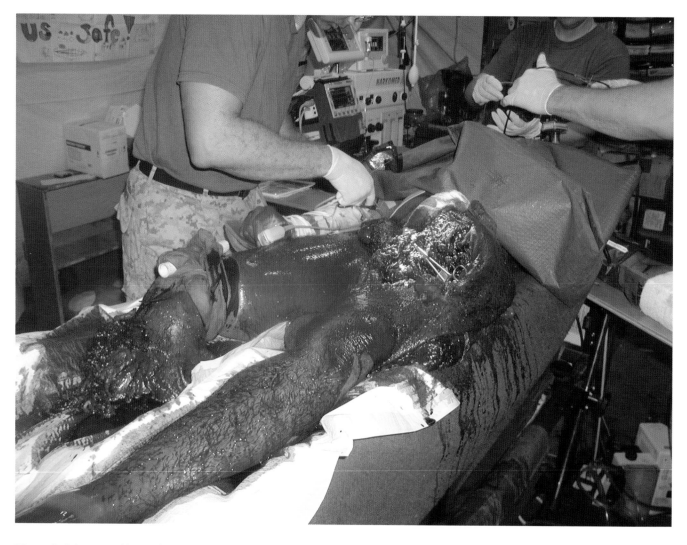

Figure 9. *Injury caused by a rocket-propelled grenade (RPG) resulting in a large through-and-through wound to the left thigh and traumatic amputation of the lower right leg. Note the makeshift tourniquet applied in the field.*

> Hemorrhage, much of which is considered compressible or amenable to tourniquet placement, is the leading cause of preventable combat-related death.

In Vietnam, casualties were described in the Wound Data and Munitions Effectiveness Team (WDMET) database.[22] From an analysis of the Vietnam casualties who ultimately died, but had survived until reaching medical care, a committee of surgeons deemed 8 to 17 percent of the deaths were potentially preventable with modern medical care.[21] The causes of these deaths included severe hemorrhage, burns, pulmonary edema, and sepsis. Furthermore, review of Vietnam data attributes over 2,500 deaths to extremity hemorrhage, which is potentially preventable (Fig. 9).

In the early years of the OEF and OIF (2001 to 2004), up to 15 percent of deaths were deemed potentially survivable. By far, the leading cause of these deaths was uncontrolled hemorrhage (82 percent), much of which was considered compressible or amenable to tourniquet placement.[13] Review of data has shown that over the past several wars (Korea, Vietnam, and the first Persian Gulf War), the killed in action (KIA) rate had not changed significantly.[23,24] The KIA rate refers to the percentage of casualties who die before reaching a medical facility out of all seriously injured casualties, and has been 20 to 25 percent since World War II.[24] In OEF and OIF, the KIA rate has decreased to 13.8 percent. Additionally, the case fatality rate, the percentage of severely wounded casualties who die, has decreased by half since Vietnam.[24] Of those KIA, the most common causes are severe head injury and severe thoracic trauma. However, 9 percent of those KIA die from hemorrhage from extremity wounds, 5 percent from tension pneumothorax, and 1 percent of airway obstruction. This group comprises most of the deaths considered potentially preventable (15 percent of those KIA) and has become the focus of many of the improvements in the medical system. Since many of these fatalities occur within the first couple of hours after injury, large efforts have been made to improve the early medical access and response.

# Advances in Combat Casualty Care

Since the recognition of hemorrhage as the major cause of potentially preventable death, a tremendous effort has been made to improve hemorrhage control and treatment of other survivable injuries. Rapid evacuation, expanded training, improved equipment, and a change in resuscitative and surgical techniques are some of the approaches discussed in greater detail below and in the chapters that follow.

## Advancements in Combat Casualty Care Training

The golden hour and its associated platinum ten minutes of trauma response lies in the hands of first responders. On the battlefield, this is often another soldier, a combat lifesaver, or combat medic. In World War II, Vietnam, and OEF and OIF, the vast majority of combat deaths occur before the casualty reaches a medical facility. [24]

Most medics, physicians and other medical personnel, and all Special Operations Forces (SOF) personnel undergo a Tactical Combat Casualty Care (TCCC) training course. The TCCC course was developed to teach deployed careproviders key elements of lifesaving prehospital medical care.[25] Among the core curriculum, techniques in hemorrhage control, needle thoracostomy, casualty positioning, and even on-site cricothyroidotomy are taught.[25] Tactical Combat Casualty Care was begun by the Naval Special Warfare Command in 1993 and later continued by the US Special Operations Command (USSOCOM). Much of its development came from a 1996 study outlining guidelines for combat care for Special Operations corpsmen and has since been expanded to all branches.[25]

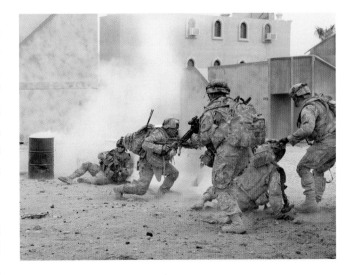

Injury care will often need to be delivered while an area is still under hostile fire, delaying the initial arrival of medical personnel and equipment (Fig. 10). Prior to evacuation, available patient care equipment is limited to what can be carried by the first responder. Equipment such as stethoscopes and

Figure 10. *US soldiers run for cover after a simulated bomb explosion during a casualty evacuation exercise in the mock village of Medina Wasl at the National Training Center (NTC), Fort Irwin, California. Image courtesy of Defense Imagery Management Operations Center (DIMOC).*

blood pressure cuffs are not available, and would not often be useful in a noisy environment. First responders must rely on basic visual and physical examination findings to dictate treatment. Casualty evacuation times are widely variable, ranging from minutes to hours, depending on the tactical situation and resources.

Given these constraints, TCCC training was designed to incorporate several principles that may depart from the standard approach to civilian trauma. These include:

- Cardiopulmonary resuscitation (CPR) is not attempted for a casualty with no signs of life

- Airway management and cervical spine immobilization are delayed until the casualty and rescuer are both removed from hostile fire

- Casualties found unconscious, but breathing, are given a nasopharyngeal airway and placed in the recovery position

- Only the minimal amount of clothing is removed to identify and treat injuries to minimize hypothermia

- Control of bleeding is paramount and takes precedence over all other efforts, including obtaining intravenous access and extrication from vehicles

- Early use of a tourniquet and hemostatic dressings are encouraged in the setting of hemorrhage

- Intravenous access is not attempted for casualties with superficial wounds, a strong radial pulse, and a normal Glasgow Coma Scale (GCS) motor score

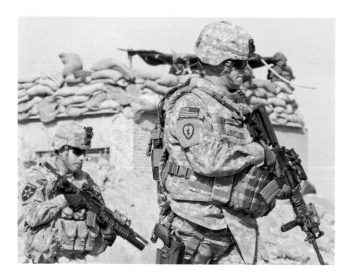

Figure 11. *US soldiers from Charlie Company, 4th Battalion, 23th Infantry Regiment conduct a foot patrol in the Helmand province of Afghanistan in January, 2010. Image courtesy of Defense Imagery Management Operations Center (DIMOC).*

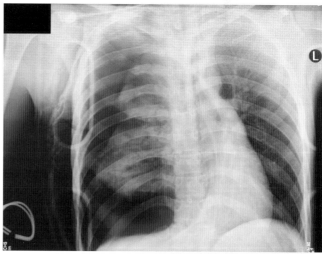

Figure 12. *Tension pneumothorax, a cause of potentially preventable battlefield death, may be treated by needle decompression.*

## Equipment Changes

### Body Armor

Expansion in the use of body armor, improvements in its surface area coverage, and enhancement of the armor's ability to deflect high-velocity projectiles are believed to explain the lower overall incidence of thoracic injury during OEF and OIF (Fig. 11).[1,9] Early studies also suggest body armor decreases the incidence of abdominal injuries.[10,26,27] Technological improvements in body armor are believed to contribute to the improvement in survival seen since Vietnam. Body armor came into widespread use during Operation Desert Storm, and its use further expanded during the current conflicts. In Vietnam, the rate of thoracic injury was 13 percent, in OEF and OIF, this rate has decreased to 5 percent.[9] Moreover, an analysis of casualties in 2004 demonstrated a rate of thoracic injury of 18 percent in those without body armor, and less than 5 percent in those wearing armor.[1] Despite the decrease in thoracic injuries, tension pneumothorax has been recognized as a potentially preventable cause of battlefield death (Fig. 12).[13,21] This resulted in the training of most SOF in the technique of needle thoracostomy. First responders now carry a large-bore needle as part of their battlefield equipment.

### Hemorrhage Control Adjuncts

Tourniquets, rarely used in the civilian sector, have become a standard part of every soldier's equipment, and all medics and SOF personnel have been trained in their use (Fig. 13). In the past, tourniquets were avoided due to concerns regarding their misuse leading to limb ischemia and lack of adequate hemorrhage control. However, this scenario typically was associated with makeshift tourniquets, such as a bandage and a stick, which were often improperly applied.

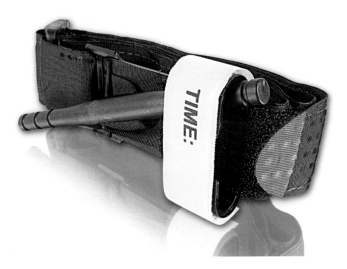

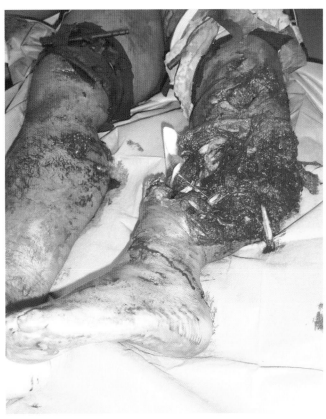

Figure 13. (Above) *The Combat Application Tourniquet®. Liberal use is recommended for uncontrolled extremity hemorrhage in the tactical environment. Image courtesy of North American Rescue, LLC.*

Figure 14. (Right) *A casualty arrives at the SSTP at Camp Taqaddum, with Combat Application Tourniquets in place. Image courtesy of CDR Subrato Deb.*

> Tourniquets save lives. Improved survival is associated with tourniquet placement before the onset of shock, while timely removal avoids complications.

Newly designed tourniquets combined with improved widespread training on tourniquet use have played a major role in improving hemorrhage control following combat injury.[28] This is especially true in battlefield or other austere environments, when access to definitive care may be delayed. At the start of OEF and OIF, there was very little tourniquet use. However, tourniquets are now applied following nearly every severe extremity injury (Fig. 14).[29] A 2008 study of severe extremity injury in an OIF Combat Support Hospital deemed that tourniquets are effective in controlling hemorrhage with no increased incidence of significant limb ischemia or early adverse outcomes.[29] Kragh et al. conducted the first prospective study of 2,838 casualties with major limb trauma admitted to a Level III Combat Support Hospital in Baghdad, and demonstrated survival benefit associated with tourniquet use.[28] Improved survival was also associated with placement of tourniquets prior to the onset of clinical signs of shock. Of the 232 patients who received 428 tourniquets (applied to 309 injured limbs), transient nerve palsy was the only adverse outcome attributed to their use.[28,30] If removed within six hours of application, tourniquets save lives without causing limb damage or secondary amputation.

> Topical hemostatic agents may be used as adjuncts in the treatment of noncompressible hemorrhage.

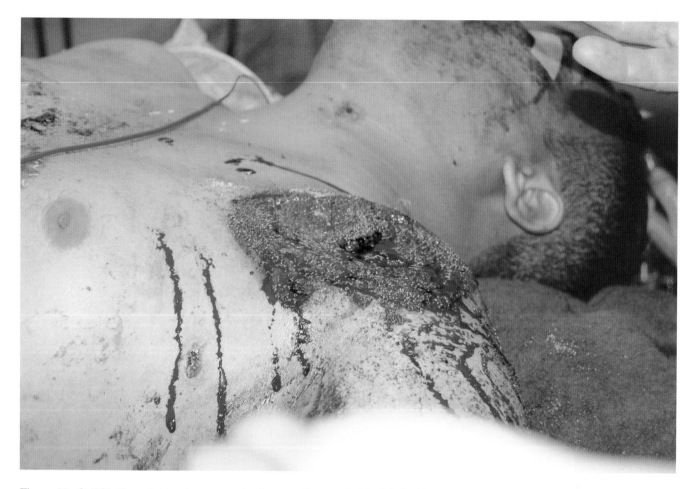

Figure 15. *QuikClot® applied to a large penetrating fragmentation wound of the left shoulder.*

Hemostatic, clot-promoting agents, such as Combat Gauze™, WoundStat™ granules, Celox™ powder, QuikClot® and HemCon™ dressings, have been used for bleeding not immediately controllable with direct pressure, pressure points, or tourniquet use (Fig. 15).[31,32,33] These hemostatic agents were developed for use in conjunction with the standard techniques of hemorrhage control, including direct pressure, elevation, and pressure point use. Some form of hemostatic dressing is now given to every individual in a combat zone. Animal models and early studies from OEF and OIF demonstrate the superiority of many of these dressings over standard gauze dressings and describe safety considerations surrounding their use.[31,32,33] A more detailed discussion of combat dressings is provided in the Damage Control Resuscitation chapter.

## *Organizational Innovations*

Beyond new products and techniques, there has been improvement in the trauma and evacuation systems at organizational levels. Since 2003, the trauma system has been organized into levels of care designed to minimize the time from injury to treatment, and to provide a continuum of care. Forward Surgical Teams are small, mobile units capable of performing a limited number of lifesaving surgeries. These FSTs have been organized into rapidly responsive and efficient units. The process of casualty evacuation from the battlefield, to the initial level of surgical care, and then on to definitive care facilities in Germany and the United States, has dramatically improved in speed and capability. These rapid evacuation systems have enabled casualties to reach forward medical facilities in minutes rather than hours. The military is now able

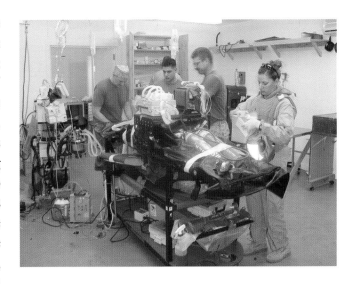

Figure 16. *An en-route-care nurse helps package a critically-injured casualty for transport in the operating room at Camp Taqaddum, Iraq.*

to transfer ventilated, critically ill patients from forward surgical sites near point-of-injury, over distances of thousands of miles while providing state-of-the-art critical care en-route (Fig. 16).

### Echelons of Care

To meet wartime needs, CCC and evacuation are organized by echelons of care. In this context, the word echelon refers to level of command and control. The medical care delivered at each echelon of the battlefield corresponds with respective levels of care (e.g., Level II care is delivered in Echelon II) (Fig. 17).

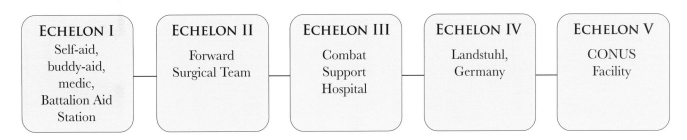

| **ECHELON I** | **ECHELON II** | **ECHELON III** | **ECHELON IV** | **ECHELON V** |
|---|---|---|---|---|
| Self-aid, buddy-aid, medic, Battalion Aid Station | Forward Surgical Team | Combat Support Hospital | Landstuhl, Germany | CONUS Facility |

Figure 17. *Evacuation chain for combat casualties.*

Trauma system activation in OEF and OIF occurs well before the combat casualty reaches the hospital. On the battlefield, the first medical responder to a casualty is usually another soldier or a combat medic, who in some instances will rapidly move the patient to a Battalion Aid Station. Care provided by the first responder through the Battalion Aid Station is considered Level I. The first response may occur when still under fire or in dangerous circumstances, and only limited equipment may be available. The combat medic assesses whether the casualty will require immediate evacuation and responds to immediately life-threatening injuries (Fig. 18). Most commonly, this includes control of hemorrhage using tourniquets as first-line therapy if care is being delivered under fire. Once the casualty and first responder are no longer under fire, hemorrhage control may be reassessed. Depending on the findings upon reassessment, hemorrhage control may either be augmented with additional tourniquets or hemostatic dressings, or controlled with a less stringent method (e.g., pressure dressing).

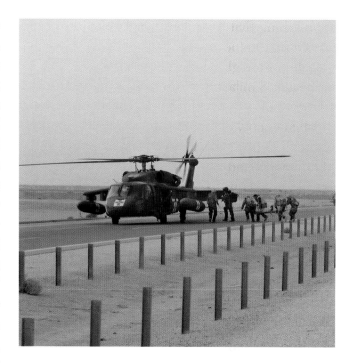

Figure 18. *Combat medics evacuate a wounded casualty on a Black Hawk helicopter. Image courtesy of the Borden Institute, Office of The Surgeon General, Washington, DC.*

Rapid evacuation systems have enabled combat casualties to reach forward medical facilities in minutes rather than hours. For patients requiring evacuation, the goal is to reach surgical care within one hour of injury.

For patients requiring evacuation, the goal is to reach surgical care within one hour of injury. Depending on the location, the casualty may initially reach either a Level II or Level III facility. Transport from point-of-injury or a Level I facility to a Level II or III facility is termed casualty evacuation (CASEVAC). A Level II facility is typically made up of a FST, capable of providing immediate, life-sustaining resuscitation and surgery until the patient can reach a higher-level facility for definitive treatment and longer-term care. Most FSTs consist of five to 20 personnel, including at least three surgeons, an orthopaedic surgeon, nurse anesthetists, critical care nurses, and technicians.[34] Forward Surgical Team personnel are capable of rapid assembly and takedown of the facility. The facility comprises two operating tables and a blood bank supplying 20 to 50 units of packed RBCs. Most FST facilities now carry plasma and recombinant factor VIIa. These FST facilities logistically support up to 30 operations before needing to resupply. The FST facilities typically do not have plain radiography capacity, but most have portable ultrasound machines.

Physicians should become proficient in the use of ultrasound for the evaluation of a combat casualty.

Forward surgical units offer a highly effective combination of proximity and capability for patients who cannot be evacuated rapidly to a Combat Surgical Hospital. Determining the ideal relationship between proximity to surgical care and the capability of the surgical unit, however, remains a challenge. In many cases, the tactical situation has permitted rapid helicopter casualty evacuation directly to a Level III facility, approaching that of transporting a civilian trauma patient to a regional Level-one trauma center in the United States. Inclement weather, the inability to land a casualty evacuation helicopter close to an active firefight, or a high volume of casualties arriving at the closest Level III facility may preclude this practice in theater. Similarly, remote combat operations may not allow timely transport of a surgical patient to a Combat Support Hospital. In these situations, the forward surgical unit's mobility and sophisticated capabilities provide valuable resources.

The physical and logistical resources required to provide life and limb-salvaging care to severely injured casualties are considerable. Managing several combat casualties over a relatively short timeframe (24 hours) can completely overwhelm a unit. The logistical support, communications, security, and ability to transfer postoperative patients are as essential to the success of these units as is their forward location. Thoughtful consideration of the tactical solution is needed to balance the benefits of enhanced proximity afforded by small and mobile forward surgical units against the disadvantages of dispersing resources and experience throughout the battlespace. Dispersion of small surgical units across the combat theater without including them in an integrated trauma system will not be effective. As noted by Dr. Ogilvie in commenting on the success of the Forward Surgical Teams used by the British 8th Army fighting the German Afrika Corps in the North African desert during World War II, "This point must be insisted on, because there is constant temptation on the part of keen medical administrative officers to push forward their surgeons beyond the point where they can do useful work, and for surgeons there to undertake more than lifesaving surgery with the splendid folly that prompted the charge of the Light Brigade."[35]

Level III facilities include Combat Support Hospitals and are significantly larger, semi-permanent hospitals capable of providing immediate patient resuscitation, temporizing and definitive surgeries, medium-term intensive care unit (ICU), and postoperative care for hundreds of patients.[1] At this level, surgical specialties including orthopedics, neurosurgery, maxillofacial surgery, urology and ophthalmology are available. All have plain radiography and fluoroscopy, and some have computed tomography (CT) capability. Level III facilities often treat host nation casualties in addition to military casualties (Fig. 19). As of 2005, there were three Army-based Combat Support Hospitals in Iraq and one in Afghanistan, as well as one Air Force Theater Hospital in Iraq. Most have five to 10 trauma bays, two to five operating rooms, and about 10 to 20 ICU beds (Fig. 20).

United States casualties requiring longer-term care are then evacuated to a Level IV facility. Nearly all US casualties in Iraq and Afghanistan are evacuated to Landstuhl Regional Medical Center in Germany, a large hospital offering all surgical specialties and rehabilitation. Finally, US casualties not expected to return to duty are ultimately evacuated back to the Continental United States (CONUS) to a Level V facility. These include Brooke Army Medical Center, Walter Reed Army Medical Center, National Naval Medical Center Bethesda, and almost all of the tri-service major medical centers.

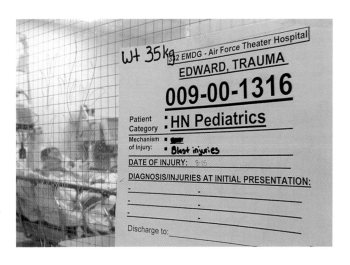

Figure 19. *Outside the room of a 14-year-old host national patient who sustained blast-related injuries and was treated at a Level III facility in Balad AB, Iraq.*

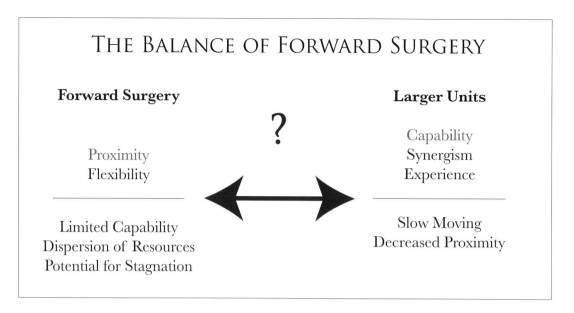

# THE BALANCE OF FORWARD SURGERY

**Forward Surgery**

**Larger Units**

**?**

Proximity
Flexibility

Capability
Synergism
Experience

Limited Capability
Dispersion of Resources
Potential for Stagnation

Slow Moving
Decreased Proximity

Figure 20. *Important considerations in casualty evacuation (CASEVAC). The prime objective is to stabilize and transport the wounded from the battlefield to the nearest appropriate medical facility available, in the most expedient fashion.*

## Patient Evacuation and Transport

"The stated vision of the JTTS was to ensure that every soldier, marine, sailor, or airman injured on the battlefield has the optimal chance for survival and maximal potential for functional recovery. In other words, to get the right patient to the right place at the right time."[1] The rapid and efficient evacuation of a large number of casualties, including those with critical injuries, has been one of the major advances in OEF and OIF. Most severely injured casualties can be rapidly transported from the field by helicopter via casualty evacuation (CASEVAC), or between Level II and Level III care facilities as a medical evacuation (MEDEVAC) (Fig. 21). The CASEVAC system is designed for speed over medical capability. The helicopter may not contain medical equipment and the crew may have little or no medical training. Medical evacuation crews have medical training and fly in designated helicopters with some medical equipment.[36] Helicopters are equipped with both a flight crew and medical team, and critically ill casualties are accompanied by an

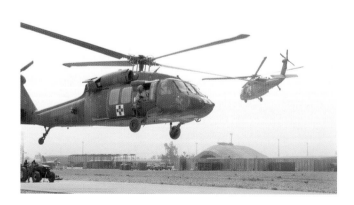

Figure 21. *A pair of Army Black Hawk helicopters take off from Balad AB to perform a MEDEVAC. The MEDEVAC crews are a critical link in the chain of events to ensure casualties in Iraq are transported to the next level of care within one hour of being injured. Image courtesy of Defense Imagery Management Operations Center (DIMOC).*

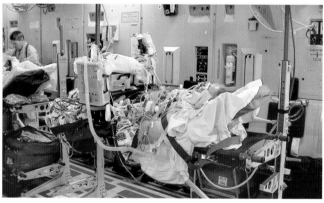

Figure 22. *USAF Critical Care Air Transport Teams (CCATTs) have enabled the movement of critically ill patients, even in the midst of ongoing resuscitation.*

en-route-care nurse who manages the patient during transport from Level I or II to Level III. Casualties are transported from the battlefield to the nearest medical facility (usually a Level II facility) either by ground transport or helicopter. Distance, weather, ground conditions, availability, number of casualties and severity of injury are among the factors used to determine which mode of transport will be used.[37]

The US Marine Corps utilizes en-route-care (critical care nurses) to provide ongoing management of ventilated, critically ill patients during transport from a forward unit to Level III care. These nurses belong to the forward unit and are not part of the air transport unit. After completion of transfer to Level III facilities they return to their originating unit. En-route nursing care is an indispensable link as patients move from Level I through Level III facilities. During the three busiest periods of First Marine Expeditionary Force (I MEF) Operations in Iraq (2003, 2004, and 2006) more than 600 en-route-care missions, moving 675 patients, were flown from Level II to Level III facilities. This accounted for 16 percent of all combat casualties during that time. Virtually all (99.5 percent) of the patients arrived safely at Level III. There were four patients who arrived unstable and all had severe injuries. All four were nonpreventable deaths on review (unpublished data, USMC 2008). Unfortunately, this was not always the case for patients transported without nursing care. Although further refinements and increased training for en-route-care between Level II and III units are necessary, this practice is an important step forward in CCC.

An aeromedical evacuation system was developed during OEF and OIF for long-range transportation. This system has transported thousands of casualties by fixed-wing aircraft since its inception.[38] In Vietnam, transporting an injured casualty back to the United States typically took well over a month. With the advancements in aeromedical transport in OEF and OIF, most casualties reach Germany or the United States within 36 hours of injury.[4,36,38] This rapid transfer of care carries the risk of losing key information along the way. Communication between the transport team and receiving careproviders is critically important during such transfers. The medical capabilities of aeromedical aircraft and personnel have significantly advanced, and these aircraft function as a 'mobile ICU' (Fig. 22).

> With advancements in aeromedical transport during OEF and OIF, most casualties reach Germany or the United States within 36 hours of injury.

Transport of the most critically ill patients is conducted by Critical Care Air Transport Teams (CCATTs). Each CCATT is staffed with at least one physician and two critical care nurses, with the capability to transport critically ill ventilated patients for eight to 12 hours at a time, to a higher level of care. The CCATTs were developed in 1994 by the US Air Force and allow for postoperative transport of patients to Level IV and V hospitals where continuing intensive care, secondary operations, and rehabilitation can occur. Evacuation out of theater to Level IV and V facilities is termed air evacuation (AIREVAC). This enables Combat Support Hospitals in Iraq and Afghanistan to preserve their ICU and surgical resources.

Since casualties with injuries not allowing them to return to duty will rapidly move through the system and rarely spend significant time at any specific level of care, communication of key information concerning their injuries and treatment is essential for optimal care. This is most problematic in an immature theater where communications and bandwidth are limited. Under these circumstances, multiple methods of transferring information have been utilized. These include paper records, writing on patients or dressings, and direct verbal transfer by accompanying medical personnel (Fig. 23). Additionally, items such as handheld portable dictaphones and even memory sticks with downloaded photos of injuries and paper records have been tried with varying success. In a mature theater with established communication capability, availability of the Joint Patient Tracking Application (JPTA) – a web-based application that allows users to obtain real-time information, e-mail, and direct phone communication – have simplified transferring medical information and providing feedback to forward units on outcomes.[1]

## Damage Control Strategies

Beyond new products and training, there has been a significant change in the management of critically injured patients reaching a medical facility, termed damage control resuscitation (DCR). Damage control resuscitation emphasizes resuscitation with

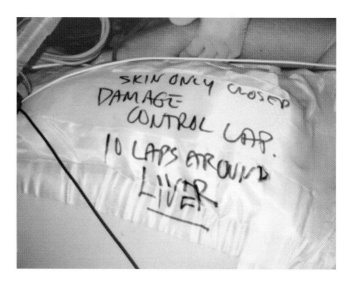

Figure 23. *Improvised patient information communication strategy. Patient information is written directly onto the dressing of a patient emerging from a damage control laparotomy. Image courtesy of the Borden Institute, Office of The Surgeon General, Washington, DC.*

hemostatic blood products and focuses on rapid control of bleeding and immediately life-threatening injuries. Its counterpart, damage control surgery (DCS) focuses only on immediately critical surgical interventions and delays more definitive care of injuries until the patient can be stabilized. In conjunction, these practices aim to prevent the lethal triad of acidosis, hypothermia, and coagulopathy.

### Damage Control Resuscitation

The recognition of hemorrhage as the primary cause of preventable combat death led to significant changes in the initial resuscitation of severely injured patients.[13,21] Most death due to hemorrhage occurs within six to 24 hours of injury. This makes hemorrhage control, reversing coagulopathy, and restoring tissue perfusion critical. Advanced Trauma and Life Support (ATLS) curriculum recommends aggressive resuscitation with crystalloids both in the prehospital and hospital settings.[39] Moreover, when a massive transfusion is required, conventional practice involves transfusion of packed RBCs first, with addition of platelets and clotting factors only after the transfusion of a full blood volume (e.g., five liters).[39]

Conventional resuscitation practices have been significantly influenced by recent CCC experiences in OEF and OIF. Upon arriving at a hospital setting, many severely injured casualties are already coagulopathic. One-third or more of combat casualties present with an international normalized ratio (INR) of 1.5 or greater.[40] Aggressive resuscitation with crystalloid and packed red cells worsens coagulopathy through dilution, promotion of hypothermia, and worsening of acidosis.[40] This lethal triad of acidosis, hypothermia, and coagulopathy has a downward spiral effect characterized by acidosis and hypothermia worsening coagulopathy, leading to progressive hemorrhaging, which itself worsens all three conditions (Fig. 24). Each of the three conditions has been shown to be an independent predictor of mortality in severely injured casualties.[40]

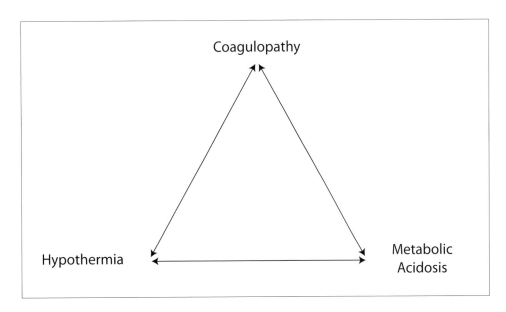

Figure 24. *The lethal triad of acidosis, hypothermia, and coagulopathy. Acidosis and hypothermia worsen coagulopathy, leading to progressive hemorrhage and worsening of all three arms of the triad.*

With conventional resuscitation practices, aggressive resuscitation with crystalloid solutions worsens coagulopathy through hemodilution, promotion of hypothermia, and worsening of acidosis. In contrast, DCR emphasizes resuscitation with hemostatic blood products, rapid control of bleeding and immediately life-threatening injuries, prevention of hypothermia, permissive hypotension, and minimal use of crystalloids.

Typical crystalloid fluids, including 0.9% normal saline and lactated Ringer's solution, have a pH of 5.5 and 6.6, respectively.[41] They are often infused in large quantities through large peripheral intravenous catheters in prehospital and early resuscitative settings. These crystalloid fluids cause a lowering of blood pH and a dilutional effect on the platelets and clotting factors needed to control bleeding. Despite attempts at warming these crystalloid fluids prior to infusion, they are rarely administered at body temperature and frequently contribute to patient hypothermia. Prolonged transport times between initial injury and arrival to medical care further potentiate the risk for hypothermia in combat casualties. Acidosis results primarily from production of lactate and other metabolic byproducts due to anaerobic metabolism, a result of inadequate tissue perfusion during patient shock. While crystalloids lower pH, massive transfusion of blood products is thought to promote acidemia as well.[42] Stored RBCs are thought to have a pH of 7.15 or lower.[43] Transfusion of large quantities of stored RBCs may have a profound lowering effect on body pH.

The goal of DCR is to reverse the three components of the lethal triad and rapidly control hemorrhage. Damage control resuscitation applies to both initial resuscitative efforts as well as the first 24 to 48 hours of postoperative ICU care. Novel aspects of DCR include permissive hypotension, minimal use of crystalloids, rapid transfusion of blood products in an RBC-to-plasma-to-platelet ratio of 1:1:1, aggressive prevention of hypothermia with warm blankets and fluids, use of fresh whole blood (FWB) when available, and the use of new products, including hemostatic agents and recombinant factor VIIa, when appropriate for severe hemorrhage.[44]

An important aspect of DCR is early recognition of critically ill combat casualties who will require massive transfusion and are susceptible to the aforementioned issues surrounding resuscitation. Limited blood product availability, lab capability, and personnel at forward resuscitative or surgical sites create the need for judicious utilization of resources. The rapid and precise recognition of casualties requiring DCR has been aided by injury pattern recognition. Casualties who present with any of the injury patterns shown in Table 3 are likely to need massive transfusion and should be treated by DCR techniques.

| RAPID RECOGNITION OF CASUALTIES REQUIRING DCR BY INJURY PATTERN |
| --- |
| • Truncal, axillary, neck, or groin bleeding not controlled by tourniquets or hemostatic dressings |
| • Major proximal traumatic amputations or mangled extremity |
| • Multiple long-bone or pelvic fractures |
| • Large soft-tissue injuries with uncontrolled bleeding |
| • Large hemothorax (greater than 1,000 milliliters) |
| • Large hemoperitoneum |

Table 3. *Injury patterns as predictors of massive transfusion.*

## *Permissive Hypotension*

Trauma patients suffering from severe injury, such as limb amputation, often arrive at medical care facilities with minimal bleeding. Once resuscitation is initiated, patients start rebleeding, often uncontrollably. Since rate of hemorrhage has a direct relationship with mean arterial pressure, it is postulated that lower blood pressures may slow the rate of hemorrhage, allow for clotting to occur, and help preserve blood volume.[44] Thus, some degree of hypotension may be protective in preventing further hemorrhage in critically injured patients. This must be weighed against the effect of hypotension on end-organ perfusion leading to multiple organ dysfunction syndrome (MODS).[45]

Traditional ATLS teaching calls for two large-bore intravenous catheter insertions in the prehospital setting with immediate aggressive crystalloid replacement.[39] However, numerous animal-model studies suggest that this leads to poorer outcomes in both blunt and penetrating trauma, perhaps due to interference with normal physiologic responses to hemorrhage.[46,47,48] In combat settings, casualties now receive minimal crystalloid or blood products in the field. Combat medics practice permissive hypotension, allowing for a mild degree of hypotension (systolic blood pressure of 90 mm Hg) in patients with a normal mental status.[49,50] In the field, this translates to a palpable radial pulse in an alert patient. The goal is to prevent the conversion of controlled hemorrhagic shock to uncontrolled hemorrhagic shock in severely injured casualties before reaching definitive care.

> In a combat setting, patients without evidence of head injury who exhibit a normal mental status and a palpable radial pulse should not receive intravenous fluids.

## *Blood Product Transfusion Ratios*

Although the definition of massive transfusion varies, the term is commonly applied to a transfusion of 10 units of RBCs or greater within a 24-hour period (Figs. 25 and 26).[51] Most combat and civilian casualties do

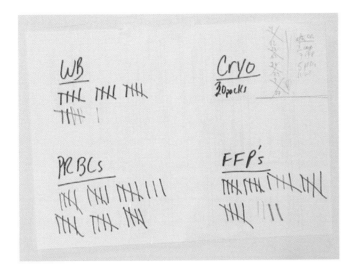

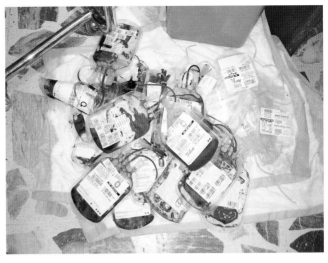

Figure 25. *Running tally of blood products administered, posted on the wall above a casualty's bed. The casualty sustained injuries from multiple transabdominal gunshot wounds.*

Figure 26. *The need for massive transfusion should be determined early. Approximately 8 percent of combat casualties require massive transfusion. Image courtesy of the Borden Institute, Office of The Surgeon General, Washington, DC.*

not require massive transfusion. In the civilian setting, it is required in only 1 to 3 percent of trauma cases. In a combat setting, the frequency is higher due to the increased incidence of penetrating trauma and blast injury. In OIF, the rate is 8 percent, compared with up to 16 percent during Vietnam.[52]

> In a combat setting, the frequency of massive transfusion is higher due to the increased incidence of penetrating trauma and blast injury.

The aim of RBC transfusion is to restore the oxygen-carrying capacity of the blood, replace lost volume, and restore tissue perfusion. For patients requiring several units of RBCs, conventional teaching was that replacement of platelets and clotting factors due to dilution was not required until the patient had been transfused a full blood volume. Thus, most massive transfusions have been heavily weighted towards RBC transfusion before other blood products were added, resulting in low plasma-to-RBC and platelet-to-RBC ratios. Multiple retrospective studies of both civilian and combat trauma patients have shown an increase in mortality, particularly in death due to hemorrhage, associated with low plasma-to-RBC and platelet-to-RBC ratios.[53,54,55] In a 2008 study by Holcomb et al., a review of 466 civilian patients requiring massive transfusion demonstrated that patients receiving higher amounts of plasma and platelet transfusion in the context of massive transfusion had decreased truncal hemorrhage. This subset of patients also had increased six-hour, 24-hour, and 30-day survival, had less ICU and ventilator days, and spent fewer days in the hospital.[55]

Blood product transfusion studies following combat-related injuries have shown the same trends. A 2008 study by Spinella et al. reviewed 708 patients in Combat Support Hospitals who required at least one unit of RBC transfusion. Each unit of RBCs transfused was associated with increased mortality, while each unit of plasma transfused was associated with increased survival.[56] Similarly, a 2007 study by Borgman et al. reviewed 246 patients at Combat Support Hospitals requiring massive transfusions and divided them into three groups based on the ratio of plasma-to-RBCs received. The three groups had the same median injury severity score of 18. The group with the lowest ratio (median 1 plasma: 8 RBC units) had significantly higher overall mortality (65 percent) and death due to hemorrhage (92.5 percent) compared to the high ratio group (median 1 plasma: 1.4 RBC units), which had a 19 percent mortality and 37 percent rate of death due to hemorrhage.[53]

Such studies have led to a paradigm shift in the provision of massive blood transfusion in combat casualties, with a low-ratio goal approaching 1:1:1 for RBCs, plasma, and platelets. This has led to significant changes in blood banking practices. For instance, since plasma is frozen, Combat Support Hospitals now pre-thaw fresh frozen plasma (FFP) daily to ensure rapid availability.

### Role of Fresh Whole Blood

With the advent of a low-ratio goal (e.g., 1:1:1) for massive blood product transfusion in combat casualties, the ideal blood replacement in the context of hemorrhage may be whole blood, rather than component transfusion.[57,58,59] Whole blood contains the most physiologic ratio of red cells, platelets, clotting factors, and fibrinogen. Secondarily, one unit of whole blood contains overall less volume than the equivalent in blood components, which can be important in patients receiving massive transfusion who are at high risk of third-spacing fluids and developing pulmonary edema. A retrospective study of 354 patients with traumatic hemorrhagic shock receiving blood transfusion found both one-day and 30-day survivals were higher in the fresh whole blood cohort as compared to the component therapy group.[57]

In addition to the problems associated with dilutional effects when RBCs alone are transfused, the age of stored RBCs is also associated with an increase in mortality.[60] The average lifespan of an RBC is 120 days, and this is traditionally the maximum storage time for a unit of frozen RBCs. As red cells age, an increasing number of cells will die or become damaged and release intracellular products. In animal models, transfusion of stored RBCs has been shown to cause release of inflammatory mediators and result in higher infection rates.[61] In addition, as red cells age, their oxygen-carrying capacity per unit diminishes and the restoration of tissue perfusion decreases, which may have adverse clinical effects.[62]

Recent investigation has given significant attention to the use of warm fresh whole blood (FWB) for massive transfusion required in a combat setting. The use of FWB started during World War I, initially out of necessity due to limited supplies of blood components in combat hospital settings. Transfusion practices have been revised during OEF and OIF to increase the safety and efficiency of the process.[44] When the number and severity of casualties exceeded the ability of blood banks to keep up with transfusion requirements, walking blood banks were established to rapidly increase the supply of available blood in disaster scenarios (Fig. 27). Whole blood donated by military personnel, prescreened and blood-typed, can be rapidly cross-matched and available for use within hours without being divided into components. Though initially developed out of necessity, the use of warm FWB is now under investigation as a potentially superior approach compared to component therapy for massive transfusion.[57,63]

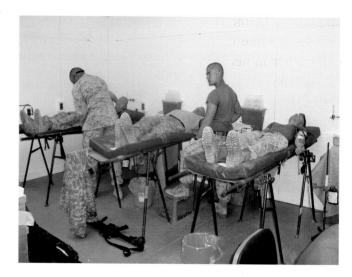

Figure 27. *Military personnel donate blood at the Walking Blood Bank, Camp Taqaddum, Iraq in 2006.*

Whole blood donated by military personnel, prescreened and blood-typed, can be rapidly cross-matched and available for use within hours without being divided into components.

### Role of Recombinant Factor VIIa

Recombinant factor VIIa has been under study for its use in severe hemorrhage.[64,65] Currently, recombinant factor VIIa (rFVIIa) is Food and Drug Administration (FDA) approved for severe bleeding in patients with factor VII deficiency. It is, however, being used off-label for patients with normal coagulation systems with life-threatening hemorrhage. Its first use in trauma was reported in 1999, and it is now used in military and civilian settings for trauma patients and for intraoperative hemorrhage.[64,65] Its off-label use has not yet been standardized and transfusion criteria, dosing, and redosing guidelines are still under investigation. Animal studies have indicated prolonged survival times and earlier control of hemorrhage associated with its use, and human case reports suggest that fewer blood products are required in hemorrhaging patients who receive rFVIIa.[64,65,66] Early randomized control trials of rFVIIa for bleeding control during various surgical procedures and in coagulopathic populations did not show reduction in mortality or transfusion requirements.[67,68,69] A 2005 randomized controlled trial of the use of rFVIIa versus placebo found rFVII demonstrated a reduction in the transfusion requirements for blunt trauma patients receiving rFVIIa, and a similar but nonsignificant trend in the penetrating trauma group.[64] Other types of studies, such as case series, meta-analyses and post-hoc analyses of randomized controlled trials have demonstrated trends (albeit statistically insignificant) toward improved outcomes.[70,71,72] Concerns regarding the use of rFVIIa are mainly related to the possibility of promoting thromboembolic complications. This was not observed in the 2005 randomized controlled trial, but has been reported in retrospective reviews.[73] Currently, in combat settings, rFVIIa is judiciously used in patients with life-threatening bleeding requiring massive transfusion.

## Damage Control Surgery

During the past 20 years, a new approach to trauma surgery known as damage control surgery (DCS) has been developed. Damage control surgery has been practiced in both civilian and combat settings, and is currently implemented in OEF and OIF. Traditional teaching advocates aiming for a single, definitive operation to repair traumatic injuries. Such an approach stems from the concern that an incomplete operation, or the need for multiple operations, could threaten a patient's overall stability and recovery. However, some definitive repairs of complex injury patterns may take hours to complete. In casualties who arrive in hemorrhagic shock, the lethal triad of coagulopathy, acidosis, and hypothermia may not be completely reversed before and during operative repair of injury. In these patients, metabolic derangements may continue to worsen in the OR, even after control of hemorrhage is achieved. Such patients may have a poorer outcome if subjected to a long, complex operation before physiologic parameters are restored.[74,75]

The principle of DCS is to minimize initial operative time in critically injured casualties by focusing only on the immediately critical actions. These critical actions are: (1) control of hemorrhage; (2) prevention of contamination and gastrointestinal soilage; and (3) protection from further injury. Injuries to the bowel requiring primary anastomosis, or other time-consuming repairs, are left for the subsequent operation(s) (Figs. 28, 29, and 30). Packing is often left in the abdomen. The abdomen is left open and sealed at the skin with a vacuum-assisted dressing to prevent abdominal compartment syndrome. Orthopedic injuries are treated with splinting or external fixation, and vascular injuries may be temporized with temporary intralumenal vascular shunts.[74,75,76]

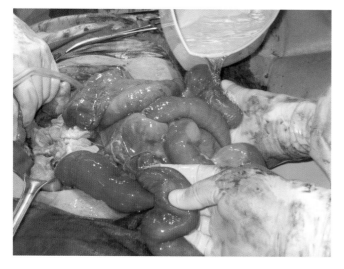

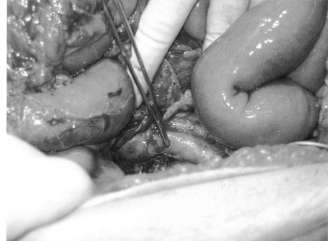

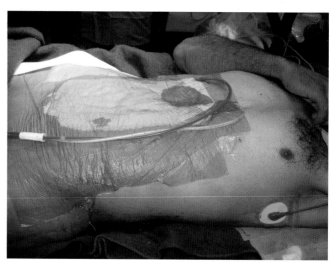

Figure 28. (Top Left) *This was a gunshot wound to the right back creating a large defect in the psoas muscle, laceration of the inferior vena cava (IVC) and destruction of the ascending colon and proximal transverse colon. The patient underwent control and repair of the IVC, packing of the retroperitoneal psoas defect (white pads seen in photo), and stapled resection of the right colon with blind ends left. Distal end of resected colon is seen under suction catheter tip. The proximal resected end was the distal ileum, which is being held in the foreground.*

Figure 29. (Top Right) *Repaired inferior vena cava.*

Figure 30. (Bottom Right) *Completed temporary vacuum-assisted dressing abdominal closure. The bowel and abdominal cavity were irrigated and decontaminated before temporary abdominal closure. The casualty underwent damage control resuscitation – receiving PRBCs, FWB, and rFVIIa – and was transported to a Level III facility less than three hours after his arrival.*

> In damage control surgery, an abbreviated operation is performed to control hemorrhage and contain gastrointestinal soilage. After a period of postoperative resuscitation in the ICU, patients may return to the operating room for a definitive procedure.

Following an abbreviated operation, patients are taken to the ICU to reverse the lethal triad through resuscitation and restoration of physiologic parameters. Here, crystalloids and transfusion are continued as needed to restore tissue perfusion and correct acidosis, and the patient is warmed and treated with vasoactive agents if needed. While the aim is to return to the OR in 24 to 48 hours, the definitive operation should not take place until the metabolic derangements are largely reversed. Several complications, including hemodynamic instability, organ failure, or acute respiratory distress syndrome (ARDS) may delay the timing of the second operation. In the definitive operation, abdominal packing and clots are removed and the abdomen is reexplored and washed out. Additional debridement, repair of shunted vascular injuries, anastomosis of bowel, and abdominal closure are performed at this subsequent operation.[74,75]

The timing of definitive surgical repair and abdominal wall closure will often vary based on injury type, severity, status (military or civilian), and nationality of the patient. For example, many US service members will undergo definitive abdominal wall closure following AIREVAC to rearward Level IV or V facilities, while host nation patients typically receive definitive surgical care at the Combat Support Hospital.[77] The combat trauma experience of the US Army 102nd FST in Afghanistan consisted of performing 112 surgeries on 90 patients over a seven-month period. Trauma accounted for 78 percent of surgical cases. Sixty-seven percent of these surgeries were performed on Afghan militia and civilians, 30 percent on US soldiers, and 3 percent on other coalition forces. Mechanisms of injury included gunshot wounds (34 percent), blasts (18 percent), motor vehicle crashes (14 percent), stab wounds (5 percent), and other trauma (7 percent).[77]

The three-step process of abbreviated operative repair, ICU resuscitation, and definitive operative repair of DCS follows the fundamental principle of treating the most immediate life-threats first. While DCR and DCS include several departures from classic ATLS teaching, the basic philosophy of prioritizing injury is the same.[74,75]

# Summary

The greatest honor we can pay to war casualties is to use their sacrifice to improve and optimize medical care. The lessons learned from OEF and OIF and prior conflicts have led to numerous advances in combat casualty and civilian trauma care. The CCC environment is vastly different from civilian trauma care settings. Thus, the approach to a combat casualty must take into account many additional logistical factors beyond the type and mechanism of injury. These include: what is the fastest way to reach a medical facility?, who is available to assist upon arrival?, is the area free of hostile fire?, will adequate personnel, blood products, and equipment be available for all those injured?, and, if not, how should casualties be prioritized? Awareness of local and support CCC capacity is as critical to improving patient survival rates as are initial airway, breathing, and circulation interventions.

The recognition of hemorrhage as the major cause of preventable death has led to a paradigm shift in the approach to the bleeding patient. Hemorrhage must be immediately and aggressively addressed with direct pressure, tourniquets, hemostatic agents, and rapid evacuation to a CCC facility. Resuscitation must be geared toward preventing and treating the downward spiral of the lethal triad of acidosis, hypothermia, and coagulopathy. Surgical intervention is directed towards rapid control of hemorrhage and contamination, rather than definitive repair of injury. Combat casualty care continues to evolve. The JTTS and the promotion of peer-reviewed scientific research during the current conflicts is a relatively new phenomenon that fosters investigation and innovation. The many improvements developed from the lessons of prior wars are now saving lives, and the efforts to continue learning will offer the best chance of survival and recovery to those we care for in the future.

# Case Study

The following is a copy of the Level II treatment summary from the record of a casualty from OIF that demonstrates most of the aspects of the prior discussions. It details the treatment from appropriate rapid initial care according to the TCCC guidelines, to utilization of DCR and DCS procedures on a critically injured casualty. The treatment summary illustrates how the continuum of care across the different levels of care leads to the survival of a casualty who in prior conflicts undoubtedly would have died.

*Casualty # 0822*

26-year-old male presented in class IV hemorrhagic shock about 25 minutes after wounding from a sniper round to abdomen. Treatment in field consisted of abdominal dressing over wound and single intravenous catheter access with limited fluid resuscitation. Initial evaluation in Shock Trauma Platoon (STP) revealed entrance wound to right flank with exit out anterior abdominal wall just to right of umbilicus with eviscerated omentum. Initial vital signs: blood pressure (BP) of 80/40, heart rate (HR) of 148, respiratory rate (RR) of 26, and pulse oximeter oxygen saturation ($SpO_2$) of 98 percent. Additional intravenous access was obtained, blood sent for labs, and antibiotics started and patient taken immediately to the operating room (less than five minutes). Walking blood bank (WBB) activated.

## Operative Findings:
- 2,000 milliliters hemoperitoneum with gross fecal contamination
- Large central zone I and right zone II retroperitoneal hematoma with active bleeding
- Abdominal cavity packed and aortic control at hiatus obtained (aortic cross clamp time of 55 minutes)
- Right medial visceral rotation performed
- Grade 5 (pulverized) right colon injury noted
- Multiple lacerations to inferior vena cava from confluence to just inferior to the right renal vein; the aorta is negative for injury
- Grade 3 laceration to third portion duodenum with ischemia

## Initial Labs:
pH = 7.1  Base Deficit = -16  Hematocrit = 28 percent

## Procedures:
- Initial attempt at inferior vena cava venorraphy but multiple lacerations posteriorly (probable torn lumbars) quickly led to oversew and ligation
- Simple whipstitch closure of duodenum to stop contamination and bleeding
- Stapled resection right colon with blind ends
- Packing right retroperitoneal psoas wound
- Washout peritoneum with rewarming
- Vacuum-pack closure abdominal dressing
- Bilateral lower extremity four compartment fasciotomies (for ligated inferior vena cava and one-hour ischemia time)

## Resuscitation by Anesthesia:
- Three liters normal saline
- Six units PRBCs
- 24 units FWB
- 7.2 milligrams rFVIIa

## Packaged for En-Route-Care:
- VS: BP = 115/61 mm Hg   HR=147   RR=12 (ventilated)   $SpO_2$=100 percent
- Departed to Level III facility less than four hours after arrival at STP
- En-route-care interventions: blood administration, sedation and paralytics, ventilator management; departing end-tidal carbon dioxide ($EtCO_2$) = 52 mm Hg

*Notes from Joint Patient Tracking Application (JPTA) at Level III Facility:*
Findings from original STP facility: Gunshot wound to right flank exited near navel. On exploratory laparotomy, patient had a long tear from the confluence of the inferior vena cava to just below the right renal vein. Inferior vena cava oversewn and ligated proximally and distally. Grade 3 injury to the third portion of the duodenum was oversewn. The aorta was cross-clamped at the hiatus (total aortic cross-clamp time was 55 minutes). Right colon with grade 5 injury: colon was resected distal ileum to mid-transverse with blind ends. Gross fecal contamination in peritoneum. Two laparotomy pads packed in right retroperitoneum. One Kerlex™ packing along anterior abdominal wall to exit wound. Vacuum-pack closure of abdomen, bilateral four compartment fasciotomies of lower extremities for ligated inferior vena cava and approximate one hour of ischemia time. Patient received six units of PRBCs, 24 units of FWB, 7.2 milligrams of rFVIIa.

*Vital Signs Upon Arrival:*
BP = 153/74 mm Hg   HR=108   RR=15   SpO$_2$=100 percent

*Level III Facility Admit Note:*
Patient was noted to be hemodynamically stable, sedated, and on the ventilator. His abdomen was dressed open and with a negative-pressure dressing (supplied by Jackson Pratts). The right lateral abdomen wound was noted. No other injuries were noted. The coagulation studies were normal and his hematocrit was normal. His base excess was +1. He appeared well-resuscitated. Given the large amount of blood loss at the original operation, will allow further time for hemostasis and he had just recently been taken from the OR. If he remains stable, will reexplore early this a.m.

*Next Day Note:*
Procedure Note: (1) Abdominal reexploration; (2) Segmental resection of proximal third portion of duodenum; (3) Side-to-side duodenoduodenostomy; (4) Pyloric exclusion; (5) Roux-en-Y gastrojejeunostomy; (6) Retrograde duodenostomy tube; (7) Jejeunostomy feeding tube; and (8) Stamm gastrostomy.

*Postoperative Day Three Note:*
Patient stable and now off ventilator. Tolerating tube feeds. Fasciotomies closed today. Jackson Pratt (JP) with minimal drainage. Labs normal. Ready for transfer in a.m.

# References

1. Eastridge BJ, Jenkins D, Flaherty S, et al. Trauma system development in a theater of war: experiences from Operation Iraqi Freedom and Operation Enduring Freedom. J Trauma 2006;61(6):1366-1373.

2. Eastridge BJ, Owsley J, Sebesta J, et al. Admission physiology criteria after injury on the battlefield predict medical resource utilization and patient mortality. J Trauma 2006;61(4):820-823.

3. Government Accountability Office (GAO). 2009. Iraq and Afghanistan: availability of forces, equipment, and infrastructure should be considered in developing U.S. strategy and plans. GAO-09-380T, Feb.12.

4. Ling GS, Rhee P, Ecklund JM. Surgical innovations arising from the Iraq and Afghanistan wars. Annu Rev Med 2010;61:457-468.

5. Burns BD, Zuckerman S. The Wounding Power of Small Bomb and Shell Fragments. London, England: British Ministry of Supply, Advisory Council on Scientific Research and Technical Development, 1942.

6. Beebe GW, DeBakey ME. Location of hits and wounds. In: Battle casualties. Springfield, IL: Charles C. Thomas; 1952. p. 165-205.

7. Reister FA. Battle Casualties and Medical Statistics: U.S. Army Experience in the Korean War. Washington, DC: The Surgeon General, Department of the Army; 1973.

8. Hardaway RM 3rd. Viet Nam wound analysis. J Trauma 1978;18(9):635-643.

9. Owens BD, Kragh JF Jr, Wenke JC, et al. Combat Wounds in Operation Iraqi Freedom and Operation Enduring Freedom. J Trauma 2008;64(2):295-299.

10. Zouris JM, Walker GJ, Dye J, et al. Wounding patterns for U.S. Marines and sailors during Operation Iraqi Freedom, Major Combat Phase. Mil Med 2006;171(3):246-252.

11. Owens BD, Kragh JF Jr, Macaitis J, et al. Characterization of extremity wounds in Operation Iraqi Freedom and Operation Enduring Freedom. J Orthop Trauma 2007;21(4):254-257.

12. Peoples GE, Gerlinger T, Craig R, et al. Combat casualties in Afghanistan cared for by a single Forward Surgical Team during the initial phases of Operation Enduring Freedom. Mil Med 2005;170(6):462-468.

13. Holcomb JB, McMullin NR, Pearse L, et al. Causes of death in the U.S. Special Operations Forces in the global war on terrorism: 2001-2004. Ann Surg 2007;245(6):986-991.

14. Marshall TJ Jr. Combat casualty care: the Alpha Surgical Company experience during Operation Iraqi Freedom. Mil Med 2005;170(6):469-472.

15. Chambers LW, Green DJ, Gillingham BL, et al. The experience of the US Marine Corps' Surgical

Shock Trauma Platoon with 417 operative combat casualties during a 12 month period of Operation Iraqi Freedom. J Trauma 2006;60(6):1155-1161.

16. Trunkey DD. History and development of trauma care in the United States. Clin Orthop Relat Res 2000; May (374):36-46.

17. King B, Jatoi I. The Mobile Army Surgical Hospital (MASH): a military and surgical legacy. J Natl Med Assoc 2005;97(5):648-656.

18. Eastridge BJ, Costanzo G, Jenkins D, et al. Impact of joint theater trauma system initiatives on battlefield injury outcomes. Am J Surg 2009;198(6):852-857.

19. Snethen B. Trauma registry system crunch time, improves battlefield care. Military Health System 2009 Jul 15 [cited 2009 Sept 21]. Available from: URL: http://www.health.mil/Press/Release.aspx?ID=820.

20. Court-Brown CM, Rimmer S, Prakash U, et al. The epidemiology of open long bone fractures. Injury 1998;29(7):529-534.

21. Blood CG, Puyana JC, Pitlyk PJ, et al. An assessment of the potential for reducing future combat deaths through medical technologies and training. J Trauma 2002;53(6):1160-1165.

22. Wound Data and Munitions Effectiveness Team. The WDMET Study. Original data from the Uniformed Services University of the Health Sciences, Bethesda, MD 20814 – 4799; summary volumes available from: Defense Documentation Center, Cameron Station, Alexandria, VA 22304-6145; 1970.

23. Directorate for information operations and reports [database on the Internet]: Department of Defense. Available from: URL: http://www.whs.mil.

24. Holcomb JB, Stansbury LG, Champion HR, et al. Understanding combat casualty care statistics. J Trauma 2006;60(2):397-401.

25. Butler FK Jr, Holcomb JB, Giebner SD, et al. Tactical combat casualty care 2007: evolving concepts and battlefield experience. Mil Med 2007;172(11 Suppl):1-19.

26. Chambers LW, Rhee P, Baker BC, et al. Initial experience of US Marine Corps forward resuscitative surgical system during Operation Iraqi Freedom. Arch Surg 2005;140(1):26-32.

27. Mabry RL, Holcomb JB, Baker AM, et al. United States Army Rangers in Somalia: an analysis of combat casualties on an urban battlefield. J Trauma 2000;49(3):515-529.

28. Kragh J, Walters TJ, Baer DG, et al. Survival with emergency tourniquet use to stop bleeding in major limb trauma. Ann Surg 2009;249(1):1-7.

29. Beekley AC, Sebesta JA, Blackbourne LH, et al. Prehospital tourniquet use in Operation Iraqi Freedom: effect on hemorrhage control and outcomes. J Trauma 2008;64(2 Suppl):S28-37.

30. Kragh JF Jr, Walters TJ, Baer DG, et al. Practical use of emergency tourniquets to stop bleeding in major limb trauma. J Trauma 2008;64(2 Suppl):S38-49; discussion S49-50.

31. Wedmore I, McManus JG, Pusateri AE, et al. A special report on the chitosan-based hemostatic dressing: experience in current combat operations. J Trauma 2006;60(3):655-658.

32. Ahuja N, Ostomel TA, Rhee P, et al. Testing of modified zeolite hemostatic dressings in a large animal model of lethal groin injury. J Trauma 2006;61(6):1312-1320.

33. Rhee P, Brown C, Martin M, et al. QuikClot use in trauma for hemorrhage control: case series of 103 documented uses. J Trauma 2008;64(4):1093-1099.

34. Eastridge BJ, Stansbury LG, Stinger H, et al. Forward Surgical Teams provide comparable outcomes to combat support hospitals during support and stabilization operations on the battlefield. J Trauma 2009;66(4 Suppl):S48-50.

35. Ogilvie WH. War surgery in Africa. Br J Surg 1944;31(124):313-324.

36. Carlton PK Jr, Jenkins DH. The mobile patient. Crit Care Med 2008;36(7 Suppl):S255-257.

37. Beninati W, Meyer MT, Carter TE. The critical care air transport program. Crit Care Med 2008;36(7 Suppl)S370-376.

38. Harman DR, Hooper TI, Gackstetter GD. Aeromedical evacuations from Operation Iraqi Freedom: a descriptive study. Mil Med 2005;170(6):521-527.

39. Alexander RH, Proctor HJ. Advanced trauma life support program for physicians. 8th ed. American College of Surgeons. Chicago; 2008.

40. Niles SE, McLaughlin DF, Perkins JG, et al. Increased mortality associated with the early coagulopathy of trauma in combat casualties. J Trauma 2008;64(6):1459-1463.

41. Physicians Desk Reference online. Available from: URL: http://www.pdr.net/home/pdrHome.aspx.

42. Hakala P, Hiippala S, Syrjala M, et al. Massive blood transfusion exceeding 50 units of plasma poor red cells or whole blood: the survival rate and the occurrence of leukopenia and acidosis. Injury 1999; 30(9):619-622.

43. Keidan I, Amir G, Mandel M, et al. The metabolic effects of fresh versus old stored blood in the priming of cardiopulmonary bypass solutions for pediatric patients. J Thorac Cardiovasc Surg 2004;127(4):949-952.

44. Beekley AC. Damage control resuscitation: a sensible approach to the exsanguinating surgical patient. Crit Care Med 2008;36(7 Suppl):S267-274.

45. Seely AJ, Christou NV. Multiple organ dysfunction syndrome: exploring the paradigm of complex nonlinear systems. Crit Care Med 2000;28(7):2198-2200.

46. Sondeen JL, Coppes VG, Holcomb JB. Blood pressure at which rebleeding occurs after resuscitation in swine with aortic injury. J Trauma 2003;54(5 Suppl):S110–117.

47. Bickell WH, Bruttig SP, Millnamow GA, et al. The detrimental effects of intravenous crystalloid after aortotomy in swine. Surgery 1991;110(3):529–536.

48. Bickell WH, Bruttig SP, Millnamow GA, et al. Use of hypertonic saline/dextran versus lactated Ringer's solution as a resuscitation fluid after uncontrolled aortic hemorrhage in anesthetized swine. Ann Emerg Med 1992;21(9):1077–1085.

49. Rhee P, Koustova E, Alam HB. Searching for the optimal resuscitation method: recommendations for the initial fluid resuscitation of combat casualties. J Trauma 2003;54(5 Suppl):S52–62.

50. US Department of Defense (US DoD). Shock and Resuscitation. In: Emergency War Surgery, Third United States Revision. Washington, DC: Department of the Army, Office of the Surgeon General, Borden Institute; 2004. p. 7.1-7.12.

51. Malone DL, Hess JR, Fingerhut A. Massive transfusion practices around the globe and a suggestion for a common massive transfusion protocol. J Trauma 2006;60(6 Suppl):S91-96.

52. Perkins JG, Cap AP, Weiss BM, et al. Massive transfusion and nonsurgical hemostatic agents. Crit Care Med 2008;36(7 Suppl):S325-339.

53. Borgman MA, Spinella PC, Perkins JG, et al. The ration of blood products transfused affects mortality in patients receiving massive transfusions at a combat support hospital. J Trauma 2007;63(4):805-813.

54. Gunter OL Jr, Au BK, Isbell JM, et al. Optimizing outcomes in damage control resuscitation: identifying blood product ratios associated with improved survival. J Trauma 2008;65(3):527-534.

55. Holcomb JB, Wade CE, Michalek JE, et al. Increased plasma and platelet to red blood cell rations improves outcome in 466 massively transfused civilian trauma patients. Ann Surg 2008;248(3):447-458.

56. Spinella PC, Perkins JG, Grathwohl KW, et al. Effect of plasma and red blood cell transfusions on survival in patients with combat related traumatic injuries. J Trauma 2008;64(2 Suppl):S69-77.

57. Spinella PC, Holcomb JB. Resuscitation and transfusion principles for traumatic hemorrhagic shock. Blood Rev 2009;23(6):231-240.

58. Armand R, Hess JR. Treating coagulopathy in trauma patients. Transfus Med Rev 2003;17(3):223-231.

59. Kauvar DS, Holcomb JB, Norris GC, et al. Fresh whole blood transfusion: a controversial military

practice. J Trauma 2006;61(1):181-184.

60. Spinella PC, Carroll CL, Staff I, et al. Duration of red blood cell storage is associated with increased incidence of deep vein thrombosis and in hospital mortality in patients with traumatic injuries. Crit Care 2009;13(5):R151. Epub 2009 Sep 22.

61. Blajchman MA, Bordin JO. Mechanisms of transfusion-associated immunosuppression. Curr Opin Hematol 1994;1(6):457-461.

62. Vandromme MJ, McGwin G Jr, Weinberg JA. Blood transfusion in the critically ill: does storage age matter? Scand J Trauma Resusc Emerg Med 2009;17(1):35-41.

63. Spinella PC. Warm fresh whole blood transfusion for severe hemorrhage: U.S. military and potential civilian applications. Crit Care Med 2008;36(7 Suppl):S340-345.

64. Boffard KD, Riou B, Warren B, et al. Recombinant factor VIIa as adjunctive therapy for bleeding control in severely injured trauma patients: two parallel randomized, placebo-controlled, double-blind clinical trials. J Trauma 2005;59(1):8-18.

65. Spinella PC, Perkins JG, McLaughlin DF, et al. The effect of recombinant activated factor VII on mortality in combat-related casualties with severe trauma and massive transfusion. J Trauma 2008;64(2):286-293.

66. Lynn M, Jerokhimov I, Jewelewicz D, et al. Early use of recombinant factor VIIa improves mean arterial pressure and may potentially decrease mortality in experimental hemorrhagic shock: a pilot study. J Trauma 2002;52(4):703-707.

67. Raobaikady R, Redman J, Ball JA, et al. Use of activated recombinant coagulation factor VII in patients undergoing reconstruction surgery for traumatic fracture of pelvis or pelvis and acetabulum: a double-blind, randomized, placebo-controlled trial. Br J Anaesth 2005;94(5):586-591.

68. Lodge JP, Jonas S, Oussoultzoglou E, et al. Recombinant coagulation factor VIIa in major liver resection: a randomized, placebo-controlled, double-blind clinical trial. Anesthesiology 2005;102(2):269–275.

69. Bosch J, Thabut D, Bendtsen F, et al. Recombinant factor VIIa for upper gastrointestinal bleeding in patients with cirrhosis: a randomized, double-blind trial. Gastroenterology 2004;127(4):1123-1130.

70. Rizoli SB, Boffard KD, Riou B, et al. Recombinant activated factor VII as an adjunctive therapy for bleeding control in severe trauma patients with coagulopathy: subgroup analysis from two randomized trials. Crit Care 2006;10(6):R178.

71. Dutton RP, McCunn M, Hyder M, et al. Factor VIIa for correction of traumatic coagulopathy. J Trauma 2004;57(4):709-719.

72. Khan AZ, Parry JM, Crowley WF, et al. Recombinant factor VIIa for the treatment of severe postoperative

and traumatic hemorrhage. Am J Surg 2005;189(3):331-334.

73. O'Connell KA, Wood JJ, Wise RP, et al. Thromboembolic adverse events after use of recombinant human coagulation factor VIIa. JAMA 2006;295(3):293-298.

74. Blackbourne LH. Combat damage control surgery. Crit Care Med 2008;36(7 Suppl):S304-310.

75. Lee JC, Peitzman AB. Damage-control laparotomy. Curr Opin Crit Care 2006;12(4):346-350.

76. Rasmussen TE, Clouse WD, Jenkins DH, et al. Echelons of care and the management of wartime vascular injury: a report from the 332nd EMDG/Air Force Theater Hospital, Balad Air Base, Iraq. Perspect Vasc Surg Endovasc Ther 2006;18(2):91-99.

77. Beekley AC, Watts DM. Combat trauma experience with the United States Army 102nd Forward Surgical Team in Afghanistan. Am J Surg 2004;187(5):652-654.

# WEAPONS EFFECTS
*Chapter 2*

**Contributing Authors**
Sidney B. Brevard, MD, MPH, FACS, COL, US Air Force
Howard Champion, MD, FRCS, FACS
Dan Katz, MD

All figures and tables included in this chapter have been used with permission from Pelagique, LLC, the UCLA Center for International Medicine, and/or the authors, unless otherwise noted.

**Disclaimer**
The opinions and views expressed herein belong solely to those of the authors. They are not nor should they be implied as being endorsed by the United States Uniformed Services University of the Health Sciences, Department of the Army, Department of the Navy, Department of the Air Force, Department of Defense, or any other branch of the federal government.

# Table of Contents

# Introduction

Understanding modern warfare, including the types of weapons employed and the mechanisms and patterns of injury they cause, is critical to providing optimal combat casualty care (CCC). Certain types of weapons (e.g., improvised explosive devices) inflict patterns of injury that are repeatedly encountered by military careproviders. By recognizing these patterns and understanding the pathophysiology behind resultant injuries, CCC providers will be better prepared to treat the injured.

The Joint Theater Trauma Registry (JTTR) is a database used to track medical treatment information on troops injured in Operation Enduring Freedom (OEF) and Operation Iraqi Freedom (OIF). Data are collected at various points as injured troops receive medical treatment in-theater and at each medical facility overseas and in the United States (US). The information recorded is extensive and includes patient demographics, mechanism of injury, type of personal protective equipment (e.g., body armor, goggles, helmet) used, body regions injured, and more.[1]

A query of the JTTR database for wounds sustained between October 2001 and January 2005 revealed the following distribution of injuries: extremities (54 percent), head and neck (29 percent), abdomen (11 percent), and chest (6 percent).[2] This injury pattern differs from that of previous conflicts, which had a higher proportion of thoracic injuries and fewer head and neck injuries.[2,3,4,5,6] This shift is likely due to enhanced body armor that protects the chest and reduces mortality.[2] Enhancements in personal protective equipment (PPE) and the shift from conventional warfare to "a complex mix of conventional, set-piece battles, and campaigns against shadowy insurgents and terrorists" contribute to current wounding patterns, which differ from those of previous conflicts (i.e., World War II, Korea, and Vietnam).[7]

> The JTTR database for wounds sustained in OEF and OIF between October 2001 and January 2005 reveals the following distribution of injuries: extremities (54 percent), head and neck (29 percent), abdomen (11 percent), and chest (6 percent).

The increase in explosion-related injuries and concomitant decrease in gunshot-related injuries in the past century and a half of US conflicts is summarized in Figure 1. This trend has accelerated substantially during recent years. This is illustrated by increases in explosion-related OEF and OIF casualties from 56 percent in 2003 to 2004 to 76 percent in 2006 and in the number of surgeries for fragment wounds from 48 percent in OIF I (2003) to 62 percent in OIF II (2004 to 2005) performed by US Navy/Marine Corps Forward Surgical Teams in OIF.[8,9]

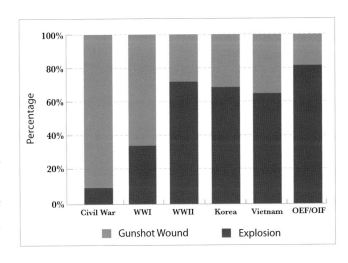

Figure 1. *Primary mechanisms of injury in United States wars.[2] Data sources: Civil War,[10] WWI and WWII,[11] Korea,[5] Vietnam,[6] OEF/OIF.[2]*

# Weapons

The primary mechanisms of combat injury in OEF and OIF are small arms (pistols, shotguns, rifles, machine guns) and explosives (mortars, landmines, rocket-propelled grenades [RPGs], and improvised explosive devices [IEDs]). As of 2009, combat casualty statistics for hostile actions indicate that explosive devices are responsible for 80 percent of injuries and 81 percent of deaths in OEF, and for 86 percent of injuries and 90 percent of deaths in OIF.[12] These mechanisms and their effects are discussed below, followed by an overview of blast injury.

# Small Arms

Current combat casualty statistics for hostile actions indicate that gunshot wounds are responsible for 22 percent of injuries and 27 percent of deaths in OEF, and for 8 percent of injuries and 19 percent of deaths in OIF.[12] Small arms are easily available in Iraq, which has an estimated combined military and civilian arsenal of seven to eight million firearms containing machine guns, submachine guns, sniper and assault rifles (including AK-47s and AK-47-style models such as the AKM), shotguns, pistols, and carbines.[13]

The degree of tissue damage resulting from small arms fire in OEF and OIF is highly variable. Combat casualty careproviders need to treat each patient's wound(s) individually. Wide surgical exploration of all bullet wounds is no longer routinely recommended.[14] Minimal tissue debridement is typically required for wounds resulting from small arms fire. As a bullet travels through tissue, a temporary cavity is created. Tissue damage in this temporary cavity is usually limited and may heal on its own without debridement.[15] Inelastic tissues, such as the brain and liver, will exhibit the most damage resulting from temporary cavitation. Elastic soft-tissue, such as lung, skeletal muscle, nerves, and blood vessels, may show minimal damage.[15] There may be cases when a bullet strikes bone or another structure and is deflected. In these cases, the damage could be more extensive and require larger debridement. Therefore, each case should be carefully evaluated and managed individually.[14]

> The degree of tissue damage resulting from small arms fire is highly variable. Wide surgical exploration of all bullet wounds is no longer routinely recommended.

# Explosives

## *Physics*

With the prevalence of explosive weapons in use in Iraq and Afghanistan, it is important that CCC providers have a basic working knowledge of the physics behind explosions. Explosions are the result of chemical conversion of a liquid or solid into a gas with generation of energy. Explosives are classified as low- or high-order based on velocity of detonation (i.e., the interval between activation and release of the explosive energy). Knowing the type of explosive that caused a casualty's injuries is important because low- and high-

| LOW-ORDER EXPLOSIVES | HIGH-ORDER EXPLOSIVES |
|---|---|
| • Dynamite<br>• Gunpowder | • Ammonium nitrate<br>• Nitroglycerin<br>• 2,4,6-trinitrotoluene (TNT)<br>• Pentaerythritol tetranitrate (PETN)<br>• Cyclotrimethylene trinitramine (RDX)<br>• Cyclotetramethylene tetranitramine (HMX)<br>• Nitrocellulose |

Table 1. *Examples of low- and high-order explosives.*

order explosives exhibit different patterns of injury and thus warrant different treatment considerations (Table 1).[16,17]

## Low-Order

Low-order explosives, which include gunpowder and dynamite, produce their effect through a relatively slow burning process called conflagration.[18] The readily combustible substances in low-order explosives are used primarily for propelling projectiles, but also take the form of pipe bombs and petroleum-based bombs (e.g., Molotov cocktails). The blast wave generated by a low-order explosive typically has a speed of less than 2,000 meters-per-second (m/sec). Low-order explosives have secondary, tertiary, quaternary, and sometimes quinary effects (see classifications described later). Importantly, they do not have the primary blast effects characteristic of high-order explosives.

## High-Order

Single-compound high-order explosives include ammonium nitrate, nitroglycerin, 2,4,6-trinitrotoluene (TNT), pentaerythritol tetranitrate (PETN), cyclotrimethylene trinitramine (RDX), cyclotetramethylene tetranitramine (HMX), and nitrocellulose. These compounds may be combined to form mixed-compound explosives, such as dynamite, composition C4, ammonium nitrate/fuel oil (ANFO), and sheet explosives.[19] Commonly-used polymer-bonded high explosives (Gelignite, Semtex) have one and one-half times the power of TNT.

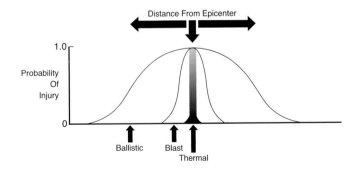

Figure 2. *As a blast wave travels away from the site of detonation, it rapidly loses both pressure and velocity. Combat blast injuries patterns often depend on the proximity of the individual to the site of detonation. Image courtesy of the Borden Institute, Office of The Surgeon General, Washington, DC.*

High-order explosives react very quickly and generate heat and energy almost instantaneously. Products of the explosive reaction occupy a greater volume than that filled by the original reactants. This results in a supersonic, superheated rise in pressure called a blast wave, which moves at speeds of 3,000 to 8,000 m/sec.[20] The blast front is the leading edge of the blast wave and has a shattering effect known as brisance. As the blast wave travels away from the site of detonation, it rapidly loses both pressure and velocity.[18,21] The duration and magnitude of the blast wave's peak depend on a host of factors, including the type of explosive used and the conducting medium.

The blast wave propels fragments with enormous force, generates environmental debris, and often causes intense thermal radiation. Its effects vary with distance from the detonation site (Figs. 2 and 3). High-order explosives are often used in military ordnance and their characteristic brisance can crush soft-tissue and bone and propel debris at ballistic speeds (fragmentation). Unlike low-order explosives, high-order explosives create blast overpressure injuries (barotrauma). As the blast wave passes, a temporary relative vacuum is created as gases continue to expand from their point of origin, and a transient blast wind may travel immediately behind the blast front. In the vicinity adjacent to an explosion, this force can cause traumatic amputation, evisceration, or total disintegration of a body. The blast wind may also cause injury by accelerating the speed of debris and fragments that subsequently strike the victim, or by displacing the victim against a stationary object.[19] These types of injuries are discussed in detail below.

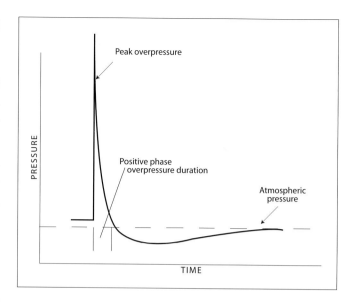

Figure 3. *Idealized blast overpressure waveform. An explosion creates a nearly instantaneous expansion of gas that compresses the surrounding medium (air or water) generating a blast wave. As it travels away from the site of detonation, the blast wave rapidly loses its pressure and velocity with distance and time.*

Low-order explosives have secondary, tertiary, quaternary, and sometimes quinary effects. Importantly, they do not have the primary blast effects characteristic of high-order explosives. High-order explosives can create significant overpressure injuries, especially at close range.

## Devices

Explosive devices, including artillery, mortars, rockets, grenades, and RPGs are responsible for more than 3,600 deaths and almost 31,000 injuries of US troops in the current conflicts in Afghanistan and Iraq.[12] Explosive devices are the weapon of choice of terrorists and insurgents, and are becoming ubiquitous in combat theaters and civilian venues alike. The major categories of explosives are landmines and unexploded ordnance, RPGs, and, most commonly, IEDs.

### Antipersonnel Landmines and Unexploded Ordnances

Landmines and unexploded ordnances (UXOs) are often discussed together because it can sometimes be difficult to separate the injuries clinically. Landmines are a form of ordnance that are placed on or under ground and explode when triggered, generally by electromagnetic waves or direct pressure (e.g., being stepped upon).[22] Unexploded ordnances include bombs, grenades, missiles, rockets, and mortar and artillery shells that were fired or dropped and did not explode.[23]

Injuries from landmines and UXOs are a risk for civilian and military personnel alike and are a worldwide problem. Landmines and UXOs are common in both Iraq and Afghanistan. Because it has been involved in intense conflict for decades, Iraq is considered one of the most heavily landmine and UXO-contaminated countries in the world. Landmines and UXOs are particularly prevalent in the north along Iraq's border with Iran and in the central and southern regions as well.[24] In Afghanistan, the International Committee of the Red Cross reports that there are 10 million landmines and more than 50 different types of landmines, and that the most heavily mined areas are along the border with Pakistan and around the cities of Kabul and Kandahar.[25] There are sections of Bagram Air Base, Afghanistan that are still not clear of landmines and are cordoned off to prevent troops from accidentally entering that area. Many of the landmine and UXO victims treated at US military medical facilities are civilians.

A recent report from the US Centers for Disease Control and Prevention (CDC) compiled data from several sources to evaluate landmine and UXO injuries in Afghanistan over a six-year period.[26] Major findings included the following: (1) almost all of the injuries were sustained by men; (2) more than half of the injured were under the age of 18 (one-third were between the ages of 10 and 14); (3) children were twice as likely to be injured by UXOs as adults, although the case-fatality rate (7 percent) was the same for both; and (4) adult males were more likely to be injured by landmines as they traveled for work or military activity, whereas children were more likely to be injured while playing with a newly found object that turned out to be an UXO.[27] These trends were confirmed in later studies.[23]

Landmines and UXOs cause injury through the blast effects described below (i.e., primary blast effect, secondary fragments, tertiary [whole-body propulsion], and quaternary [burns]).[28] The three main types of conventional antipersonnel landmines are blast or static, bounding fragmentation, and directional fragmentation; each has an associated pattern of injury (Table 2).

| TYPE OF MINE | HOW CONCEALED | HOW DETONATED | PRIMARY AREAS OF WOUNDING |
|---|---|---|---|
| Blast or static | Buried just below ground surface | Pressure (e.g., being stepped upon) | Foot, upper leg, lower leg |
| Fragmentation<br>• *Bounding* | Buried just below surface with fuse protruding, or laid on surface | Fuse or tripwire | All |
| • *Directional* | Laid on surface | Electrical charge, timed fuse, or tripwire | All |

Table 2. *Categories of Antipersonnel Landmines. Adapted from Bellamy, 1991[10] and the International Committee of the Red Cross.[29]*

## Blast (Static) Landmines

Static landmines are small mines planted and designed to activate when a person steps on them (Fig. 4). Many of these devices are designed to injure but not kill an individual.[30] However many are lethal, either due to the immediate injury or to subsequent uncontrolled hemorrhage. There are classically two patterns of

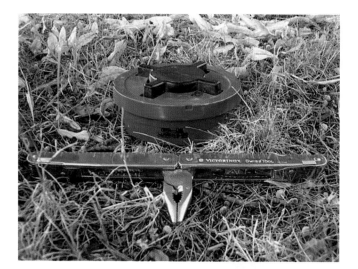

Figure 4. (Right) *Example of static landmine. Image courtesy of the United Nations Mine Action Service.*

Figure 5. (Below) *Static landmines detonate when stepped on, resulting in partial or complete lower limb amputation, most commonly at the midfoot or distal tibia. Debris may be driven up along fascial planes with tissue stripped from the bone. Image courtesy of the Borden Institute, Office of The Surgeon General, Washington, DC. Illustrator: Bruce Maston.*

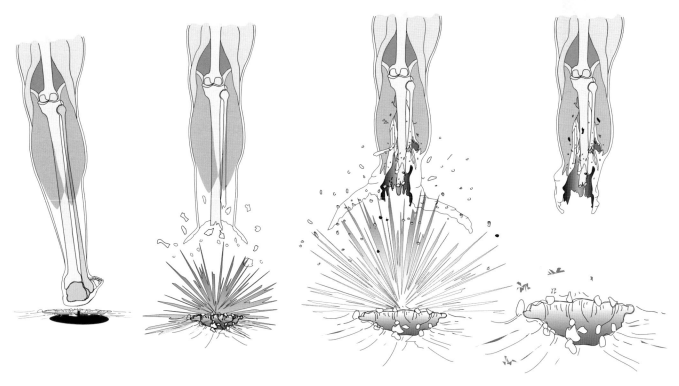

injury: (1) complete or near-complete amputation of the foot (Fig. 5); and (2) random penetrating fragment injuries along the tissue and fascial planes of the lower leg (Fig. 6).[31] When these types of mines explode, particles of the dirt in which they were buried, debris, clothing, bone, and mine fragments can be driven by the blast up the leg into the upper or mid-calf causing gross contamination.[10,15]

## Fragmentation Landmines

The two types of fragmentation landmines are bounding and directional fragmentation landmines (Fig. 7). The bounding type of antipersonnel mine is so named because it bounds upward and then explodes mid-air at approximately torso level. Upon detonation, this type of mine propels hundreds of fragments in all directions (as far as hundreds of meters), inflicts injuries higher in the body (e.g., torso, upper extremities, neck, or head) compared to static mines, and has the highest mortality of any landmine type.[15] Perhaps the

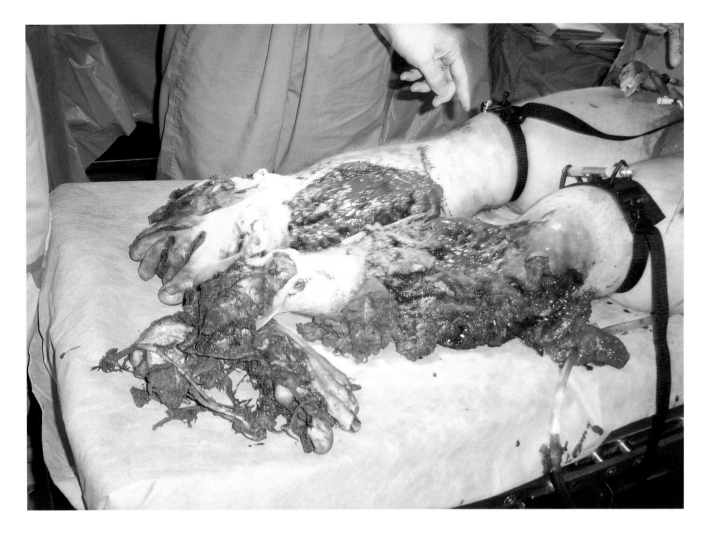

Figure 6. (Above) *A landmine blast leads to an umbrella effect in which the soft tissues, vessels, and nerves are stripped from the bone. This results in a more proximal injury than may be clinically apparent. Image courtesy of the Borden Institute, Office of The Surgeon General, Washington, DC.*

Figure 7. (Right) *When triggered, fragmentation mines project a lethal shower of metallic fragments in all directions. The bounding types are projected upwards, prior to exploding mid-air at approximately torso level. Image courtesy of the United Nations Mine Action Service.*

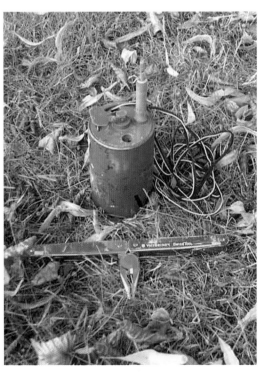

best-known type of bounding mine is the M16A2 or "Bouncing Betty," which was developed in the 1930s and widely used during World War II.[10,32]

## Directional Fragmentation Landmines

Upon detonation, directional fragmentation landmines project fragments in a single direction to cause multiple wounds both high and low on the body.[15] A commonly used directional fragmentation mine is the Claymore mine, which is placed above-ground and can spray 700 circular pellets over an arc

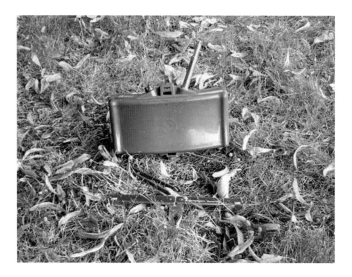

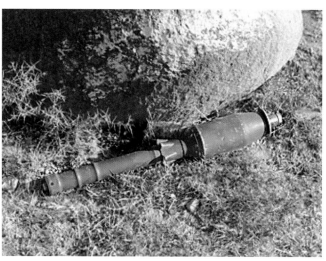

Figure 8. *Directional fragmentation landmines project fragments in a single direction to cause multiple wounds, both high and low on the body. Image courtesy of the United Nations Mine Action Service.*

Figure 9. *A rocket-propelled grenade (RPG). The high-explosive warhead is affixed to a rocket motor and stabilized in flight by fins. Image courtesy of the United Nations Mine Action Service.*

of 60 degrees (Fig. 8).[15] Lethal injuries occur within 50 meters from the point of detonation, and nonlethal fragmentation injuries can occur as far as 300 meters away.[10]

## Rocket-Propelled Grenades

Rocket-propelled grenades (RPGs) are muzzle-loaded, shoulder-fired weapons that are primarily used against armored vehicles and ground personnel (Fig. 9). The various types of RPGs can fire fragmentation and high-explosive (e.g., high-explosive antitank [HEAT]) rounds and have a lethal blast radius of four meters.[33] Ground troops are sometimes injured when anti-vehicle rounds are aimed at adjacent structures, resulting in structural collapse and generation of multiple fragments. Because they are inexpensive and easy to transport and operate, RPGs are the weapon of choice for insurgents in many former Soviet-supported countries, including Iraq and Afghanistan. They can be found in almost 40 countries throughout the world.[34] Although RPG effects vary case-by-case, they frequently cause devastating injuries.[33]

## Improvised Explosive Devices

Improvised explosive device (IED) attacks have become a mainstay in the current conflicts. IED attacks are most often used in insurgency and terrorist operations. They have been responsible for 40 to 60 percent of military casualties (wounded and killed) in Iraq between 2006 and mid-2009, and 50 to 75 percent in Afghanistan.[35,36] The incidence of IED-related injuries will vary depending on the phase of military operations. The decline in IED-related casualties in Iraq has been partly attributed to the increase in mine-resistant ambush protected (MRAP) vehicles sent to Iraq.[36] The sharp increase in IED-related casualties in Afghanistan has been attributed to "expanded military operations, a near-doubling of the number of troops since the beginning of the year and a Taliban offensive that has included a proliferation of roadside bombings."[37] Pentagon sources indicate that the number of IEDs in Afghanistan has increased 350 percent since 2007, with a subsequent increase in the number of IED-related combat injuries and deaths of more than 700 and 400 percent, respectively.[38]

IEDs are defined as devices that are placed or fabricated in an improvised manner incorporating destructive, lethal, noxious, pyrotechnic, or incendiary chemicals and are designed to destroy, incapacitate, harass, or distract (Fig. 10).[39] They may incorporate military weapons, such as artillery shells or antitank mines, but are usually devised from non-military components.

IEDs vary in size, shape, form, and explosive power. They are easy to make and use, can be housed in almost any type of container, and can be hidden almost anywhere. The various types of IEDs use a range of explosive materials and are concealed, deployed, and detonated in different ways:

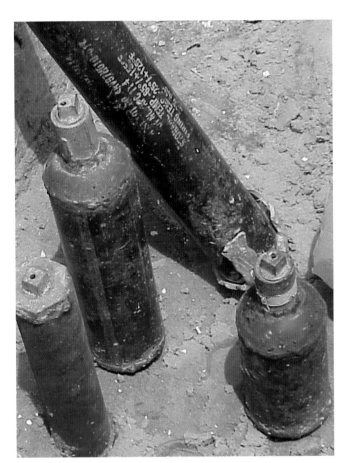

Figure 10. *IEDs are defined as devices that are placed or fabricated in an improvised manner incorporating destructive, lethal, noxious, pyrotechnic, or incendiary chemicals and are designed to destroy, incapacitate, harass, or distract. Image courtesy of the United Nations Mine Action Service.*

- Casings, ranging in size from a cigarette pack to a large vehicle, are used to hide the IED and possibly provide fragmentation. Small or large packages, including 120-mm and larger artillery or mortar projectiles with armor-piercing capability, are often placed in potholes covered with dirt, behind cinder blocks or sand piles to direct the blast, hidden in garbage bags or animal carcasses, or thrown in front of vehicles.

- Common hardware such as ball bearings, bolts, nuts, or nails can be used to enhance the fragmentation. Propane tanks, fuel cans, and battery acid have been added to IEDs to increase their blast and thermal effects. The damaging effects of IEDs can be maximized via coupling (linking one munition to another), boosting (stacking one munition upon another), and daisy-chaining (many munitions physically and temporally linked together length-wise).

- Triggers can be command-detonated by a remote device such as a cell phone, car alarm, toy car remote, or garage door opener, or with a time-delay device to allow the bomber to escape or to target military forces operating in a pattern. The initiator almost always includes a blasting cap and batteries as a power source for the detonator.

- Person-borne or victim-actuated devices (suicide bombs), typically using a powerful explosive with enhanced fragmentary effects, are employed to kill or maim as many people as possible. These are concealed in clothing worn by the assailant and hand-detonated.

- Vehicle-borne devices can vary in size from 100 to 1,000 pounds, depending on the size of the vehicle. The explosive charge can include mortar and artillery rounds, rocket mortars, warheads, and PE4 explosives. These can be concealed in vehicles of all types (cars, trucks, donkey carts). They can be deployed singly or in multiple vehicles. A lead vehicle is used to slow traffic and is followed by the main explosive device to maximize casualties. Detonation is by a command firing system.

- IEDs can be engineered to overcome IED detection measures through rolling (i.e., a target vehicle rolls over an initial unfused munition and then triggers a second trailing munition, which in turn detonates the initial munition). This sequencing positions the second (and most damaging) explosion directly under the target vehicle.

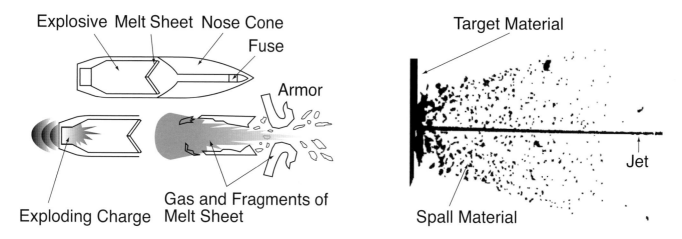

Figure 11. *Shaped-charge round:* (Left) *Disruptive mechanisms of the shaped-charge warhead include the jet of the charge itself and the debris knocked off from the inside face of the armored plate.* (Right) *Diagram taken from photograph of an actual detonation of a shaped-charged warhead against the armor plate caused by antitank land mines.*
*Image courtesy of the Borden Institute, Office of The Surgeon General, Washington, DC.*
*Illustrator: Bruce Maston.*

Improvised explosive device (IED) attacks have become a mainstay in OEF and OIF. They have been responsible for 40 to 60 percent of military casualties (wounded and killed) in Iraq between 2006 and mid-2009, and 50 to 75 percent in Afghanistan.

## Antitank Munitions

In Iraq, there has been a trend away from small bombs (e.g., concealed in containers such as soft drink cans) to large rocket propellant or shaped-charges with armor-piercing capability.[40] Heavily armored vehicles are less susceptible to smaller, home-made roadside IEDs, and newer vehicle designs such as the MRAP provide enhanced protection to occupants from even larger IEDs. Antitank munitions are categorized as: (1) shaped-charges; (2) kinetic energy rounds; and (3) antitank landmines.[15]

### *Shaped-Charge*

Shaped-charges have various degrees of armor-piercing capability (Fig. 11). High-explosive antitank (HEAT) rounds are composed of explosive charges packed around a reverse cone (this is the concept behind the anti-armor warhead of an RPG) (Fig. 12). If the charge is able to defeat the armor of the vehicle, injury to the occupants occurs via two methods. The initial potentially catastrophic injuries (including burns) are caused by the jet of the shaped-charge after it penetrates the vehicle's armor. Next, as the weapon strikes the armor, small pieces of irregularly shaped debris (spall) break away from the interior of the vehicle and are propelled into the occupants.

A commonly used shaped-charge variant is the explosively formed projectile (EFP) (Figs. 13 and 14). This IED variant consists of a cylindrical casing, such as a metal pipe. The side facing the target is closed with a concave-shaped metal plate facing inward, and the explosive charge is placed behind the metal plate.[41] On detonation, the concave plate is propelled out of the casing, becoming a high-speed aerodynamic penetrator (velocity can exceed 1,500 m/sec). This bullet or rod-shaped projectile easily pierces vehicle armor, causing catastrophic damage to vehicle occupants and other personnel in its path.[42]

The increased use and effects of EFPs are illustrated in a review of IED injuries seen in a British field hospital in 2006.[42] All casualties had injuries from roadside bombs directed at Coalition vehicles. Almost all (91 percent) of the explosions were caused by an EFP, and EFPs were responsible for all deaths. Main findings included the following:

- Most casualties (87 percent in survivors and nonsurvivors) had extremity injuries
- Most casualties had injuries to several regions of the body (e.g., 2.6 mean areas injured in survivors and 4.7 in nonsurvivors)
- All casualties had open wounds
- More than half of casualties (53 percent) had fractures
- There was little primary blast injury; only two casualties were thought to have died directly from a primary blast mechanism (blast lung)
- Only 15 percent of casualties had burns; no burns covered more than five percent total body surface area (TBSA)
- Approximately half of the survivors required immediate operative intervention at the field hospital

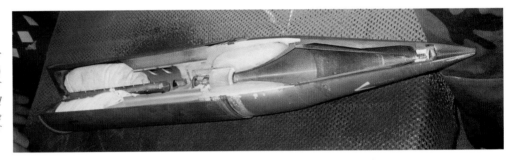

Figure 12. *Cross-section image of a high-explosive antitank (HEAT) round. Note the reverse cone of metal liner in the mid-section and the exploding charge at the base of the round. Image courtesy of Wikimedia Commons.*

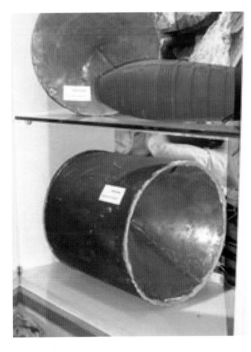

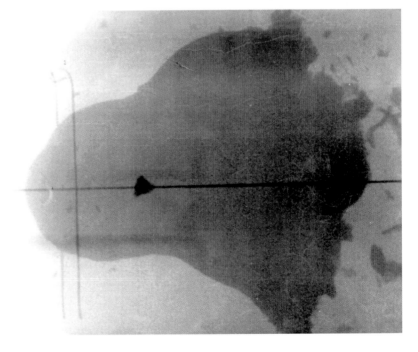

Figure 13. (Left) *An explosively formed projectile is an IED variant consisting of a cylindrical casing, closed with a concave-shaped metal plate facing inward, and an internal explosive charge. On detonation, the concave plate is propelled out of the casing and can inflict catastrophic injury. Image courtesy of Defense-Update.com.*

Figure 14. (Right) *X-ray of explosively formed projectile (EFP) detonation. Image courtesy of Applied Research Associates, Inc.*

> Explosively formed projectiles (EFPs) generate "all or nothing" wounding patterns whereby casualties experience either catastrophic injuries or relatively minor wounds.[42] Significant EFP attacks cause multiple injuries in each survivor, including a high incidence of open wounds, extremity injuries, and fractures.

### Kinetic Energy Rounds

Kinetic energy rounds are shaped like darts and are made from hard metals such as depleted uranium. Like shaped-charges, these weapons inflict damage by direct penetration of the vehicle or by generating spall. Warfighters with wounds caused by depleted uranium fragments should undergo standard wound care. Although there is a potential long-term risk from chronic exposure to depleted uranium, it does not justify extensive procedures to remove the fragments.[43]

### Antitank Landmines

Antitank landmines are being modified and used as buried IEDs in OEF and OIF. Often, as described previously, more than one mine will be linked together to enhance the level of destruction.[14]

## Explosion-Related Injury

### Patterns

Explosive devices produce the ultimate polytrauma (i.e., a wide range of injury types to many body regions caused by the full range of injury mechanisms).[44] Explosions produce patterns of injury that are distinct from those of other mechanisms.[45] The simultaneous combination of different injury mechanisms (below) produces a complex array of injuries that must be understood to produce the best patient outcomes. In comparison with trauma patients whose injuries were not caused by explosions, bombing victims have lower states of consciousness as well as increased hypotension, injury severity, presence of multiple injuries, need for surgery, use of critical care services, length of hospital stay (LOS), and mortality.[45]

> Explosive devices produce a complex array of injuries that must be understood to produce the best patient outcomes.

Military Casualties

A report that examined victims of close-proximity IED blasts of a variety of types (antipersonnel and antitank, including 105 to 120 mm mortars, 155 mm artillery-round IEDs, and a VS-1.6 antitank mine) revealed complex injuries in all cases and a 50 percent mortality rate despite the fact that all had been wearing Kevlar helmets, ballistic eye protection, and full body armor.[46] Some were injured on foot patrol, and some were in vehicles. The aforementioned report demonstrates the complexity of IED-related injuries.[42] The types of injuries produced by antitank weapons are shown in Figure 15 and include:

A. Translational blast injury (tertiary blast injury) can occur as the vehicle and its occupants are suddenly propelled upward causing blunt injury to occupants.
B. Toxic gases (a form of quaternary blast injury) can cause significant inhalation injury.
C. Primary blast injury can cause injury to the ears, lung, bowel, brain, and other organs.
D. Ballistic injury from the weapon and resultant debris fragments as the vehicle armor is defeated also occurs (secondary blast injury), as do thermal injuries resulting from flammable materials within the vehicle (quaternary blast injury).

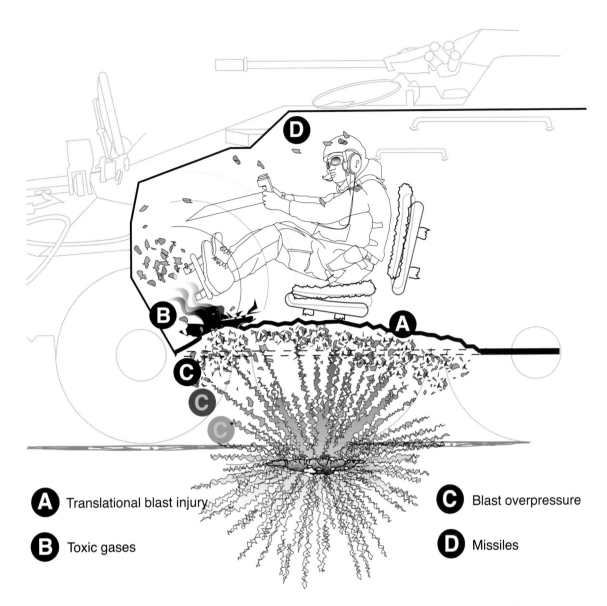

A Translational blast injury

B Toxic gases

C Blast overpressure

D Missiles

Figure 15. *Injuries sustained as a result of defeated armor: (A) translational blast injury, (B) toxic gases, (C) blast overpressure, and (D) penetrating missile wounds.*
*Adapted image courtesy of the Borden Institute, Office of The Surgeon General, Washington, DC.*
*Illustrator: Bruce Maston.*

## Civilian Casualties

Following an explosion in the civilian sector (e.g., open market bombing), most patients with lethal injuries will die immediately. Although the majority of survivors do not have life-threatening injuries, approximately 10 to 15 percent of casualties will have critical injuries and may be saved with appropriate management.[47,48,49]

Morbidity and mortality are generally dictated by the size of the explosive charge, whether the explosion occurs within a confined space, and whether it causes structural collapse.[50] Patterns of injury unique to blast include the following:[51]

- Most injuries are noncritical soft-tissue or skeletal injuries
- Head injury predominates as a cause of death (50 to 70 percent)
- The incidence of head injuries is disproportionate to exposed total body surface area (TBSA)
- Most blast lung injury kills immediately

In Israeli reviews, victims of terrorist bomb attacks, when compared to victims of non-terrorist trauma, have been shown to: (1) sustain more severe injuries, as measured by Injury Severity Score (ISS) (ISS greater than 16 in 74 percent versus 10 percent) and median intensive care unit (ICU) LOS (5 days versus 3 days);[52] (2) commonly have a combination of blunt and penetrating injuries (85 percent versus 15 percent)[53] and injuries to several areas of the body (three or more body regions injured in 28 percent versus 6 percent patients);[52] and (3) have injuries that are more likely to be fatal (mortality 6 percent versus 2 to 3 percent).[52,53] As demonstrated repeatedly among civilian populations that have been dealing with terrorism for years, terrorist bomb attacks produce injuries that are more complex, more severe, more lethal, and occur in a greater number of body regions than non-bomb-associated injuries.[45,54]

> In civilian sector explosions, most patients with lethal injuries die immediately. Although the majority of survivors do not have life-threatening injuries, some 10 to 15 percent of casualties with critical injuries may be saved with appropriate treatment.

## Potentiators

A variety of strategies are used to increase the wounding and killing potential of explosives. These include: (1) increasing the size of the charge and amount of explosive; (2) increasing the number and type of secondary fragments (e.g., packing the devices with metal objects or pieces of concrete); (3) adding harmful substances such as chemicals, animal feces, or bacterial contaminants to produce infection; (4) planting explosives under vehicles to generate secondary fragments; and (5) adding incendiary substances such as petroleum products. Secondary explosions are often initiated by fuel-air explosives that disperse and ignite a spray of aerosol fuel, or by cluster bombs that distribute bomblets over a wide area.

The damage of the initial explosion is compounded by deploying snipers, subsequent bombs, or a remotely-detonated explosion to damage rescuers and first responders and vastly enhance the chaos. These tactics were used in Northern Ireland and are common in Iraq and Israel. Precise timing and location are also used to maximize the numbers of injured and dead.[47] Responders at the scene must be aware of these tactics and their effects, especially as recent data show increased coordination of terrorist attacks, including secondary attacks on first responders at the scene of an explosion, and increased variability in IEDs, including the introduction of chemical IEDs.[55]

Perhaps one of the most effective potentiators is the planting of explosives in confined spaces. Explosions that take place in confined spaces (e.g., buses and buildings) have patterns of injury that differ from those in open spaces (e.g., markets). Confined-space (closed-space) explosions generally produce more primary blast injury (discussed below) and penetrating injuries than explosions in open areas (open-space). The pressure

| | OPEN-SPACE | CLOSED-SPACE |
|---|---|---|
| Deaths | 8 percent | 49 percent |
| Injuries | | |
| • Primary blast injury | 34 percent | 77 percent |
| • Burns, TBSA | 18 percent | 31 percent |
| • Injury severity: median Injury Severity Score (ISS) | 4 (minor) | 18 (moderate/severe) |

Table 5. *Comparison of open- and closed-space bombing deaths and injuries. Adapted from Leibovici, 1996.*[58]

wave associated with high-order explosive detonation reflects off doors, ceilings, and walls in confined spaces, lasts longer, and comprises what is termed a "quasi-static" exposure to overpressure effects.[56]

> In OEF and OIF, most explosions are open-space bombings, and most injuries and deaths are from explosive fragments (secondary blast injury).

Israeli studies show significantly increased morbidity and mortality among those in confined-space bombings compared to those in open-space attacks.[57,58,59,60] In a 1996 study, an 8 percent mortality rate was observed among open-air (open-space) bombings versus 49 percent in bus bombings (Table 5).[58] An earlier study showed high percentages of primary blast injuries in bus bombings. In this study, 76 percent of victims had tympanic membrane perforation, 38 percent had blast lung, and 14 percent had abdominal blast injury.[57]

| BLAST INJURY EFFECTS | MECHANISM OF INJURY |
| --- | --- |
| Primary | Injury caused by the effect of the blast wave on the body. Primary blast injury occurs principally in the gas-filled organs and results from extreme pressure differentials developed at body surfaces. Organs most susceptible include the middle ear, lung, brain, and bowel. |
| Secondary | Injury caused by flying debris and fragments, propelled mostly by the blast winds generated by an explosion. Most commonly produces penetrating injury to the body. At very close distance to the explosion, debris and fragments may cause limb amputation or total body disruption. This is the most common mechanism of injury from blast. |
| Tertiary | Injury results from victim being propelled through space by the blast wind and impacting a stationary object. |
| Quaternary | Injury suffered as a result of other effects of bomb blasts, including crush injury from a collapsed structure, inhalation of toxic gases and debris, thermal burns, and exacerbation of prior medical illnesses. |
| Quinary | Injury resulting from contamination via biological and chemical agents, radioactive materials, or contaminated tissue from attacker or other person at the scene. |

Table 6. *Categories of blast injury effects with corresponding mechanisms of injury.*

When the confined space is a building, the force of the blast may break windows, producing thousands of glass shards, and buckle the walls, floor, and ceiling, resulting in partial or complete building collapse and subsequent crush injuries.[61] Studies contrasting open-space bombings with bombings involving buildings (closed-space) show a much higher mortality rate in the latter. For example, all deaths and almost all (96 percent) injuries in the 1996 Khobar Towers bombing in Saudi Arabia occurred inside the buildings; and in the 1995 Oklahoma City bombing, 87 percent of those in the collapsed section of the Murrah Building died, compared with 5 percent of those in the uncollapsed section.[48,62]

In OEF and OIF, most explosions are open-space bombings and most injuries and deaths are from fragments.[44,63]

## Categories

Blast injuries are categorized as having primary, secondary, tertiary, quaternary, and quinary effects, each with its own mechanism of injury (Table 6).

### Primary Blast Injury

Primary blast injuries result when the pressure wave interacts with the body, especially the gas-containing organs, via spalling, implosion, acceleration-deceleration, or initiation of pressure differentials.[31]

- ◆ "Spalling, or spallation, occurs when particles from a more dense substance are thrown into a less dense substance at their interface."[31] Spall is a flake or small particles that are broken off a larger solid body and can be produced by a variety of mechanisms, including projectile impact (Fig. 16).
- ◆ Implosion is the momentary contraction of gas pockets that occurs when the blast wave moves through the tissue. The pressure differential may force blood and fluid into the previously air-filled spaces, as seen with pulmonary contusion and hemorrhage in blast lung injury.[31]
- ◆ Acceleration-deceleration, or shear injury, occurs when movement of the body wall in the direction of the blast wave displaces the internal structures. Because the structures accelerate at different rates, shearing or disruption may occur.
- ◆ The pressure differential between the inside and outside of the body induced by the blast wave produces injuries.[31]

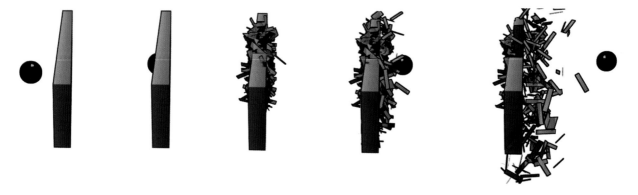

Figure 16. *Spall is debris generated when particles from a more dense substance are thrown into a less dense substance at their interface. In this illustration, the ball impacts a metallic plate and knocks off material from the inside surface into the air. Adapted image courtesy of Wikimedia Commons.*

> Survival after a primary blast injury is dependent on the energy of the blast, whether it occurred in an open or enclosed (closed) space, and the distance of the individual from the point of detonation (standoff distance).[20] The main sites of primary blast injury are the ears, lungs, intestinal tract, and brain.[64,65]

### *Ears*

A powerful blast wave can overwhelm the extremely delicate structures within the ear, causing tympanic membrane rupture, fracture or dislocation of the ossicles, and permanent inner ear damage. Rupture of the tympanic membrane is a common injury following an explosive blast.[66] Further, the tympanic membranes are the structures that are injured at the lowest pressure, and thus have been used as a sentinel for other, more serious injuries.[64] Recent reports have disputed the reliability of tympanic membrane rupture as a sensitive screening tool for primary blast injury detection.[21,66] The absence of tympanic membrane rupture does not exclude other types of blast injury. An increase in pressure of as little as five pounds per square inch (psi) may cause eardrum rupture, 15 psi carries a 50 percent chance, and 30 to 40 psi will almost certainly rupture the eardrum.[67] Recent data from OEF and OIF with explosion-related injuries indicated an approximate 15 to 16 percent incidence of tympanic membrane rupture.[21,66] The most common symptoms reported by the patients experiencing an audiovestibular injury are hearing loss (60 percent), tinnitus (49 percent), otalgia (26 percent), and dizziness (15 percent).[68,69]

> Rupture of the tympanic membrane is a common injury following an explosive blast. Its absence may not be adequate to rule out primary blast injury and does not exclude other types of blast injury.

During the secondary survey in the initial evaluation of a blast victim, the tympanic membranes should be evaluated. Improvised explosive device detonations typically propel debris into the external auditory canal. The debris should be carefully removed to allow full visualization of the ear canal. The external auditory canal should not be blindly irrigated because this can result in pain and vertigo in patients with perforated tympanic membranes.[70] If debris is noted in the external auditory canal or behind the ruptured tympanic membrane, topical antibiotic eardrops, such as a fluoroquinolone, are recommended to prevent infection.[64,70] The presence of cerebrospinal fluid or blood in the external auditory canal or hemotympanum is suggestive of a basilar skull fracture.

Most (80 to 90 percent) tympanic membrane perforations heal spontaneously. The larger the perforation, however, the lower the probability that it will heal spontaneously.[21] Perforations involving more than 30 percent of the surface area of the tympanic membrane are significantly less likely to heal spontaneously than smaller perforations (Fig. 17).[70] Spontaneous healing also varies with the location of the rupture. Central tympanic membrane ruptures have the least likelihood of healing spontaneously, whereas inferior perforations are the most likely.[21]

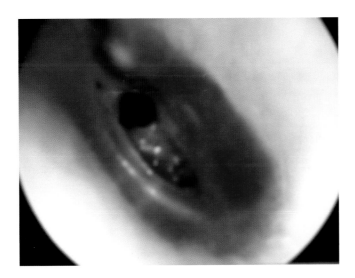

Figure 17. *Tympanic membrane perforation. Image courtesy of Gene Liu, MD, Cedars-Sinai Medical Center.*

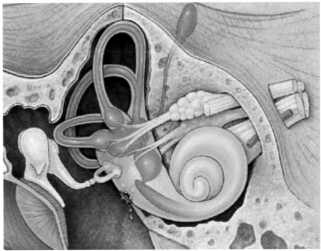

Figure 18. *Blast effect can cause inner ear injuries, such as the perilymphatic fistula shown here, and ruptures of the saccule, utricle, and basilar membrane. In the middle ear, the ossicles may fracture or disarticulate, independent of a tympanic membrane perforation. Image courtesy of Timothy Hain, MD, Northwestern University.*

Besides rupturing the tympanic membrane, the blast can also cause middle ear damage, such as fracture of the ossicles or disarticulation of the ossicular chain.[68] Although these usually occur in conjunction with tympanic membrane perforation, they can occur independently. Injury to the inner ear, such as perilymphatic fistulae in the oval window and ruptures of the saccule, utricle, and basilar membrane, may also occur (Fig. 18). Sensorineural hearing loss may be seen with loss of hair cell integrity. Similarly, damage to the vestibular apparatus may occur and manifest as vertigo.[19]

Consultation with the otolaryngology service should be performed when greater than 50 percent tympanic membrane perforation occurs or if other audiovestibular symptoms are noted. All blast injury patients requiring inpatient care should have audiometric testing when possible.[21,71] The management guidelines used at Balad Air Base in Iraq are presented in Table 7. Hearing protection has been shown to significantly reduce the incidence of tympanic membrane rupture, and its use should be encouraged in combatants who are deployed in high-risk environments.[72]

## Lungs

The lungs are also vulnerable to primary blast effects. Explosions can cause a variety of thoracic injuries including pulmonary contusion, pneumothorax, pneumomediastinum, air emboli, hemothorax, and subcutaneous emphysema (Fig. 19).[64] An external force acting on the chest wall may compress the lungs slowly enough to allow air contained in the alveoli to be expelled through the trachea. However, when a significant blast wave impacts the chest wall, there is little time for pressure equilibration. The pressure

| CONSULTATION | INDICATIONS | |
| --- | --- | --- |
| | ABSOLUTE | RELATIVE |
| Otolaryngology | Vertigo lasting greater than three days | Tympanic membrane rupture greater than 50 percent |
| | Presence of clear otorrhea | Debris in the external auditory canal that does not resolve with topical antibiotics |
| | Discolored otorrhea that persists despite seven days of topical antibiotic therapy | Inability to visualize the tympanic membrane despite removal of debris from the external auditory canal |
| Audiology | An average hearing threshold greater than 30dB at frequencies of 500, 1000, and 2000Hz | Significant communication problems |
| | A hearing threshold greater than 35dB at frequencies of 500, 1000, or 2000Hz | Tinnitus significantly affecting quality of life |
| | A hearing threshold greater than 55dB at frequencies of 3000 or 4000Hz | |
| | New-onset asymmetrical hearing loss | |

Table 7. *Management guidelines for otolaryngology and audiology consultations used at Balad Air Base, Iraq. Adapted from Depenbrock, 2008.*[70]

differentials that develop at the interface between media of different densities tear the alveolar walls, disrupt the alveolar–capillary interface, and cause the emphysematous spaces to fill with blood, resulting in primary blast injury to the lung (blast lung).[19] Pressures of 30 to 40 psi are associated with possible lung injury, and at 80 psi, a 50 percent chance of lung injury exists.[67] As a point of reference, pressures in the 100 to 200 psi range may be lethal, and when psi exceeds 200 to 250, death is almost certain.[67]

> Lungs are vulnerable to primary blast effects. Explosions can cause a variety of intrathoracic injuries including pulmonary contusion, pneumothorax, pneumomediastinum, air emboli, hemothorax, and subcutaneous emphysema.

Pulmonary manifestations vary greatly depending on the size of the blast wave. The mildest form of this tissue disruption was noted to be pleural and subpleural petechiae in animal studies.[73,74] The classic chest radiograph demonstrates bilateral central infiltrates and has been described as a butterfly or batwing pattern (Fig. 20). This pattern is probably caused by reflection of the blast wave off of the mediastinal structures within the thoracic cavity. Additionally, the central location of the infiltrates helps differentiate this from the more classic lateral infiltrates seen with pulmonary contusion (Fig. 21).[75]

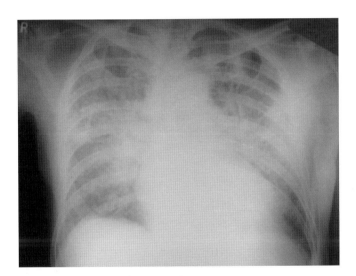

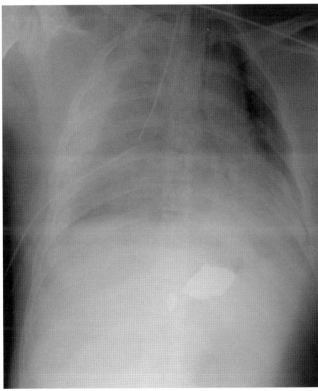

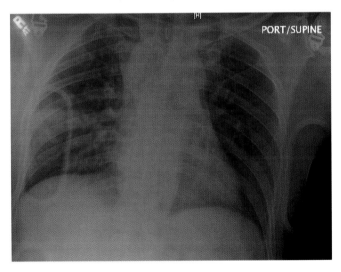

Figure 19. (Top Right) *Chest radiograph demonstrating pneumothorax, hemothorax, and a penetrating fragment, following an IED explosion.*

Figure 20. (Top Left) *The classic chest radiograph seen with primary blast injury to the lung demonstrates a butterfly or batwing pattern.*

Figure 21 (Bottom Left) *Chest radiograph demonstrating a peripherally located pulmonary contusion resulting from blast injury.*

| INDICATIONS & REQUIREMENTS | BLAST LUNG INJURY CATEGORIES | | |
|---|---|---|---|
| | MILD | MODERATE | SEVERE |
| **Indications** | | | |
| Radiographic infiltrates | Unilateral | Asymmetrical and bilateral | Diffuse |
| PaO$_2$ to FiO$_2$ Ratio (mm Hg) | >200 | 60 to 200 | <60 |
| Bronchopleural fistula | No | Yes | Yes |
| **Requirements** | | | |
| Positive pressure ventiliation (PPV) requirement | Unlikely for respiratory problem | Highly likely but usually conventional methods | Universal and unconventional methods common |
| Positive end-expiratory pressure (PEEP) requirement (cm H$_2$O) | <5 if PPV needed | 5 to 10 usually needed | >10 commonly needed |

Table 8. *Severity categories for blast lung injury based upon radiographic appearance, oxygen requirement, and the presence of bronchopleural fistula. Adapted from Pizov, 1999.*[80]

The incidence of blast lung in OEF and OIF has been low because open-space explosions predominate. When blast lung occurs in patients, it has high associated morbidity and its treatment is resource-intensive.[76,77,78] Primary blast injury to the lung may not be immediately obvious upon external examination.[79] Symptoms of blast lung can manifest within the first few minutes following a blast or can develop and evolve over a period of hours to days.[21,57,75,80,81] Blast lung has been shown to have the following characteristics:

- Symptoms include dyspnea, chest pain, hemoptysis, and cough[19]
- Clinical signs include cyanosis, tachypnea, rapid or shallow breathing, crackles, diminished breath sounds, dullness to percussion, increased resonance, retrosternal crunch, subcutaneous crepitus, and tracheal deviation[19]
- Hypoxemia and hypercarbia[81]
- Rapid respiratory deterioration with progressive hypoxia[58]
- Progressive need for ventilation with high FiO$_2$[58]
- Progressive haziness in serial chest radiographs[58]
- Hemodynamic instability[58]
- Pulmonary edema with frothing at the mouth, frequently lethal[64]

Enclosed-space (closed-space) bombings should raise the index of suspicion for blast lung and other primary blast injuries.[53] Patients with blast lung require supportive care with special emphasis on ensuring adequate oxygenation and ventilation. Standard ventilator management with initial use of positive end-expiratory pressure of 10 centimeters (cm) water is acceptable.[18] However, advanced ventilatory methods, such as independent lung ventilation, high-frequency jet ventilation, nitric oxide inhalation, and extracorporeal membrane oxygenation, may also be of value.[47,80,82] Intravenous fluids should be administered judiciously to minimize capillary leak and pulmonary edema. Patients should be monitored closely for development of pneumothorax. The clinical efficacy of prophylactic antibiotics and steroids in blast lung injury is undetermined.[64] Published blast lung injury severity categories, based on radiographic appearance, oxygen requirement, and the presence of bronchopleural fistula, may be helpful in determining which patients require positive pressure mechanical ventilation and positive end-expiratory pressure (Table 8).[80] While ear protection has been shown to offer some protection of the tympanic membrane against primary blast injury, thoracic body armor may not have the same protective effect on the lungs.[64,83]

### Solid and Hollow Organs

A blast wave can cause rapid compression and expansion of air in gas-filled organs, which often results in contusions, perforations, or intramural hemorrhage. When air emboli fill the pulmonary and coronary vessels, early death often occurs.[54] Delayed rupture of the intestinal tract can occur secondary to significant ischemia and infarction within the mesentery.[64] While the gastrointestinal tract is particularly susceptible to primary blast injury, especially the colon, primary blast injury of hollow organs in OEF and OIF is rarely encountered.[84,85,86,87]

Solid organs, principally the liver, spleen, and kidney, have a relatively uniform liquid density. When a blast wave impacts these organs, little compression occurs, and significant injury to the tissue is less likely to occur.[19,88] Solid intraabdominal organs are more likely to be injured through secondary or tertiary mechanisms. However, blast waves can cause shear forces to develop at points of attachments of organs or at the surfaces of the organs. In the former case, an organ may tear off of its point of attachment, while in the latter case, subcapsular petechiae, contusions, lacerations, or rupture may occur.[19]

Patients may present with a variety of abdominal signs and symptoms including pain, nausea, vomiting, hematemesis, melena, and signs of peritoneal irritation.[21] Patients with overt hemodynamic instability should undergo immediate exploratory laparotomy for presumed active hemorrhage from the intestinal mesentery or a solid organ injury.[89] More stable patients can be evaluated using computed tomography (CT) imaging. Ritenour noted that "CT evidence of blast injury includes pneumoperitoneum, free intraperitoneal fluid not consistent with blood, and a sentinel clot seen on bowel wall or mesentery."[21] Intestinal contusion, submucosal hematoma, and mesenteric hematoma can also be seen on CT imaging following blast injury.[89]

> The gastrointestinal tract is particularly susceptible to primary blast injury, especially the colon. Significant ischemia and infarction within the mesentery following primary blast injury can lead to delayed rupture of the intestinal tract.

### Brain

The prevalence of traumatic brain injury (TBI) among combat casualties is higher in the current conflicts than in previous wars. This is primarily because many patients with previously lethal injuries are now surviving, largely due to enhanced helmets that prevent or reduce penetrating head trauma, advances in battlefield medicine, and rapid evacuation to a well-honed system of care.[90] Thus, TBI has become the current signature injury of combat, much as shell shock was the signature injury of World War I.[65,91] Traumatic brain injury potentially affects up to one-third of OEF and OIF combatants and approximately 320,000 reported experiencing symptoms that may be related to TBI during deployment.[92] Of patients admitted to Walter Reed Army Medical Center (WRAMC) between 2003 and 2005 who had been exposed to explosive blasts, 59 percent were found to have symptoms that may relate to TBI. Of these, 56 percent had moderate/severe TBI and 44 percent had mild TBI.[93,94] In contrast, only 20 percent of civilian TBIs are moderate/severe.[95] It is difficult to determine which explosion-related TBIs can be attributed to primary blast effects alone, even in cases where no fragment injuries are present.[96] In a recent study of 2003 to 2008 OIF casualties with head trauma, 48 percent had closed head injury that was attributed to primary and/or tertiary blast injury mechanisms.[97] Kinetic energy following blasts causes shearing in the central nervous system, resulting in both focal and diffuse axonal injury, air embolism, and cranial fractures with associated sinus cavity involvement.[64,89,98] Cognitive and biochemical changes occur in animals exposed to blasts (oxidative stress in the hippocampus), and electroencephalographic changes, punctuate hemorrhages, and chromatolysis have been seen in the brains of human blast victims.[21,88,99,100] The authors of the aforementioned studies could not reliably differentiate between injury mechanisms due to lack of specifics about the individual explosions and/or coexistence of blunt trauma mechanisms (e.g., vehicle incidents). The exact mechanism(s) of brain injury from blast overpressure remains unclear.[44,101,102,103,104,105]

> Traumatic brain injury has become the current signature injury of combat. It is difficult to determine which explosion-related TBI-type symptoms can be attributed to primary blast alone, as opposed to other blunt trauma-related TBI. The exact mechanism(s) of brain injury from blast overpressure remains unclear.

Patients can present with a variety of signs and symptoms ranging from a headache to coma. Clinical findings may include fatigue, headache, back or generalized pain, vertigo, paralysis (transient or persistent), and altered mental status.[21,99] Psychological symptoms include excitability, irrationality, amnesia, apathy, lethargy, poor concentration, insomnia, psychomotor agitation, depression, or anxiety.[21,104]

Cumulative and long-term effects of mild TBI on US troops are beginning to be a cause for concern. In one study, 44 percent of soldiers suffering mild TBI with loss of consciousness (LOC) met the criteria for post-traumatic stress disorder (PTSD) on evaluation three to four months after returning home.[65] Twenty-seven percent of soldiers who were simply dazed after a blast subsequently reported PTSD symptoms. Many soldiers reported significant problems with their general health, poor work habits, and a variety of symptoms. A study by Hoge "concluded that PTSD and depression were mediators of the relationship between mild TBI and physical health problems."[65] The Defense and Veterans Brain Injury Center (DVBIC), the lead agency in investigating TBI in the military, publishes updated data on military TBI. Their recommendations have included pre-deployment neurocognitive testing and the use of the Brief TBI Screen (BTBIS) in the post-deployment process.

Clinical Practice Guidelines (CPGs) published by the Joint Theater Trauma System (JTTS) provide algorithms for TBI evaluation at Level I (medic at point of wounding), Level II (Forward Surgical Team [FST]), and Level III (Combat Support Hospital [CSH]).[106,107] For mild TBI (GCS score of 13 to 15), Level I and II facility careproviders should perform the standard physical examination and use the Military Acute Concussion Evaluation (MACE) for assessment (MACE form available through the Defense and Veterans Brain Injury Center). Level III facility evaluation is often more comprehensive and may involve further neurocognitive testing following MACE performance.[108] Patients with a head injury and a GCS score of nine to 12 are classified as having moderate head injuries, and patients with GCS scores lower than nine are considered to have severe TBI. The lower the GCS score within this range, the higher the chance of death and the lower the chance that the patient will return to independent living (Fig. 22).

Blast effects to the brain can result in neurocognitive changes that may not manifest as obvious physical symptoms requiring treatment. Possible injury to the brain may be manifested in other ways, which can be assessed using the MACE scale. Individuals who have "seen stars" or are "just not themselves" may have suffered a mild TBI. In an effort to decrease the possibility of exposure to sequential concussive brain injury, warfighters who have been exposed to explosive blasts should be tested using MACE. Scores lower than 25 warrant further evaluation and treatment. As a preventive measure, it is recommended that these individuals only return to light duty in an effort to decrease the possibility of a subsequent exposure to a blast or vehicle crash while their brains recover.[106]

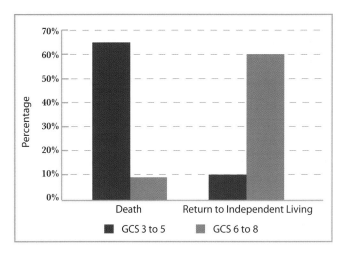

Figure 22. *Prognosis for OEF/OIF combatants with severe TBI (GCS score less than 9). Data source: Joint Theater Trauma Registry (JTTR).*

### Eyes

Although primary blast injury to the eye is rare because of the uniform density of the eye, it occasionally occurs in the form of globe rupture, retinitis, and hyphema.[64] The most common sign of primary blast injury to the eye is subconjunctival hemorrhage.[74] Injuries to the eye are more commonly caused by secondary blast fragments (e.g., splinters of glass and other debris), many of which are preventable with simple eye protection equipment.

### Extremities

Primary blast injury resulting in amputation is rare and often part of a pattern of lethal injuries.[109] As the blast wave impacts an extremity, tremendous pressure differentials may shatter the bone, and the near-simultaneous blast wind may subsequently avulse the extremity. On the whole, avulsions are observed mainly along the shaft of long bones and are most common among dead or dying victims. In one study, traumatic amputations due to primary blast primarily occurred in the upper third of the tibia.[110] These amputation injuries have a high risk for exsanguination, and the limbs are rarely reattachable.[19]

Secondary Blast Injury

The overpressurization wave created by the primary blast is followed by a negative-pressure phase. This generates a blast wind that propels debris and objects with ballistic speed and force to create multiple penetrating injuries.[31] Although they are termed secondary blast injuries, these are the predominant explosion-related injuries in survivors.[63,111]

> The greatest diagnostic challenges for clinicians at all levels of care in the aftermath of explosions are the large numbers of casualties and multiple penetrating injuries.[44]

### Primary and Secondary Fragments

Flying fragments and debris from the explosive and its surrounding environment are differentiated as primary and secondary fragments. In conventional military ordnance, primary fragments typically consist of bits of the exploding weapon. In IEDs, primary fragments include the shell casing as well as items packed into the explosive to increase wounding potential, such as nails, bolts, ball bearings, or other small, sharp items (Fig. 23). The effectiveness of this technique has been demonstrated. For example, following a suicide bomb attack in Israel, the bodies of all those who died immediately after the blast and all with severe injury (ISS greater than 16) were "saturated with steel spheres."[112]

All explosives generate secondary fragments that consist of debris from manufactured (e.g., metal from vehicle interiors, shattered furniture, splinters of window glass) and natural environments (e.g., rocks, dirt).[113] Dust and tiny grains of dirt can become embedded in the skin, causing a characteristic, dusky, tattooed effect.[114] Among all fragment types, glass causes a disproportionate amount of secondary injury. Of the 95 percent of survivors of the 1996 Khobar Towers bombing with fragment injuries, 88 percent were injured by glass (primarily from windows).[62]

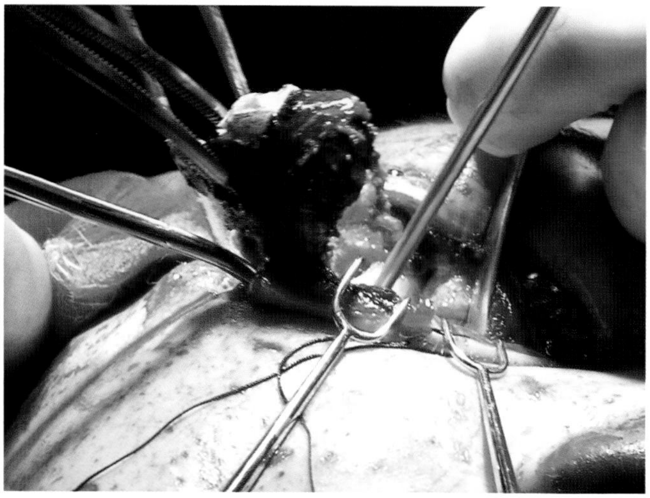

Figure 23. *A combat casualty undergoing removal of metallic shrapnel embedded in his right periorbital region following an IED blast.*

## Fragment Physics

Fragment projectiles differ from bullet projectiles in that they are scattered (not channeled through a barrel), are irregularly shaped, and have different velocities upon impact.[31] After detonation, aerodynamic drag is exerted on the fragments, which then strike the body as both high- and low-velocity projectiles.[31] Initial velocities of primary fragments can be as high as 1800 m/sec, but under 600 m/sec appears to be the upper limit of survivability.[15,115] Low-velocity fragments may tumble or shimmy, crush large areas of tissue, and fragment further to exacerbate the injuries.[116,117,118] This is counter to the previously held notion that the higher the velocity of a missile, the more tissue damage there will be.[15] In addition, fragments contaminate wounds with environmental debris. All of these factors likely account for the differences in fragment and bullet injuries, even though both are caused by small missiles propelled at great speeds.[31]

## Fragment Wounds

The distinguishing feature of most explosion-related injuries is the presence of multiple penetrating fragment injuries to several regions of the body (Fig. 24).[44,119] Because fragment wounds can be so numerous (e.g., 30 to 40 in a single patient), CCC providers can find it difficult to determine which wound(s) requires high-priority evaluation. The body region involved and associated clinical findings determine clinical impact and treatment priorities.[119]

Because of the protection offered by body armor, military personnel have a high incidence of fragment injuries to the head, extremities, and the junctions between the torso, arms, neck, and legs. These should be managed in the same way as other penetrating injuries. Meticulous wound inspection and debridement are important in the management of such injuries. Secondary blast injury also frequently results in facial and ocular injuries.[21,64] The eyes are particularly vulnerable to secondary blast injuries largely caused by minute bits of shattered glass or metal. As many as 10 percent of all blast injury survivors have significant eye injuries from projectiles, with signs and symptoms that include pain, irritation, sensation of a foreign body, changes in visual acuity, swelling, and contusions.[17] Most such eye injuries are preventable with appropriate eye protection. Among survivors of the September 11, 2001 attacks on the World Trade Center, 26 percent had ocular injuries.[120]

---

The distinguishing feature of most explosion-related injuries is the presence of multiple penetrating fragment injuries, or fragment wounds, to several regions of the body. Injuries and deaths from fragments occur much further from the point of detonation than do those associated with the primary blast.

---

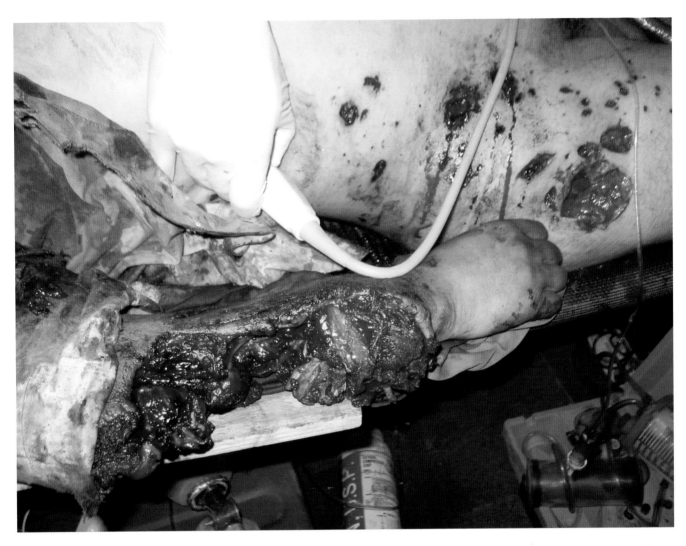

Figure 24. *A casualty seen at Camp Taqaddum, Iraq in 2004, with fragmentation wounds from an IED blast. The distinguishing feature of most explosion-related injuries is the presence of multiple individual injuries in several regions of the body. Image courtesy of Harold Bohman, MD, CAPT, MC, US Navy.*

Although prior literature advocated extensive debridement of fragment wound tracts, recent experience shows that this is no longer required. This is because: (1) high-velocity projectiles often do not cause temporary cavitation; (2) elastic soft-tissue generally heals without excision if the blood supply is intact; and (3) antibiotics play a larger role in mitigating infection.[121] In cases involving multiple fragments, it is not recommended to attempt to extract every fragment, but instead to remove those that pose a threat to life or health. The potential damage that could be caused by removing a fragment or through extensive wound exploration or debridement must be weighed against the damage that might result from not removing it. For example, in casualties with low-velocity penetrating head injury, debridement was limited to minimize risk of causing additional neurologic injury, with no apparent adverse affects on outcome.[122]

### Fragment Range

Risk of fragment injury occurs over a much wider radius than blast overpressure. Thus, in an open-space explosion, the primary mechanism of injury is fragment penetration.[119] The safe standoff distance for fragments has been noted to exceed that for blast overpressure by a factor of 100. Injuries and deaths from fragments occur much further from the point of detonation than do those associated with the primary blast

| | MORBIDITY AND MORTALITY | |
|---|---|---|
| DISTANCE FROM BLAST | PRIMARY BLAST INJURY | SECONDARY BLAST INJURY |
| 0 to 50 feet | Death, eardrum rupture | Death |
| 50 to 80 feet | Eardrum rupture | Death |
| 80 to 130 feet | Temporary hearing threshold shift | Injury |
| 130 to 1800 feet | None | Injury |

Table 9. *Blast injury effects based on distance from open-space blast explosion (155-mm shell). Adapted from Champion, 2009.*[44]

(Table 9).[47,119] Following the 1998 terrorist bombing of the US Embassy in Nairobi, fragment injuries were sustained by people as far as two kilometers from the point of detonation.[18] Secondary injury is largely penetrating, but victims can experience nonpenetrating injuries as well. For example, the low-velocity fragments responsible for all Khobar Towers bombing injuries caused penetrating, blunt, and crush injuries.[62] A large proportion of blunt injuries, however, are caused by tertiary blast effects.

> In an open-space explosion, the primary mechanism of injury is fragment penetration.
> Injuries and deaths from fragments occur much further from the point of detonation than do those associated with the primary blast.[119]

Tertiary Blast Injury

Tertiary blast injuries are caused by propulsion and displacement of the blast victim, of large fragments, or of surrounding structures such as a building or vehicle. The subsequent impact of victims upon structures or structures upon victims causes blunt and penetrating injuries that include crush, impalement, and other injuries whose severities vary with the degree of fragmentation and structural collapse.[64]

Although most tertiary blast injuries comprise soft-tissue wounds or fractures that are not immediately life-threatening, complete structural collapse is rarely survivable.[123] This was illustrated in the examples of the Khobar Towers and Oklahoma City bombings.[16] Individuals inside vehicles sustaining an IED blast can also experience tertiary blast injuries as the vehicle is propelled upward against the occupants or as the occupants are projected within the vehicle. In blast injury tests on vehicles, the vast majority of the injuries were tertiary. For undercarriage blasts, lower limbs were crushed, and in roadside blasts, occupants sustained severe head and side-thoracic impacts. These results are not dissimilar from those observed in data from OEF/OIF.

Crush syndrome, or traumatic rhabdomyolysis, often follows structural collapse and entrapment causing crush injury. Severe muscle damage, prolonged ischemia, and cell death can result in release of myoglobin, urates, and potassium. Myoglobinuria produces dark amber urine that will test positive for hemoglobin on urine dipstick analysis. Significant rhabdomyolysis can cause hypovolemia, metabolic acidosis, hyperkalemia, hypocalcemia, and coagulopathy.[124] Early and aggressive fluid resuscitation to ensure adequate renal perfusion and urinary output is vital in preventing renal failure.[124,125]

> Crush syndrome, or traumatic rhabdomyolysis, often follows structural collapse and body entrapment.

Myoglobinuria produces dark amber urine that will test positive for hemoglobin on urine dipstick analysis. Significant rhabdomyolysis can cause the following:

- hypovolemia,
- metabolic acidosis,
- hyperkalemia,
- hypocalcemia, and
- coagulopathy.

Osmotic diuretics (mannitol) and intravenous sodium bicarbonate are commonly advocated as adjuncts to prevent renal failure.[124] Alkalinization of the urine with intravenous sodium bicarbonate is thought to decrease intratubular precipitation of myoglobin in the kidneys.[124] Mannitol has been suggested to minimize intratubular pigment deposition, act as a renal vasodilator, and act as a free-radical scavenger.[124,126,127,128] It is worth noting that some authors feel that there is no clear clinical data showing benefit with either of these agents over simple fluid resuscitation.[124,129] Compartment syndromes can also develop in association with a crush injury or over-resuscitation and are discussed in later chapters.

Alkalinization of the urine with intravenous sodium bicarbonate is thought to decrease intratubular precipitation of myoglobin in the kidneys. Mannitol has been suggested to
- minimize intratubular pigment deposition,
- act as a renal vasodilator, and
- act as a free-radical scavenger.

## Quaternary Blast Injury

Quaternary blast injury encompasses blast sequelae that include, but are not limited to, burns, inhalation injury, and asphyxiation.[119] Burns are a form of quaternary blast injury in OEF and OIF and more frequently occur when victims are trapped in a burning vehicle or building than because of the blast fireball (which lasts for milliseconds). Burns that immediately follow an explosion result from exposure to the intense heat of the blast and indicate close proximity to the point of detonation.[123]

An analysis of OEF and OIF casualties with significant burns treated at the US Army Institute of Surgical Research (USAISR) between 2003 and 2005 revealed increases in burn frequency, extent, and severity.[130] Findings included:

- Burns caused by explosions increased from 18 percent to 69 percent
- Total body surface area burned increased from 15 percent (± 12 percent) to 21 percent (± 23 percent)
- Injury severity scores (ISS) increased from minor (8 ±11) to moderate/severe (17 ±18)[130]

Inhalation injury is especially prevalent with building collapse.

As illustrated in the 1993 World Trade Center bombing, 93 percent of victims suffered acute and chronic inhalation injuries

Burns were caused primarily by IEDs (55 percent), car bombs (16 percent), and RPGs (15 percent) and were largely sustained in unprotected areas of the body. The hands and face were the most frequently burned areas, and only one-third (36 percent) of burned patients resumed full military duty. The study also revealed an increase in the frequency of inhalation injury in the current conflicts from 5 percent to 26 percent.[130]

Inhalation injury is especially prevalent with building collapse, as illustrated in the 1993 World Trade Center bombing, in which 93 percent of victims suffered acute and chronic inhalation injuries.[113]

> Burns are a form of quaternary blast injury and occur more frequently when victims are trapped in a burning vehicle or building, rather than due to a blast fireball.

## Quinary Blast Injury

Quinary effects largely refer to contamination of tissues resulting from the release of chemical, biological agents, or radioactive materials upon detonation of an explosive device. A unique type of quinary injury encountered in OEF and OIF is that inflicted by human-remains-shrapnel, or pieces of bone from suicide bombers or other victims that cause penetrating injuries and increase the risk of transmission of blood-borne diseases such as hepatitis or human immunodeficiency virus (HIV).[87,131,132,133]

> These agents are classified as
> - nerve
> - blister (vesicant), and
> - choking agents.
>
> Indications of nerve agent exposure include a variety of autonomic and neuromuscular signs and symptoms, for example.
> - pinpoint pupils,
> - muscular twitching,
> - unexplained nasal secretion,
> - hypersalivation,
> - tightness of the chest,
> - shortness of breath,
> - nausea,
> - abdominal cramps,
> - seizures,
> - paralysis, and
> - respiratory failure.

Chemical agents may be inhaled or absorbed through the skin, and can induce coughing, itching, skin, and eye inflammation.[119] These agents are classified as nerve, blister (vesicant), and choking agents. Indications of nerve agent exposure include a variety of autonomic and neuromuscular signs and symptoms (e.g., pinpoint pupils, muscular twitching, unexplained nasal secretion, hypersalivation, tightness of the chest, shortness of breath, nausea, abdominal cramps, seizures, paralysis, and respiratory failure). Immediate intramuscular injection of atropine, combined if possible with pralidoxime chloride (2-PAM), is recommended.[134] Blister agents cause a spectrum of injury to exposed surfaces (e.g., skin, eyes, and mucous membranes) and result in symptoms over varying timeframes (minutes to several hours). Immediate decontamination by removal of contaminated clothing and irrigation of exposed surfaces with large amounts of water is first-line therapy.[134,135,136] Choking agents cause coughing, tightness in the chest, vomiting, headache, and lacrimation.[134] Treatment consists of removing the patient from the offending agent and providing supportive care. All of these effects can exacerbate preexisting conditions.[64] Exposure to radiation released in an explosion will result in a variety of effects that are largely determined by the size and type of explosion, which radioactive elements are involved, length of exposure, and other factors.[137] While discussion of chemical and biological

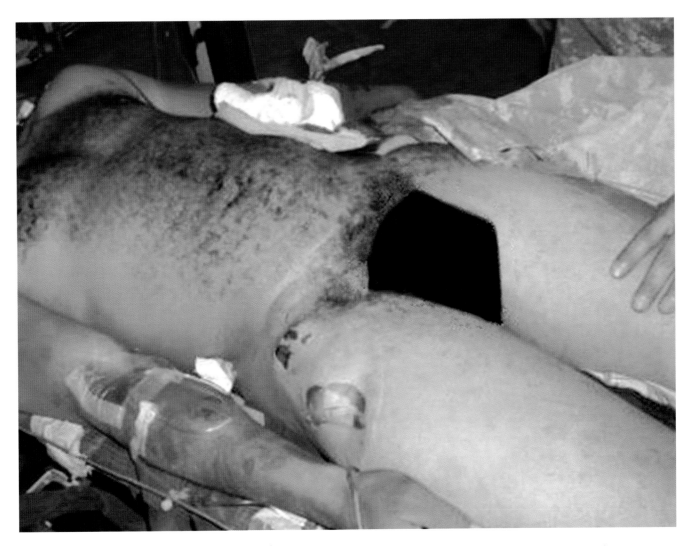

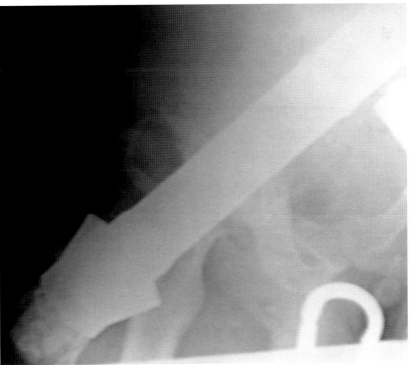

Figure 25. (Above) *Unexploded ordnance tenting the subcutaneous tissue of the right thigh, having traversed the pelvis in a left-to-right trajectory. The extruding tail of the rocket is demarcated by the arrow. Image courtesy of the Borden Institute, Office of The Surgeon General, Washington, DC.*

Figure 26. (Right) *A radiograph of the UXO embedded in the pelvis and femur confirms the warhead is not attached to the rocket. Image courtesy of the Borden Institute, Office of The Surgeon General, Washington, DC.*

agents and radiation threats is beyond the scope of this chapter, CCC providers should have a decontamination plan in place to avoid secondary contamination of their combat care facility and themselves.

> Know your environment, and have a decontamination plan in place to avoid secondary contamination of yourself and your combat care facility.

## Management Considerations

While damage-control practices will need to be applied to explosion-related injury management by CCC providers, the polytrauma that ensues in bomb explosions creates management challenges.[79] Patients with concurrent brain and hemorrhaging solid organ injuries often need to undergo immediate damage control surgery prior to delineation of a brain injury via CT imaging.[79] Advanced ventilatory strategies (e.g., permissive hypercapnia, high-frequency oscillatory ventilation) may often be required to manage lung overpressure injuries.[79] The coagulopathy that often accompanies blast injury will need to be rapidly recognized and appropriately managed.[79] Finally, the crystalloid and blood product requirements in patients with multiple injuries that include burns, head, and pulmonary injuries must be balanced against the risks (among others) of dilutional coagulopathy and compartment syndromes.[45,138]

## Embedded Unexploded Ordnance

The management of intracorporeal unexploded ordnances (UXOs) represents a unique challenge for CCC providers. Mortars, rockets, and grenades that fail to trigger may become embedded in a casualty without exploding (Figs. 25 and 26). Due to the extensive time and resources needed to appropriately manage these casualties and the potential for collateral damage from premature detonation, military recommendations include initially triaging such patients as nonemergent, isolating them from others, and operating on them last.[15,139]

> Military recommendations include:
> ♦ initially triaging such patients as nonemergent,
> ♦ isolating them from others, and
> ♦ operating on them last.

According to Lien, "the fuse is the key to understanding unexploded ordnance."[139] A fuse serves as a trigger for an explosive device and may be set off by impact, electromagnetically, or as a function of time or distance traveled. Care should be taken to minimize manipulation or movement of the UXO and casualty. If helicopter transport is necessary, the patient should be flown independent of other patients, and the flight crew should be kept to a minimum and protected with body armor.[140] Diagnostic and therapeutic

> Electrical equipment, such as:
> ♦ electrocautery,
> ♦ surgical saws or drills,
> ♦ blood warmers,
> ♦ monitors,
> ♦ defibrillators,
> ♦ ultrasound, or
> ♦ computed tomography imaging,
> should be avoided until the unexploded ordinance is removed.

medical equipment can trigger a fuse and inadvertently cause an explosion. Electrical equipment, such as electrocautery, surgical saws or drills, blood warmers, monitors, defibrillators, ultrasound, or computed tomography imaging should be avoided until the UXO is removed.[15] Some of these diagnostic and treatment adjuncts may radiate electrical fields, cause severe vibration, or result in elevated temperatures that may arm the fusing mechanism.[139]

> Plain radiography is considered safe and is used to identify the type of munition and fuse, as well as to define the surgical approach to embedded UXOs.[139] As part of preoperative planning, the explosive ordnance disposal (EOD) team should be notified and present to assist in the proper handling and disposal of the UXO.

Traditional recommendations for removal of UXOs include the use of regional or spinal anesthesia and departure of operating room personnel except for the operating surgeon.[15] Recent case reports from OEF and OIF have suggested that general anesthesia allows for a more controlled environment, and that having the appropriate, rather than minimal, number of assistants in the operating room can lead to the most successful outcomes.[140] Operating room staff should wear protective gear, including body armor, ballistic eye protection, and a helmet. Sandbags should be positioned around the patient. Gentle technique and en-bloc resection of the UXO minimizes manipulation and the inherent risk of detonating the device. If embedded in an extremity, amputation should be considered.[15,140]

# Conclusions

Understanding modern warfare, including the types of weapons employed and the mechanisms and patterns of injury they cause, is critical to providing optimal CCC. The primary mechanisms of combat injury in OEF and OIF are small arms and explosives. Explosion-related injuries account for a majority of the injuries and deaths in OEF and OIF. Improvised explosive device attacks have become a mainstay in the current conflicts. Explosive devices produce the ultimate polytrauma (i.e., a wide range of injury types to many body regions caused by the full range of injury mechanisms). Explosions produce patterns of injury

> Understanding modern warfare, including the types of weapons employed and the mechanisms and patterns of injury they cause, is critical to providing optimal combat casualty care.

that are distinct from those of other mechanisms. In an open-space explosion, the primary mechanism of injury is fragment penetration. Injuries and deaths from fragments occur much further from the point of detonation than do those associated with the primary blast. The simultaneous combination of different blast injury mechanisms produces a complex array of injuries. Combat casualty care providers must fully understand these complex injuries and their management to ensure optimal patient outcomes.

# References

1. Eastridge BJ, Jenkins D, Flaherty S, et al. Trauma system development in a theater of war: experiences from Operation Iraqi Freedom and Operation Enduring Freedom. J Trauma 2006;61(6):1366-1372; discussion 1372-1373.

2. Owens BB, Kragh JF Jr, Wenke JC, et al. Combat wounds in Operation Iraqi Freedom and Operation Enduring Freedom. J Trauma 2008;64(2):295-299.

3. Burns BD, Zuckerman S. The wounding power of small bomb and shell fragments. London, England: British Ministry of Supply, Advisory Council on Scientific Research and Technical Development; 1942.

4. Beebe GW, DeBakey ME. Location of hits and wounds. In: Battle casualties: incidence, mortality, and logistic considerations. Springfield, IL: Charles C Thomas; 1952. p. 165-205.

5. Reister FA. Battle casualties and medical statistics: U.S. Army experience in the Korean War. Washington, DC: The Surgeon General, Department of the Army; 1973.

6. Hardaway RM. Viet Nam wound analysis. J Trauma 1978;18(9):635-643.

7. Shanker T. Pentagon to outline shift in war planning strategy. The New York Times, 2009 June 22.

8. Kelly JF, Ritenour AE, McLaughlin DF, et al. Injury severity and causes of death from Operation Iraqi Freedom and Operation Enduring Freedom: 2003-2004 versus 2006. J Trauma 2008;64(2 Suppl):S21-26; discussion S26-27.

9. Brethauer SA, Choo A, Chambers LW, et al. Invasion vs insurgency: US Navy/Marine Corps forward surgical care during Operation Iraqi Freedom. Arch Surg 2008;143(6):564-569.

10. Bellamy RF, Zajtchuk R. The weapons of conventional land warfare. In: Bellamy RF, Zajtchuk R, editors. Conventional warfare: ballistic, blast, and burn injuries. Washington, DC: The Borden Institute; 1991. p. 1-52.

11. Beebe GW, DeBakey ME. Death from wounding. In: Battle casualties: incidence, mortality, and logistic considerations. Springfield, IL: Charles C Thomas; 1952. p. 74-147.

12. US Department of Defense (US DoD). DoD personnel and military casualty statistics. Global War on Terrorism by Reason: October 7, 2001 through October 31, 2009. DoD, Statistical Information Analysis Division (SIAD), Defense Manpower Data Center (DMDC) [cited 2009 Nov 4]. Available from: URL: http://siadapp.dmdc.osd.mil/personnel/CASUALTY/gwot_reason.pdf.

13. Amnesty International. Blood at the crossroads: making the case for global arms trade treaty. London, UK: Amnesty International Publications 2008 [cited 2009 Oct 28]. Available from: URL: http://www.amnesty.org/en/library/asset/ACT30/011/2008/en/19ea0e74-8329-11dd-8e5e-3ea85d15a69/act300112008en.pdf.

14. Santucci RA, Chang YJ. Ballistics for physicians: Myths about wound ballistics and gunshot injuries. J Urol 2004;171(4):1408-1414.

15. US Department of Defense (US DoD). Weapons Effects and Parachute Injuries. In: Emergency War Surgery, Third United States Revision. Washington, DC: Department of the Army, Office of the Surgeon General, Borden Institute; 2004. p. 1.1-1.14.

16. Arnold JL, Halpern P, Tsai MC, et al. Mass casualty terrorist bombings: a comparison of outcomes by bombing type. Ann Emerg Med 2004;43(2):263-273.

17. Centers for Disease Control and Prevention (CDC). Explosions and blast injuries: A primer for clinicians. 2006 [cited 2009 Nov 5]. Available from: URL: http://www.bt.cdc.gov/masscasualties/explosions.asp.

18. Wightman JM, Gladish SL. Explosions and blast injuries. Ann Emerg Med 2001;37(6):664-678.

19. Votey SR, UCLA Emergency Medicine Multimedia Education Working Group. Chemical, Biological, Radiological, Nuclear, Explosives: Emergency Preparedness for Medical Care Providers. Multimedia CD-ROM. California Hospital Bioterrorism Preparedness Committee and California Emergency Medical Services Authority, 2004.

20. Eastridge BJ. Things that go boom: injuries from explosives. J Trauma 2007;62(6 Suppl):S38.

21. Ritenour AE, Baskin TW. Primary blast injury: Update on diagnosis and treatment. Crit Care Med 2008;36(7 Suppl):S311-317.

22. Butler DK. Landmines and UXO. The Leading Edge 1997;16(10):1460-1461.

23. Surrency AB, Graitcer PL, Henderson AK. Key factors for civilian injuries and death from exploding landmines and ordnance. Inj Prev 2007;13(3):197-201.

24. Human Rights Watch. Landmines in Iraq: Questions and Answers. Human Rights News, Arms Division Homepage. 2002 Dec [cited 2009 Oct 30]. Available from: URL: http://www.hrw.org/legacy/campaigns/iraq/iraqmines1212.htm.

25. Afghanistan ICRC Mine Data Collection Programme – Details [cited 2001 May 25]. Available from: URL: http://www.icrc.org.

26. Centers for Disease Control and Prevention (CDC). Injuries associated with landmines and unexploded ordnance—Afghanistan, 1997-2002. JAMA 2003;52(36):859-862.

27. Injuries associated with landmines and unexploded ordnance—Afghanistan, 1997-2002. MMWR 2003;52:859-862.

28. Hamdan TA. Missile injuries of the limbs: an Iraqi perspective. J Am Acad Orthop Surg 2006;14(10 Spec No.):S32-36.

29. International Committee of the Red Cross (ICRC). Book I: Weapon Contamination. Geneva: ICRC; 2007 Aug [cited 2009 Nov 2]. Available from: URL: http://www.scribd.com/doc/22010755/Book-I-Weapon-contamination-environment.

30. Office of the Secretary of Defense (OSD). Landmines. Force Health Protection and Readiness. 2009 [cited 2009 Nov 1]. Available from: URL: http://fhp.osd.mil/factsheetDetail.jsp?fact=14.

31. Covey DC. Blast and fragment injuries of the musculoskeletal system. J Bone Joint Surg Am 2002;84-A(7):1221-1234.

32. German Mine 35/44 Bouncing Betty. European Center of Military History 2009 Feb 22 [cited 2009 Nov 1]. Available from: URL: http://www.eucmh.com/2009/02/22/schrapnellmine-3544-bouncing-betty/.

33. Woebkenberg BJ, Devine J, Rush R, et al. Nonconventional uses of the rocket-propelled grenade and its consequences. Mil Med 2007;172(6):622-624.

34. RPG-7: The famous RPG-7 is in use with over 40 countries. Military Factory 2009 Jul 7 [cited 2009 Nov 2]. Available from: URL: http://www.militaryfactory.com/smallarms/detail.asp?smallarms_id=10.

35. Wilson C. CRS Report for Congress – Improvised Explosive Devices (IEDs) in Iraq and Afghanistan: Effects and Countermeasures. Order Code RS22330, 2008.

36. Vanden Brook T. IEDs now cause 75% of Afghanistan casualties. USA Today 2009 Apr 4.

37. Tyson AS. U.S. combat injuries rise sharply. The Washington Post 2009 Oct 31;Sect A1, A7.

38. Shaunessy L, Hornick E, Starr B. Detecting IEDs: a daunting challenge for U.S. military. Joint IED Defeat Organization (JIEDDO) 2009 Oct 27 [cited 2009 Nov 4]. Available from: URL: https://www.jieddo.dod.mil/article.aspx?ID=685.

39. US Marine Corps. Field Medical Service Technician Student Manual—2008 Web Edition. Camp LeJeune, NC; 2008: FMST 1206, Improvised Explosive Devices. Available at: http://www.operationalmedicine.org/TextbookFiles/FMST_20008/FMST_1206.htm. Accessed May 14, 2012.

40. Anderson JW. Bigger, stronger homemade bombs now to blame for half of U.S. deaths. The Washington Post 2005 Oct 21.

41. Morrison JJ, Mahoney PF, Hodgetts T. Shaped charges and explosively formed penetrators: Background for clinicians. J R Army Med Corps 2007;153(3):184-187.

42. Ramasamy A, Harrisson SE, Clasper JC, et al. Injuries from roadside improvised explosive devices. J Trauma 2008;65(4):910-914.

43. McDiarmid MA, Engelhardt SM, Oliver M, et al. Health surveillance of Gulf War I veterans exposed to depleted uranium: updating the cohort. Health Phys 2007;93(1):60-73.

44. Champion HR, Holcomb JB, Young LA. Injuries from explosions: Physics, biophysics, pathology, and required research focus. J Trauma 2009;66(5):1468-1477.

45. Kluger Y, Peleg K, Daniel-Aharonson L, et al. The special injury pattern in terrorist bombings. J Am Coll Surg 2004;199(6):875-879.

46. Nelson TJ, Clark T, Stedje-Larsen ET, et al. Close proximity blast injury patterns from improvised explosive devices in Iraq: A report of 18 cases. J Trauma 2008;65(1):212-217.

47. Stein M, Hirshberg A. Medical consequences of terrorism: The conventional weapon threat. Surg Clinic North Am 1999;79(6):1537-1552.

48. Mallonee S, Shariat S, Stennies G, et al. Physical injuries and fatalities resulting from the Oklahoma City bombing. JAMA 1996;276(5):382-387.

49. Quenemoen LE, Davis YM, Malilay J, et al. The World Trade Center bombing: injury prevention strategies for high-rise building fires. Disasters 1996;20(2):125-132.

50. Phillips YY, Richmond DR. Primary blast injury and basic research: a brief history. In Bellamy RF, Zajtchuk R, editors. Conventional warfare: ballistic, blast, and burn injuries. Washington, DC, Office of the Surgeon General, Department of the Army; 1989. p. 221-240.

51. Frykberg ER, Tepas JJ 3rd. Terrorist bombings. Lessons learned from Belfast to Beirut. Ann Surg 1988;208(5):569-576.

52. Almogy G, Rivkind AI. Surgical lessons learned from suicide bombing attacks. J Am Coll Surg 2006;202(2):313-319.

53. Aschkenasy-Steuer G, Shamir M, Rivkind A, et al. Clinical review: The Israeli experience: conventional terrorism and critical care. Crit Care 2005;9(5):490-499.

54. Kluger Y. Bomb explosions in acts of terrorism – detonation, wound ballistics, triage and medical concerns. Isr Med Assoc J 2003;5(4):235-240.

55. National Counterterrorism Center (NCTC). 2007 Report on Terrorism. 2008 [cited 2008 Sept 2]. Available from: URL: http://wits.nctc.gov/Reports.do?page=5.

56. Cooper GJ, Maynard RL, Cross NL, et al. Casualties from terrorist bombings. J Trauma 1983;23(11):955-967.

57. Katz E, Ofek B, Adler J, et al. Primary blast injury after a bomb explosion in a civilian bus. Ann Surg 1989;209(4):484-488.

58. Leibovici D, Gofrit ON, Stein M, et al. Blast injuries: Bus versus open-air bombings—a comparative study of injuries in survivors of open-air versus confined-space explosions. J Trauma 1996;41(6):1030-1035.

59. Kluger Y, Kashuk J, Mayo A. Terror bombings—mechanisms, consequences, and implications. Scand J Surg 2004;93(1):11-14.

60. Mayo A, Kluger Y. Terrorist bombing. World J Emerg Surg 2006;1:1-33.

61. Federal Emergency Management Agency (FEMA). Explosive blast. In Primer to Design Safe Schools Projects in Case of Terrorist Attacks. Washington, DC: FEMA; 2003. p. 4-1–4-13.

62. Thompson D, Brown S, Mallonee S, et al. Fatal and non-fatal injuries among U.S. Air Force personnel resulting from the terrorist bombing of the Khobar Towers. J Trauma 2004;57(2):208-215.

63. Wade CE, Ritenour AE, Eastridge BJ, et al. Explosion injuries treated at combat support hospitals in the global war on terrorism. In: Elsayed N, Atkins J, editors. Explosion and blast-related injuries: effects of explosion and blast from military operations and acts of terrorism. Amsterdam; Boston: Elsevier; 2008. p. 41-72.

64. DePalma RG, Burris DG, Champion HR, et al. Blast injuries. N Engl J Med 2005;352(13):1335-1342.

65. Hoge CW, McGurk D, Thomas JL, et al. Mild traumatic brain injury in U.S. soldiers returning from Iraq. N Engl J Med 2008;358(5):453-463.

66. Harrison CD, Bebarta VS, Grant GA. Tympanic Membrane Perforation After Combat Blast Exposure in Iraq: A Poor Biomarker of Primary Blast Injury. J Trauma 2009;67(1):210-211.

67. Owen-Smith M. Bomb blast injuries: In an explosive situation. Nurs Mirror 1979;149(13):35-39.

68. Chait RH, Casler J, Zajtchuk JT. Blast injury to the ear: Historical perspective. Ann Otol Rhinol Laryngol 1989;140(Suppl):9-12.

69. Cave KM, Cornish EM, Chandler DW. Blast injury to the ear: Clinical update from the global war on terror. Mil Med 2007;172(7):726-730.

70. Depenbrock P. Tympanic membrane perforation in IED blasts. J Spec Oper Med 2008;8:51-53.

71. Kronenberg J, Ben-Shoshan J, Modan M, et al. Blast injury and cholesteatoma. Am J Otol 1988;9(2):127-130.

72. Xydakis MS, Bebarta VS, Harrison CD, et al. Tympanic-membrane perforation as a marker of concussive brain injury in Iraq. N Engl J Med 2007;357(8):830-831.

73. Sharpnak D, Johnson A, Philips Y. The pathology of primary blast injury. In: Bellamy R, Zatchuk R, editors. Conventional warfare: ballistic, blast, and burn injuries. Washington, D.C.: Office of the Surgeon General of the US Army, 1991. p. 271-294.

74. Mayorga MA. The pathology of primary blast overpressure injury. Toxicology 1997;121(1):17-28.

75. Avidan V, Hersch M, Armon Y, et al. Blast lung injury: clinical manifestations, treatment, and outcomes. Am J Surg 2005;190(6):927-931.

76. de Ceballos JP, Turegano-Fuentes F, Perez-Diaz D, et al. 11 March 2004: The terrorist bomb explosions in Madrid, Spain—an analysis of the logistics, injuries sustained and clinical management of casualties treated at the closest hospital. Crit Care 2005;9(1):104-111.

77. Aharonson-Daniel L, Klein Y, Peleg K. ITG. Suicide bombers form a new injury profile. Ann Surg 2006;244(6):1018-1023.

78. Goh SH. Bomb blast mass casualty incidents: initial triage and management of injuries. Singapore Med J 2009;50(1):101-106.

79. Kashuk JL, Halperin P, Caspi G, et al. Bomb explosions in acts of terrorism: evil creativity challenges our trauma systems. J Am Coll Surg 2009;209(1):134-140.

80. Pizov R, Oppenheim-Eden A, Matot I, et al. Blast lung injury from an explosion on a civilian bus. Chest 1999;115(1):165-172.

81. Cohn SM. Pulmonary contusion: Review of the clinical entity. J Trauma 1997;42(5):973-979.

82. Halpern P, Tsai MC, Arnold JL, et al. Mass-casualty, terrorist bombings: Implications for emergency department and hospital emergency response (Part II). Prehosp Disaster Med 2003;18(3):235-241.

83. Mellor SG, Cooper GJ. Analysis of 828 servicemen killed or injured by explosion in Northern Ireland 1970-84: The Hostile Action Casualty System. Br J Surg 1989;76(10):1006-1010.

84. Irwin RJ, Lerner MR, Bealer JF, et al. Shock after blast wave injury is caused by a vagally mediated reflex. J Trauma 1999;47(1):105-110.

85. Guzzi LM, Argyros G. The management of blast injury. Eur J Emerg Med 1996;3(4):252-255.

86. Yang Z, Wang Z, Tang C, et al. Biological effects of weak blast waves and safety limits for internal organ injury in the human body. J Trauma 1996;40(3 Suppl):S81-84.

87. Singer P, Cohen JD, Stein M. Conventional terrorism and critical care. Crit Care Med 2005;33(1 Suppl):S61-65.

88. Born CT. Blast trauma: The fourth weapon of mass destruction. Scand J Surg 2005;94(4):279-285.

89. Mellor SG. The pathogenesis of blast injury and its management. Br J Hosp Med 1988;39(6):536-539.

90. Grady D. The wounded: The survivors – Surviving multiple injuries; struggling back from war's once-deadly wounds. New York Times 2006 Jan 22.

91. Henry M. Jackson Foundation for the Advancement of Military Medicine, Inc. The Defense and Veterans Brain Injury Center—Providing care for soldiers with traumatic brain injury. 2006 [cited 2009 Jan 4]. Available from: URL: http://www.hjf.org/research/featureDVBIC.html.

92. Tanielian T, Jaycox LH, editors. Invisible Wounds of War: Psychological and Cognitive Injuries, Their Consequences, and Services to Assist Recovery. Santa Monica, CA: Rand Corporation; 2008.

93. Okie S. Traumatic brain injury in the war zone. N Engl J Med 2005;352(20):2043-2047.

94. Warden DL, Ryan LM, Helmick KM, et al. War neurotrauma: The Defense and Veterans Brain Injury Center (DVBIC) experience at Walter Reed Army Medical Center (WRAMC). J Neurotrauma 2005;22:1178.

95. Brain Injury Association of America (BIAA). Traumatic brain injury in the United States: A call for public/private cooperation. McLean, VA: BIAA; 2007.

96. Taber KH, Warden DL, Hurley RA. Blast-related traumatic brain injury: What is known? J Neuropsychiatry Clin Neurosci 2006;18(2):141-145.

97. Bell RS, Vo AH, Neal CJ, et al. Military traumatic brain and spinal column injury: A 5-year study of the impact blast and other military grade weaponry on the central nervous system. J Trauma 2009;66(4 Suppl):S104-111.

98. Cernak I, Wang Z, Jiang J, et al. Ultrastructural and functional characteristics of blast injury-induced neurotrauma. J Trauma 2001;50(4):695-706.

99. Guy RJ, Glover MA, Cripps NP. Primary blast injury: pathophysiology and implications for treatment. Part III: Injury to the central nervous system and limbs. J R Nav Med Serv 2000;86(1):27-31.

100. Trudeau DL, Anderson J, Hansen LM, et al. Findings of mild traumatic brain injury in combat veterans with PTSD and a history of blast concussion. J Neuropsychiatry Clin Neurosci 1998;10(3):308-313.

101. Belanger HG, Kretzmer T, Yoash-Gantz R, et al. Cognitive sequelae of blast-related versus other mechanisms of brain trauma. J Int Neuropsychol Soc 2009;15(1):1–8.

102. Wilk JE, Thomas JL, McGurk DM, et al. Mild traumatic brain injury (concussion) during combat: lack of association of blast mechanism with persistent postconcussive symptoms. J Head Trauma Rehabil 2010;25(1):9–14.

103. Cernak I, Savic J, Malicevic Z, et al. Involvement of the central nervous system in the general response to pulmonary blast injury. J Trauma 1996;40(3 Suppl):S100-104.

104. Cernak I, Savik J, Ignjatovic D, et al. Blast injury from explosive munitions. J Trauma 1999;47(1):96-103.

105. Ling G, Bandak F, Armonda R, et al. Explosive blast neurotrauma. J Neurotrauma 2009;26(6):815–825.

106. Joint Theater Trauma System (JTTS) Clinical Practice Guideline. Management of mild traumatic brain injury (mTBI)/concussion in the deployed setting. 2008 Nov 21 [cited 2009 Nov 12]. Available from: URL: http://www.usaisr.amedd.army.mil/cpgs.html.

107. Joint Theater Trauma System (JTTS) Clinical Practice Guideline. Management of patients with severe head trauma. 2009 Feb 13 [cited 2009 Nov 12]. Available from: URL: http://www.usaisr.amedd.army.mil/cpgs.html.

108. Defense and Veterans Brain Injury Center (DVBIC). Military Acute Concussion Evaluation (MACE). 2007 Jul [cited 2007 Jul 13]. Available from: URL: http://www.dvbic.org/pdfs/DVBIC_pocket_card.pdf.

109. Centers for Disease Control and Prevention. Blast Injuries: Fact Sheets for Professionals. National Center for Injury Prevention and Control 2008 [cited 2008 Dec 22]. Available from: URL: http://emergency.cdc.gov/masscasualties/blastinjuryfacts.asp.

110. Hull JB, Cooper GJ. Pattern and mechanism of traumatic amputation by explosive blast. J Trauma 1996;40(3 Suppl):S198-205.

111. Linsky R, Miller A. Types of explosions and explosive injuries defined. In: Keyes DC, editor. Medical response to terrorism: preparedness and clinical practice. Philadelphia, PA: Lippincott Williams & Wilkins; 2005. p. 198-211.

112. Kluger Y, Mayo A, Hiss J, et al. Medical consequences of terrorist bombs containing spherical metal pellets: analysis of a suicide terrorism event. Eur J Emerg Med 2005;12(1):19-23.

113. Arnold JL, Tsai MC, Halpern P, et al: Mass-casualty, terrorist bombings: epidemiological outcomes, resource utilization, and time course of emergency needs (Part I). Prehosp Disaster Med 2003;18(3):220-234.

114. Crane J. Explosive injury. In: Payne-James J, Byard RW, Corey TS, et al, editors. Encyclopedia of forensic and legal medicine. London: Elsevier; 2005. p. 98-110.

115. Bowyer GW, Cooper GJ, Rice P. Small fragment wounds: biophysics and pathophysiology. J Trauma 1996; 40(3 Suppl):S159-164.

116. Fasol R, Irvine S, Zilla P. Vascular injuries caused by anti-personnel mines. J Cardiovasc Surg 1989;30(3):467-472.

117. Amato JJ, Billy LJ, Gruber RP, et al. Vascular injuries. An experimental study of high and low velocity missile wounds. Arch Surg 1970;101(2):167-174.

118. Fackler ML. Wound ballistics. A review of common misconceptions. JAMA 1988;259(18):2730-2736.

119. Champion HR, Baskin T, Holcomb JB. Injuries from explosives. In: McSwain NE, Salomone J, editors. Basic and advanced pre-hospital trauma life support, military edition. 2nd ed. St. Louis, MO: Mosby, National Association of Emergency Medical Technicians; 2006.

120. Boodram B, Torian L, Thomas P, et al. Rapid assessment of injuries among survivors of the terrorist attack on the World Trade Center—New York City, September 11, 2001. MMWR 2002 Jan 11 [cited 2009 Nov 13];51(01);1-5. Available from: URL: http://www.cdc.gov/mmwr/preview/mmwrhtml/mm5101a1.htm.

121. Wedmore IS, McManus JG Jr, Coakley TA. Penetrating and explosive injury patterns. In: Schwartz RB, McManus JG, Swienton RE, editors. Tactical emergency medicine. Philadelphia, PA: Lippincott, Williams & Wilkins; 2008. p. 63-73.

122. Amirjamshidi A, Abbassioun K, Rahmat H. Minimal debridement or simple wound closure as the only surgical treatment in war victims with low-velocity penetrating head injuries. Indications and management protocol based upon more than 8 years follow-up of 99 cases from Iran-Iraq conflict. Surg Neurol 2003;60(2):105-110.

123. Frykberg ER. Explosions and blast injury. In: Shapira SC, Hammond JS, Cole LA, editors. Essentials of terror medicine. New York: Springer; 2009. p. 171-193.

124. Huerta-Alardin AL, Varon J, Marik PE. Bench-to-bedside review: Rhabdomyolysis – an overview for clinicians. Crit Care 2005;9(2):158-169.

125. Abassi ZA, Hoffman A, Better OS. Acute renal failure complicating muscle crush injury. Semin Nephrol 1998;18(5):558-565.

126. Zager RA. Rhabdomyolysis and myohemoglobinuric acute renal failure. Kidney Int. 1996;49(2):314-326.

127. Shilliday I, Allison ME. Diuretics in acute renal failure. Ren Fail 1994;16(1):3-17.

128. Odeh M. The role of reperfusion-induced injury in the pathogenesis of the crush injury. N Engl J Med 1991;324(20):1417-1422.

129. Homsi E, Barreiro MF, Orlando JM, et al. Prophylaxis of acute renal failure in patients with rhabdomyolysis. Ren Fail 1997;19(2):283-288.

130. Kauvar DS, Wolf SE, Wade CE, et al. Burns sustained in combat explosions in Operations Iraqi and Enduring Freedom (OIF/OEF explosion burns). Burns 2006;32(7):853-857.

131. Braverman I, Wexler D, Oren M. A novel mode of infection with hepatitis B: penetrating bone fragments due to the explosion of a suicide bomber. Isr Med Assoc J 2002;4(7):528-529.

132. Leibner ED, Weil Y, Gross E, et al. A broken bone without a fracture: traumatic foreign bone implantation resulting from a mass casualty bombing. J Trauma 2005;58(2):388-390.

133. Wong JM, Marsh D, Abu-Sitta G, et al. Biological foreign body implantation in victims of the London July 7th suicide bombings. J Trauma 2006;60(2):402-404.

134. Federation of American Scientists (FAS). Types of chemical weapons. 2008 [cited 2008 Dec 30]. Available from: URL: http://www.fas.org/programs/ssp/bio/chemweapons/cwagents.html.

135. Chemical & biological attacks, detection, & response FAQ. KI4U, Inc., 2008 [cited 2008 Dec 30]. Available from: URL: http://www.ki4u.com/chemical_biological_attack_detection_response.htm.

136. Centers for Disease Control and Prevention. Chemical categories: A to Z [cited 2008 Dec 30]. Available from: URL: http://www.bt.cdc.gov/agent/agentlistchem-category.asp.

137. DeGarmo B. Radiological terrorism: the 'dirty bomb.' 2003 [cited 2008 Dec 31]. Available from: URL: bioterrorism.slu.edu/bt/products/ahec_rad/ppt/Dirty%20Bomb.ppt.

138. Kashuk JL, Moore EE, Johnson JL, et al. Postinjury life threatening coagulopathy: is 1:1, fresh frozen plasma: packed red blood cells the answer? J Trauma 2008;65(2):261-270; discussion 270-271.

139. Lein B, Holcomb J, Brill S, et al. Removal of unexploded ordnance from patients: a 50-year military experience and current recommendations. Mil Med 1999;164(3):163-165.

140. Nessen SC, Lounsbury DE, Hetz SP, editors. Removal of an Unexploded Ordnance. In: War Surgery in Afghanistan and Iraq: A Series of Cases, 2003-2007. Washington, DC: Department of the Army, Office of the Surgeon General, Borden Institute; 2008. p. 373-376.

# FUNDAMENTALS OF COMBAT CASUALTY CARE

*Chapter 3*

**Contributing Authors**
Robert T. Gerhardt, MD, MPH, FACEP, FAAEM, LTC, US Army
Robert L. Mabry, MD, FACEP, MAJ(P), US Army
Robert A. De Lorenzo, MD, MSM, FACEP, COL, US Army
Frank K. Butler, MD, FACS, CAPT, US Navy (Ret)

All figures and tables included in this chapter have been used with permission from Pelagique, LLC, the UCLA Center for International Medicine, and/or the authors, unless otherwise noted.

Use of imagery from the Defense Imagery Management Operations Center (DIMOC) does not imply or constitute Department of Defense (DOD) endorsement of this company, its products, or services.

**Disclaimer**
The opinions and views expressed herein belong solely to those of the authors. They are not nor should they be implied as being endorsed by the United States Uniformed Services University of the Health Sciences, Department of the Army, Department of the Navy, Department of the Air Force, Department of Defense, or any other branch of the federal government.

# Table of Contents

# Introduction

Over the past century, an evolution in combat casualty care (CCC) has occurred. As the current century unfolds, we expect even more remarkable advances as increasing resources are focused on the out-of-hospital phases of emergency care. In addition to the development of new resuscitation strategies, surgical techniques, pharmaceuticals and other adjuncts, the military and emergency medicine communities continue to champion innovation in first responder and combat medic training and seek the means to provide effective medical direction to the incipient "Combat Emergency Medical Services (EMS) system."[1]

From its earliest days, the process of evacuating the sick and wounded from the battlefield resulted in displays of great sacrifice, bravery, and all too often, tragic errors of both omission and commission. In most cases, current practices have evolved from the on-the-job experiences of CCC providers. Clinical and treatment data in the out-of-hospital arena remain sparse, with minimal granularity consisting of occasional after-action reports bolstered by sporadic field medical records. Civilian sector solutions and training paradigms are often extrapolated and applied to the tactical setting, but translate into suboptimal tactical and clinical outcomes.[2]

## Leading Causes of Preventable Death

The Wound Data and Munitions Effectiveness Team (WDMET) study provided one of the first objective databases from which inferences regarding evacuation and en-route-care were drawn.[3] Building on the WDMET concept, the Joint Theater Trauma Registry (JTTR) was developed by the United States (US) Army Institute of Surgical Research in partnership with the US Air Force and US Navy, in response to a Department of Defense directive to capture and report battlefield injury.[4] The JTTR is designed to facilitate the collection, analysis, and reporting of CCC data along the continuum of care and to make this data accessible to healthcare providers engaged in the care of individual patients, as well as for system analysis and quality improvement. While implementation of the JTTR has been successful from the point of initial surgical intervention back to rehabilitative care, success in collection of the out-of-hospital components of the registry has been more elusive. Factors limiting consistent, systematically standardized and complete out-of-hospital data collection include: (1) legacy data collection methods (handwritten documents and antiquated field medical treatment cards); (2) lack of a complementary out-of-hospital component of the Joint Theater Trauma System; and (3) lack of a standard requirement for reporting out-of-hospital casualty care clinical records.

Recent studies confirm many of the WDMET findings, with evidence that compressible hemorrhage, tension pneumothorax, and airway and ventilatory compromise, are the leading causes of preventable death in Operation Enduring Freedom (OEF) and Operation Iraqi Freedom (OIF).[5,6] The WDMET study identified the following three conditions as primary causes of preventable death on the battlefield: (1) airway obstruction (6 percent), (2) tension pneumothorax (33 percent), and (3) hemorrhage from extremity wounds (60 percent). Analysis of autopsy records from OIF indicated a frequency of preventable battlefield death between 10 to 15 percent from airway obstruction and 33 percent for extremity hemorrhage thought to be preventable by tourniquet application.[6] In a smaller study describing 12 potentially preventable deaths in special operations forces, Holcomb et al. reported the following six conditions as potential contributors to death: noncompressible hemorrhage (eight deaths), tourniquet-amenable hemorrhage (three deaths), "non-tourniquetable" hemorrhage (two deaths), tension pneumothorax (one death), airway obstruction (one death), and sepsis (one death).[5] One death was deemed due to dual conditions. To affect survival, it is critical to recognize and treat most of these conditions within the first minutes after wounding.[7] Only combatant first responders, combat medics, and other far-forward clinicians can deliver this timely care.

---

Compressible hemorrhage, tension pneumothorax, and airway and ventilatory compromise are the leading causes of preventable death in OEF and OIF.

---

Despite the relative simplicity of the maneuvers required to treat these conditions, they remain a significant cause of mortality. This underscores the need to ensure clinical competence among CCC providers, including combatant first responders, medics, corpsmen, physicians, physician assistants and nurses, as well as an effective means of capturing clinical data in the out-of-hospital setting.[8] Gerhardt et al. recently studied the impact of deploying emergency medicine specialty-trained CCC providers including an emergency physician, an emergency medicine physician assistant, and advanced-scope-of-practice combat medics. The study demonstrated a 7.1 percent case fatality rate as compared to the concurrent theater aggregate US case fatality rate of 10.5 percent. This occurred despite a battle casualty rate nearly three times that of the contemporaneous combat theater-wide rate, an out-of-theater evacuation rate over twice that of the theater aggregate rate, and an equivalent injury severity score (ISS) to that of the theater aggregate. No deaths were attributed to airway obstruction or tension pneumothorax. One case of potentially compressible hemorrhage following traumatic lower extremity amputation resulting in death was reported.[9]

The Defense Health Board's Committee on Tactical Combat Casualty Care (TCCC) recently developed and promulgated coherent guidelines for those who engage in out-of-hospital CCC.[10] To the extent possible, the guidelines were created using literature-based evidence, rather than solely relying upon expert consensus. The importance of fully understanding TCCC principles and guidelines is underscored by the following case study.

## Case Study: Out-of-Hospital Care

A combat engineer section with attached civil affairs and medical personnel mounted in up-armored High-Mobility Multipurpose Wheeled Vehicles (HMMWVs) is conducting civil-military operational activities in a semipermissive section of a large urban center in US Central Command (CENTCOM) Area of Responsibility. The three-vehicle patrol halts along an alternate supply route after visually identifying an unexploded artillery shell. Several soldiers dismount. Moments later, the convoy comes under effective fire from a four-man team of insurgents armed with a light machine gun, a rocket-propelled grenade (RPG) launcher, and two assault rifles. One vehicle is disabled by an RPG. A second RPG is launched and strikes the unit's combat medic at an oblique angle, ricocheting off his individual body armor small arms protective insert and detonating after striking the ground near his feet. The medic sustains shrapnel wounds to the right medial thigh and right forearm, in addition to blunt chest trauma. A combat engineer is also wounded with shrapnel in his right forearm. Both casualties have brisk bleeding from their forearm wound sites. As the medical officer and other soldiers approach the wounded, the RPG gunner rises again, preparing to fire at them.

What actions should be taken in this vignette? Combatants are often faced with similar scenarios. Rapid action, decision making, and technical performance of interventions are critical. In this scenario, the appropriate immediate response would be to return effective fire to suppress or neutralize the threat (i.e., enemy combatant RPG gunner). Once the tactical situation allows, hasty (rapidly applied) tourniquets should be placed proximal to both respective forearm wounds. The tourniquets should be rapidly applied over casualties' clothing in care-under-fire scenarios. Additional casualties who are unable to ambulate independently should be extricated and moved to an area of cover.

Upon reaching the relative safety of cover, the CCC provider should assess casualties for airway patency, adequate ventilation, type and severity of chest trauma, and tourniquet efficacy. A brief survey of the casualties for additional (undiscovered) wounds should be quickly performed. Suspected tension pneumothorax is treated by needle thoracostomy. If tactical conditions permit, previously applied tourniquets should be reassessed for efficacy. Such tourniquets should be more deliberately positioned

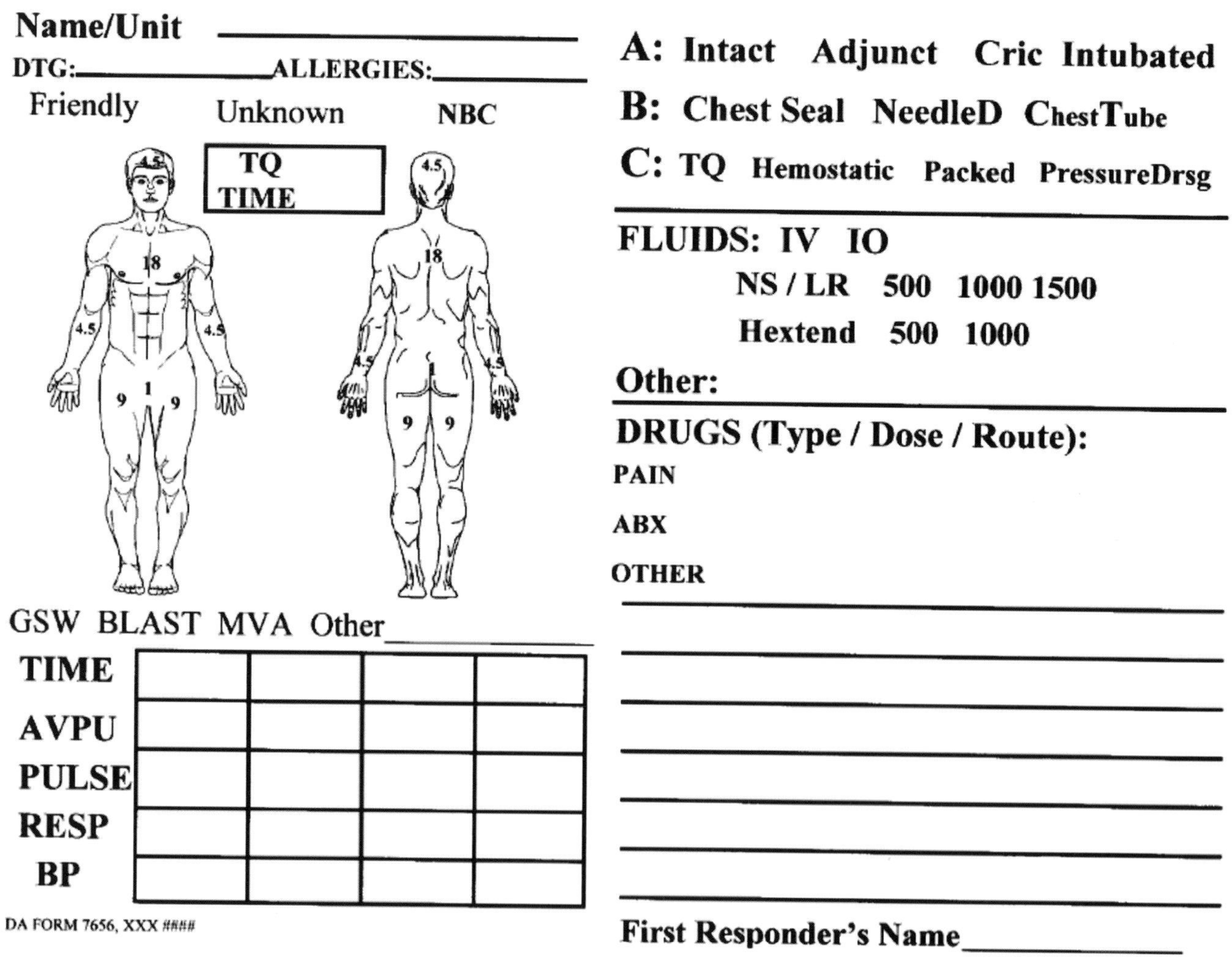
Name/Unit ____________
DTG:____________ ALLERGIES:____________
Friendly Unknown NBC
TQ TIME

GSW BLAST MVA Other____________

| TIME | | | | |
|---|---|---|---|---|
| AVPU | | | | |
| PULSE | | | | |
| RESP | | | | |
| BP | | | | |

DA FORM 7656, XXX ####

A: Intact Adjunct Cric Intubated
B: Chest Seal NeedleD ChestTube
C: TQ Hemostatic Packed PressureDrsg
FLUIDS: IV IO
NS / LR 500 1000 1500
Hextend 500 1000
Other:
DRUGS (Type / Dose / Route):
PAIN
ABX
OTHER
First Responder's Name____________

Figure 1. *TCCC casualty treatment card (DA 7656).*

directly proximal to the wound over bare skin. If, upon further examination of the casualty, a tourniquet is believed unnecessary, extremity wounds can be treated with standard or hemostatic wound dressings. This is followed by administration of prophylactic antibiotics and analgesics. During the ongoing process of assessment and tactical field care, appropriate tactical evacuation should be arranged. The CCC provider should continue to monitor and treat casualties during casualty evacuation. A TCCC casualty treatment card (DA 7656) should be completed at the earliest possible juncture, and it should be submitted to the appropriate authority (Fig. 1). Lastly, upon arrival at the receiving facility or upon transfer to the evacuation conveyance, the CCC provider should verbally sign over care (e.g., briefly summarize injuries and care) of casualties to receiving medical personnel.

## Combat Versus Civil Sector Out-of-Hospital Care

While some similarities exist, out-of-hospital care in combat settings often radically differs from civil sector practice in the US. Beyond the challenges of individual patient care, harsh weather conditions, and austere settings, out-of-hospital careproviders face unique tactical challenges. For example, in civilian sector emergency medical services (EMS), a typical motor vehicle collision scene might include an ambulance crew routinely consisting of two or even three emergency medical technicians (EMTs), with at least one being an EMT-Paramedic. Often, firefighters will be present, providing additional capabilities. Ambulances will be stocked with a wide array of basic and advanced life support devices, monitors, and pharmaceuticals. First responders will have telecommunication capacity and some form of medical direction for decision support and destination guidance. In the majority of cases, significant resources will be brought to bear upon one or two patients. In addition, civilian sector out-of-hospital careproviders do not typically face hostile gunfire and are able to fully focus on patient care.

Though some similarities exist, out-of-hospital care in combat settings often differs radically from civil sector practice in the US.

In contrast to the aforementioned scenario, one may envision a combat medic or other careprovider responding to casualties after a roadside bomb detonates adjacent to their convoy. After exiting his or her vehicle, the first responder proceeds on foot to the scene. Usually, all available medical equipment is carried by the medics themselves in a rucksack or otherwise harnessed to them. There is likely to be only one medic assisting casualties that were injured by a combination of high-explosive ordnance, vehicle fires, or small-arms fire. The medic is appropriately focused on patient care but must also be cognizant that the overarching priorities are the combat unit's integrity and mission. While working, the medic may become the target of hostile fire and may have to return fire.

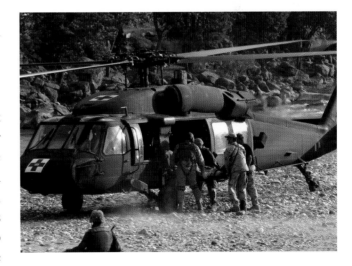

Figure 2. *Medical evacuation (MEDEVAC) of an injured soldier onto a UH-60 Black Hawk helicopter in Afghanistan. Evacuations tend to be longer in distance, duration, and complexity as compared to civilian settings. Image courtesy of Defense Imagery Management Operations Center (DIMOC).*

As highlighted previously, TCCC poses additional unique challenges compared to civilian practice. Combat casualty careproviders are more likely to encounter mass- and multiple-casualty-incidents and patients with catastrophic wounds. The epidemiology of wounding in OEF and OIF reveals a high incidence of penetrating trauma and blast-related mechanisms of injury.[11,12] Casualty evacuations tend to be longer in distance, duration, and complexity as compared to civilian settings. Such conditions combine to make CCC extremely challenging (Fig. 2).

> As compared to civilian practice, TCCC providers are more likely to encounter penetrating trauma, blast-related mechanisms of injury, and mass- and multiple-casualty-incidents while facing more complex casualty evacuation scenarios.

In addition to the individual challenges of CCC, several systemic issues pose significant obstacles to the optimization of CCC in the modern battlespace. The most pressing of these issues is a lack of effective clinical data collection in the forward setting and the need for adaptation of clinical operating guidelines (COG) and scope of practice for out-of-hospital practitioners. Outcomes research in EMS is sparse in both the civilian sector and combat settings. Randomized, controlled, prospective trials are the exception rather than the rule.[13] Much of what is available comes in the form of case reports or series focusing on single aspects of out-of-hospital CCC or case series resulting from individual engagements.[14] A primary challenge facing military medical leaders is the development and implementation of an effective, sustainable, and physically hardy system for documenting and sharing the equivalent of what would be a routine patient care report (PCR). Until the advent of such a system, critical elements of out-of-hospital CCC will lag behind civil sector EMS. This lack of out-of-hospital clinical data presents a formidable obstacle to implementing a civilian sector EMS-style medical direction model with its component process improvement mechanisms, including field medical treatment record review.

Future steps include: (1) organizing and training the military's out-of-hospital enlisted CCC providers to a level approaching that of special operations advanced tactical practitioners; (2) optimally utilizing military emergency medicine-trained practitioners (including emergency physicians and specialty-trained physician assistants, and certified emergency nurses); and (3) developing true emergency medical direction capability. Reflecting the success of civil sector EMS and trauma systems, the future military EMS medical direction capability should encompass retrospective process improvement program management as well as online decision support to far-forward practitioners.[7] In the interim, it is incumbent on individual CCC providers to make the best effort possible to document and forward clinical data pertaining to the casualties they treat, the interventions they performed, and the resulting outcomes.

## Tactical Combat Casualty Care (TCCC)

The inadequacy of applying a civilian trauma model to tactical situations has long been recognized.[15,16,17] The TCCC program was initiated by the Naval Special Warfare Command in 1993, and later continued by the US Special Operations Command (USSOCOM). This effort developed a set of tactically appropriate battlefield trauma care guidelines that provide CCC providers with trauma management strategies that combine good medicine with good small-unit tactics.[15] Tactical Combat Casualty Care guidelines recognize that trauma care in the tactical environment has three goals: (1) treat the casualty; (2) prevent additional casualties; and (3) complete the mission.

The first TCCC course was taught in 1996 in the Undersea Medical Officer course sponsored by the Navy Bureau of Medicine and Surgery (BUMED). Shortly thereafter, this training was mandated for all US Navy Sea-Air-Land (SEAL) naval special warfare corpsmen.[15] Since that time, TCCC has gradually gained acceptance in US and foreign military forces.[15,16,17,18,19,20,21,22,23] It has also found acceptance in the civilian law enforcement medical community.[24] Preliminary evidence from the current conflicts in Afghanistan and Iraq supports the contention that in the hands of clinically and tactically competent CCC providers, TCCC contributes to casualty survival.[25]

> Tactical Combat Casualty Care is divided into three phases: (1) care-under-fire, (2) tactical field care, and (3) tactical evacuation care.

Trauma care measures proposed in the original TCCC guidelines are outlined in Table 1. The overarching goal of the TCCC initiative is the combination of good tactics with good medicine. As the name implies, TCCC is practiced during combat missions. TCCC is divided into three phases: (1) care-under-fire, (2) tactical field care, and (3) tactical evacuation care. In care-under-fire, CCC providers and their units are presumed to be under effective hostile fire, and the care they are capable of providing is very limited. In the tactical field care phase, CCC providers and their patients are no longer under effective hostile fire, and more extensive care can be provided. In the tactical evacuation care phase, casualties are transported to a medical facility by an aircraft, ground vehicle, or boat, and there is an opportunity to provide a higher level of care.

## ORIGINAL TACTICAL COMBAT CASUALTY CARE TREATMENT MEASURES

1. Early use of tourniquets to control clinically important extremity hemorrhage
2. Systemic antibiotic prophylaxis near point of injury
3. Tactically appropriate intravenous or intraosseous access and fluid resuscitation
4. Improved battlefield analgesia (intravenous or intramuscular opiates)
5. Nasopharyngeal airways as first-line airway devices
6. Surgical airways for maxillofacial trauma with an obstructed airway
7. Aggressive diagnosis and treatment of tension pneumothorax via needle decompression
8. Incorporation of input from CCC providers into TCCC guidelines
9. Employment of tactically and clinically-relevant scenarios into TCCC training

Table 1. *Original Tactical Combat Casualty Care treatment measures.*

## *Care-Under-Fire Issues*

The first phase of the TCCC paradigm is composed of two verbs: care and fire. This implies the unpleasant realities that one's unit has come under attack by hostile personnel who have made the unit the target of effective fire by one or more lethal weapon systems, and, as a result, someone has been wounded. The essential initial action is to return effective fire toward the threat with the specific intent of neutralizing or otherwise preventing hostile personnel from continuing to place effective fire on the CCC provider or their unit. Until this is accomplished, the CCC provider will be unable to render effective medical care, and the careprovider, fellow warfighters, or existing casualties could be further wounded or killed. A summary of actions conducted during the care-under-fire phase includes: (1) returning effective fire toward the source of hostile engagement; (2) tactical movement of the casualty and careprovider to an area of cover and concealment; (3) and the rapid assessment for sources of massive extremity hemorrhage amenable to placement of a tourniquet, followed by rapid tourniquet placement if practicable. Once these tasks have been accomplished and the unit is no longer under effective hostile fire, this phase of TCCC is complete (Fig. 3).

> In care-under-fire situations, the CCC provider should return effective fire, move the casualty to a safe area, rapidly assess the casualty for sources of massive extremity hemorrhage, and apply a tourniquet if necessary.

The care-under-fire phase of TCCC is often difficult for careproviders transitioning from civilian healthcare backgrounds. It is imperative that all CCC providers develop and maintain, at a minimum, basic proficiency in fundamental soldier skills prior to tactical deployment. Basic tactical warfighting skills include four fundamental components: shooting, moving, communicating, and surviving. It is important to: (1) understand how small units (squads, platoons, and companies) operate in combat; (2) know how to employ cover and concealment when moving tactically (both in vehicles and while dismounted on foot); (3) possess basic firearm marksmanship culminating in true proficiency with one's primary weapon and familiarity with other weapons used by one's unit or organization; and (4) have a working knowledge of how to locate and use the unit's radio and other available communications systems. A CCC provider should not presume the aforementioned skills will be provided by one's gaining unit. Rather, one should actively seek training and mentoring in these essential tasks prior to and during deployment.

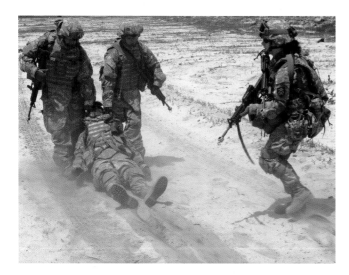

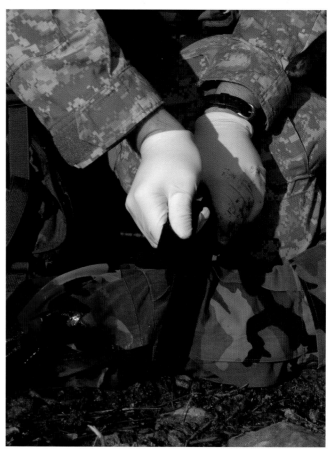

Figure 3. (Above) *After returning effective fire, casualties should be moved to an area of cover and concealment and assessed for massive extremity hemorrhage amenable to placement of a tourniquet. Image courtesy of Defense Imagery Management Operations Center (DIMOC).*

Figure 4. (Right) *Hemorrhage control is a priority in all phases of TCCC. Tourniquets or hemostatic dressings combined with direct pressure should be applied early, when indicated. Image courtesy of Defense Imagery Management Operations Center (DIMOC).*

## Tactical Field Care

### Hemorrhage Control and Tourniquet Use

Uncontrolled hemorrhage remains the largest single cause of combat deaths, accounting for over 80 percent of combat deaths.[6] Moreover, compressible hemorrhage remains a significant cause of preventable battlefield deaths.[5,6] As such, the control of hemorrhage remains a priority in all phases of TCCC and includes the employment of hasty (rapidly applied) tourniquets as the primary means of controlling significant extremity hemorrhage (Fig. 4). After the casualty is extracted from effective hostile fire, hemostatic dressings may be placed with direct pressure applied to extremity bleeding sites, distal to tourniquets. Similarly, hemostatic dressings and direct pressure are applied to sources of bleeding on the torso and other sites that are not amenable to tourniquet application.

> Uncontrolled hemorrhage remains the largest single cause of combat deaths, accounting for over 80 percent of combat deaths.

Extremity wounds that require continued tourniquet use for hemostasis should have hasty (rapidly applied) tourniquets converted to definitive (deliberate) tourniquets. This is accomplished by removing overlying clothing and armor and applying definitive tourniquets immediately proximal (two to three inches above the wound) to the hemorrhage site (e.g., mangled or amputated extremity). If required, additional tourniquets may be placed (in sequence longitudinally) proximal to the source of bleeding to reinforce the hemostatic effect. In situations where hasty tourniquets were placed in a care-under-fire scenario, reassessment of the injured extremity can now be performed in the tactical field care phase. In a hemodynamically stable patient, a tourniquet can be removed if the extremity injury was not as severe as originally judged, or hemostasis is maintained with hemostatic dressings and direct pressure. Additional information on tourniquets can be found in the Extremity Injury chapter.

### Hemostatic Agents

Operation Enduring Freedom and OIF have supported important research, development, and acquisition efforts focused on creating effective hemostatic agents for out-of-hospital setting use. The use of parenteral hemostatic agents, such as recombinant factor VIIa, has been met with controversy and conflicting clinical data, resulting in limited use.[26,27,28,29,30,31,32,33,34,35,36,37,38,39,40,41] Likewise, there is little definitive clinical data supporting the use of hemostatic dressings, despite their ubiquitous presence on the battlefield.[42,43,44,45,46,47] First-generation agents such as Zeolite (QuikClot®) and Chitosan-impregnated semi-rigid dressings (HemCon®) have given way to hemostatic-impregnated gauze (e.g., Kaolin Combat Gauze™, HemCon ChitoFlex™, CELOX Chitosan Gauze™). The current TCCC guidelines recommend Combat Gauze™ as the hemostatic agent of choice for compressible hemorrhage not amenable to tourniquet use.[10] These hemostatic agents may offer incremental benefits, particularly in cases of junctional hemorrhage (inguinal or axillary wounds) or in cavitary wound applications. At present, there is insufficient evidence to recommend specific products over others in out-of-hospital care. It should be emphasized that proper dressing and bandaging techniques and the early and appropriate use of tourniquets are the most critical elements of out-of-hospital hemorrhage control.

## Vascular Access and Fluid Resuscitation

Casualties with controlled sources of hemorrhage who have a palpable radial pulse and a normal mental status do not require immediate vascular access and resuscitative fluids in the out-of-hospital phase of care (Fig. 5).[48] Vascular access should be obtained for casualties with uncontrolled hemorrhage or in cases of presumed significant head injury (e.g., altered mental status) and significant blood loss. While peripheral intravenous access remains the criterion standard, the emergence of intraosseous devices has provided a viable alternative.[49] Requiring minimal training to achieve and maintain proficiency, common intraosseous devices in current military use employ the sternal manubrium, tibial tuberosity, lateral humeral head, or iliac crest as access sites and permit administration of resuscitation fluids, blood products, and many pharmaceuticals (Fig. 6).[50,51,52,53]

> Casualties with controlled sources of hemorrhage who have a palpable radial pulse and a normal mental status do not require immediate vascular access and resuscitative fluids in the out-of-hospital phase of care.

The optimal type and volume of intravenous solution to employ in acute hemorrhagic shock in the out-of-hospital tactical setting is still a subject for debate. Described by Beecher as a result of combat surgical experience in World War II and resurfacing with the work of Bickell et al. in 1994, the concept of hypotensive resuscitation has regained traction in the military CCC community.[49,54,55] The evidence in support of specific volumes and types of intravenous resuscitation fluids for use in combat is limited. Existing data does support logistical arguments favoring a hypotensive resuscitation scheme including the use of colloids due to decreased carrying weight and space requirements.[56] Hetastarch 6% in lactated electrolyte solution and 7% hypertonic saline (HTS) have been studied as fluid resuscitation solutions.[48,57] These resuscitation solutions effectively restore intravascular volume, minimize inappropriate immune response and cellular injury, and improve overall survival in the absence of blood products.[57] Of note, colloids such as hydroxyethyl starch have been known to increase coagulopathy (in vitro) by impairing von Willebrand factor activity in plasma.[58] The only trauma clinical trial involving Hextend® to date uncovered

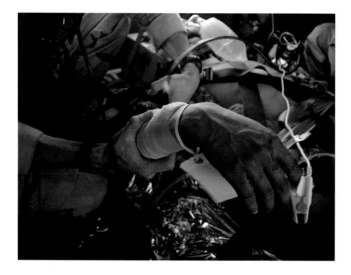

Figure 5. *Casualties with controlled sources of hemorrhage who have a palpable radial pulse and a normal mental status do not require immediate vascular access and resuscitative fluids in the out-of-hospital phase of care. Image courtesy of Defense Imagery Management Operations Center (DIMOC).*

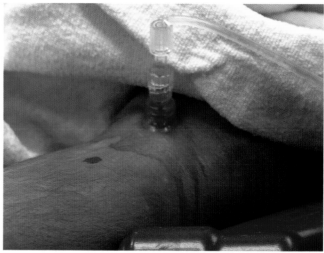

Figure 6. *If immediate vascular access is needed and a standard intravenous line cannot be established, intraosseous access should be obtained. All resuscitative medications and blood products can be infused via an intraosseous needle.*

no clinical signs of coagulopathy in the Hextend®-resuscitated group as compared to the control group.[59]

As a practical matter, hypertonic saline solutions are not readily available commercially for use as intravascular volume replacement, whole blood and fresh frozen plasma are currently impractical in tactical settings, and hemoglobin-based oxygen carriers are still under development. As of this printing, the current TCCC recommendation for intravascular fluid resuscitation is the use of Hextend® (6% Hetastarch in Lactated Electrolyte Injection) in 500 milliliter aliquots, with a maximum administration of 1,000 milliliters.[10] Similarly, the recommended resuscitation endpoints for combat casualties are evolving. Reasonable endpoints include a palpable radial pulse or a systolic blood pressure of 90 mm Hg and improved mental status in non-head-injured patients.[49]

## Acute Airway Obstruction and Ventilatory Support

Recent analyses of preventable deaths in OEF and OIF revealed 10 to 15 percent of casualties were deemed to have acute airway obstruction or ventilatory failure as a proximate cause of death.[6,60,61] To further underscore the need for out-of-hospital phase early airway support, a subanalysis of the Registry of Emergency Airways at Combat Hospitals (REACH) study by Adams et al. reported that 76 of 1,622 subjects (5 percent) arrived at a Combat Support Hospital (CSH) without a definitive airway, despite needing one.[62]

> Ten to 15 percent of preventable deaths in OEF and OIF were attributed to acute airway obstruction or ventilatory failure.[60,61]

The CCC provider must be able to provide basic and advanced airway support and control. This includes use of basic airway adjuncts (oral and nasopharyngeal airways), providing bag-valve-mask ventilatory support, establishing definitive airways (endotracheal intubation and cricothyroidotomy), and using a portable mechanical ventilator. While rapid sequence direct laryngoscopic orotracheal intubation remains the criterion standard for advanced airway management in the civil sector, its efficacy and continued role in the out-of-hospital setting remains the subject of debate.[63,64,65,66] Furthermore, this intervention does not translate well into the tactical environment, unless performed by practitioners who are proficient in its execution.[9,62] According to TCCC guidelines, surgical cricothyroidotomy (provided careproviders are trained in its performance) is the preferred method for establishing a definitive airway during tactical field care or the tactical evacuation phase.[1,9,10,17] This recommendation assumes careproviders in the field lack the necessary equipment, pharmaceutical agents, or training to perform rapid-sequence orotracheal intubation.

Alternative methods of securing a definitive airway in the tactical environment include standard laryngoscopic orotracheal intubation, blind insertion airway devices, such as laryngeal tube devices, or esophageal gastric tube airways. Laryngeal-mask airways (LMA) are considered a temporizing airway measure as opposed to a definitive airway. While they are among the easiest-to-use, they are limited by their inability to be firmly secured in place and provide definitive airway protection. Lastly, the recent advent of video-based laryngoscopic devices (such as Glidescope® and RES-Q-SCOPE®) may offer a viable option for orotracheal intubation in field and transport settings; however, data confirming efficacy in this setting is lacking.[67,68,69]

Ensuring combat casualties have a secure and patent airway is strongly recommended during the tactical field care phase prior to tactical evacuation. In circumstances where this is impossible or impractical, the practitioner's goal will shift toward attempting to prevent airway compromise en route, as the environment in most evacuation conveyances is suboptimal at best for advanced airway placement. In the event that unanticipated airway compromise occurs during evacuation, the practitioner must rapidly assess the likely cause and attempt to mitigate it. Simple suctioning and jaw-thrust maneuvers may suffice. If these initial interventions fail, the practitioner may be forced to perform an advanced airway maneuver. Under such circumstances, the decision whether to perform surgical cricothyroidotomy or to employ alternative methods of securing an airway will have to be made, taking into consideration the patient's unique anatomy, conditions in the vehicle (vibration, kinetics, visibility, maneuver room), available airway supplies, and skill of the CCC provider.

### Tension Pneumothorax

Traumatic pneumothorax is a potentially life-threatening condition and may rapidly progress to tension pneumothorax, an immediate life-threat. Likewise, an accumulating hemothorax or hemopneumothorax may cause similar cardiovascular collapse due to both ongoing hemorrhage, as well as the introduction of tension physiology.

Tension pneumothorax, hemodynamically significant hemothorax, or tension hemopneumothorax should be suspected in the setting of blunt or penetrating thoracic trauma when a combination of the following

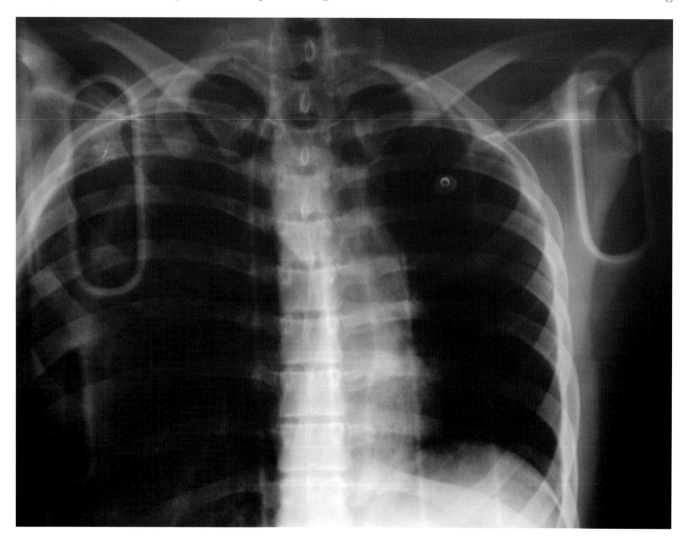

Figure 7. *Immediate needle thoracentesis should be performed in cases of suspected tension pneumothorax.*

clinical findings are present: progressive respiratory distress, hypotension, contralateral tracheal deviation, hyperresonance or dullness on percussion of the affected hemithorax, asymmetric chest wall rise with inhalation, or ipsilateral or bilateral decreased breath sounds upon auscultation. Under such conditions a needle thoracentesis should be performed. A 14-gauge intravenous catheter with a minimum length of eight centimeters (3.25 inch needle/catheter unit) is placed in the second intercostal space along the midclavicular line.[10,70,71] The recently revised recommendation to use a longer needle is based on data indicating a larger chest wall thickness in military personnel.[71] Tube thoracostomy should follow needle thoracentesis at the earliest possible juncture. Chest tube insertion in the setting of a pneumothorax is strongly recommended in advance of tactical evacuation, particularly if casualties will be transported by air. If this is not practicable, placement of a three-way stopcock for serial decompression or repeated needle thoracentesis may be required. The casualty should be closely monitored for recurrence of tension pneumothorax (Fig. 7).

## Spinal Injury Precautions

In the current conflicts in Afghanistan and Iraq, spinal trauma is an increasing source of morbidity often leading to spinal cord injury and paralysis.[72] Cervical, thoracic, and lumbar spinal injuries (along with multiple spinal level injuries) are encountered in combat casualties injured by gunfire, explosions, motor vehicle accidents, and falls.[73,74,75,76]

Although recently challenged in cases of penetrating spinal trauma, spinal immobilization is a fundamental tenet of out-of-hospital EMS practice in the civil sector.[77] The employment, methods, and point of initiation of spinal immobilization in combat settings differ by necessity from civil sector practice. Factors influencing this phenomenon include tactical considerations, the effect of individual body armor on both spinal immobilization and alignment, and the logistical challenges associated with the movement of a properly immobilized patient through the tactical evacuation chain.

> By necessity, the employment, methods, and point of initiation of spinal immobilization in combat settings differ from civil sector practice.

There is insufficient literature to provide definitive guidelines on spinal immobilization in tactical settings.[78] First responders will need to use their best judgment in such settings. When a CCC provider suspects spinal trauma, tactically sound attempts at maintaining the casualty's spinal column in as near-neutral a position as possible should be attempted during care-under-fire and initial extrication. Individual body armor, though in itself a potential source of spinal misalignment, should remain on the casualty for as long as there continues to be a realistic threat of further engagement by hostile ordnance (Fig. 8). When tactical conditions allow, individual body armor should be removed or loosened to facilitate further casualty examination. If suspicion for spinal injury persists after secondary survey, and tactical conditions permit, individual body armor should be removed and spinal immobilization measures instituted. Spinal injury precautions should then be maintained throughout tactical evacuation (Fig. 9).

> Spinal immobilization techniques used in a combat setting mirror those found in the civilian sector.

## Traumatic Brain Injury

Blunt and penetrating head injuries are common occurrences in OEF and OIF, despite the advent of Kevlar-based helmets.[6] The continued use of roadside bombs by enemy combatants has accelerated efforts

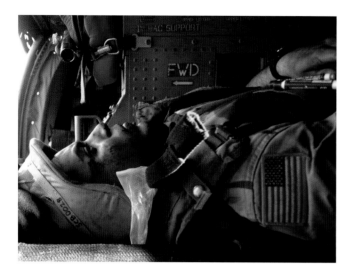

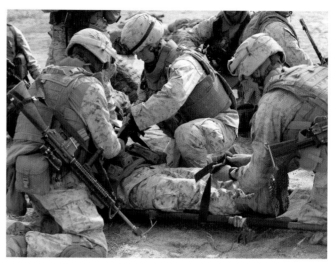

Figure 8. *An injured US Army soldier aboard a UH-60 Black Hawk MEDEVAC helicopter as he is airlifted to a Level III facility. Individual body armor should remain on the casualty for as long as there continues to be a realistic threat of further engagement by hostile ordnance. Image courtesy of Defense Imagery Management Operations Center (DIMOC).*

Figure 9. *Spinal immobilization applied during a training drill. Image courtesy of Defense Imagery Management Operations Center (DIMOC).*

to improve both diagnostic and therapeutic approaches to traumatic brain injury. Civilian research studies have established that patients suffering severe head injuries complicated by episodes of transient hypoxia or hypotension in the prehospital phase of care have worse outcomes.[79] As such, out-of-hospital careproviders should attempt to prevent episodes of hypoxemia and hypotension in patients with traumatic brain injuries. Casualties with head injuries who manifest signs of hemorrhagic shock should undergo interventions directed towards hemorrhage control, optimization of airway and ventilatory status, and restoration of adequate tissue perfusion. The goal of airway and ventilatory support in the tactical setting is to maintain adequate tissue oxygenation and normal ventilation. Patients should have their partial pressure of oxygen in arterial blood ($PaO_2$) maintained at or above 60 mm Hg (pulse oximeter reading greater than 90 percent oxygen saturation) and partial pressure of carbon dioxide ($PCO_2$) values in the normal range of 35 to 40 mm Hg.[79] While endpoints of fluid resuscitation in the tactical setting include a palpable radial pulse or improved mental status in non-head-injured patients, alternative strategies may be indicated in patients with suspected traumatic brain injury. More aggressive fluid resuscitation may be required to minimize secondary brain injury from hypotension (defined as systolic blood pressure less than 90 mm Hg). The ability to meet these parameters in a tactical field care setting is complicated by numerous factors.

| In patients with suspected head injury, more aggressive fluid resuscitation strategies may be necessary to minimize secondary brain injury from cerebral hypoperfusion resulting from systemic hypotension. |
| --- |

Patients with blunt head injuries are at risk for coexisting cervical spine injury.[80,81,82] Hence, spinal immobilization or at least maintenance of neutral spinal alignment is recommended at the earliest possible juncture during the tactical field care phase. Similar to casualties with other causes for potential closed-space gas collection, patients with suspected intracranial injury should be transported with the minimal possible increase in altitude and should be positioned in a neutral supine position.[83] Early post-traumatic seizures have been observed in 5 to 30 percent of severe head injury patients and may exacerbate secondary brain injury.[84,85] Seizures occurring in the tactical setting may be controlled initially with benzodiazepines administered via intramuscular, intravenous, intraosseous, or rectal routes. Airway control and breathing support in the setting of head trauma and seizures are important because the administration of benzodiazepines may hasten or exacerbate hypotension and ventilatory insufficiency.

A final consideration in the tactical care of head injury patients is the potential need for neurosurgical intervention and the availability of such services within range of evacuation assets. The determination of whether to seek the nearest resuscitative surgical care versus overflight to more comprehensive medical treatment facilities is a complex decision. These decisions can be made by communicating with Level III careproviders, ideally prior to evacuation of the combat casualty.

## Hypothermia Prevention and Management

Hypothermia is recognized as an independent factor contributing to increased morbidity and mortality in trauma patients.[86] In the combat casualty, hypothermia may occur due to prolonged prehospital time, cold fluid administration, environmental factors, and trauma-related bleeding and hypoperfusion. Arthurs et al. found that 18 percent of casualties presenting to a CSH in OIF were hypothermic (temperature less than 36°C).[87] Keeping a patient warm, especially early in tactical field care, will minimize subsequent hypothermia and resultant cold coagulopathy. This may be accomplished using passive external means, such as blankets, vehicle heating systems, hats and hoods to minimize heat loss from the head and scalp, and by ensuring that wet clothing or dressings are replaced. The recent fielding of the Hypothermia Prevention and Management Kit (HPMK®), which is composed of a disposable weather-resistant bag, insulating liner, chemical heat packet, and a heat-radiant cap, has capitalized on several effective field-expedient

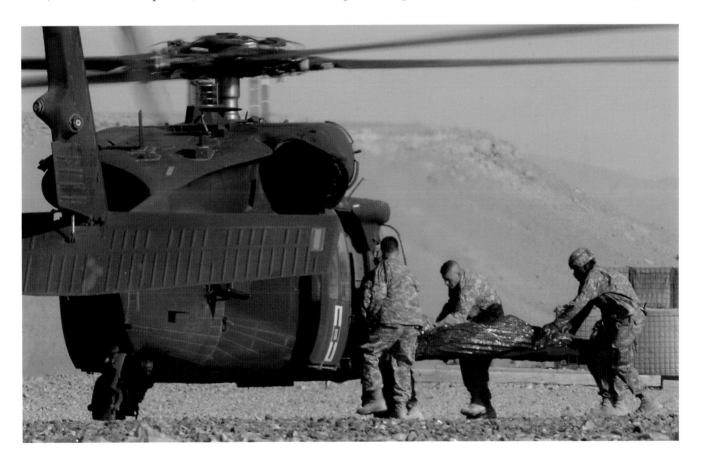

Figure 10. *A US casualty being loaded onto a UH-60Q Black Hawk helicopter in Afghanistan. Note casualty is covered in a solar blanket. Image courtesy of Defense Imagery Management Operations Center (DIMOC).*

treatments developed by tactical practitioners (Fig. 10). Many alternative hypothermia prevention devices exist (e.g., Thermal Angel®, ChillBuster®, Blizzard Survival Blanket).

The CCC provider should be cognizant of the relative temperatures of intravenous fluids being administered to casualties. Ideally, intravenous fluids are delivered at body temperature. Infusing cold fluids will hasten hypothermia and initiate cold coagulopathy. Potential tactical countermeasures include storage of small volume intravenous fluids on the body (in the axilla against the torso), field-expedient insulation of intravenous tubing using rolled paper or cloth, and placement of the intravenous infusion set along with the casualty in a sleeping bag or similar cover.

## Infection Prophylaxis

It is a widely held belief in military medical circles that combat wounds are more likely to become infected than corresponding wounds occurring in the civilian sector setting. Gerhardt et al. presented data that both lent credence to this notion and also provided evidence in support of copious wound irrigation and systemic antibiotic prophylaxis of combat wounds in a population of subjects not requiring surgical intervention.[88] In this study, infections developed within 48 hours in 7 percent of subjects receiving systemic antibiotic prophylaxis versus 40 percent without antibiotic prophylaxis. Infections developed within 48 hours in 4.5 percent of cases undergoing wound irrigation versus 55 percent of cases that did not undergo irrigation. Further analysis demonstrated that the lowest infection rates were associated with the combination of systemic antibiotic prophylaxis and irrigation. The high frequency of complex combat wounds, delays in evacuation to definitive care, and the logistical difficulty associated with irrigation at the point of injury support the current TCCC guideline encouraging early systemic antibiotic prophylaxis after wounding through the use of combat pill packs on the battlefield.[10]

> Evidence supports the use of systemic antibiotic prophylaxis and copious wound irrigation in the management of combat wounds.

Tactical Combat Casualty Care recommendations for systemic antibiotic prophylaxis include moxifloxacin (400 milligrams by mouth once daily) for patients who are able to tolerate oral administration, or intravenous cefotetan (2 grams every 12 hours) or ertapenam (1 gram intravenously or intramuscularly once daily).[10] Of note, the author (RG) has utilized oral levofloxacin or intramuscular/intravenous ceftriaxone to good effect. An additional factor in favor of these latter antibiotics is the widespread availability of these agents throughout the current battlespace.

## Pain Management

Despite decades of dogma to the contrary, numerous studies have demonstrated that the judicious use of analgesic agents does not significantly alter the physical examination or impede medical diagnosis.[89] The timely and adequate relief of pain is both humane and often the only effective treatment that may be offered to a casualty.[83] In addition, recent evidence supports the contention that the failure to address acute pain in the setting of combat wounds may increase the incidence of both post-traumatic stress disorder and chronic regional pain syndromes.[90,91]

> Use of analgesics does not significantly alter physical examination or medical diagnosis.

In the setting of mild, particularly musculoskeletal injuries, a nonsteroidal antiinflammatory drug (NSAID) may be administered. For more severe wounds, or if a NSAID fails to provide adequate relief, opioid analgesics (e.g., morphine sulfate) provide potent acute analgesia. Intramuscular use of opiates is discouraged, due to unpredictability of absorption and bioavailability. Oral or intravenous preparations are recommended. As of this writing, oral transmucosal fentanyl citrate (OTFC) is emerging as a potential solution for tactical analgesia (800 micrograms transbuccally). Although this is an off-label use of this medication and the Food and Drug Administration (FDA) has issued a black box warning that states that oral transmucosal fentanyl citrate should not be used except for breakthrough pain in opioid-tolerant patients, this medication has been used safely in combat.[92] Current TCCC recommendations for combat pill packs include meloxicam (15 milligrams by mouth once daily). Meloxicam was selected due to its lack of a sulfa moiety, which could prove hazardous in cases of sulfa-allergic casualties.[10]

## Air Medical Evacuation Considerations

Air medical transport can adversely affect medical conditions characterized by gas trapped in a fixed space such as untreated pneumothorax. Lower ambient atmospheric pressures at altitude cause intrapleural gas to expand with a resultant increased compression of the heart and contralateral lung. The practical effect of Boyle's law ($P_1 V_1 = P_2 V_2$; P denotes the pressure of the system, and V denotes the volume of the gas) on a casualty with an untreated simple pneumothorax undergoing air evacuation via an unpressurized compartment is development of a tension pneumothorax after ascent to altitude. The same may be said for other trapped-gas clinical conditions. As a result, it is recommended that patients suspected or known to have a pneumothorax receive decompression of the affected anatomical space prior to transport.[83] If decompression is not performed, evacuation should be conducted via routes that minimize elevation within the confines of the tactical situation. Although little scientific evidence exists for such cases, avoiding ascent to altitudes in excess of 5,000 feet above mean sea level has been recommended.[93] In cases where a unit is operating in alpine terrain (routinely above 5,000 feet mean sea level), the authors' recommend minimizing further ascent, to the extent possible. Air medical transport-related barometric complications also include pneumocephalus, pneumoperitoneum, and overexpansion of endotracheal and Foley catheter tube cuffs filled with air.[83] Endotracheal tube and Foley catheter cuffs should be filled with crystalloid solutions or sterile water prior to evacuation, mitigating the risk of cuff overexpansion. Occlusive dressings covering thoracic puncture wounds should be checked periodically while en route and should be vented as clinically indicated.

## *Tactical Evacuation Care*

Once casualties arrive at a company combat casualty collection point or equivalent element, evacuation becomes the responsibility of the gaining medical unit. As such, each Battalion Aid Station is equipped with an ambulance squad and charged with transport of casualties from casualty collection point to Battalion Aid Station. Likewise, each Brigade Support Medical Company (BSMC) possesses ambulance platoons to transport patients from the Battalion Aid Station to the Brigade Support Medical Company and to coordinate ambulance exchange points in settings where distances or terrain separating medical treatment facilities are prohibitive. In addition to these unit-level assets, combat divisions possess Medical Companies (Air Ambulance), more commonly known as MEDEVAC units. These units are often allocated to subordinate medical units, or staged at Level III facilities such as CSHs.

There will be circumstances when the evacuation capabilities of maneuver units are temporarily overwhelmed. It is under these circumstances that nonstandard vehicles may be employed for casualty evacuation. While often necessary in mass-casualty-incidents, this form of transportation should be considered a last resort. This is because of the relative difficulty involved in adequately securing patients for transport and the probable lack of en-route-care resulting from the absence of medics assigned to the casualty evacuation (CASEVAC) vehicles.

After initial triage and stabilization, casualties in the tactical setting are categorized for evacuation.[83] Traditionally, the primary objectives of air medical evacuation have been speed and access. While quantitative data are lacking, the transport time interval between point of injury to damage control resuscitation and damage control surgery is perceived as critical to the survival of combat casualties in OEF and OIF. Designated MEDEVAC precedence categories (urgent, urgent surgical, priority, routine, and convenience) are used to determine evacuation priorities and should not be confused with US/NATO mass casualty triage categories (immediate, delayed, minimal, expectant, and urgent surgical) (Fig. 11).

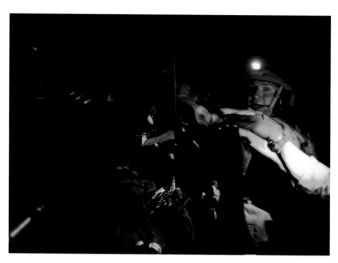

Figure 11. *A severely wounded service member aboard an HC-130P Hercules aircraft flying over Afghanistan en route to a CSH. Image courtesy of Defense Imagery Management Operations Center (DIMOC).*

> The transport time interval between point of injury to damage control resuscitation and damage control surgery is critical to the survival of combat casualties in OEF and OIF.

The urgent evacuation category is reserved primarily for casualties requiring immediate care who should be evacuated within a maximum time interval of one hour. An urgent surgical subcategory exists for casualties deemed to be at the greatest severity who require rapid evacuation for lifesaving surgical interventions to prevent death. Under current US and Coalition doctrine, urgent patients receive MEDEVAC if weather and tactical conditions allow. Priority evacuation is conducted mainly for delayed category casualties requiring transport to higher level care within four hours in order to avoid deterioration to an urgent condition or to avoid undue pain or disability. This category usually is transported via ground assets, although air transport may be used under some conditions. Routine evacuation is reserved for casualties triaged as minimally injured, and generally is performed by standard ground or waterborne assets within 24 hours of the initial event. Convenience denotes cases where medical evacuation is performed for convenience rather than necessity. It is worth noting that a recent requirement placed by the Office of the Secretary of Defense now mandates a one-hour evacuation for urgent casualties.

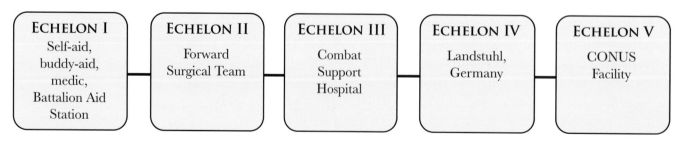

Figure 12. *Evacuation chain for combat casualties.*

Another challenge to the evacuation system is the ability to deliver effective, advanced en-route-care (Fig. 12). Traditionally, MEDEVAC platforms have been staffed with combat medics or their sister-service counterparts. Training and experience levels vary widely, as does the capability to provide or continue advanced lifesaving interventions such as ventilatory, circulatory, or pharmacological support.[94,95] Given the limited scope of practice of Army flight medics who staff MEDEVAC aircraft, the need to augment the MEDEVAC crew with an advanced practice medic or credentialed provider should be anticipated if critically injured patients will be transported.[94,95]

The US military refers collectively to the effects of the operational milieu as mission, equipment, terrain and weather, time, troops (both US and enemy combatants), and civilians (METT-TC) on the battlefield.[96] All of these factors possess the potential to impact, either positively or negatively, an evacuation plan. Combat casualty careproviders

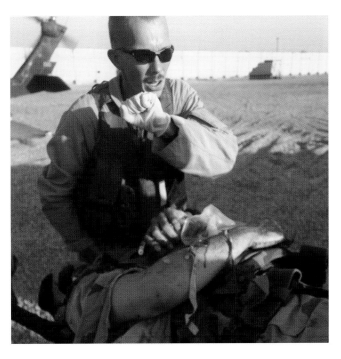

Figure 13. *A US casualty with a neck injury is loaded onto a UH-60 Black Hawk MEDEVAC helicopter at a landing zone in Camp Victory, Iraq. Image courtesy of Defense Imagery Management Operations Center (DIMOC).*

must be aware of these issues as they affect both tactical and medical operations. Operational areas may be broad and deep, resulting in significantly greater distances required for evacuation. These conditions compound the standard risks inherent in tactical evacuation and en-route-care. As a result, evacuation planning and coordination among first responders, destination facilities, evacuation assets, and maneuver elements become critical for mission success and casualty survival.

Important time-distance considerations in casualty evacuation and en-route-care include:
1. Location, number, and type of elements supported
2. Their internal (organic) medical support and evacuation assets
3. Location of echelon II and III combat health support units in your respective Area of Responsibility (AOR)
4. Terrain features affecting potential evacuation routes
5. Analysis of adversary locations, capabilities and limitations, and prior conduct toward noncombatant medical units
6. US or Coalition maneuver and support elements available to escort or otherwise assist the evacuation mission
7. Friendly evacuation assets available to you, including dedicated medical evacuation vehicles and aircraft, nonstandard vehicles, potential crew members, and nonmedical attendants
8. Your source of launch authority

The METT-TC information forthcoming from the requesting unit is most readily obtained by receipt of a standard MEDEVAC request, usually composed in a nine-line format. An example of a standard MEDEVAC request appears in Table 2.

## NATO NINE-LINE MEDEVAC REQUEST

1. Location of landing zone (LZ) for casualty collection (eight digit MGRS grid coordinates)
2. Radiofrequency, call sign, and suffix of requesting element
3. Number of patients by precedence:
   - A - Urgent
   - B - Urgent surgical
   - C - Priority
   - D - Routine
   - E - Convenience
4. Special equipment required:
   - A - None
   - B - Hoist
   - C - Extrication equipment
   - D - Ventilator
   - E - Other (specify)
5. Number of casualties by type
   - A - Litter
   - B - Ambulatory
   - C - Escort
6. Security at LZ / pick-up site
   - N - No enemy troops in area
   - P - Possible enemy troops – approach with caution
   - E - Enemy troops in area
   - X - Enemy troops in area – armed escort required
7. Method of marking LZ* / pick-up site
   - A - Panels (VS-17 or similar)
   - B - Pyrotechnic
   - C - Smoke
   - D - None
   - E - Other (specify)
   - *Methods may be listed by local tactical standard operating procedures
8. Casualty nationality and status
   - A - Coalition military
   - B - Coalition civilian
   - C - Non-Coalition forces
   - D - Non-Coalition civilian
   - E - Opposing forces detainee
   - F - Child
9. Pick-up zone terrain obstacles

Table 2. *NATO nine-line MEDEVAC request.*

Air medical evacuation is the primary method for urgent and urgent surgical casualties, and may be appropriate for priority casualties (Fig. 13). The decision to employ MEDEVAC support is complicated by many variables and must take into account the vulnerability of rotary wing aircraft to virtually any modern weapons system.[83] This risk is amplified in urban terrain or mountains where flight paths and landing zones often intersect closely with terrain features of similar or greater elevation, providing optimal battle positions to engage the aircraft with hostile fire. A sobering thought to be considered by anyone requesting MEDEVAC is the possibility that both the casualty and the MEDEVAC crew might perish as the result of hostile fire or marginal flight conditions.[83] As such, these resources should be used carefully, and the decision to employ MEDEVAC should be made with input by competent clinical and tactical operators with a minimum of emotion. Appropriate indications for air medical evacuation are outlined in Table 3.

## INDICATIONS FOR AIR MEDICAL EVACUATION

1. Casualties meeting criteria for urgent evacuation (loss of life, limb, or eyesight within two hours)
2. Casualties meeting priority evacuation criteria, but for whom other means of evacuation will cause deterioration
3. Circumstances in which the organic (internal) medical capabilities of the supported unit have been rendered ineffective (e.g., mass-casualty-incident, medical element neutralized by hostile action)
4. Risk of loss of evacuation aircraft and air crew is considered manageable by launch authority

Table 3. *Indications for air medical evacuation.*

# Health Services Support (HSS): Echelons, Levels, and Roles of Care

Nearly two decades after the end of the Cold War the US and its Allies are facing new and emerging threats. Military operations are often conducted in an expeditionary fashion employing minimal permanent footprints in host or target nations and often involve nonpermissive or forced initial entry operations. The physical environment for most current conflicts has shifted from remote to urban. Emphasis has also shifted from major theater wars to full-spectrum operations, including simultaneous combat and stability and peacekeeping operations. Retired Marine Corps General Charles Krulak summarized this concept as "the Three Block War." [97,98] New paradigms have been developed for defining, identifying, and mitigating threats to the US and its Allies.[98]

Traditionally, the US Army divided CCC and evacuation into five levels corresponding to the command and control echelons of the battlespace (Fig. 12). Echelons I to III compose the combat zone, while echelon IV consists of the communications zone, and echelon V is the zone of the interior, or US Homeland. The medical care delivered at each echelon of the battlefield is referred to as respective levels of care. Thus, at echelon I (unit level), one would encounter Level I medical care, comprising self- and buddy-aid, initial treatment by a combat lifesaver, and emergency medical treatment by a healthcare specialist (known more commonly as a combat medic). In most cases, Level I care also encompasses company casualty collection points and Battalion Aid Station care. Doctrinally, the evacuation of casualties from the Battlefield Aid Stations would progress to echelon II (division level), with its corresponding Level II care, which focuses primarily at the Brigade Support Medical Company. Level II care includes advanced trauma management by physicians and physician assistants. Level II facilities are equipped with limited plain radiography and laboratory services and, in some instances, may be supplied with blood products for emergency transfusion. In addition, the Brigade Support Medical Company is also the primary site of attachment for Forward Surgical Teams (FSTs), which are capable of conducting forward resuscitative surgical interventions aimed primarily at hemostasis of non-compressible hemorrhage, such as intraabdominal or intrathoracic wounds.

> Traditionally, the US Army divided CCC and evacuation into five levels corresponding to the command and control echelons of the battlespace. The medical care delivered at each echelon of the battlefield is referred to as respective levels of care.

While the traditional system describes Army CCC doctrine, the Navy and Marine Corps possess additional out-of-hospital units. These include Forward Surgical Companies, Forward Resuscitative Surgical Systems (FRSS), and Shock Trauma Platoons (STP) (Fig. 14). The Forward Resuscitative Surgical Systems share some similarities with the Army Forward Surgical Teams but have several notable differences, including self-sustainability and the assignment of an emergency physician to the unit. The Shock Trauma Platoons consist of two emergency physicians, physician assistants, an emergency nurse, and several medical corpsmen (the Navy equivalent of the combat medic). Both the Forward Resuscitative Surgical Systems and Shock Trauma Platoons are capable of augmenting

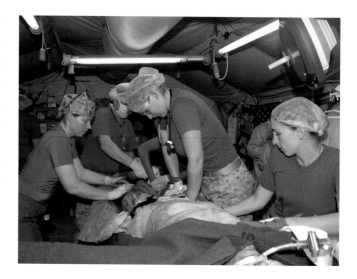

Figure 14. *Medical care at a Forward Resuscitative Surgical System. Image courtesy of Harold Bohman, MD, CAPT, MC, US Navy.*

a Battalion Aid Station or Brigade Support Medical Company in mass-casualty circumstances, such as might be expected during an amphibious assault or vertical envelopment (helicopter or Vertical Take-Off and Landing [VTOL]) entry operation.[99] The Forward Resuscitative Surgical Systems and Shock Trauma Platoons may also be combined into a hybrid entity known as a Surgical Shock Trauma Platoon (SSTP), representing perhaps the most robust forward medical capability within the Department of Defense. Lastly, the Air Force maintains Mobile Field Surgical Teams (MFST) as part of its modular Expeditionary Medical System (EMEDS), possessing resuscitative surgical capability, emergency care, and a preventive medicine cell (Fig. 15).[100]

If required, evacuation continues to echelon III (corps level), where the Level III Army CSHs, Navy Expeditionary Medical Facilities (EMF), and Air Force Theater Hospitals (AFTH) conduct both resuscitative and definitive surgery to save life, limb, and eyesight. If more complex surgical intervention or prolonged convalescence is required, casualties may be evacuated to echelon IV (communications zone level), where regional medical centers provide Level IV tertiary care and convalescence for up to two weeks. These facilities are currently located in Germany and Hawaii. The most severely injured, requiring extensive rehabilitation and convalescent care, are evacuated to echelon V (zone of interior or continental US). Here they receive Level V care at Army, Navy, and Air Force medical centers, and in the event of medical discharge, at Department of Veterans Affairs medical facilities.

| Army Echelon I/II CHS | USN/USMC Echelon I/II CHS | USAF Echelon I/II CHS |
|---|---|---|
| ✓Front-loaded for unit level basic life support care | ✓BALANCED and PROGRESSIVE levels of care | ✓Minimal Echelon I/II CHS (EXCEPT AFSOC) |
| ✓Often, this care CANNOT be rendered due to METT-TC | ✓Advanced life support / emergency careproviders far-forward | ✓Advanced life support/ emergency careproviders forward deployable |
| ✓No true advanced life support care until FST/CSH | ✓Self-sustaining resuscitative surgery far-forward | ✓Self-sustaining resuscitative surgery far-forward |
| ✓EVAC care MAY be a step-down in scope of practice | ✓Advanced life support "CASEVAC" support available | ✓Advanced life support "CASEVAC" support available |
| ✓LEGACY "medic-to-surgeon" mentality | ✓WEAKNESS: No dedicated tactical MEDEVAC | ✓WEAKNESS: Generally are not deployed forward of facilities capable of resuscitative surgery and secure airstrip |
| ARMY is exclusively responsible for tactical MEDEVAC in joint operations models | USN/USMC model likely represents the optimal current model for forward CHS, but is difficult to sustain in terms of personnel | USAF has MOST ADVANCED forward CHS capability— an "underutilized" resource? |

Figure 15. *Attributes of Echelon I/II combat health support (CHS) units in branches of the US military.*

This complex description of echelons of the battlefield and levels of health care has recently undergone further revision in order to meet North Atlantic Treaty Organization (NATO) standards.[101] Utilizing Roles of Care, the NATO system simplifies the levels of care based upon the availability and sophistication of surgical intervention. Under the NATO system, Role I medical treatment encompasses out-of-hospital and presurgical care analogous to Level I and Level II (absent forward surgical attachments). Role II also encompasses out-of-hospital care but incorporates forward resuscitative surgical capability and advanced resuscitative techniques, thus requiring the presence of a Forward Surgical Team, Forward Resuscitative Surgical System, or Mobile Field Surgical Team. Role III represents theater hospitalization, correlating directly to Level III. Finally, in the NATO system, Levels IV and V are combined into Role IV, representing continued surgical, recuperative, and rehabilitative care outside of the combat zone.

# Mass-Casualty-Incident Management

## US and NATO Military Mass-Casualty Triage Systems

In US military parlance, a mass-casualty-incident is defined as a casualty-producing event that overwhelms the existing medical capacity of the receiving facility or of the unit providing medical support in the out-

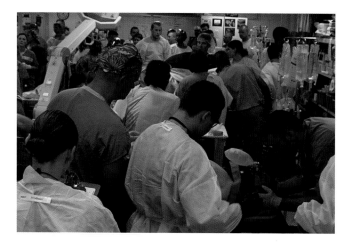

Figure 16. *Multiple-casualty-incident at a Level III facility.*

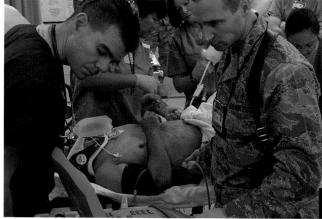

Figure 17. *Use of portable ultrasonography at a Level III facility.*

of-hospital setting. After initial collection, sorties of casualties who arrive in numbers sufficient to initially overwhelm the treatment and evacuation resources are triaged for priority of treatment (Fig. 16). The US military mass-casualty triage process comprises immediate, delayed, minimal, expectant, and urgent surgical categories. This is similar to the NATO triage system, which is partly based upon Medical Emergency Triage Tags (METTAG) methodology. Unlike METTAG, the US/NATO system adds a fifth urgent surgical category, which has been used to describe surgical patients who need an operation but can wait a few hours. It is important to note that urgent surgical patients who receive the appropriate initial categorization (e.g., urgent surgical) and intervention may be sufficiently stabilized and retriaged to a lower subsequent category (e.g., delayed). This US/NATO triage categorization should not be confused with MEDEVAC precedence categories (urgent, urgent surgical, priority, routine, and convenience) that are used to determine evacuation priorities.[102]

> Similar to the NATO triage system, the US military mass-casualty triage process comprises immediate, delayed, minimal, expectant, and urgent surgical categories.

Beekley et al. recorded a series of "lessons learned" in mass-casualty triage conducted at surgical facilities in Iraq, which may have some application in the out-of-hospital setting.[103] They included the observation that the requirement to perform triage in close proximity to the medical treatment facility can complicate the process. Likewise, the type of evacuation platform upon which casualties arrive may adversely affect the triage process. While Beekley et al. may have been referring to variation in numbers of casualties-per-sortie, what is of equal import is that the arrival of large sorties of casualties in high-capacity conveyances (such as flatbed trucks and buses) generally equates to a relative lack of en-route-care and minimal casualty triage. Beekley et al. also emphasized the importance of retriaging at progressive treatment sites as well as after time elapses, particularly in situations where significant delays in access to surgical intervention may occur. Lastly, Beekley et al.'s observations regarding the utility of focused abdominal sonography in trauma (FAST) as a triage tool resonated with similar anecdotal experiences by forward practitioners. While ultrasound use near point of injury is logistically and tactically undesirable, it has been successfully employed at Battalion Aid Stations, casualty collection points, and MEDEVAC landing zones, particularly in cases of prolonged delays in evacuation. In addition to traditional FAST applications, McNeil et al.[104] employed ultrasound for assessment of long-bone fractures. Potential additional uses include ocular assessment for intracranial pressure elevation, thoracic ultrasound for pneumothorax, and vascular assessments for diagnosis and access (Fig. 17).

The authors' practical experience with current NATO triage methodology has been satisfactory, but its effectiveness is dependent upon the practitioner being facile with the common types of injuries and associated respective triage categories. Anecdotal reports from the field indicate that many CCC providers, and in particular those with less clinical experience, tend to overtriage patients. Alternatively, overtriage may arise from the desire to not underestimate a casualty's injuries or from personal motivation to secure expeditious evacuation for patients who are acquaintances or close personal friends. While laudable, this practice should be avoided as it poses the potential to deplete limited MEDEVAC resources and may place MEDEVAC crews and aircraft in excessive danger for what might amount to relatively minor and otherwise survivable injuries.

### Alternative Mass-Casualty Triage Systems

Alternatives to the US/ NATO and METTAG systems include but are not limited to the Simple Triage And Rapid Treatment (START®) triage system, the International Committee for the Red Cross (ICRC) method, and the Sort, Assess, Lifesaving Interventions, Triage/Treat/Transport (SALT) system. The START® methodology incorporates a very brief assessment (spontaneous respiration, presence of peripheral pulses, level of consciousness) and simple interventions (noninvasive airway maneuvers, tourniquets) to triage casualties into one of five color-coded categories: immediate (red), delayed (yellow), minimal (green), expectant/ salvageable (blue), and expectant/unsalvageable (black). The blue category represents casualties who might be saved, but who require such intense resource allocation that they would likely cause the death of other more salvageable casualties due to neglect. It is theorized that this additional category may provide a better means of staging expectant patients for care once resources become available; in addition, it may ease the process of triaging casualties to expectant status, as at least semantically, the blue category differs from the black category.

The ICRC system reflects the austerity and remoteness often encountered by ICRC personnel, as well as the limitations of healthcare systems in many developing countries. While the ICRC recognizes and references a METTAG variant (immediate, delayed, minimal, expectant), they have also employed a simpler, two-tiered system for settings where no surgical care is available locally. This methodology simply divides casualties by the determination of whether they require surgical intervention. Those needing surgery and who are anticipated to survive a journey are transported to the nearest available surgical facility, while nonsurgical and expectant casualties are provided care by existing local resources.

Most recently, the US Centers for Disease Control and Prevention convened an expert consensus panel to develop an optimized mass-casualty triage scheme.[105] The resulting product, referred to as the SALT system (Sort, Assess, Lifesaving Interventions, Triage/Treat/Transport), provides a model for a standardized, all-hazards model for triage. The model also integrates adult, child, and special populations into the single protocol. If implemented widely, it possesses the potential to improve interoperability and standardization of triage. Trials of relative efficacy and accuracy, along with the international community's response to this method, remain to be observed before recommendations regarding adoption of the SALT system for tactical medical use may be offered.

# Reprise and Conclusion of Case Study

While the team is packaging the casualties for tactical evacuation, the medical officer observes, acquires, and engages the RPG gunner with small-arms fire, neutralizing him. The remaining insurgents disengage after receiving fire from the convoy's crew-served weapons (M-2 heavy machine guns). Hasty tourniquets are applied to bleeding extremity wounds on both casualties, followed by performance of rapid secondary surveys. Both casualties possess patent airways and are conscious. The casualty with blunt thoracic trauma has clinical signs of multiple rib fractures, but no flail segment is present, there is no jugular venous distention, the trachea is midline, and the affected hemithorax is resonant upon percussion. The casualties are loaded into an operating HMMWV escorted by the medical officer. After hastily attaching the disabled HMMWV to an operating vehicle via a tow rope, the convoy proceeds at top speed to the nearest forward operating base where the casualties are further stabilized. On arrival at the Battalion Aid Station, the staff radios a nine-line MEDEVAC request. The casualty with the isolated penetrating wound to the forearm receives a hemostatic dressing and direct pressure, which provides adequate hemostasis. The other casualty receives a tube thoracostomy, with approximately 30 milliliters of blood drained after placement. Both receive intravenous morphine and ceftriaxone, and both are packaged on stretchers with warm blankets. Tactical Combat Casualty Care casualty cards (DA Form 7656) are prepared and appended with clinical and treatment data. Subsequently, they undergo air MEDEVAC to a CSH. Both survive, are evacuated to the continental US, and eventually return to duty with their unit prior to rotation home.

## Future Directions

The practice of out-of-hospital CCC is poised for dramatic change. Senior military leadership, military medical thought leaders, and combat casualty researchers have arrived at a collective agreement that the out-of-hospital phase of care (Roles I and II) is the place where the next "great leap" in casualty survival will be realized. Innovations in technology, training, medical direction, and communications will occur. Future solutions may include field-deployable blood components and procoagulants designed to prevent or mitigate traumatic coagulopathy and improve tissue oxygenation. These first steps toward a system of remote damage control resuscitation hold great promise and may decrease prehospital mortality and postoperative multiorgan system failure. The development of tactical medical information systems is an area of intense focus. The eventual goal is reliably capturing out-of-hospital physiologic and therapeutic data. This data will improve training and support of CCC providers, as well as help to define future research agendas. Perhaps most exciting is the potential for developing integrated and graduated out-of-hospital CCC. This would combine professional medical oversight and real-time decision support with skilled resuscitation teams and critical care air transport capability for MEDEVAC units. While integration and implementation of this "Combat EMS System" will prove challenging, the successes of past and current CCC providers – coupled with the aforementioned research and development foci – may set the conditions for this "next great leap."

# References

1. Gerhardt RT, Hermstad EL, Oakes M, et al. An experimental predeployment training program improves self-reported patient treatment confidence and preparedness of Army combat medics. Prehosp Emerg Care 2008;12(3):359-365.

2. Butler F. Tactical combat casualty care: combining good medicine with good tactics. J Trauma 2003;54(5 Suppl):S2–3.

3. Bellamy RF. The causes of death in conventional land warfare: implications for casualty care research. Mil Med 1984;149(2):55-62.

4. Eastridge BJ, Jenkins D, Flaherty S, et al. Trauma system development in a theater of war: experiences from Operation Iraqi Freedom and Operation Enduring Freedom. J Trauma 2006;61(6):1366-1373.

5. Holcomb JB, McMullin NR, Pearse L, et al. Causes of Death in U.S. Special Operations Forces in the global war on terrorism 2001–2004. Ann Surg 2007;245(6):986–991.

6. Kelly JF, Ritenour AE, McLaughlin DF, et al. Injury severity and causes of death from Operation Iraqi Freedom and Operation Enduring Freedom: 2003-2004 versus 2006. J Trauma 2008;64(2 Suppl):S21–27; discussion S26-27.

7. Gerhardt, RT, Adams BD, De Lorenzo RA, et al. Panel synopsis: pre-hospital combat health support 2010: what should our azimuth be? J Trauma 2007;62(6 Suppl):S15-16.

8. De Lorenzo RA. Improving combat casualty care and field medicine: focus on the military medic. Mil Med 1997;162(4):268-272.

9. Gerhardt RT, De Lorenzo RA, Oliver J, et al. Out-of-hospital combat casualty care in the current war in Iraq. Ann Emerg Med 2009;53(2):169-174.

10. Tactical Combat Casualty Care Guidelines. 2009 Nov [cited 2010 May 31]. Available from: URL: http://www.usaisr.amedd.army.mil/tccc/TCCC%20Guidelines%20091104.pdf.

11. Owens BD, Kragh JF Jr, Wenke JC, et al. Combat wounds in operation Iraqi Freedom and operation Enduring Freedom. J Trauma 2008;64(2):295-299.

12. Eastridge BJ, Costanzo G, Jenkins D, et al. Impact of joint theater trauma system initiatives on battlefield injury outcomes. Am J Surg 2009;198(6):852-857.

13. Sayre MR, White LJ, Brown LH, et al. National EMS Research Agenda. Prehosp Emerg Care 2002;6(3 Suppl):S1–43.

14. Cloonan CC. "Don't just do something, stand there!": to teach or not to teach, that is the question—intravenous fluid resuscitation training for Combat Lifesavers. J Trauma 2003;54(5 Suppl):S20–25.

15. Butler FK, Hagmann J, Butler EG. Tactical combat casualty care in special operations. Mil Med 1996;161 (Suppl):3-16.

16. Richards TR. Commander, Naval Special Warfare Command letter 1500 Ser 04/03/41;9 April 1997.

17. Butler FK Jr, Holcomb JB, Giebner SD, et al. Tactical combat casualty care 2007: evolving concepts and battlefield experience. Mil Med 2007;172(11 Suppl): 1-19.

18. Butler FK Jr. Tactical medicine training for SEAL mission commanders. Mil Med 2001;166(7):625-631.

19. De Lorenzo RA. Medic for the millennium: the U.S. Army 91W health care specialist. Mil Med 2001;166(8): 685-688.

20. Pappas CG. The Ranger medic. Mil Med 2001;166(5):394-400.

21. Allen RC, editor. Pararescue medication and procedure handbook. 2nd ed. Air Force Special Operations Command Publication; 2001.

22. Malish RG. The preparation of a special forces company for pilot recovery. Mil Med 1999;164(12):881-884.

23. Krausz MM. Resuscitation Strategies in the Israeli Army. Presentation to the Institute of Medicine Committee on Fluid Resuscitation for Combat Casualties, 1998.

24. McSwain NE, Frame S, Paturas JL, editors. Prehospital trauma life support manual. 4th ed. St. Louis, MO: Akron, Mosby; 1999.

25. Tarpey M. Tactical combat casualty care in Operation Iraqi Freedom. US Army Med Dep J 2005:38-41.

26. Benharash P, Bongard F, Putnam B. Use of recombinant factor VIIa for adjunctive hemorrhage control in trauma and surgical patients. Am Surg 2005;71(9):776-780.

27. Dutton RP, McCunn M, Hyder M, et al. Factor VIIa for correction of traumatic coagulopathy. J Trauma 2004;57(4):709-718.

28. Felfernig M; European rFVIIa Trauma Study Group. Clinical experience with recombinant activated factor VII in a series of 45 trauma patients. J R Army Med Corps 2007;153(1):32-39.

29. Ganguly S, Spengel K, Tilzer LL, et al. Recombinant factor VIIa: unregulated continuous use in patients with bleeding and coagulopathy does not alter mortality and outcome. Clin Lab Haematol 2006;28(5):309-312.

30. Harrison TD, Laskosky J, Jazaeri O, et al. "Low-dose" recombinant activated factor VII results in less blood and blood product use in traumatic hemorrhage. J Trauma 2005;59(1):150-154.

31. McMullin NR, Kauvar DS, Currier HM, et al. The clinical and laboratory response to recombinant factor VIIA in trauma and surgical patients with acquired coagulopathy. Curr Surg 2006;63(4):246-251.

32. Perkins JG, Schreiber MA, Wade CE, et al. Early versus late recombinant factor VIIa in combat trauma patients requiring massive transfusion. J Trauma 2007;62(5):1095-1099.

33. Boffard KD, Riou B, Warren B, et al. Recombinant factor VIIa as adjunctive therapy for bleeding control in severely injured trauma patients: two parallel randomized, placebo-controlled, double-blind clinical trials. J Trauma 2005;59(1):8-15.

34. Thomas GO, Dutton RP, Hemlock B, et al. Thromboembolic complications associated with factor VIIa administration. J Trauma 2007;62(3):564-569.

35. Aledort LM. Comparative thrombotic event incidence after infusion of recombinant factor VIIa versus VIII inhibitor bypass activity. J Thromb Haemost 2004;2(10):1700-1708.

36. O'Connell KA, Wood JJ, Wise RP, et al. Thromboembolic adverse events after use of recombinant human coagulation factor VIIa. JAMA 2006;295(3):293-298.

37. Levy JH, Fingerhut A, Brott T, et al. Recombinant factor VIIa in patients with coagulopathy secondary to anticoagulant therapy, cirrhosis, or severe traumatic injury: review of safety profile. Transfusion 2006;46(6):919-933.

38. Stanworth SJ, Birchall J, Doree CJ, et al. Recombinant factor VIIa for the prevention and treatment of bleeding in patients without haemophilia. Cochrane Database Syst Rev 2007;(2):CD005011.

39. Diringer MN, Skolnick BE, Mayer SA, et al. Risk of thromboembolic events in controlled trials of rFVIIa in spontaneous intracerebral hemorrhage. Stroke 2008;39(3):850-856.

40. Hsia CC, Chin-Yee IH, McAlister VC. Use of recombinant activated factor VII in patients without hemophilia: a meta-analysis of randomized control trials. Ann Surg 2008;248(1):61-68.

41. Zangrillo A, Mizzi A, Biondi-Zoccai G, et al. Recombinant activated factor VII in cardiac surgery: a meta-analysis. J Cardiothorac Vasc Anesth 2009;23(1):34-40. Epub 2008.

42. Achneck HE, Sileshi B, Jamiolkowski RM, et al. A comprehensive review of topical hemostatic agents: efficacy and recommendations for use. Ann Surg 2010;251(2):217-228.

43. Cox ED, Schreiber MA, McManus J, et al. New hemostatic agents in the combat setting. Transfusion 2009;49 (Suppl 5):248S-255S.

44. Perkins JG, Cap AP, Weiss BM, et al. Massive transfusion and nonsurgical hemostatic agents. Crit Care Med 2008;36(7 Suppl):S325-339. Erratum in: Crit Care Med. 2008;36(9):2718.

45. Pusateri AE, Holcomb JB, Kheirabadi BS, et al. Making sense of the preclinical literature on advanced hemostatic products. J Trauma 2006;60(3):674-682.

46. Wedmore I, McManus JG, Pusateri AE, et al. A special report on the chitosan-based hemostatic dressing: experience in current combat operations. J Trauma 2006;60(3):655-658.

47. Neuffer MC, McDivitt J, Rose D, et al. Hemostatic dressings for the first responder: a review. Mil Med 2004;169(9):716-720.

48. Rhee P, Koustova E, Alam HB. Searching for the optimal resuscitation method: recommendations for the initial fluid resuscitation of combat casualties. J Trauma 2003;54(5 Suppl):S52-62.

49. National Association of Emergency Medical Technicians. Tactical field care. In: NAEMT, editors. PHTLS prehospital trauma life support: military version. 6th ed. St. Louis, MO: Mosby/JEMS; 2006. p. 521-523.

50. Gerritse BM, Scheffer GJ, Draaisma JM. Prehospital intraosseous access with the bone injection gun by a helicopter-transported emergency medical team. J Trauma 2009;66(6):1739-1741.

51. Fowler R, Gallagher JV, Isaacs SM, et al. The role of intraosseous vascular access in the out-of-hospital environment (resource document to NAEMSP position statement). Prehosp Emerg Care 2007;11(1):63-66.

52. Vojtko M, Hanfling D. The sternal IO and vascular access – any port in a storm. Air Med J 2003;22(1):32-34; discussion 34-35.

53. Dubick MA, Holcomb JB. A review of intraosseous vascular access: current status and military application. Mil Med 2000;165(7):552-559.

54. Beecher HK. The management of traumatic shock. In: Beecher HK, editor. Resuscitation and anesthesia for wounded men. 6th ed. Springfield, IL: Banerstone House; 1949.

55. Bickell WH, Wall MJ Jr, Pepe PE, et al. Immediate versus delayed fluid resuscitation for hypotensive patients with penetrating torso injuries. N Engl J Med 1994;331(17):1105-1109.

56. Pearce FJ, Lyons WS. Logistics of parenteral fluids in battlefield resuscitation. Mil Med 1999;164(9):653-655.

57. Alam HB, Rhee P. New developments in fluid resuscitation. Surg Clin N Am 2007;87(1):55-72, vi.

58. Treib J, Baron JF, Grauer MT, et al. An international view of hydroxyethyl starches. Intensive Care Med 1999;25(3):258-268.

59. Ogilvie MP, Pereira BM, McKenney MG, et al. First report on safety and efficacy of hetastarch solution for initial fluid resuscitation at a level I trauma center. J Am Coll Surg 2010;210(5):870-880, 880-882.

60. Kelly JF, Ritenour AE, McLaughlin DF, et al. Injury severity and causes of death from Operation Iraqi Freedom and Operation Enduring Freedom: 2003–2004 versus 2006. J Trauma 2008;64(2 Suppl):S21–26; discussion S26–27.

61. Mabry RL, Edens JW, Pearse L, Kelly JF, Harke H. Fatal airway injuries during Operation Enduring Freedom and Operation Iraqi Freedom. Prehosp Emerg Care 2010;14(2, Apr 6):272–277.

62. Adams BD, Cuniowski PA, Muck A, et al. Registry of emergency airways at combat hospitals. J Trauma 2008;64(6):1548-1554.

63. Cady CE, Weaver MD, Pirrallo RG, et al. Effect of emergency medical technician-placed combitubes on outcomes after out-of-hospital cardiopulmonary arrest. Prehosp Emerg Care 2009;13(4):495-499.

64. Strote J, Roth R, Cone DC, et al. Prehospital endotracheal intubation: the controversy continues (Conference Proceedings). Am J Emerg Med 2009;27(9):1142-1147.

65. Davis DP, Ochs M, Hoyt DB, et al. Paramedic-administered neuromuscular blockade improves prehospital intubation success in severely head-injured patients. J Trauma 2003;55(4):713-719.

66. Lockey D, Davies G, Coats T. Survival of trauma patients who have prehospital tracheal intubation without anaesthesia or muscle relaxants: observational study. BMJ 2001;323(7305):141.

67. Stroumpoulis K, Pagoulatou A, Violari M, et al. Videolaryngoscopy in the management of the difficult airway: a comparison with the Macintosh blade. Eur J Anaesthesiol 2009;26(3):218-222.

68. Bjoernsen LP, Lindsay B. Video laryngoscopy in the prehospital setting. Prehosp Disaster Med 2009;24(3):265-270.

69. Bjoernsen LP, Parquette BT, Lindsay MB. Prehospital use of video laryngoscope by an air medical crew. Air Med J 2008;27(5):242-244.

70. Givens ML, Ayotte K, Manifold C. Needle thoracostomy: implications of computed tomography chest wall thickness. Acad Emerg Med 2004;11(2):211-213.

71. Harcke HT, Pearse LA, Levy AD, et al. Chest wall thickness in military personnel: implications for needle thoracentesis in tension pneumothorax. Mil Med 2007;172(12):1260-1263.

72. Bell RS, Vo AH, Neal CJ, et al. Military traumatic brain and spinal column injury: a 5-year study of the impact blast and other military grade weaponry on the central nervous system. J Trauma 2009;66(4 Suppl):S104-111.

73. Weaver FM, Burns SP, Evans CT, et al. Provider perspectives on soldiers with new spinal cord injuries returning from Iraq and Afghanistan. Arch Phys Med Rehabil 2009;90(3):517-521.

74. Hammoud MA, Haddad FS, Moufarrij NA. Spinal cord missile injuries during the Lebanese civil war. Surg Neurol 1995;43(5):432-442.

75. Kahraman S, Gonul E, Kayali H, et al. Retrospective analysis of spinal missile injuries. Neurosurg Rev 2004;27(1):42–45.

76. Splavski B, Vrankovic D, Saric G, et al. Early management of war missile spine and spinal cord injuries: experience with 21 cases. Injury 1996:27(10):699-702.

77. Haut ER, Kalish BT, Efron DT, et al. Spinal immobilization in penetrating trauma: more harm than good? J Trauma 2010;68(1):115-120; discussion 120-121.

78. Kwan I, Bunn F, Roberts I. Spinal immobilisation for trauma patients. Cochrane Database Syst Rev 2001;(2):CD002803.

79. Assessment: oxygenation and blood pressure. In: Badjatia N, Carrey N, Crocco TJ, editors. Guidelines for prehospital management of traumatic brain injury. 2nd ed. New York, NY: Brain Trauma Foundation; 2007. p. 16-25.

80. Tian HL, Guo Y, Hu J, et al. Clinical characterization of comatose patients with cervical spine injury and traumatic brain injury. J Trauma 2009;67(6):1305-1310.

81. Mulligan RP, Friedman JA, Mahabir RC. A nationwide review of the associations among cervical spine injuries, head injuries, and facial fractures. J Trauma 2010;68(3):587-592.

82. Iida H, Tachibana S, Kitahara T, et al. Association of head trauma with cervical spine injury, spinal cord injury, or both. J Trauma 1999;46(3):450-452.

83. Gerhardt RT. Tactical En Route Care. Principles and Direction of Air Medical Transport. Air Medical Physician Association, 2006.

84. Agrawal A, Timothy J, Pandit L, et al. Post-traumatic epilepsy: an overview. Clin Neurol Neurosurg 2006;108(5):433–439.

85. Vespa PM, Nuwer MR, Nenov V, et al. Increased incidence and impact of nonconvulsive and convulsive seizures after traumatic brain injury as detected by continuous electroencephalographic monitoring. J Neurosurg 1999;91(5):750-760.

86. Gentilello LM, Jurkovich GJ, Stark MS, et al. Is hypothermia in the victim of major trauma protective or harmful? A randomized, prospective study. Ann Surg 1997;226(4):439-447; discussion 447-449.

87. Arthurs Z, Cuadrado D, Beekley A, et al. The impact of hypothermia on trauma care at the 31st combat support hospital. Am J Surg 2006;191(5)610-614.

88. Gerhardt RT, Matthews JM, Sullivan SG. The effect of systemic antibiotic prophylaxis and wound irrigation on penetrating combat wounds in a "return-to-duty" population. Prehosp Emerg Care 2009;13(4):500-504.

89. Ducharme J. Acute pain and pain control: state of the art. Ann Emerg Med 2000;35(6):592-603. [Erratum in Ann Emerg Med 2000 Aug;36(2):171].

90. Holbrook TL, Galarneau MR, Dye JL. et al. Morphine use after combat injury in Iraq and post-traumatic stress disorder. N Engl J Med 2010;362(2):110-117.

91. Joshi GP, Ogunnaike BO. Consequences of inadequate postoperative pain relief and chronic persistent postoperative pain. Anesthesiol Clin North America 2005;23(1):21-36.

92. Kotwal RS, O'Connor KC, Johnson TR, et al. A novel pain management strategy for combat casualty care. Ann Emerg Med 2004;44(2):121-127.

93. US Department of Defense (US DoD). Aeromedical Evacuation. In: Emergency War Surgery, Third United States Revision. Washington, DC: Department of the Army, Office of the Surgeon General, Borden Institute; 2004. p. 4.1-4.9.

94. Gerhardt RT, McGhee JS, Cloonan C, et al. U.S. Army MEDEVAC in the new millennium: a medical perspective. Aviat Space Environ Med 2001;72(7):659-664.

95. De Lorenzo RA. Military and civilian emergency aeromedical services: common goals with different approaches. Aviat Space Environ Med 1997;68(1):56-60.

96. Joint Publication 1-02. U.S. Department of Defense. Department of Defense Dictionary of Military and Associated Terms. Defense Technical Information Center; 2003.

97. Joint Publication 4-02. U.S. Joint Chiefs of Staff, U.S. Department of Defense. Doctrine for health service support in joint operations. U.S. Government Printing Office, Washington, D.C.; 2001.

98. Krulak CC. The strategic corporal: leadership in the three block war. Marines Magazine 1999.

99. Headquarters, US Marine Corps. Report No. I5921C4A-1. Table of Manpower Requirements, Headquarters and Service Company, Medical Battalion, Force Service Support Group, Fleet Marine Force. USMC, Quantico, VA, 1999.

100. Nix RE, Onofrio K, Konoske PJ, et al. Report No. 04-34. The Air Force Mobile Forward Surgical Team (MFST): Using the Estimating Supplies Program to Validate Clinical Requirement. U.S. Navy Bureau of Medicine and Surgery, Naval Health/Research Center, 2004.

101. Rödig E. NATO Joint Medical Support – Reality and Vision. Research and Technology Office, North Atlantic Treaty Organization, RTO-MP-HFM-109, 2004 [cited 2010 Feb 1]. Available from: URL: http://ftp.rta.nato.int/public/Pubfulltext/RTO/MP/RTO-MP-HFM-109///MP-HFM-109-$KN2.pdf.

102. US Department of Defense (US DoD). Triage. In: Emergency War Surgery, Third United States Revision. Washington, DC: Department of the Army, Office of the Surgeon General, Borden Institute; 2004. p. 3.1-3.10.

103. Beekley AC, Martin MJ, Spinella PC, et al. Predicting resource needs for multiple and mass casualty events in combat: lessons learned from combat support hospital experience in Operation Iraqi Freedom. J Trauma 2009;66(4 Suppl):S129-137.

104. McNeil CR, McManus J, Mehta S. The accuracy of portable ultrasonography to diagnose fractures in an austere environment. Prehosp Emerg Care 2009;13(1):50-52.

105. Lerner EB, Schwartz RB, Coule PL, et al. Mass casualty triage: an evaluation of the data and development of a proposed national guideline (Review). Disaster Med and Pub Health Prep 2008;2(Suppl 1):S25-34.

# DAMAGE CONTROL RESUSCITATION
*Chapter 4*

**Contributing Authors**
Jeremy G. Perkins, MD, FACP, LTC, MC, US Army
Alec C. Beekley, MD, FACS, LTC, MC, US Army

All figures and tables included in this chapter have been used with permission from Pelagique, LLC, the UCLA Center for International Medicine, and/or the authors, unless otherwise noted.

## Disclaimer

# Table of Contents

# Introduction

Hemorrhage accounts for 30 to 40 percent of all fatalities, second only to traumatic brain injury as a cause of death following trauma.[1,2,3] Hemorrhagic death is the leading preventable cause of mortality in combat casualties and typically occurs within six to 24 hours of injury.[4,5,6,7,8,9,10] Patients who die from hemorrhage enter a "vicious bloody cycle" characterized by the lethal triad of hypothermia, acidosis, and coagulopathy.[11]

> Hemorrhagic death is the leading preventable cause of mortality in combat casualties and typically occurs within six to 24 hours of injury. Causes of death from massive hemorrhage include compressible extremity hemorrhage (due to amputation or vascular injury), noncompressible proximal extremity hemorrhage (axillary or groin vascular injuries), and truncal hemorrhage (from solid organ, pelvic fracture, and thoracic injuries).

Damage control resuscitation (DCR) is a strategy that seeks to prevent or mitigate hypothermia, acidosis, and coagulopathy through combined treatment paradigms. Damage control resuscitation comprises early hemorrhage control, hypotensive resuscitation (permissive hypotension), hemostatic resuscitation (minimization of crystalloid fluids and fixed ratio blood product transfusion), prevention or alleviation of hypothermia (through warming measures), and amelioration of acidosis through judicious use of blood products and hemodynamic resuscitation endpoints.[12,13,14,15,16] In short, the goal of DCR is to stop hemorrhage and prevent or reverse the three components of the lethal triad.

The majority of trauma patients arriving at hospitals in both civilian and military settings will not require transfusion and are not coagulopathic on arrival. However, an important subset of severely injured casualties will manifest coagulopathy on arrival.[17,18] These patients are more likely to require massive transfusion, defined as infusion of 10 or greater units of red blood cells (RBCs), in the first 24 hours following injury. Traumatic coagulopathy exacerbates bleeding from injury, and aggressive resuscitation can cause patients to spiral into the "bloody vicious cycle" in which coagulopathy leads to further hemorrhage and worsening

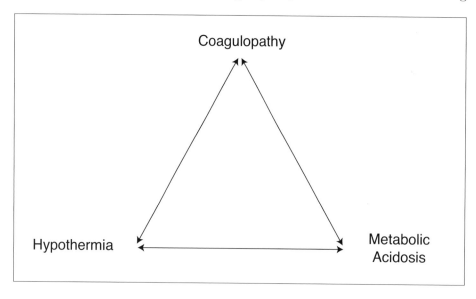

Figure 1. *The lethal triad.*

acidosis, in turn prompting additional fluid resuscitation and transfusion (Fig. 1). Such resuscitation can then contribute to more profound coagulopathy resulting from hemodilution and hypothermia. When such coagulopathy is present, it is associated with increased mortality.[17,18] Acidosis, hypothermia, and coagulopathy have been collectively termed the "lethal triad."[19]

> Massive transfusion is defined as infusion of 10 or greater units of RBCs in the first 24 hours after injury. Massive blood transfusion is infrequent in civilian trauma, occurring in only 2 to 13 percent of trauma admissions. Due to a higher rate of penetrating injury in combat casualties, massive transfusion occurred in approximately 8 percent of OIF casualties.

Causes of death from massive hemorrhage include compressible extremity hemorrhage (due to amputation or vascular injury), noncompressible proximal extremity hemorrhage (axillary or groin vascular injuries), and truncal hemorrhage (from solid organ, pelvic fracture, and thoracic injuries).[5] Patients with the aforementioned injuries may benefit from DCR in parallel with damage control surgical management.[5] Both damage control strategies are used to treat the acute traumatic problems of hemorrhage and coagulopathy. They are intended to prevent the complications that can occur following extensive operations and infusion of large volumes of fluids and blood products.

### DCR LESSONS LEARNED IN OEF AND OIF AS OF 2010

- Rapid control of compressible hemorrhage should be initiated with direct pressure, tourniquets, or hemostatic dressings.
- There should be rapid identification and surgical control of noncompressible and major vascular hemorrhage sites.
- The use of crystalloid and colloid solutions should be minimized in hemodynamically stable patients.
- Patients requiring DCR should be identified early using rapid bedside measures or tests.
- The early delivery of plasma and platelet transfusion in fixed ratios to red blood cells approaching 1:1:1 should be considered.
- Until surgical control of bleeding has been achieved, continued transfusion should be based primarily on the clinical condition of the patient rather than on laboratory values.
- Advanced bedside coagulation studies (e.g., thromboelastography) are available at some Level III care facilities and may provide better guides to a patient's blood product needs than standard laboratory values such as prothrombin time (PT) and activated partial thromboplastin time (aPTT).
- The use of low-dose vasopressin and other vasopressors as an adjunct to DCR is a treatment option that requires further validation.
- Adjuncts for control of nonsurgical bleeding (e.g., recombinant factor VIIa or antifibrinolytics) can be considered but remain controversial.
- Damage control resuscitation can be terminated once clinical hemorrhage is controlled and validated endpoints of resuscitation, such as clearance of serum lactate or base deficit, have been achieved.

Table 1. *DCR lessons learned in OEF and OIF.*

# Damage Control Resuscitation: Lessons Learned

This chapter will address the key components of DCR, including: (1) preventing the need for massive transfusion through external hemorrhage control to prevent exsanguination; (2) predicting the need for massive transfusion of blood products; (3) current recommendations for massive transfusion and management of the anticipated complications; and (4) adjuncts to resuscitation and transfusion that are frequently employed in damage control settings. An overview of DCR lessons learned over the course of Operation Enduring Freedom (OEF) and Operation Iraqi Freedom (OIF) is provided in Table 1.

# Preventing the Need for Massive Transfusion

Ideally, traumatic hemorrhage is controlled prior to hemodynamic compromise resulting from exsanguination. A series of preventive measures and prehospital treatment techniques have been instituted in both military and civilian trauma settings to rapidly control hemorrhage. The tools and techniques discussed below may prevent or slow ongoing blood loss, decrease the number of blood products required, and ultimately prevent unnecessary deaths.

## *Hemorrhage Control Techniques*

Hemorrhage sites are either anatomically compressible and amenable to tourniquet control, compressible but not amenable to tourniquet control (e.g., axillary or groin vascular injuries), or completely noncompressible (e.g., truncal injuries) (Fig. 2). Patients with noncompressible hemorrhage sources should receive the highest priority for evacuation to a hospital, as there are few tools available to prehospital careproviders to manage such bleeding. Compressible hemorrhage sites are amenable to direct digital pressure, which can be instituted by first responders as the initial hemorrhage control intervention. Attempts to reinforce saturated dressings with large stacks of gauze or additional dressings (in lieu of manual compression) should be avoided, as this technique dissipates the pressure applied directly to the bleeding site and may delay identification of ongoing bleeding (Fig. 3).

> Hemorrhage sites are either anatomically compressible and amenable to tourniquet control, compressible but not amenable to tourniquet control (e.g., axillary or groin vascular injuries), or completely noncompressible (e.g., truncal injuries). Tourniquet application, direct pressure, or hemostatic dressings applied to the wound site should be favored over pressure point control and extremity elevation for the initial control of hemorrhage.

Direct pressure to arteries proximal to bleeding sites and elevation of the affected extremity above the level of the heart should be considered as second-line adjunctive hemorrhage control interventions, and they are not currently recommended for use by the Committee on Tactical Combat Casualty Care for any phases of care.[20] Applying direct pressure to arteries proximal to the bleeding site may control arterial inflow, but it will not control venous hemorrhage. Associated injuries (e.g., fractures) and patient transportation considerations often make extremity elevation problematic. Hence, tourniquet application, direct pressure, or hemostatic dressings applied to the wound site should be favored over pressure point control and extremity elevation for the initial control of hemorrhage.[21]

## Hemorrhage Pressure Points

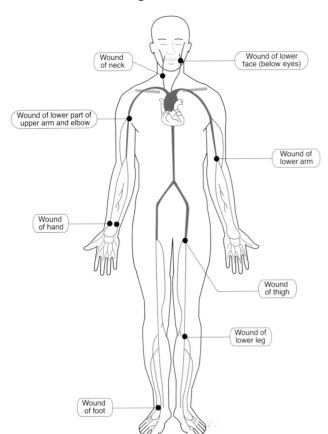

Figure 2. (Left) *Potential sites for pressure point control of hemorrhage.*

Figure 3. (Below) *A combat casualty arriving at a Level III facility following a fragmentation injury from a blast. Note the saturated layers of gauze on this limb where no tourniquet or hemostatic agents was applied.*

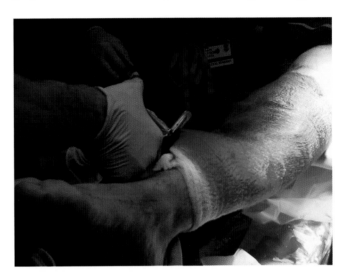

## *Tourniquets and Hemostatic Dressings*

The use of direct pressure to control hemorrhage is only a temporizing measure until a more secure and durable form of hemorrhage control can be employed. First responders often find it necessary to perform other tasks or treat other casualties; hence, modular tourniquets and hemostatic dressings have been developed to provide the first responder with alternative methods for hemorrhage control.

Historically, extremity tourniquets were a controversial method of last resort for extremity hemorrhage control.[22,23] Extremity tourniquets are now used as a first-line therapy for the prehospital control of extremity hemorrhage for care-under-fire scenarios (Fig. 4).[20] Expanded guidelines for tourniquet use, combined with a rapid evacuation system in OEF and OIF, have resulted in significant numbers of casualties arriving to surgical care with extremity tourniquets in place (Fig. 5). Multiple reports in the literature of tourniquet use in OEF and OIF have defined the characteristics and advantages of tourniquet use.[16, 24,25,26,27,28] These include: (1) an average prehospital tourniquet time under six hours; (2) improved hemorrhage control upon patient arrival; (3) decreased incidence of shock in those casualties treated with tourniquets; (4) improved survival; and (5) acceptably low tourniquet-related complications. Tourniquets should be applied to exsanguinating extremities as soon as possible in care-under-fire scenarios.[29] Additional information on tourniquets can be found in the Extremity Injury chapter.

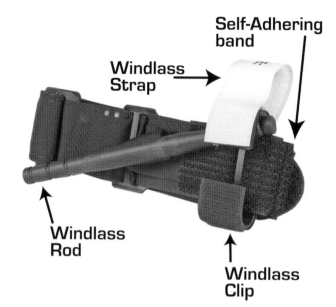

**Self-Adhering band**

**Windlass Strap**

**Windlass Rod**

**Windlass Clip**

Figure 4. (Right) *The Combat Application Tourniquet® is a one-handed tourniquet that uses a self-adhering band to fit a wide range of extremities. It incorporates a windlass system that locks into place. Image courtesy of North American Rescue, LLC.*

Figure 5. (Below) *A combat casualty who sustained bilateral lower extremity injuries from an improvised explosive device (IED) blast with right-sided tourniquet in place.*

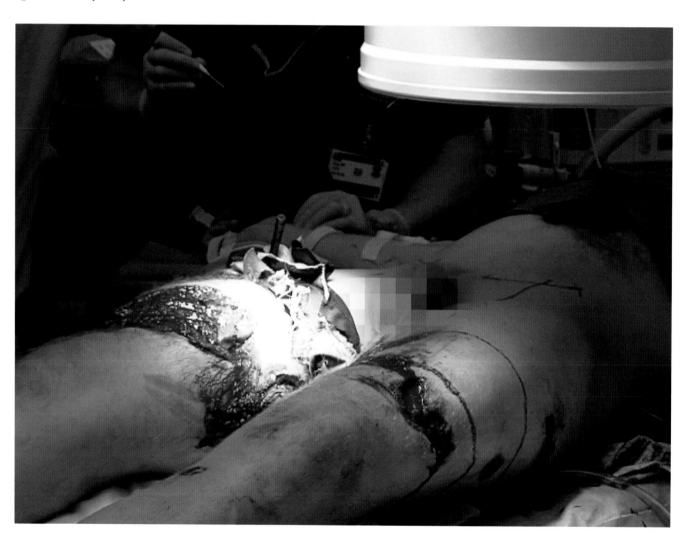

Extremity tourniquets are used as a first-line therapy for the prehospital control of extremity hemorrhage in care-under-fire scenarios. If used before onset of shock, there is 90 percent improved survival relative to use after onset of shock. Hemostatic dressings and agents are used with increased frequency, as both primary hemorrhage control measures for wounds not amenable to tourniquet control or as adjuncts to tourniquet use.

Similarly, hemostatic dressings and agents are now deployed and used with increasing frequency as both primary hemorrhage control measures for wounds not amenable to tourniquet control or as adjuncts to tourniquet use.[20,21] Animal research demonstrates the superiority of dressings such as the fibrin-impregnated bandage (produced by the American Red Cross) and chitosan dressings over standard gauze.[30] Another agent, granular zeolite [QuikClot® (Z-Medica; Wallingford, CT)], a microporous crystalline aluminosilicate hemostatic agent, is Food and Drug Administration (FDA) approved for hemostasis of external wounds (Fig. 6). Granular zeolite has been fielded by the United States (US) Marine Corps and US Army during OEF and OIF with some success.[31,32] Limitations of granular zeolite include an exothermic reaction that can cause burns, and the time-consuming removal of granules from wounds. The potential utility of these dressings has been supported by early clinical reports from OEF and OIF.[31,33]

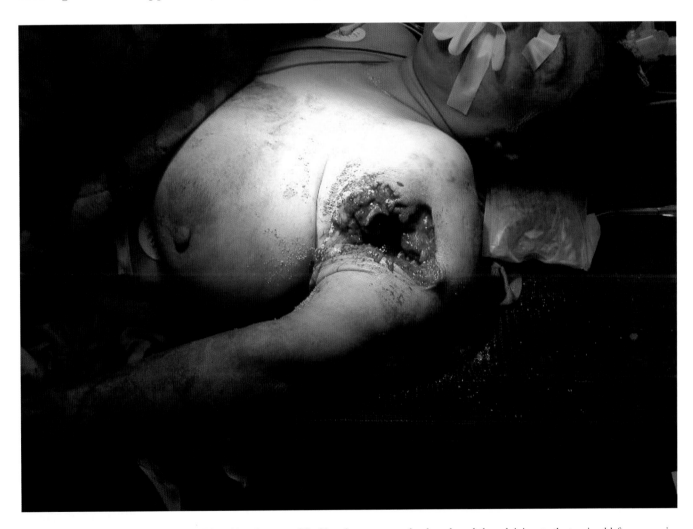

Figure 6. *This Iraqi civilian was injured by a blast fragment. The blast fragment caused a through-and-through injury to the proximal left arm causing hemorrhage that was not amenable to tourniquet use. Hemorrhage was controlled with QuikClot®. Image courtesy of Harold Bohman, MD, CAPT, MC, US Navy.*

The challenge of developing and fielding newer generations of bandages is illustrated by the recall of a granular combination of a smectite mineral and polymer in 2008 (WoundStat™ [TraumaCure, Inc; Bethesda, MD]) due to concerns over the risk of thrombosis and endothelial injury when applied to arteries. This agent had been tested by the US Army Institute of Surgical Research (USAISR) and had been shown to be more efficacious in treating animal models of arterial hemorrhage than currently deployed products.[34] Combat Gauze™ (Z-Medica, Wallingford, CT) is composed of surgical gauze impregnated with kaolin (Fig. 7). This dressing has been shown to be extremely safe and effective in a lethal animal hemorrhage model.[35] Combat Gauze™ is the current hemostatic dressing of choice for the military as recommended by the Committee on Tactical Combat Casualty Care.[20] It is important to note that clinical experience with Combat Gauze™ is limited, and there are currently no publications on its use in humans. Further clinical experience with hemostatic agents and dressings will be required to fully define their clinical benefits and risks.

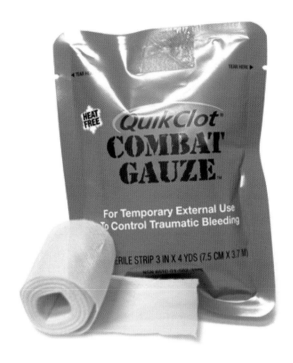

Figure 7. *Combat Gauze™, a kaolin-impregnated surgical gauze, is the current hemostatic dressing of choice. The gauze is tightly packed into the wound, then pressure is held directly over the bleeding source until hemorrhage stops. Image courtesy of Combat Medical Systems™.*

## Preventing Hypothermia

Hypothermia is defined as mild when the core body temperature is 32°C to 35°C, moderate when the core body temperature is 28°C to 32°C, and severe when the core body temperature is below 28°C.[36] Hypothermia is associated with an increased risk of uncontrolled bleeding and mortality in trauma patients.[36,37] Severe trauma-related hypothermia has been associated with 100 percent mortality.[38] Trauma patients in hemorrhagic shock have uncoupling of normal metabolic pathways, resulting in the loss of the ability to maintain temperature homeostasis. Factors such as cold or wet weather, prolonged extrication or scene time, intoxication, infusion of cold or room temperature fluids, and convective heat losses (e.g., open helicopter door during flight) can worsen hypothermia. Both civilian and military trauma centers have linked the presence of hypothermia on arrival to increased mortality.[39,40,41]

Hypothermia in combat casualties was identified as a theater-wide trauma system challenge in OIF.[42,43] Simple hypothermia prevention measures were disseminated to the combat medics on the battlefield. These measures included emphasis on external hemorrhage control as the first priority, limiting removal of clothing to areas of the body requiring treatment, wrapping casualties in wool or solar blankets, and using in-line fluid warmers such as the Thermal Angel® (Estill Medical Technologies, Inc., Dallas, Texas) (Fig. 8).

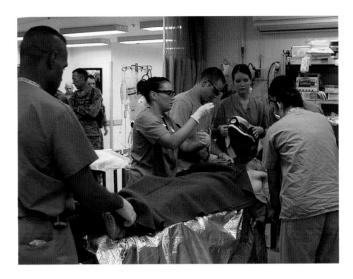

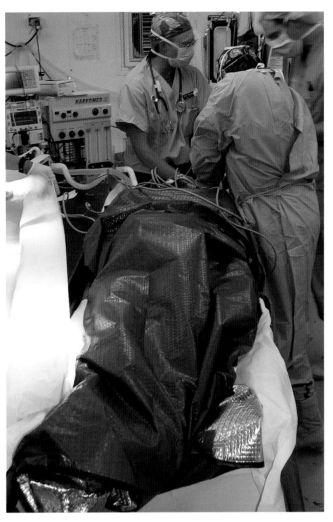

Figure 8. (Above) *A combat casualty arriving at a Level III facility. Hypothermia prevention measures include wrapping the casualty in wool and solar blankets, and limited removal of clothing.*

Figure 9. (Right) *Active rewarming and stabilization of the patient in an intensive care unit (ICU) using a solar blanket, warmed fluids, and a warm humidified ventilator circuit. Image courtesy of the Borden Institute, Office of The Surgeon General, Washington, DC.*

> Prevention and treatment of hypothermia at initial care facilities include the use of standardized heat-loss prevention kits, forced-air warming blankets, fluid warmers and rapid infusers, maintenance of warmed trauma suites and operating rooms, and warm humidified ventilator circuits.

Measures to prevent and treat hypothermia at initial care facilities have included the use of standardized heat-loss prevention kits (e.g., solar blankets, heated blankets, and body bags), the use of forced-air warming blankets, the use of fluid warmers and rapid infusers, the maintenance of warmed trauma suites and operating rooms, and the use of warm humidified ventilator circuits (Fig. 9).[15,44,45,46,47,48,49] Since institution of these performance improvement measures, the incidence of hypothermia in patients arriving at Combat Support Hospitals (CSHs) has fallen from 7 percent to below 1 percent.[43] Since severe hypothermia has become a rarity in OEF and OIF, active core body rewarming measures, such as continuous arteriovenous rewarming and body cavity lavage of warmed fluids, are less frequently needed.[50,51] While cardiopulmonary bypass may be used in extreme cases of hypothermia for controlled active rewarming in some civilian trauma centers, it is not available in Level III care facilities in Iraq or Afghanistan.

# Predicting the Need for Massive Transfusion

Despite marked advances in the prehospital management of hemorrhage, patients with noncompressible sources of bleeding will still arrive in the trauma bay with uncontrolled hemorrhage. Effective DCR often requires the early delivery of coagulation factors, soon after patient arrival to the resuscitation area.[4] Since coagulation factor replacement is needed by only a small fraction of trauma patients, rapid identification of such patients is critical.[4,52] Clinical and laboratory parameters are used to predict the need for massive transfusion in such patients.[53]

> Penetrating mechanisms of injury, particularly involving the trunk, predict the need for massive transfusion in combat casualties. Systemic hypotension is a useful and validated predictor for the need for both emergent intervention and transfusion in the arriving trauma patient.

## *Mechanism of Injury*

Penetrating mechanisms, particularly involving the trunk, predict the need for massive transfusion in

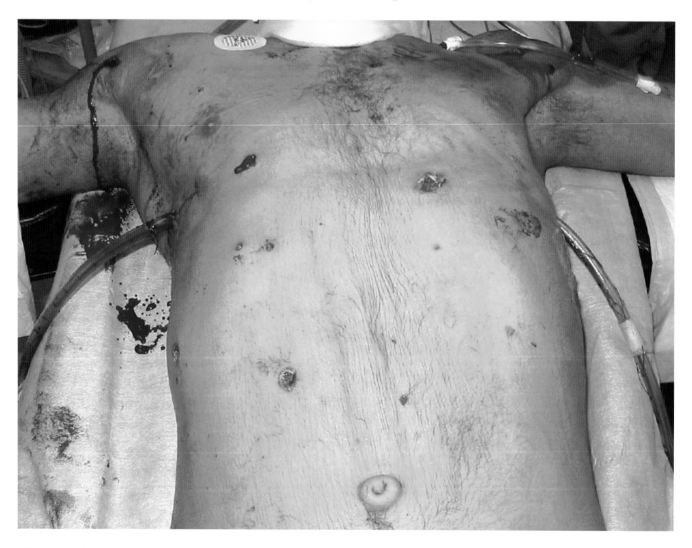

Figure 10. *This host national was admitted to a CSH with hypotension and multiple fragment entry wounds to his chest and abdomen. This patient is at elevated risk for requiring massive transfusion. Image courtesy of the Borden Institute, Office of The Surgeon General, Washington, DC.*

combat casualties and for emergent intervention in civilian trauma patients (Fig. 10).[52,54] This contrasts with blunt mechanisms of injury, which are poor predictors of the need for trauma team activation or emergent intervention.[54,55] The presence of penetrating wounds in combat casualties is frequently obvious and dramatic, as with high-velocity penetrating abdominal wounds with associated evisceration, multiple proximal limb amputations, and penetrating buttock or pelvic wounds (Fig. 11). Combat casualty care (CCC) providers are usually able to visually appreciate the extent of tissue destruction and anticipate associated anatomic and physiologic derangements in such casualties.

## Bedside Clinical Findings

Heart rate alone is an insufficient predictor of the need for emergency interventions for management of hemorrhage.[56] A core body temperature below 36°C (96°F) on arrival has been shown in both civilian and military trauma patients to be associated with worse outcomes.[39,41,57] Furthermore, several investigators have correlated the presence of hypothermia with injury severity and the requirement for blood transfusion.[58,59,60]

Systemic hypotension is a useful and validated predictor of the need for both emergent intervention and

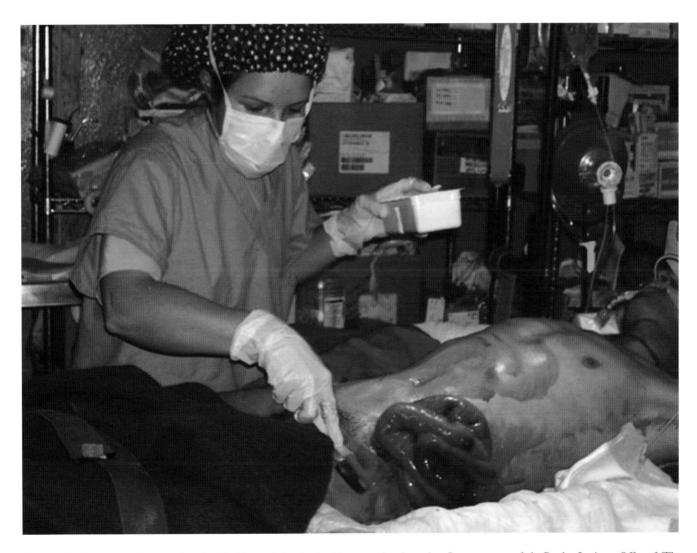

Figure 11. *Host national who sustained a blast injury to his flank with traumatic evisceration. Image courtesy of the Borden Institute, Office of The Surgeon General, Washington, DC.*

transfusion in the arriving trauma patient.[54,61,62,63] Systolic blood pressure has been combined with other variables to create trauma scores, such as the Revised Trauma Score (RTS).[64,65,66,67] Although not perfect, these scores are superior to any single test alone and have emerged as useful and accurate predictors of mortality and the requirement for massive transfusion.[68] Rapid manual bedside tests such as the radial pulse character and Glasgow Coma Scale (GCS) motor score have also been shown to predict the need for lifesaving interventions.[69] In Holcomb's study, trauma patients with a weak or absent radial pulse combined with an abnormal GCS verbal or motor score on arrival had an 88 percent probability of requiring a lifesaving intervention.[69] On the basis of simplicity, rapidity, and relative accuracy, these techniques are helpful in both the prehospital and initial hospital management of trauma patients.[69,70]

While hypotension historically has been defined as a systolic blood pressure (SBP) below 90 mm Hg, recently this value has been challenged. Eastridge and colleagues recently evaluated data from the National Trauma Data Bank and found that an admission SBP value below 110 mm Hg was associated with higher mortality rates.[71] Every 10 mm Hg drop in SBP below 110 mm Hg was associated with a 4.8 percent increase in mortality, up to a maximum of 26 percent mortality at a systolic blood pressure of 60 mm Hg. The authors also noted that base deficits began to rise below a SBP of 118 mm Hg. These findings imply that some trauma patients may have systemic tissue hypoperfusion despite systolic blood pressures well above 90 mm Hg.

## Laboratory Testing

The role of clinical laboratory testing in predicting the need for massive transfusion remains in evolution. Admission labs associated with the need for massive transfusion include a base deficit greater than six, an international normalized ratio (INR) of 1.5 or greater, and a hemoglobin value of less than 11 grams (g) per deciliter.[52,72,73] In a more recent study, McLaughlin et al. found that a heart rate greater than 105 beats per minute, a SBP less than 110 mm Hg, a pH value less than 7.25, and a hematocrit value of less than 32 percent were all independent predictors of massive transfusion in combat casualties.[74] This preliminary study awaits further validation. Patients with any of these values, particularly in combination with hypotension, diminished GCS score, or obvious physical exam findings, should be considered for immediate transition from a standard resuscitation mode to a damage control resuscitation mode.[63]

> Admission labs associated with the need for massive transfusion include a base deficit greater than six, an international normalized ratio of 1.5 or greater, and a hemoglobin value of less than 11 g per deciliter. Such laboratory tests are generally available at Level II facilities.

Laboratory tests generally available at Level II facilities (Forward Surgical Teams and Forward Resuscitative Surgical Systems) include arterial blood gas, complete blood count analysis, PT and INR. At Level III facilities, PT and INR are routinely available, and even thromboelastography is available at some CSHs in Iraq and Afghanistan. Thromboelastography provides real-time graphic evidence of clot formation in whole blood and may be a better method of detecting coagulopathy in trauma patients.[75,76]

## Newer Technologies for Predicting the Need for Massive Transfusion

The utility of novel applications of continuous, noninvasive monitors linked to computer software are under study as tools to provide an early warning of systemic hypoperfusion. These technologies include the measure of heart rate complexity, arterial pulse pressure, and tissue oxygenation as measured by near-infrared spectroscopy.[77,78,79,80,81,82,83,84] Loss of heart rate variability has predicted the need for lifesaving interventions and increased mortality in trauma patients.[85,86,87] Decreased tissue oxygen saturation detected by continuous near-infrared spectroscopy has predicted the development of multiple organ failure and the need for massive transfusion.[88] While these technologies will not replace clinical judgment, they may add objective data to help careproviders maximize patient outcomes while minimizing resource utilization.

# Transfusion of Blood Products

For most casualties, current resuscitation guidelines published in the American College of Surgeons Advanced Trauma Life Support (ATLS) course and elsewhere are sufficient for managing blood and fluid losses. However, the frequent need for massive transfusion of blood products in OEF and OIF has prompted critical reassessment of the appropriateness of these standard resuscitation and transfusion practices for this subset of casualties with exsanguinating hemorrhage. Military careproviders have found that massively bleeding patients may actually be harmed by standard approaches (Beekley A, MD, FACS, LTC, MC, US Army, personal communication, January 13, 2010). There is mounting evidence that these patients require an approach that begins treating all the physiologic derangements of massive blood loss as soon as possible after injury (Beekley A, MD, FACS, LTC, MC, US Army, personal communication, January 13, 2010). This realization has strongly influenced current damage control resuscitation practices, which are described in detail below.

> Military careproviders have found that massively bleeding patients may be harmed by standard approaches to resuscitation. Such casualties require an approach that immediately treats all physiologic derangements associated with massive blood loss.

## *Massive Blood Transfusion*

Massive blood transfusion requires extensive blood banking resources and is associated with high mortality.[89,90,91,92,93,94] The most frequently used definition of massive transfusion is replacement of a patient's entire blood volume or 10 or more units of blood transfused in 24 hours.[95,96] Massive blood transfusion is infrequent in civilian trauma, occurring in only 2 to 13 percent of trauma admissions.[93,97] Due to a higher rate of penetrating injury in combat casualties, massive transfusion occurred in approximately 8 percent of OIF admissions and in as many as 16 percent during the Vietnam War.[98,99]

Resuscitation of exsanguinating patients is a challenging problem that is exacerbated when clear massive transfusion protocols have not been developed.[100] Although many institutions have massive transfusion protocols in place, adherence to such guidelines requires strong collaboration and effective communication between providers in the emergency department, operating room, ICU, and blood bank.[101] A study by Dente et al. demonstrated that the institution of a massive transfusion protocol in a civilian trauma center reduced early coagulopathy and decreased mortality in blunt trauma patients.[102]

## *Red Blood Cells*

Patients requiring blood can safely receive uncrossmatched Type O blood until type-specific products are available.[103,104,105] Although type-specific uncrossmatched blood has also been used successfully for massive transfusion, acute hemolytic reactions have been reported.[106,107,108]

## Fresh Frozen Plasma

Fresh frozen plasma (FFP) has been recognized as an important component in preventing and treating coagulopathy in trauma.[14,109,110,111] A donor unit of whole blood (approximately 450 milliliters) is separated into several components, with the plasma comprising approximately 250 milliliters (ml) of the liquid portion of blood containing water, electrolytes, and proteins (and lacking red blood cells, leukocytes, and platelets) (Fig. 12). The plasma proteins include the major clotting factors and intrinsic anticoagulants. In addition to the coagulation factors, the plasma found in one unit of whole blood also contains approximately 500 milligrams (mg) of fibrinogen (approximately equal to the amount of fibrinogen found in two units of cryoprecipitate).[112] While most clotting factors are stable at normal concentrations in plasma, some factors including factor V and factor VIII, termed labile factors, degrade over time; this degradation accelerates while plasma is stored in the liquid state (hence, why plasma is stored in a frozen state).

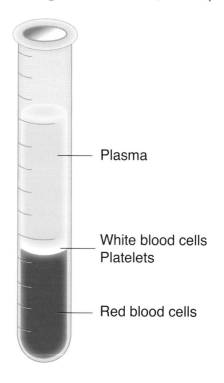

Figure 12. *Blood may be transfused as whole blood, or separated into its components via centrifugation.*

Transfusion of fixed ratios of FFP to RBCs has been proposed as a strategy to manage coagulopathy, particularly with rapid exsanguination and absent lab testing. Data from combat casualties in OIF support the use of plasma transfusion, showing a 65 percent mortality for patients who receive less than one unit of FFP for every four units of RBCs compared to a 19 percent mortality with more than one unit of FFP for every two units of RBCs.[113] While the optimal FFP to RBC ratio is unknown, mathematical models for FFP transfusion have been developed that support clinical data, suggesting that a ratio of 2:3 to as high as 1:1 (units of FFP to RBC) would be appropriate.[114,115]

> The optimal FFP to RBC ratio is unknown. Both mathematical models and clinical data for FFP transfusion favor a ratio of 2:3 to as high as 1:1 (units of FFP to RBC).

It has been suggested that FFP should be transfused early in the resuscitation to prevent dilutional coagulopathy.[73,94,96] Unfortunately, thawing of FFP is time-consuming, and patients often receive more blood or crystalloids in place of FFP, further exacerbating coagulopathy. Once patients have been stabilized, fixed FFP to RBC ratios are less critical, and standard transfusion strategies for plasma may be more appropriate. Standard transfusion criteria for plasma products include an INR greater than or equal to 1.5 or prolonged R-time on thromboelastography in the presence of active bleeding, or in a patient at high-risk for recurrent bleeding.[75]

All studies to date examining plasma, as well as other products including whole blood, platelets, and fibrinogen, have been retrospective and cannot be used to make definitive conclusions about the best care for trauma casualties. With retrospective analyses, there is the influence of survival bias that excludes patients dying quickly before being able to receive products such as plasma or platelets. It remains possible that patients received products such as plasma or platelets because they survived as opposed to surviving because they received the products.[116] A recent study by Watson et al. even linked administration of FFP with a higher subsequent risk of developing multiple organ failure and acute respiratory distress syndrome.[117] Further prospective study evaluating the use of blood products in fixed ratios is warranted prior to drawing any definitive conclusions.

## Platelets

Retrospective civilian data have supported the use of platelets in patients requiring massive transfusion.[92,109,118] Apheresis platelets (aPLT) have been available in Iraq since November 2004. Apheresis is the process of removing select components such as platelets from blood and returning remaining components to the blood. Emerging data from OIF have shown an improved survival at 24 hours in patients receiving a high platelet ratio greater than or equal to 1:8 apheresis platelet unit per stored red blood cell unit (aPLT to RBC) as compared to patients receiving a medium ratio (less than 1:8 to 1:16 aPLT to RBC), and patients receiving the lowest ratio of platelets (less than 1:16 aPLT to RBC) (24-hour survival 95 percent, 87 percent, and 64 percent, respectively).[116] The survival benefit for the high and medium ratio groups persisted at 30 days as compared to the lowest ratio group (75 percent and 60 percent versus 43 percent). On multivariate regression, the aPLT to RBC ratio was independently associated with improved survival at 24 hours and at 30 days.[116] A single unit of apheresis platelets is approximately equal to six units of pooled platelets. To simplify massive transfusion protocol strategies, the current Joint Theater Trauma System guidelines recommend transfusion of 1:1:1 pooled platelets to FFP to RBC (or 1:6:6 apheresis platelets to FFP to RBC) for patients requiring or anticipated to require massive transfusion.

As with plasma, once patients have been stabilized, platelet transfusion in a fixed ratio with RBCs may be less critical, and standard transfusion strategies for platelets may be more appropriate. The commonly recommended platelet transfusion threshold is a platelet count below 50,000/μL in patients with active bleeding.[119] In cases of high-energy multisystem trauma or central nervous system bleeding frequently seen in combat casualties, a higher platelet transfusion threshold of 100,000/μL has been recommended.[120]

## Fibrinogen

Fibrinogen depletion develops earlier than other coagulation factor deficiencies.[121] Fibrinogen ratios examined in OIF casualties, and fibrinogen to RBC ratios of less than 0.2 g fibrinogen per RBC unit were associated with a higher mortality.[122] Given that there are 0.4 g of fibrinogen in one unit of FFP, administration of FFP in appropriate ratios (1:2 to 1:1) exceeds this fibrinogen ratio. Most deployed medical units do not have the capability to check fibrinogen in the laboratory, although thromboelastography is available at some Level III CSHs and can detect hypofibrinoginemia. Clot strength, as measured by the maximum amplitude on thromboelastography, is influenced by both platelet function and fibrinogen concentration. In cases where the platelet count is adequate, a decreased maximum amplitude would indicate hypofibrinoginemia.[123]

## Fresh Whole Blood

Fresh whole blood (FWB), defined as blood collected and maintained at 22°C for a maximum of 24 hours, is rarely used in civilian practice.[124] However, the military has relied upon the use of FWB in circumstances when stored blood products are unavailable.[125] As FWB contains red blood cells, plasma, and platelets in physiologic ratios and contains less total preservative solution – compared to a mixture of separate RBC, FFP, and platelet components – some have advocated that FWB is a superior resuscitation product.[126,127] In a retrospective study of 354 patients with traumatic hemorrhagic shock receiving blood transfusion, both 24-hour and 30-day survival were higher in the FWB cohort as compared to a component therapy group.[128] An increased amount (825 ml) of additives and anticoagulants were administered to the component therapy as compared to the FWB group. More recent data on combat casualties has tempered this conclusion, showing equivalence of 24-hour and 30-day survival between massively transfused patients receiving apheresis platelets compared to those receiving FWB.[276]

> In patients with hemorrhagic shock, when standard blood components such as apheresis platelets or plasma are unavailable, FWB is a lifesaving alternative.

# Massive Transfusion-Associated Complications

## *Electrolyte Disorders*

Hyperkalemia is a common complication with rapid or large-volume transfusion of red blood cells. Increased levels of extracellular potassium develop during the storage of red blood cells with concentrations averaging 12 milliequivalents (mEq) per liter at seven days and increasing to 32 mEq per liter after 21 days of storage.[129] Massive transfusion of senescent red blood cells could produce ventricular arrhythmia and cardiac standstill.[130,131] Some authors have theorized that effects of hyperkalemia may be mitigated by infusing blood into lines farther away from the right atrium to permit greater mixture of blood before arrival to the heart.[125] Fresher blood may also be requested from the blood bank or may be considered as an institutional policy for massively transfused patients. Once massive transfusion-associated hyperkalemia develops, it is treated in a conventional manner based on the clinical scenario (e.g., intravenous calcium, dialysis, dextrose and insulin infusion, bicarbonate, and diuretics).

> Hyperkalemia, due to extracellular potassium build-up in stored red blood cells, and hypocalemia, due to the binding of ionized calcium by citrate, may cause cardiovascular toxicity following large-volume transfusions.

Massive transfusion-associated hypocalcemia results from the presence of citrate as an anticoagulant in blood products (and subsequent citrate binding of serum ionized calcium), particularly in those with high plasma content such as FFP and platelets.[132,133] Citrate metabolism may be dramatically impaired in patients with hypoperfusion states, hypothermia, and advanced liver disease. This can produce citrate toxicity with resultant hypocalcemic tetany, prolonged QT interval on electrocardiogram, decreased myocardial contractility, hypotension, narrowed pulse pressure, and elevated end-diastolic left ventricular and central venous pressures.[134] If hypocalcemia is anticipated based on the clinical features, electrocardiographic changes, or ionized calcium levels, it may be managed with intravenous calcium chloride or calcium gluconate.

## *Massive Transfusion-Associated Coagulopathy*

Coagulopathy is frequently present on admission in severely injured patients, particularly with brain or penetrating trauma injuries, and is associated with increased mortality.[17,52,94,135,136,137] Coagulopathy leads to further hemorrhage and worsening physiologic derangements, in turn prompting additional fluid resuscitation and transfusion that can exacerbate coagulopathy, particularly if not appropriately managed, leading to the "bloody vicious cycle."[11]

Absent laboratory testing, clinical factors such as severe injury, shock, and hypothermia can predict coagulopathic bleeding.[118] Coagulopathy may be clinically recognized as abnormal microvascular bleeding of uninjured mucosal or serosal surfaces, or by prolonged bleeding at sites of vascular access and wound tissue surfaces following control of vascular bleeding.[138] At times, coagulopathy may not be recognized immediately and can be further obscured by standard clinical laboratory tests that fail to reflect clinically observed (in vivo) coagulopathy.[139] The laboratory values that are most frequently abnormal in the setting of coagulopathy are the PT time (97 percent), platelet count (72 percent), and aPTT (70 percent).[140] Notably, abnormal coagulation tests have been associated with increased mortality.[141] Thromboelastography, while less widely available at medical centers, is a method of measuring whole blood coagulation and has been proposed as a more accurate marker of coagulopathy and predictor of transfusion requirements than standard coagulation tests (Fig. 13).[75,142] More studies are needed to better define the potential role of thromboelastography as a diagnostic test and its ability to guide subsequent transfusion practices.[128]

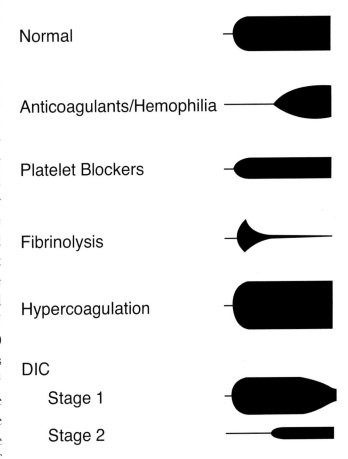

Normal

Anticoagulants/Hemophilia

Platelet Blockers

Fibrinolysis

Hypercoagulation

DIC
  Stage 1
  Stage 2

Figure 13. *Illustration of thromboelastography patterns. This method of measuring whole blood coagulation has been proposed as a more accurate marker of coagulopathy and predictor of transfusion requirements than standard coagulation tests.*

Factors contributing to coagulopathy in patients undergoing massive transfusion include systemic acidosis, hypothermia, and consumptive and dilutional coagulopathy. Acidemia, largely due to lactate production by hypoperfused tissues utilizing anaerobic metabolism, can develop during hemorrhagic shock.[143,144,145] Acidosis may both exacerbate and cause coagulopathy.[118,146,147] Clotting factors and platelet aggregation are impaired by acidosis.[148,149] There is also evidence of natural anticoagulant activation through protein C and enhanced fibrinolysis through increased tissue plasminogen activator release and plasminogen-activator inhibitor-type 1 (PAI-1) depletion in shock and acidosis.[150,151]

Coagulopathy may be present on admission in severely injured patients and is associated with increased mortality. Factors contributing to coagulopathy in patients undergoing massive transfusion include systemic acidosis, hypothermia, and consumptive and dilutional coagulopathy. Though standard coagulation tests (INR, aPTT, and platelets) are relied upon, thromboelastography may be a more accurate marker of coagulopathy and predictor of transfusion requirements.

Hypothermia impairs the coagulation system in multiple ways.[36,39,152,153,154] Hypothermia has a modest effect on coagulation factor activity with a reduction of 10 percent of clotting factor activity for each 1°C decrease in temperature.[13] It also results in a marked effect on platelet function.[13,155,156] Platelet dysfunction develops due to defects in platelet activation, adhesion, and aggregation. Normalization of body temperature has been found to reverse inhibition of thrombin generation on platelets.[157,158,159]

Consumption of factors with disseminated intravascular coagulation (DIC) has been noted in early trauma, particularly in association with extensive endothelial injury, massive soft-tissue damage, fat embolization from long-bone fractures, and brain injury.[160,161] In addition to consumption of clotting factors, there is dysregulation of coagulation through consumption of antithrombin III, acquired platelet defects, and through increased fibrinolysis from increased tissue plasminogen activator and decreased α-2 antiplasmin.[162,163,164,165,166,167]

Dilutional coagulopathy develops during DCR as a consequence of the replacement of lost whole blood with coagulation factor-poor and platelet-poor fluids like crystalloids, colloids, and stored packed red blood cells.[126,168] In addition to coagulation factor and platelet deficiencies, a lowered hematocrit may further contribute to coagulopathy as erythrocytes marginalize platelets toward the capillary wall and endothelium.[169] Local platelet concentrations along the endothelium are nearly seven times higher than the average blood concentration due to this effect.[170] Studies have shown that anemia has been correlated with increased bleeding times that are reversible with RBC transfusion.[171,172] While clotting factors and platelets can be transfused during DCR, preservatives in these solutions of stored blood products may further worsen the dilutional coagulopathy.[126]

# Damage Control Resuscitation Adjunctive Measures

## *Hypotensive Resuscitation*

The practice of hypotensive resuscitation (permissive hypotension) has been traced back to Walter Cannon, who in 1918 proposed hypotension as a method for reducing uncontrolled internal hemorrhage.[173] Hypotensive resuscitation has been described as a method to improve patient outcomes by simultaneously limiting active hemorrhage and dilutional coagulopathy by tolerating lower than normal blood pressures (e.g., systolic pressure of less than 90 mm Hg) in trauma patients.[12] The combined effect of the natural coagulation cascade, hypotension, and vessel spasm is thought to temporarily arrest traumatic hemorrhage and serves as the underlying foundation for hypotensive resuscitation.[4,12,174,175,176,177] The direct effects of hypotensive resuscitation, or the failure to employ hypotensive resuscitation, are most readily apparent in traumatic amputation patients (Fig. 14). These patients often arrive without apparent bleeding from traumatically amputated limbs, only to have rapid arterial bleeding resume once resuscitation begins and hypotension is corrected to normal systolic pressures. This bleeding can sometimes overwhelm tourniquet control.[178] This rebleeding phenomenon was well-known and previously described by World War I and II era surgeons.[179]

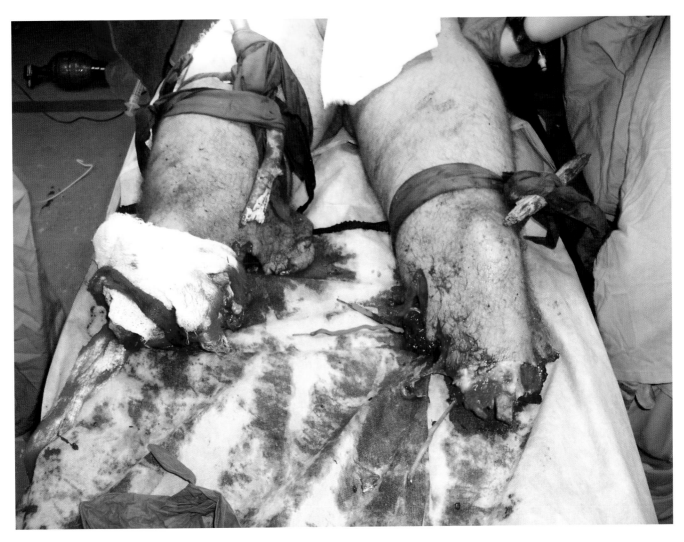

Figure 14. *Overly aggressive fluid resuscitation of patients with traumatically amputated limbs may cause nonbleeding wounds to hemorrhage profusely. Image courtesy of the Borden Institute, Office of The Surgeon General, Washington, DC.*

> Current military doctrine and training emphasize minimizing fluid and blood product delivery in prehospital settings for combat casualties who have a palpable radial pulse and normal mental status. The combined effect of the natural coagulation cascade, hypotension, and vessel spasm is thought to temporarily arrest traumatic hemorrhage and serves as the underlying foundation for hypotensive resuscitation. Such strategies are inappropriate with central nervous system injury or when cardiovascular collapse is imminent.

Several terms have been used to describe the strategy of tolerating relative hypotension in trauma victims prior to surgical hemorrhage control. These terms include hypotensive resuscitation, deliberate hypotension, and permissive hypotension. Although mixed results have been noted in studies, both animal and human clinical trials have supported the concept.[12,176,180,181,182,183,184,185,186,187,188] Current military doctrine and training emphasize minimizing fluid and blood product delivery in prehospital settings for combat casualties who have a palpable radial pulse and normal mental status.[189,190] This approach is also employed in the trauma bays with Forward Surgical Teams and CSHs to prevent unnecessary blood loss before surgical control is achieved.[190]

The challenge to providers using hypotensive resuscitation as part of their strategy is recognizing when to withhold additional fluid, but also knowing when such strategies are inappropriate, such as with central nervous system injury or when cardiovascular collapse is imminent.[191] Tissue ischemia followed by reperfusion is associated with biochemical and cellular changes resulting in complement activation and inflammatory responses.[192,193] These inflammatory responses are responsible for the development of acute lung injury and multiple organ failure, and are potentially exacerbated by the choice of resuscitation fluid.[194,195] The understanding of these processes is incomplete and an area of active research.

Patients with active hemorrhage may deteriorate quickly, and currently there are few data available to guide the hypotensive resuscitation strategy. As a general recommendation, patients are permitted to remain mildly hypotensive in two clinical circumstances. The first is the patient who is being rapidly transported to an operating room with the anticipation that surgical control of hemorrhage will be obtained quickly. Volume administration prior to hemorrhage control has the potential to raise the SBP sufficiently to overcome the natural hemostatic mechanisms. The second circumstance is for the patient with noncompressible hemorrhage who is a great distance from an operating room, either geographically or temporally. These patients may reach a temporary stable state where natural hemostatic mechanisms have slowed or stopped ongoing hemorrhage. Large volumes may overwhelm this natural hemostasis and cause exsanguination during transport. In both cases, the goal should be transfer to an operating room at the earliest possible time.

## *Optimal Use of Crystalloid and Colloid Solutions*

Crystalloids and colloids greatly intensify dilutional effects if given in significant quantities (greater than 20 ml per kilogram). In addition to dilutional effects, colloids such as hydroxyethyl starch (HES) are also known to increase coagulopathy by impairing von Willebrand factor activity in plasma.[196,197] Moreover, a preventable cause of iatrogenic acidemia involves the choice of resuscitation fluid. The two most commonly used isotonic crystalloid solutions in emergency departments and prehospital settings are lactated Ringer's solution and normal saline. Both of these fluids possess pH ranges as low as 4.5 for normal saline (NS) and 6.0 for lactated Ringer's (LR) solution.

> Crystalloids and colloids greatly intensify hemodilutional effects if given in significant quantities (greater than 20 ml per kilogram). The low pH values of normal saline and lactated Ringer's solution contribute to iatrogenic acidemia when administered in large volumes.

In a fairly extensive review of animal research, case reports, case series, and clinical studies, Ho and colleagues demonstrated that use of large amounts of normal saline in trauma patients with shock contributes to metabolic acidosis, which also can significantly worsen coagulopathy.[198] This effect was not demonstrated with lactated Ringer's solution. Several other recent animal studies have demonstrated superiority of lactated Ringer's solution over normal saline as a resuscitation fluid in hemorrhagic shock.[199,200,201] Nevertheless, the choice of lactated Ringer's solution as a resuscitation fluid, particularly for severely injured patients undergoing damage control surgery and massive transfusion, has other drawbacks. Lactated Ringer's solution in large volumes provides little or no direct contribution to improve coagulation or oxygen-carrying capacity, relative to early use of blood products. More recently, lactated Ringer's solution has also been found to dramatically activate the immune system and potentially contribute to secondary cellular injury.[190,202,203,204,205] Use of this fluid may be detrimental in patients with uncontrolled hemorrhage.[176,180,181]

## Vasoactive Agents

Exogenous catecholamines and other vasopressor agents (e.g., vasopressin) are used frequently as adjuncts to the resuscitation of patients with severe hemorrhagic shock. Although previous data on the employment of vasopressors in hemorrhagic shock are mixed, recent animal studies reveal potentially favorable results with the use of low-dose vasopressin in resuscitation after brain injury or hemorrhage and blunt pulmonary contusion or hemorrhage.[206,207,208,209,210,211,212,213,214,215,216,217,218,219,220,221] Other investigators have shown that vasopressin becomes deficient in advanced stages of hemorrhagic and vasodilatory shock and hence is an appropriate target for replacement.[222] A recent review article by Cohn suggests that low-dose vasopressin in severe hemorrhagic shock can lower resuscitation volumes and potentially improve morbidity and mortality.[223] Overall, the multiple publications analyzing the effects of low-dose vasopressin in various clinical settings have resulted in conflicting results.[217,218,219,224,225,226,227,228,229,230,231] Further well-designed clinical trials in trauma patients are necessary to better define the role of vasoactive agents (e.g., vasopressin) as adjuncts to resuscitation.

> While exogenous catecholamines and other vasopressor agents are frequently used during resuscitation of patients with severe hemorrhagic shock, further studies are necessary to establish their efficacy.

## Nonsurgical Hemostatic Agents

### Topical Sealants

Topical hemostatic sealants are used as adjuncts for local hemostasis in cases where conventional measures for bleeding control fail. Agents such as FLOSEAL™, GELFOAM®, and SURGICEL® are useful adjuncts to standard hemorrhage control techniques in patients undergoing cardiac, vascular, and spinal surgery.[232,233,234]

### Recombinant Factor VIIa

While recombinant factor VIIa (rFVIIa) is currently only approved for the management of bleeding in patients with congenital Factor VII deficiency and hemophilia A or B with inhibitors, this agent has been extensively used off-label in trauma. Further interest was spurred following a series of experimental animal liver trauma studies that showed prolongations in survival and decreased blood loss with its use.[235,236,237,238,239] These studies coincided with a number of subsequent case reports and case series of rFVIIa use in trauma and uncontrolled hemorrhage suggesting decreased blood loss or decreased transfusion requirements for patients.[98,240,241,242,243,244,245,246,247,248,249,250,251,252,253,254,255,256,257,258,259,260]

> As of 2009, there is no evidence of improved major clinical outcomes (e.g., decreased mortality) as a direct result of using rFVIIa in the management of trauma patients.

The only randomized trial of rFVIIa in trauma patients (published in 2005) randomized 301 patients with blunt or penetrating injuries to receive placebo or rFVIIa after the eighth unit of blood.[261] This trial showed a reduction of 2.6 units of RBC transfusions for the blunt trauma subgroup and a similar though non-significant trend in the penetrating injury subgroup receiving factor rVIIA. While trends toward reductions in mortality and critical complications were seen, no statistically significant results were documented.[261] The CONTROL study, a randomized double-blind trial whose purpose was to evaluate the safety and effectiveness of rFVIIa in severely injured trauma patients, was discontinued at Phase III because a preplanned futility analysis predicted a very low likelihood of reaching a successful outcome on the primary efficacy endpoints.[262] As of 2010, there is no evidence of improved major clinical outcomes (e.g., decreased mortality) as a direct result of using rFVIIa in the management of trauma patients.

The potential for thromboembolic complications associated with rFVIIa has received considerable attention. Meta-analyses of randomized, controlled trials have shown mixed results while multiple studies have suggested that thromboemboli are an apparent complication.[263,264,265,266,267,268,269]

## Antifibrinolytics

As hyperfibrinolysis is a contributor to the coagulopathy of trauma, antifibrinolytics have the potential to reduce blood loss and improve outcomes in traumatic bleeding. Antifibrinolytic agents have been noted to reduce blood loss in patients with both normal and exaggerated fibrinolytic responses to surgery.[270] The most extensively evaluated agents are aprotinin, epsilon aminocaproic acid, and tranexamic acid. The Food and Drug Administration suspended marketing of aprotinin in November 2007 due to reports of increased mortality in coronary bypass surgery.[271] While aminocaproic acid is approved by the FDA for enhancing hemostasis in states of hyperfibrinolysis, and tranexamic acid is approved for hemophilia patients undergoing tooth extraction, a Cochrane Review of antifibrinolytic drugs in acute traumatic injury revealed no studies of sufficient quality to assess the benefits in this population.[272,273,274] There is currently a major ongoing international trial, CRASH-2: Clinical Randomization of an Antifibrinolytic in Significant Hemorrhage (NCT00375258), to evaluate the use of tranexamic acid compared to placebo in trauma patients.[275] Until these results are available, there is little role for the prophylactic or empiric use of antifibrinolytics in acute trauma.

# Conclusions

The resuscitation of severely injured trauma patients will continue to remain a complex and multifaceted problem. The recent large numbers of combat casualties requiring massive transfusion, an unfortunate by product of modern war, has enabled both the military and civilian trauma communities to formulate an evolving DCR strategy. Ongoing and future research are needed to further refine and validate: (1) novel prehospital therapies for the treatment of noncompressible hemorrhage; (2) technologies to rapidly assess the physiologic status of injured patients; (3) methods to select patients for damage control approaches; (4) the optimal content and proper sequence of administration of resuscitation products; and (5) novel approaches to managing patients at or near the limits of physiologic reserve.

# References

1. Baker CC, Oppenheimer L, Stephens B, et al. Epidemiology of trauma deaths. Am J Surg 1980;140(1):144-150.

2. Sauaia A, Moore FA, Moore EE, et al. Epidemiology of trauma deaths: a reassessment. J Trauma 1995;38(2):185-193.

3. Shackford SR, Mackersie RC, Holbrook TL, et al. The epidemiology of traumatic death. A population-based analysis. Arch Surg 1993;128(5):571-575.

4. Holcomb JB, Jenkins D, Rhee P, et al. Damage control resuscitation: directly addressing the early coagulopathy of trauma. J Trauma 2007;62(2):307-310.

5. Kelly JF, Ritenour AE, McLaughlin DF, et al. Injury severity and causes of death from Operation Iraqi Freedom and Operation Enduring Freedom: 2003-2004 versus 2006. J Trauma 2008;64(2 Suppl):S21-26.

6. Acosta JA, Yang JC, Winchell RJ, et al. Lethal injuries and time to death in a level I trauma center. J Am Coll Surg 1998;186(5):528-533.

7. Demetriades D, Murray J, Charalambides K, et al. Trauma fatalities: time and location of hospital deaths. J Am Coll Surg 2004;198(1):20-26.

8. Peng R, Chang C, Gilmore D, et al. Epidemiology of immediate and early trauma deaths at an urban level I trauma center. Am Surg 1998;64(10):950-954.

9. Stewart RM, Myers JG, Dent DL, et al. Seven hundred fifty-three consecutive deaths in a level I trauma center: the argument for injury prevention. J Trauma 2003;54(1):66-70.

10. Wudel JH, Morris JA Jr, Yates K, et al. Massive transfusion: outcome in blunt trauma patients. J Trauma 1991;31(1):1-7.

11. Kashuk JL, Moore EE, Millikan JS, et al. Major abdominal vascular trauma – a unified approach. J Trauma 1982;22(8):672-679.

12. Bickell WH, Wall MJ Jr, Pepe PE, et al. Immediate versus delayed fluid resuscitation for hypotensive patients with penetrating torso injuries. N Engl J Med 1994;331(17):1105-1109.

13. Hess JR, Lawson JH. The coagulopathy of trauma versus disseminated intravascular coagulation. J Trauma 2006;60(6 Suppl):S12-19.

14. Cotton BA, Gunter OL, Isbell J, et al. Damage control hematology: the impact of a trauma exsanguination protocol on survival and blood product utilization. J Trauma 2008;64(5):1177-1182.

15. Dubick MA, Brooks DE, Macaitis JM, et al. Evaluation of commercially available fluid-warming devices for use in forward surgical and combat areas. Mil Med 2005;170(1):76-82.

16. Kragh JF Jr, Walters TJ, Baer DG, et al. Practical use of emergency tourniquets to stop bleeding in major limb trauma. J Trauma 2008;64(2 Suppl):S38-49.

17. Brohi K, Singh J, Heron M, et al. Acute traumatic coagulopathy. J Trauma 2003;54(6):1127-1130.

18. MacLeod JB, Lynn M, McKenney MG, et al. Early coagulopathy predicts mortality in trauma. J Trauma 2003;55(1):39-44.

19. Blackbourne LH. Combat damage control surgery. Crit Care Med 2008;36(7 Suppl):S304-310.

20. Committee on Tactical Combat Casualty Care. Tactical Field Care. 2009. (Accessed January 12, 2010, at http://www.health.mil/Pages/Page.aspx?ID=34.)

21. Committee on Tactical Combat Casualty Care. Care Under Fire. 2009. (Accessed January 12, 2010, at http://www.health.mil/Pages/Page.aspx?ID=34.)

22. Husum H, Gilbert M, Wisborg T, et al. Prehospital tourniquets: there should be no controversy. J Trauma 2004;56(1):214-215.

23. Navein J, Coupland R, Dunn R. The tourniquet controversy. J Trauma 2003;54(5 Suppl):S219-220.

24. Beekley AC, Sebesta JA, Blackbourne LH, et al. Prehospital tourniquet use in Operation Iraqi Freedom: effect on hemorrhage control and outcomes. J Trauma 2008;64(2 Suppl):S28-37.

25. Brodie S, Hodgetts TJ, Ollerton J, et al. Tourniquet use in combat trauma: UK military experience. J R Army Med Corps 2007;153(4):310-313.

26. Kragh JF Jr, Baer DG, Walters TJ. Extended (16-hour) tourniquet application after combat wounds: a case report and review of the current literature. J Orthop Trauma 2007;21(4):274-278.

27. Lakstein D, Blumenfeld A, Sokolov T, et al. Tourniquets for hemorrhage control on the battlefield: a 4-year accumulated experience. J Trauma 2003;54(5 Suppl):S221-S225.

28. Mabry RL. Tourniquet use on the battlefield. Mil Med 2006;171(5):352-356.

29. Kragh JF Jr, Walters TJ, Baer DG, et al. Survival with emergency tourniquet use to stop bleeding in major limb trauma. Ann Surg 2009;249(1):1-7.

30. Kheirabadi BS, Acheson EM, Deguzman R, et al. Hemostatic efficacy of two advanced dressings in an aortic hemorrhage model in swine. J Trauma 2005;59(1):25-34.

31. Rhee P, Brown C, Martin M, et al. QuikClot use in trauma for hemorrhage control: case series of 103

documented uses. J Trauma 2008;64(4):1093-1099.

32. McManus J, Hurtado T, Pusateri A, et al. A case series describing thermal injury resulting from zeolite use for hemorrhage control in combat operations. Prehosp Emerg Care 2007;11(1):67-71.

33. Wedmore I, McManus JG, Pusateri AE, et al. A special report on the chitosan-based hemostatic dressing: experience in current combat operations. J Trauma 2006;60(3):655-658.

34. Kheirabadi BS, Edens JW, Terrazas IB, et al. Comparison of new hemostatic granules/powders with currently deployed hemostatic products in a lethal model of extremity arterial hemorrhage in swine. J Trauma 2009;66(2):316-326.

35. Kheirabadi BS, Scherer MR, Estep JS, et al. Determination of efficacy of new hemostatic dressings in a model of extremity arterial hemorrhage in swine. J Trauma 2009;67(3):450-459; discussion 459-460.

36. Peng RY, Bongard FS. Hypothermia in trauma patients. J Am Coll Surg 1999;188(6):685-696.

37. Gentilello L, Jurkovich GJ. Hypothermia. In: Ivatury RR, Cayten CG, editors. The textbook of penetrating trauma. Media, PA: Williams & Wilkins; 1996. p. 995-1006.

38. Jurkovich GJ, Greiser WB, Luterman A, et al. Hypothermia in trauma victims: an ominous predictor of survival. J Trauma 1987;27(9):1019-1024.

39. Arthurs Z, Cuadrado D, Beekley A, et al. The impact of hypothermia on trauma care at the 31st combat support hospital. Am J Surg 2006;191(5):610-614.

40. Gentilello LM, Jurkovich GJ, Stark MS, et al. Is hypothermia in the victim of major trauma protective or harmful? A randomized, prospective study. Ann Surg 1997;226(4):439-447.

41. Martin RS, Kilgo PD, Miller PR, et al. Injury-associated hypothermia: an analysis of the 2004 National Trauma Data Bank. Shock 2005;24(2):114-118.

42. Beekley AC. United States military surgical response to modern large-scale conflicts: the ongoing evolution of a trauma system. Surg Clin North Am 2006;86(3):689-709.

43. Eastridge BJ, Jenkins D, Flaherty S, et al. Trauma system development in a theater of war: experiences from Operation Iraqi Freedom and Operation Enduring Freedom. J Trauma 2006;61(6):1366-1372.

44. Kober A, Scheck T, Fulesdi B, et al. Effectiveness of resistive heating compared with passive warming in treating hypothermia associated with minor trauma: a randomized trial. Mayo Clin Proc 2001;76(4):369-375.

45. Watts DD, Roche M, Tricarico R, et al. The utility of traditional prehospital interventions in maintaining thermostasis. Prehosp Emerg Care 1999;3(2):115-122.

46. Steele MT, Nelson MJ, Sessler DI, et al. Forced air speeds rewarming in accidental hypothermia. Ann Emerg Med 1996;27(4):479-484.

47. Roizen MF, Sohn YJ, L'Hommedieu CS, et al. Operating room temperature prior to surgical draping: effect on patient temperature in recovery room. Anesth Analg 1980;59(11):852-855.

48. Lloyd EL, Frandland JC. Letter: accidental hypothermia: central rewarming in the field. Br Med J 1974;4(5946):717.

49. Slovis CM, Bachvarov HL. Heated inhalation treatment of hypothermia. Am J Emerg Med 1984;2(6):533-536.

50. Gentilello LM, Rifley WJ. Continuous arteriovenous rewarming: report of a new technique for treating hypothermia. J Trauma 1991;31(8):1151-1154.

51. Gentilello LM, Cobean RA, Offner PJ, et al. Continuous arteriovenous rewarming: rapid reversal of hypothermia in critically ill patients. J Trauma 1992;32(3):316-325.

52. Schreiber MA, Perkins J, Kiraly L, et al. Early predictors of massive transfusion in combat casualties. J Am Coll Surg 2007;205(4):541-545.

53. Park MS, Martini WZ, Dubick MA, et al. Thromboelastography as a better indicator of hypercoagulable state after injury than prothrombin time or activated partial thromboplastin time. J Trauma 2009;67(2):266-275.

54. Lehmann RK, Arthurs ZM, Cuadrado DG, et al. Trauma team activation: simplified criteria safely reduces overtriage. Am J Surg 2007;193(5):630-634.

55. Shatney CH, Sensaki K. Trauma team activation for 'mechanism of injury' blunt trauma victims: time for a change? J Trauma 1994;37(2):275-281.

56. Brasel KJ, Guse C, Gentilello LM, et al. Heart rate: is it truly a vital sign? J Trauma 2007;62(4):812-817.

57. Gentilello LM. Advances in the management of hypothermia. Surg Clin North Am 1995;75(2):243-256.

58. Bernabei AF, Levison MA, Bender JS. The effects of hypothermia and injury severity on blood loss during trauma laparotomy. J Trauma 1992;33(6):835-839.

59. Ferrara A, MacArthur JD, Wright HK, et al. Hypothermia and acidosis worsen coagulopathy in the patient requiring massive transfusion. Am J Surg 1990;160(5):515-518.

60. Luna GK, Maier RV, Pavlin EG, et al. Incidence and effect of hypothermia in seriously injured patients. J Trauma 1987;27(9):1014-1018.

61. Holcomb JB, Niles SE, Miller CC, et al. Prehospital physiologic data and lifesaving interventions in trauma patients. Mil Med 2005;170(1):7-13.

62. Eastridge BJ, Malone D, Holcomb JB. Early predictors of transfusion and mortality after injury: a review of the data-based literature. J Trauma 2006;60(6 Suppl):S20-25.

63. Eastridge BJ, Owsley J, Sebesta J, et al. Admission physiology criteria after injury on the battlefield predict medical resource utilization and patient mortality. J Trauma 2006;61(4):820-823.

64. Champion HR, Sacco WJ, Carnazzo AJ, et al. Trauma score. Crit Care Med 1981;9(9):672-676.

65. Champion HR, Gainer PS, Yackee E. A progress report on the trauma score in predicting a fatal outcome. J Trauma 1986;26(10):927-931.

66. Champion HR, Sacco WJ, Copes WS, et al. A revision of the Trauma Score. J Trauma 1989;29(5):623-629.

67. Sacco WJ, Champion HR, Gainer PS, et al. The Trauma Score as applied to penetrating trauma. Ann Emerg Med 1984;13(6):415-418.

68. Cancio LC, Wade CE, West SA, et al. Prediction of mortality and of the need for massive transfusion in casualties arriving at combat support hospitals in Iraq. J Trauma 2008;64(2 Suppl):S51-55.

69. Holcomb JB, Salinas J, McManus JM, et al. Manual vital signs reliably predict need for life-saving interventions in trauma patients. J Trauma 2005;59(4):821-828.

70. McManus J, Yershov AL, Ludwig D, et al. Radial pulse character relationships to systolic blood pressure and trauma outcomes. Prehosp Emerg Care 2005;9(4):423-428.

71. Eastridge BJ, Salinas J, McManus JG, et al. Hypotension begins at 110 mm Hg: redefining "hypotension" with data. J Trauma 2007;63(2):291-297.

72. Davis JW, Parks SN, Kaups KL, et al. Admission base deficit predicts transfusion requirements and risk of complications. J Trauma 1996;41(5):769-774.

73. Ketchum L, Hess JR, Hiippala S. Indications for early fresh frozen plasma, cryoprecipitate, and platelet transfusion in trauma. J Trauma 2006;60(6 Suppl):S51-58.

74. McLaughlin DF, Niles SE, Salinas J, et al. A predictive model for massive transfusion in combat casualty patients. J Trauma 2008;64(2 Suppl):S57-63.

75. Plotkin AJ, Wade CE, Jenkins DH, et al. A reduction in clot formation rate and strength assessed by thromboelastography is indicative of transfusion requirements in patients with penetrating injuries. J Trauma 2008;64(2 Suppl):S64-68.

76. Jeger V, Zimmermann H, Exadaktylos AK. Can RapidTEG accelerate the search for coagulopathies in the patient with multiple injuries? J Trauma 2009;66(4):1253-1257.

77. Batchinsky AI, Cooke WH, Kuusela T, et al. Loss of complexity characterizes the heart rate response to experimental hemorrhagic shock in swine. Crit Care Med 2007;35(2):519-525.

78. Batchinsky AI, Cancio LC, Salinas J, et al. Prehospital loss of R-to-R interval complexity is associated with mortality in trauma patients. J Trauma 2007;63(3):512-518.

79. Cohn SM, Crookes BA, Proctor KG. Near-infrared spectroscopy in resuscitation. J Trauma 2003;54(5 Suppl):S199-202.

80. Cohn SM. Near-infrared spectroscopy: potential clinical benefits in surgery. J Am Coll Surg 2007;205(2):322-332.

81. Convertino VA, Cooke WH, Holcomb JB. Arterial pulse pressure and its association with reduced stroke volume during progressive central hypovolemia. J Trauma 2006;61(3):629-634.

82. Convertino VA, Ryan KL. Identifying physiological measurements for medical monitoring: implications for autonomous health care in austere environments. J Gravit Physiol 2007;14(1):P39-42.

83. Cooke WH, Rickards CA, Ryan KL, et al. Autonomic compensation to simulated hemorrhage monitored with heart period variability. Crit Care Med 2008;36(6):1892-1899.

84. Santora RJ, McKinley BA, Moore FA. Computerized clinical decision support for traumatic shock resuscitation. Curr Opin Crit Care 2008;14(6):679-684.

85. Cancio LC, Batchinsky AI, Salinas J, et al. Heart-rate complexity for prediction of prehospital lifesaving interventions in trauma patients. J Trauma 2008;65(4):813-819.

86. Cooke WH, Salinas J, McManus JG, et al. Heart period variability in trauma patients may predict mortality and allow remote triage. Aviat Space Environ Med 2006;77(11):1107-1112.

87. Cooke WH, Salinas J, Convertino VA, et al. Heart rate variability and its association with mortality in prehospital trauma patients. J Trauma 2006;60(2):363-370.

88. Cohn SM, Nathens AB, Moore FA, et al. Tissue oxygen saturation predicts the development of organ dysfunction during traumatic shock resuscitation. J Trauma 2007;62(1):44-54.

89. Como JJ, Dutton RP, Scalea TM, et al. Blood transfusion rates in the care of acute trauma. Transfusion 2004;44(6):809-813.

90. Harvey MP, Greenfield TP, Sugrue ME, et al. Massive blood transfusion in a tertiary referral hospital. Clinical outcomes and haemostatic complications. Med J Aust 1995;163(7):356-359.

91. Sawyer PR, Harrison CR. Massive transfusion in adults. Diagnoses, survival and blood bank support. Vox Sang 1990;58(3):199-203.

92. Cinat ME, Wallace WC, Nastanski F, et al. Improved survival following massive transfusion in patients who have undergone trauma. Arch Surg 1999;134(9):964-968.

93. Huber-Wagner S, Qvick M, Mussack T, et al. Massive blood transfusion and outcome in 1062 polytrauma patients: a prospective study based on the Trauma Registry of the German Trauma Society. Vox Sang 2007;92(1):69-78.

94. Phillips TF, Soulier G, Wilson RF. Outcome of massive transfusion exceeding two blood volumes in trauma and emergency surgery. J Trauma 1987;27(8):903-910.

95. Hewitt PE, Machin SJ. ABC of transfusion. Massive blood transfusion. BMJ 1990;300(6717):107-109.

96. Malone DL, Hess JR, Fingerhut A. Massive transfusion practices around the globe and a suggestion for a common massive transfusion protocol. J Trauma 2006;60(6 Suppl):S91-96.

97. Malone DL, Dunne J, Tracy JK, et al. Blood transfusion, independent of shock severity, is associated with worse outcome in trauma. J Trauma 2003;54(5):898-905.

98. Perkins JG, Schreiber MA, Wade CE, et al. Early versus late recombinant factor VIIa in combat trauma patients requiring massive transfusion. J Trauma 2007;62(5):1095-1099.

99. Collins JA. Problems associated with the massive transfusion of stored blood. Surgery 1974;75(2):274–295.

100. Geeraedts LM Jr, Demiral H, Schaap NP, et al. 'Blind' transfusion of blood products in exsanguinating trauma patients. Resuscitation 2007;73(3):382-388.

101. Gonzalez EA, Moore FA, Holcomb JB, et al. Fresh frozen plasma should be given earlier to patients requiring massive transfusion. J Trauma 2007;62(1):112-119.

102. Dente CJ, Shaz BH, Nicholas JM, et al. Improvements in early mortality and coagulopathy are sustained better in patients with blunt trauma after institution of a massive transfusion protocol in a civilian level I trauma center. J Trauma 2009;66(6):1616-24.

103. Crosby WH, Akeroyd JH. Some immunohematologic results of large transfusions of group O blood in recipients of other blood groups; a study of battle casualties in Korea. Blood 1954;9(2):103-116.

104. Lefebre J, McLellan BA, Coovadia AS. Seven years experience with group O unmatched packed red blood cells in a regional trauma unit. Ann Emerg Med 1987;16(12):1344-1349.

105. Schwab CW, Civil I, Shayne JP. Saline-expanded group O uncrossmatched packed red blood cells as

an initial resuscitation fluid in severe shock. Ann Emerg Med 1986;15(11):1282-1287.

106. Blumberg N, Bove JR. Un-cross-matched blood for emergency transfusion. One year's experience in a civilian setting. JAMA 1978;240(19):2057-2059.

107. Gervin AS, Fischer RP. Resuscitation of trauma patients with type-specific uncrossmatched blood. J Trauma 1984;24(4):327-331.

108. Camp FR Jr, Dawson RB. Prevention of injury to multiple casualties requiring resuscitation following blood loss. Mil Med 1974;139:893-898.

109. Holcomb JB, Wade CE, Michalek JE, et al. Increased plasma and platelet to red blood cell ratios improves outcome in 466 massively transfused civilian trauma patients. Ann Surg 2008;248(3):447-458.

110. Maegele M, Lefering R, Paffrath T, et al. Red-blood-cell to plasma ratios transfused during massive transfusion are associated with mortality in severe multiple injury: a retrospective analysis from the Trauma Registry of the Deutsche Gesellschaft fur Unfallchirurgie. Vox Sang 2008;95(2):112-119.

111. Sperry JL, Ochoa JB, Gunn SR, et al. An FFP:PRBC transfusion ratio >/=1:1.5 is associated with a lower risk of mortality after massive transfusion. J Trauma 2008;65(5):986-993.

112. Hoffman M, Jenner P. Variability in the fibrinogen and von Willebrand factor content of cryoprecipitate. Implications for reducing donor exposure. Am J Clin Pathol. 1990;93(5):694-697.

113. Borgman MA, Spinella PC, Perkins JG, et al. The ratio of blood products transfused affects mortality in patients receiving massive transfusions at a combat support hospital. J Trauma 2007;63(4):805-813.

114. Hirshberg A, Dugas M, Banez EI, et al. Minimizing dilutional coagulopathy in exsanguinating hemorrhage: a computer simulation. J Trauma 2003;54(3):454-463.

115. Ho AM, Dion PW, Cheng CA, et al. A mathematical model for fresh frozen plasma transfusion strategies during major trauma resuscitation with ongoing hemorrhage. Can J Surg 2005;48(6):470-478.

116. Perkins JG, Cap AP, Spinella PC, et al. An evaluation of the impact of apheresis platelets used in the setting of massively transfused trauma patients. J Trauma 2009;66(4 Suppl):S77-85.

117. Watson GA, Sperry JL, Rosengart MR, et al. Inflammation and host response to injury investigators. Fresh frozen plasma is independently associated with a higher risk of multiple organ failure and acute respiratory distress syndrome. J Trauma 2009;67(2):221-227; discussion 228-230.

118. Cosgriff N, Moore EE, Sauaia A, et al. Predicting life-threatening coagulopathy in the massively transfused trauma patient: hypothermia and acidoses revisited. J Trauma 1997;42(5):857-861.

119. Contreras M. Consensus conference on platelet transfusion: final statement. Vox Sang 1998;75(2):173-174.

120. Stainsby D, MacLennan S, Thomas D, et al. British Committee for Standards in Haematology. Guidelines on the management of massive blood loss. Br J Haematol 2006;135(5):634-641.

121. Hiippala ST, Myllyla GJ, Vahtera EM. Hemostatic factors and replacement of major blood loss with plasma-poor red cell concentrates. Anesth Analg 1995;81(2):360-365.

122. Stinger HK, Spinella PC, Perkins JG, et al. The ratio of fibrinogen to red cells transfused affects survival in casualties receiving massive transfusions at an army combat support hospital. J Trauma 2008;64(2 Suppl):S79-85.

123. Mallett SV, Cox DJ. Thromboelastography. Br J Anaesth 1992;69(3):307-313.

124. MacLennan S, Murphy MF. Survey of the use of whole blood in current blood transfusion practice. Clin Lab Haematol 2001;23(6):391-396.

125. Perkins JG, Cap AP, Weiss BM, et al. Massive transfusion and nonsurgical hemostatic agents. Crit Care Med 2008;36(7 Suppl):S325-339.

126. Armand R, Hess JR. Treating coagulopathy in trauma patients. Transfus Med Rev 2003;17(3):223-231.

127. Kauvar DS, Holcomb JB, Norris GC, et al. Fresh whole blood transfusion: a controversial military practice. J Trauma 2006;61(1):181-184.

128. Spinella PC, Holcomb JB. Resuscitation and transfusion principles for traumatic hemorrhagic shock. Blood Rev 2009;23(6):231-240.

129. Ellison N. Transfusion therapy; anesthesia and perioperative care of the combat casualty. In: Zajtchuk R, Grande CM, editors. Textbook of military medicine. Falls Church, VA: Borden Institute; 1995. p. 330.

130. Stewart HJ, Shepard EM, Horger EL. Electrocardiographic manifestations of potassium intoxication. Am J Med 1948;5(6):821-827.

131. Smith HM, Farrow SJ, Ackerman JD, et al. Cardiac arrests associated with hyperkalemia during red blood cell transfusion: a case series. Anesth Analg 2008;106(4):1062-1069.

132. Salant W, Wise LE. The action of sodium citrate and its decomposition in the body. J Biol Chem 1918;28:27-58.

133. Sihler KS, Napolitano LM. Complications of massive transfusion. Chest 2010;137(1):209-220.

134. Bunker JP, Bendixen HH, Murphy AJ. Hemodynamic effects of intravenously administered sodium citrate. N Engl J Med 1962;266:372-377.

135. Faringer PD, Mullins RJ, Johnson RL, et al. Blood component supplementation during massive transfusion of AS-1 red cells in trauma patients. J Trauma 1993;34(4):481-485.

136. MacLeod J, Lynn M, McKenney MG, et al. Predictors of mortality in trauma patients. Am Surg 2004;70(9):805-810.

137. Mitchell KJ, Moncure KE, Onyeije C, et al. Evaluation of massive volume replacement in the penetrating trauma patient. J Natl Med Assoc 1994;86(12):926-929.

138. Ordog GJ, Wasserberger J. Coagulation abnormalities in traumatic shock. Crit Care Med 1986;14(5):519.

139. Tieu BH, Holcomb JB, Schreiber MA. Coagulopathy: its pathophysiology and treatment in the injured patient. World J Surg 2007;31(5):1055-1064.

140. Aasen AO, Kierulf P, Vaage J, et al. Determination of components of the plasma proteolytic enzyme systems gives information of prognostic value in patients with multiple trauma. Adv Exp Med Biol 1983;156 (Pt B):1037-1047.

141. Hess JR, Lindell AL, Stansbury LG, et al. The prevalence of abnormal results of conventional coagulation tests on admission to a trauma center. Transfusion 2009;49(1):34-39.

142. Kheirabadi BS, Crissey JM, Deguzman R, et al. In vivo bleeding time and in vitro thromboelastography measurements are better indicators of dilutional hypothermic coagulopathy than prothrombin time. J Trauma 2007;62(6):1352-1359.

143. Collins JA, Simmons RL, James PM, et al. The acid-base status of seriously wounded combat casualties. I. Before treatment. Ann Surg 1970;171(4):595-608.

144. Cannon WB, Frasen J, Cowel EM. The preventive treatment of wound shock. JAMA 1918;70:618.

145. Macleod JJR. The concentration of lactic acid in the blood in anoxemia and shock. Am J Physiol 1921;55(2):184-196.

146. Simmons RL, Collins JA, Heisterkamp CA, et al. Coagulation disorders in combat casualties. I. Acute changes after wounding. II. Effects of massive transfusion. 3. Post-resuscitative changes. Ann Surg 1969;169(4):455-482.

147. Turpini R, Stefanini M. The nature and mechanism of the hemostatic breakdown in the course of experimental hemorrhagic shock. J Clin Invest 1959;38(1, Part 1):53-65.

148. Martini WZ, Pusateri AE, Uscilowicz JM, et al. Independent contributions of hypothermia and acidosis to coagulopathy in swine. J Trauma 2005;58(5):1002-1009.

149. Meng ZH, Wolberg AS, Monroe DM III, et al. The effect of temperature and pH on the activity of

factor VIIa: implications for the efficacy of high-dose factor VIIa in hypothermic and acidotic patients. J Trauma 2003;55(5):886-891.

150. Brohi K, Cohen MJ, Ganter MT, et al. Acute traumatic coagulopathy: initiated by hypoperfusion: modulated through the protein C pathway? Ann Surg 2007;245(5):812-818.

151. Tagnon HJ, Levenson SM, Davidson CS, et al. The occurrence of fibrinolysis in shock, with observations on the prothrombin time and the plasma fibrinogen during hemorrhagic shock. Am J Med Sci 1946;211(1):88-96.

152. Johnston TD, Chen Y, Reed RL II. Functional equivalence of hypothermia to specific clotting factor deficiencies. J Trauma 1994;37(3):413-417.

153. Patt A, McCroskey BL, Moore EE. Hypothermia-induced coagulopathies in trauma. Surg Clin North Am 1988;68(4):775-785.

154. Watts DD, Trask A, Soeken K, et al. Hypothermic coagulopathy in trauma: effect of varying levels of hypothermia on enzyme speed, platelet function, and fibrinolytic activity. J Trauma 1998;44(5):846-854.

155. Kettner SC, Kozek SA, Groetzner JP, et al. Effects of hypothermia on thrombelastography in patients undergoing cardiopulmonary bypass. Br J Anaesth 1998;80(3):313-317.

156. Kettner SC, Sitzwohl C, Zimpfer M, et al. The effect of graded hypothermia (36 degrees C-32 degrees C) on hemostasis in anesthetized patients without surgical trauma. Anesth Analg 2003;96(6):1772-1776.

157. Kermode JC, Zheng Q, Milner EP. Marked temperature dependence of the platelet calcium signal induced by human von Willebrand factor. Blood 1999;94(1):199-207.

158. Wolberg AS, Meng ZH, Monroe DM III, et al. A systematic evaluation of the effect of temperature on coagulation enzyme activity and platelet function. J Trauma 2004;56(6):1221-1228.

159. Zhang JN, Wood J, Bergeron AL, et al. Effects of low temperature on shear-induced platelet aggregation and activation. J Trauma 2004;57(2):216-223.

160. Kearney TJ, Bentt L, Grode M, et al. Coagulopathy and catecholamines in severe head injury. J Trauma 1992;32(5):608-611.

161. Levi M. Disseminated intravascular coagulation. Crit Care Med 2007;35(9):2191-2195.

162. Levi M, de Jonge E, van der Poll T. Rationale for restoration of physiological anticoagulant pathways in patients with sepsis and disseminated intravascular coagulation. Crit Care Med 2001;29(7 Suppl):S90-94.

163. O'Brien JR, Etherington M, Jamieson S. Refractory state of platelet aggregation with major operations. Lancet 1971;2(7727):741-743.

164. Utter GH, Owings JT, Jacoby RC, et al. Injury induces increased monocyte expression of tissue factor: factors associated with head injury attenuate the injury-related monocyte expression of tissue factor. J Trauma 2002;52(6):1071-1077.

165. Martini WZ, Chinkes DL, Pusateri AE, et al. Acute changes in fibrinogen metabolism and coagulation after hemorrhage in pigs. Am J Physiol Endocrinol Metab 2005;289(5):E930-934.

166. Gando S, Tedo I, Kubota M. Posttrauma coagulation and fibrinolysis. Crit Care Med 1992;20(5):594-600.

167. Kushimoto S, Yamamoto Y, Shibata Y, et al. Implications of excessive fibrinolysis and alpha(2)-plasmin inhibitor deficiency in patients with severe head injury. Neurosurgery 2001;49(5):1084-1089.

168. Ho AM, Karmakar MK, Dion PW. Are we giving enough coagulation factors during major trauma resuscitation? Am J Surg 2005;190(3):479-484.

169. Eberst ME, Berkowitz LR. Hemostasis in renal disease: pathophysiology and management. Am J Med 1994;96(2):168-179.

170. Uijttewaal WS, Nijhof EJ, Bronkhorst PJ, et al. Near-wall excess of platelets induced by lateral migration of erythrocytes in flowing blood. Am J Physiol 1993;264(4 Pt 2):H1239-1244.

171. Blajchman MA, Bordin JO, Bardossy L, et al. The contribution of the haematocrit to thrombocytopenic bleeding in experimental animals. Br J Haematol 1994;86(2):347-350.

172. Valeri CR, Cassidy G, Pivacek LE, et al. Anemia-induced increase in the bleeding time: implications for treatment of nonsurgical blood loss. Transfusion 2001;41(8):977-983.

173. Cannon WB. Acidosis in cases of shock, hemorrhage and gas infection. JAMA 1918;70:531-535.

174. Bickell WH, Shaftan GW, Mattox KL. Intravenous fluid administration and uncontrolled hemorrhage. J Trauma 1989;29(3):409.

175. Bickell WH. Are victims of injury sometimes victimized by attempts at fluid resuscitation? Ann Emerg Med 1993;22(2):225-226.

176. Bickell WH, Stern S. Fluid replacement for hypotensive injury victims: how, when and what risks? Curr Opin Anaesthesiol 1998;11(2):177-180.

177. Lu YQ, Cai XJ, Gu LH, et al. Experimental study of controlled fluid resuscitation in the treatment of severe and uncontrolled hemorrhagic shock. J Trauma 2007;63(4):798-804.

178. Beekley AC, Starnes BW, Sebesta JA. Lessons learned from modern military surgery. Surg Clin North Am 2007;87(1):157-84, vii.

179. Cannon W, Frawer J, Cowell E. The preventive treatment of wound shock. JAMA 1918;70:618-621.

180. Bickell WH, Bruttig SP, Millnamow GA, et al. The detrimental effects of intravenous crystalloid after aortotomy in swine. Surgery 1991;110(3):529-536.

181. Bickell WH, Bruttig SP, Millnamow GA, et al. Use of hypertonic saline/dextran versus lactated Ringer's solution as a resuscitation fluid after uncontrolled aortic hemorrhage in anesthetized swine. Ann Emerg Med 1992;21(9):1077-1085.

182. Stern SA, Dronen SC, Birrer P, et al. Effect of blood pressure on hemorrhage volume and survival in a near-fatal hemorrhage model incorporating a vascular injury. Ann Emerg Med 1993;22(2):155-163.

183. Dutton RP, Mackenzie CF, Scalea TM. Hypotensive resuscitation during active hemorrhage: impact on in-hospital mortality. J Trauma 2002;52(6):1141-1146.

184. Dutton RP. Low-pressure resuscitation from hemorrhagic shock. Int Anesthesiol Clin 2002;40(3):19-30.

185. Dutton RP. The role of deliberate hypotension. Hosp Med 2005;66(2):72-73.

186. Holcomb JB. Fluid resuscitation in modern combat casualty care: lessons learned from Somalia. J Trauma 2003;54(5 Suppl):S46-51.

187. Sondeen JL, Coppes VG, Holcomb JB. Blood pressure at which rebleeding occurs after resuscitation in swine with aortic injury. J Trauma 2003;54(5 Suppl):S110-117.

188. Sondeen JL, Pusateri AE, Hedner U, et al. Recombinant factor VIIa increases the pressure at which rebleeding occurs in porcine uncontrolled aortic hemorrhage model. Shock 2004;22(2):163-168.

189. US Department of Defense (US DoD). Shock and Resuscitation; Controlled Resuscitation. In: Emergency War Surgery, Third United States Revision. Washington, DC: Department of the Army, Office of the Surgeon General, Borden Institute; 2004. p. 7.4-7.6.

190. Rhee P, Koustova E, Alam HB. Searching for the optimal resuscitation method: recommendations for the initial fluid resuscitation of combat casualties. J Trauma 2003;54(5 Suppl):S52-62.

191. Brain Trauma Foundation; American Association of Neurological Surgeons; Congress of Neurological Surgeons; et al. Guidelines for the management of severe traumatic brain injury. I. Blood pressure and oxygenation. J Neurotrauma 2007;24(1 Suppl):S7-13.

192. Diebel LN, Liberati DM, Lucas CE, et al. Systemic not just mesenteric lymph causes neutrophil priming after hemorrhagic shock. J Trauma 2009;66(6):1625-1631.

193. Keel M, Trentz O. Pathophysiology of polytrauma. Injury 2005;36(6):691-709.

194. Ciesla DJ, Moore EE, Johnson JL, et al. The role of the lung in postinjury multiple organ failure. Surgery 2005;138(4):749-757; discussion 757-758.

195. Rhee P, Wang D, Ruff P, et al. Human neutrophil activation and increased adhesion by various resuscitation fluids. Crit Care Med 2000;28(1):74-78.

196. Treib J, Haass A, Pindur G. Coagulation disorders caused by hydroxyethyl starch. Thromb Haemost 1997;78(3):974-983.

197. Treib J, Baron JF, Grauer MT, et al. An international view of hydroxyethyl starches. Intensive Care Med 1999;25(3):258-268.

198. Ho AM, Karmakar MK, Contardi LH, et al. Excessive use of normal saline in managing traumatized patients in shock: a preventable contributor to acidosis. J Trauma 2001;51(1):173-177.

199. Healey MA, Davis RE, Liu FC, et al. Lactated Ringer's is superior to normal saline in a model of massive hemorrhage and resuscitation. J Trauma 1998;45(5):894-899.

200. Kiraly LN, Differding JA, Enomoto TM, et al. Resuscitation with normal saline (NS) vs. lactated Ringers (LR) modulates hypercoagulability and leads to increased blood loss in an uncontrolled hemorrhagic shock swine model. J Trauma 2006;61(1):57-64.

201. Todd SR, Malinoski D, Muller PJ, et al. Lactated Ringer's is superior to normal saline in the resuscitation of uncontrolled hemorrhagic shock. J Trauma 2007;62(3):636-639.

202. Alam HB, Sun L, Ruff P, et al. E- and P-selectin expression depends on the resuscitation fluid used in hemorrhaged rats. J Surg Res 2000;94(2):145-152.

203. Alam HB, Stanton K, Koustova E, et al. Effect of different resuscitation strategies on neutrophil activation in a swine model of hemorrhagic shock. Resuscitation 2004;60(1):91-99.

204. Ayuste EC, Chen H, Koustova E, et al. Hepatic and pulmonary apoptosis after hemorrhagic shock in swine can be reduced through modifications of conventional Ringer's solution. J Trauma 2006;60(1):52-63.

205. Watters JM, Tieu BH, Todd SR, et al. Fluid resuscitation increases inflammatory gene transcription after traumatic injury. J Trauma 2006;61(2):300-308.

206. Sanui M, King DR, Feinstein AJ, et al. Effects of arginine vasopressin during resuscitation from hemorrhagic hypotension after traumatic brain injury. Crit Care Med 2006;34(2):433-438.

207. Schmittinger CA, Astner S, Astner L, et al. Cardiopulmonary resuscitation with vasopressin in a dog. Vet Anaesth Analg 2005;32(2):112-114.

208. Schwarz B, Mair P, Raedler C, et al. Vasopressin improves survival in a pig model of hypothermic

cardiopulmonary resuscitation. Crit Care Med 2002;30(6):1311-1314.

209. Schwarz B, Mair P, Wagner-Berger H, et al. Neither vasopressin nor amiodarone improve CPR outcome in an animal model of hypothermic cardiac arrest. Acta Anaesthesiol Scand 2003;47(9):1114-1118.

210. Sperry JL, Minei JP, Frankel HL, et al. Early use of vasopressors after injury: caution before constriction. J Trauma 2008;64(1):9-14.

211. Stadlbauer KH, Wagner-Berger HG, Raedler C, et al. Vasopressin, but not fluid resuscitation, enhances survival in a liver trauma model with uncontrolled and otherwise lethal hemorrhagic shock in pigs. Anesthesiology 2003;98(3):699-704.

212. Stadlbauer KH, Wagner-Berger HG, Krismer AC, et al. Vasopressin improves survival in a porcine model of abdominal vascular injury. Crit Care 2007;11(4):R81.

213. Strohmenger HU, Krismer A, Wenzel V. Vasopressin in shock states. Curr Opin Anaesthesiol 2003;16(2):159-164.

214. Voelckel WG, Lurie KG, McKnite S, et al. Comparison of epinephrine and vasopressin in a pediatric porcine model of asphyxial cardiac arrest. Crit Care Med 2000;28(12):3777-3783.

215. Voelckel WG, Lurie KG, McKnite S, et al. Comparison of epinephrine with vasopressin on bone marrow blood flow in an animal model of hypovolemic shock and subsequent cardiac arrest. Crit Care Med 2001;29(8):1587-1592.

216. Voelckel WG, Raedler C, Wenzel V, et al. Arginine vasopressin, but not epinephrine, improves survival in uncontrolled hemorrhagic shock after liver trauma in pigs. Crit Care Med 2003;31(4):1160-1165.

217. Wenzel V, Lindner KH, Prengel AW, et al. Vasopressin improves vital organ blood flow after prolonged cardiac arrest with postcountershock pulseless electrical activity in pigs. Crit Care Med 1999;27(3):486-492.

218. Wenzel V, Raab H, Dunser MW. Arginine vasopressin: a promising rescue drug in the treatment of uncontrolled haemorrhagic shock. Best Pract Res Clin Anaesthesiol 2008;22(2):299-316.

219. Wenzel V, Raab H, Dunser MW. Role of arginine vasopressin in the setting of cardiopulmonary resuscitation. Best Pract Res Clin Anaesthesiol 2008;22(2):287-297.

220. Feinstein AJ, Patel MB, Sanui M, et al. Resuscitation with pressors after traumatic brain injury. J Am Coll Surg 2005;201(4):536-545.

221. Feinstein AJ, Cohn SM, King DR, et al. Early vasopressin improves short-term survival after pulmonary contusion. J Trauma 2005;59(4):876-882.

222. Robin JK, Oliver JA, Landry DW. Vasopressin deficiency in the syndrome of irreversible shock. J Trauma 2003;54(5 Suppl):S149-154.

223. Cohn SM. Potential benefit of vasopressin in resuscitation of hemorrhagic shock. J Trauma 2007;62(6 Suppl):S56-57.

224. Krismer AC, Wenzel V, Stadlbauer KH, et al. Vasopressin during cardiopulmonary resuscitation: a progress report. Crit Care Med 2004;32(9 Suppl):S432-435.

225. Krismer AC, Wenzel V, Voelckel WG, et al. Employing vasopressin as an adjunct vasopressor in uncontrolled traumatic hemorrhagic shock. Three cases and a brief analysis of the literature. Anaesthesist 2005;54(3):220-224.

226. Wenzel V, Lindner KH, Krismer AC, et al. Repeated administration of vasopressin but not epinephrine maintains coronary perfusion pressure after early and late administration during prolonged cardiopulmonary resuscitation in pigs. Circulation 1999;99(10):1379-1384.

227. Wenzel V, Ewy GA, Lindner KH. Vasopressin and endothelin during cardiopulmonary resuscitation. Crit Care Med 2000;28(11 Suppl):N233-235.

228. Wenzel V, Lindner KH. Vasopressin and epinephrine for cardiac arrest. Lancet 2001;358(9298):2080-2081.

229. Wenzel V, Krismer AC, Arntz HR, et al. A comparison of vasopressin and epinephrine for out-of-hospital cardiopulmonary resuscitation. N Engl J Med 2004;350(2):105-113.

230. Wenzel V, Kern KB, Hilwig RW, et al. Effects of intravenous arginine vasopressin on epicardial coronary artery cross sectional area in a swine resuscitation model. Resuscitation 2005;64(2):219-226.

231. Wenzel V, Lindner KH. Vasopressin combined with epinephrine during cardiac resuscitation: a solution for the future? Crit Care 2006;10(1):125.

232. Oz MC, Cosgrove DM III, Badduke BR, et al. Controlled clinical trial of a novel hemostatic agent in cardiac surgery. The Fusion Matrix Study Group. Ann Thorac Surg 2000;69(5):1376-1382.

233. Renkens KL Jr, Payner TD, Leipzig TJ, et al. A multicenter, prospective, randomized trial evaluating a new hemostatic agent for spinal surgery. Spine 2001;26(15):1645-1650.

234. Reuthebuch O, Lachat ML, Vogt P, et al. FloSeal: a new hemostyptic agent in peripheral vascular surgery. Vasa 2000;29(3):204-206.

235. Howes DW, Stratford A, Stirling M, et al. Administration of recombinant factor VIIa decreases blood loss after blunt trauma in noncoagulopathic pigs. J Trauma 2007;62(2):311-315.

236. Jeroukhimov I, Jewelewicz D, Zaias J, et al. Early injection of high-dose recombinant factor VIIa

decreases blood loss and prolongs time from injury to death in experimental liver injury. J Trauma 2002;53(6):1053-1057.

237. Lynn M, Jerokhimov I, Jewelewicz D, et al. Early use of recombinant factor VIIa improves mean arterial pressure and may potentially decrease mortality in experimental hemorrhagic shock: a pilot study. J Trauma 2002;52(4):703-707.

238. Martinowitz U, Holcomb JB, Pusateri AE, et al. Intravenous rFVIIa administered for hemorrhage control in hypothermic coagulopathic swine with grade V liver injuries. J Trauma 2001;50(4):721-729.

239. Schreiber MA, Holcomb JB, Hedner U, et al. The effect of recombinant factor VIIa on coagulopathic pigs with grade V liver injuries. J Trauma 2002;53(2):252-257.

240. Bauza G, Hirsch E, Burke P, et al. Low-dose recombinant activated factor VII in massively transfused trauma patients with coagulopathy. Transfusion 2007;47(4):749-751.

241. Benharash P, Bongard F, Putnam B. Use of recombinant factor VIIa for adjunctive hemorrhage control in trauma and surgical patients. Am Surg 2005;71(9):776-780.

242. Brandsborg S, Sorensen B, Poulsen LH, et al. Recombinant activated factor VIIa in uncontrolled bleeding: a haemostasis laboratory study in non-haemophilia patients. Blood Coagul Fibrinolysis 2006;17(4):241-249.

243. Christians K, Brasel K, Garlitz J, et al. The use of recombinant activated factor VII in trauma-associated hemorrhage with crush injury. J Trauma 2005;59(3):742-746.

244. Dutton RP, Hess JR, Scalea TM. Recombinant factor VIIa for control of hemorrhage: early experience in critically ill trauma patients. J Clin Anesth 2003;15(3):184-188.

245. Dutton RP, McCunn M, Hyder M, et al. Factor VIIa for correction of traumatic coagulopathy. J Trauma 2004;57(4):709-718.

246. Eikelboom JW, Bird R, Blythe D, et al. Recombinant activated factor VII for the treatment of life-threatening haemorrhage. Blood Coagul Fibrinolysis 2003;14(8):713-717.

247. Felfernig M; European rFVIIa Trauma Study Group. Clinical experience with recombinant activated factor VII in a series of 45 trauma patients. J R Army Med Corps 2007;153(1):32-39.

248. Ganguly S, Spengel K, Tilzer LL, et al. Recombinant factor VIIa: unregulated continuous use in patients with bleeding and coagulopathy does not alter mortality and outcome. Clin Lab Haematol 2006;28(5):309-312.

249. Geeraedts LM Jr, Kamphuisen PW, Kaasjager HA, et al. The role of recombinant factor VIIa in the treatment of life-threatening haemorrhage in blunt trauma. Injury 2005;36(4):495-500.

250. Gowers CJ, Parr MJ. Recombinant activated factor VIIa use in massive transfusion and coagulopathy unresponsive to conventional therapy. Anaesth Intensive Care 2005;33(2):196-200.

251. Harrison TD, Laskosky J, Jazaeri O, et al. "Low-dose" recombinant activated factor VII results in less blood and blood product use in traumatic hemorrhage. J Trauma 2005;59(1):150-154.

252. Holcomb JB, Hoots K, Moore FA. Treatment of an acquired coagulopathy with recombinant activated factor VII in a damage-control patient. Mil Med 2005;170(4):287-290.

253. Martinowitz U, Kenet G, Segal E, et al. Recombinant activated factor VII for adjunctive hemorrhage control in trauma. J Trauma 2001;51(3):431-438.

254. Martinowitz U, Kenet G, Lubetski A, et al. Possible role of recombinant activated factor VII (rFVIIa) in the control of hemorrhage associated with massive trauma. Can J Anaesth 2002;49(10):S15-20.

255. Mayo A, Misgav M, Kluger Y, et al. Recombinant activated factor VII (NovoSeven): addition to replacement therapy in acute, uncontrolled and life-threatening bleeding. Vox Sang 2004;87(1):34-40.

256. McMullin NR, Kauvar DS, Currier HM, et al. The clinical and laboratory response to recombinant factor VIIA in trauma and surgical patients with acquired coagulopathy. Curr Surg 2006;63(4):246-251.

257. O'Connell NM, Perry DJ, Hodgson AJ, et al. Recombinant FVIIa in the management of uncontrolled hemorrhage. Transfusion 2003;43(12):1711-1716.

258. O'Connor JV, Stein DM, Dutton RP, et al. Traumatic hemoptysis treated with recombinant human factor VIIa. Ann Thorac Surg 2006;81(4):1485-1487.

259. O'Neill PA, Bluth M, Gloster ES, et al. Successful use of recombinant activated factor VII for trauma-associated hemorrhage in a patient without preexisting coagulopathy. J Trauma 2002;52(2):400-405.

260. Udy A, Vaghela M, Lawton G, et al. The use of recombinant activated factor VII in the control of haemorrhage following blunt pelvic trauma. Anaesthesia 2005;60(6):613-616.

261. Boffard KD, Riou B, Warren B, et al. Recombinant factor VIIa as adjunctive therapy for bleeding control in severely injured trauma patients: two parallel randomized, placebo-controlled, double-blind clinical trials. J Trauma 2005;59(1):8-15.

262. Dutton R, Hauser C, Boffard K, et al.; CONTROL Steering Committee. Scientific and logistical challenges in designing the CONTROL trial: recombinant factor VIIa in severe trauma patients with refractory bleeding. Clin Trials 2009 Oct;6(5):467-479.

263. Johansson P. Off-label use of recombinant factor VIIa for treatment of haemorrhage: results from randomized clinical trials. Vox Sang 2008;95(1):1-7. Epub 2008 Apr 23.

264. Hardy JF, Belisle S, Van der Linden P. Efficacy and safety of recombinant activated factor VII to

control bleeding in nonhemophiliac patients: a review of 17 Randomized Controlled Trials. Ann Thorac Surg 2008;86(3):1038-1048.

265. Von Heymann C, Jonas S, Spies C, et al. Recombinant activated factor VIIa for the treatment of bleeding in major abdominal surgery including vascular and urological surgery: a review and meta-analysis of published data. Crit Care 2008;12(1):R14.

266. Thomas GO, Dutton RP, Hemlock B, et al. Thromboembolic complications associated with factor VIIa administration. J Trauma 2007;62(3):564-569.

267. Aledort LM. Comparative thrombotic event incidence after infusion of recombinant factor VIIa versus VIII inhibitor bypass activity. J Thromb Haemost 2004;2(10):1700-1708.

268. O'Connell KA, Wood JJ, Wise RP, et al. Thromboembolic adverse events after use of recombinant human coagulation factor VIIa. JAMA 2006;295(3):293-298.

269. Levy JH, Fingerhut A, Brott T, Recombinant factor VIIa in patients with coagulopathy secondary to anticoagulant therapy, cirrhosis, or severe traumatic injury: review of safety profile. Transfusion 2006;46(6):919-933.

270. Porte RJ, Leebeek FW. Pharmacological strategies to decrease transfusion requirements in patients undergoing surgery. Drugs 2002;62(15):2193-2211.

271. FDA Requests Marketing Suspension of Trasylol®. U.S. Food and Drug Administration Website, U.S. Food and Drug Administration, 2007. (Accessed January 13, 2010, at http://www.fda.gov/NewsEvents/Newsroom/PressAnnouncements/2007/ucm109021.htm.)

272. Amicar® (aminocaproic acid), package insert, 2008a.

273. Cyclokapron® (tranexamic acid), package insert, 2008c.

274. Coats T, Roberts I, Shakur H. Antifibrinolytic drugs for acute traumatic injury. Cochrane Database Syst Rev 2004;(4):CD004896.

275. Roberts I. Clinical Randomisation of an Antifibrinolytic in Significant Haemorrhage, 2009. (Accessed January 12, 2010, at http://clinicaltrials.gov/ct2/show/NCT00375258.)

276. Perkins JG, Cap AP, Spinella PC, et al. Comparison of platelet transfusion as fresh whole blood versus apheresis platelets for massively transfused combat trauma patients. Transfusion, 2011;51(2):242-252.

# DAMAGE CONTROL SURGERY

*Chapter 5*

**Contributing Authors**
Brian J. Eastridge, MD, COL, MC, US Army
Lorne H. Blackbourne, MD, COL, MC, US Army
Todd Rasmussen, MD, LTC, US Air Force
Henry Cryer, MD
Alan Murdock, MD, LTC, US Air Force

**Disclaimer**

# Table of Contents

# Introduction to Damage Control

Damage control surgery techniques have evolved within the continuum of military and civilian trauma care since the Napoleonic Wars. Though civilian trauma surgeons now uniformly embrace the relatively contemporary label "damage control," the techniques have firm foundation within the history of military medicine.[1] In the later part of the 18th century during the Napoleonic campaign, the French surgeon Larrey succinctly alluded to the rationale for expedited battlefield procedures: "When a limb is so much injured by a gunshot wound that it cannot be saved, it should be amputated immediately. The first 24 hours is the only period during which the system remains tranquil, and we should hasten during this time, as in all dangerous diseases, to adopt the necessary remedy."[2] Military historical references to the techniques of damage control surgery in the United States (US) appear around the time of the Civil War (Fig. 1).[3] In World War II, the Second Auxiliary Surgery Group treated over 22,000 combat wounded soldiers, including 8,800 "severely wounded," during a two-year interval from 1943 to 1945.[4] The ensuing 912-page report and scientific publications that were consequent to the operation yielded insight into the surgical treatment of thoracic injury; the reactive

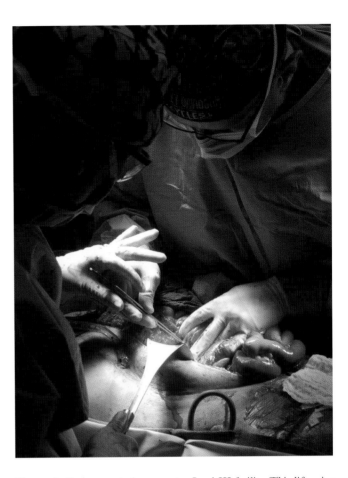

Figure 1. *Damage control surgery at a Level III facility. This lifesaving surgical paradigm now includes thoracic, vascular, orthopedic, and neurosurgical procedures.*

lung injury associated with severe trauma denoted "the wet lung of trauma," which we now know as acute respiratory distress syndrome (ARDS); and the utility of techniques aimed at the "correction of profound physiologic disturbances which immediately endanger life" is now described by the moniker, damage control. In the Vietnam War, it was recognized in several case series that temporizing surgical procedures often demonstrated a survival advantage when compared to definitive surgical therapy.[5] Though apparently temporarily forgotten after the Vietnam War, the technique reappeared in the hallmark publication by Stone in 1983, which advocated abbreviated celiotomy in patients with abdominal injury with associated coagulopathy and hypothermia.[6] Since that time, many reported successes with similar salvage techniques have been cited.[7,8,9,10] Within the last decade, a number of authors have also described the expansion of this lifesaving surgical practice to include thoracic, vascular, orthopedic, and neurosurgical procedures.[11,12,13,14]

# General Principles of Damage Control

Modern day concepts of damage control have been honed in the civilian sector resulting in survival rates of 50 percent in severely injured patients in hemorrhagic shock.[15,16,17,18,19,20,21,22] Damage control as it is currently practiced is simply defined as the rapid initial control of hemorrhage and contamination with packing and a temporary closure, followed by physiologic resuscitation in the intensive care unit (ICU), and subsequent reexploration and definitive repair once normal physiology has been restored (Fig. 2). From a military perspective, damage control concepts apply to all body regions, with an emphasis on abbreviated and focused surgery on patients expected to survive, thus conserving resources and allowing definitive care at the next level of care.

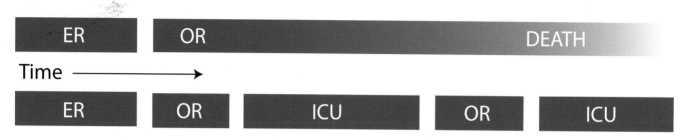

Figure 2. *Damage control procedures are defined by an abbreviated surgery, followed by resuscitation in the ICU, with subsequent reexploration and definitive repair once normal physiology has been restored. This approach has led to improved patient survival.*

Rapidly achieving these objectives in severely injured trauma patients is crucial to mitigating the trauma "lethal triad" of hypothermia, acidosis, and coagulopathy.[23] The acidosis results from hypovolemic shock and inadequate tissue perfusion. Hypothermia results from exsanguination and loss of intrinsic thermoregulation. Coagulopathy results from hypothermia, acidemia, platelet and clotting factors consumption, and blood loss. Coagulopathy, in turn, causes more hemorrhage and thus causes more acidosis and hypothermia; so the "bloody vicious cycle" continues. Once established, this vicious cycle is almost uniformly fatal and must be prevented using damage control principles rather than attempting to treat it once it has occurred.

> Damage control surgery is defined as the rapid initial control of hemorrhage and contamination with packing and temporary closure, followed by resuscitation in the ICU, and subsequent reexploration and definitive repair once normal physiology has been restored.

While the current principles of damage control in well-equipped trauma centers have led to improved survival, the combat environment offers challenges and adds complexity to the practice of damage control. Nonetheless, descriptions of military applications of damage control procedures have recently emerged in the trauma literature. Although these publications comprise a small series of patients, they suggest that damage control in the combat environment is as effective as it is in civilian trauma care.[24,25,26,27]

As currently configured, the military process involves the simultaneous and coordinated operation, resuscitation, and serial evacuation of the casualty, via both rotary-wing and fixed-wing aircraft, through several levels of military medical care across continents (Fig. 3). The feasibility of damage control in combat casualty care (CCC) settings is dependent upon: (1) the availability of resources to prevent and treat hypothermia, coagulopathy, and acidosis; and (2) the ability to provide supportive care pending staged reoperation or evacuation from theater with subsequent staged operation in Germany, future Level IV facilities, or the US. Central to CCC that takes place in the relatively resource-constrained environment of a theater of war is the capability of military Level II and Level III care facilities to supply blood components, including packed red blood cells, plasma, and platelets commensurate with demand

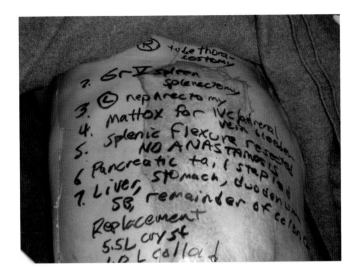

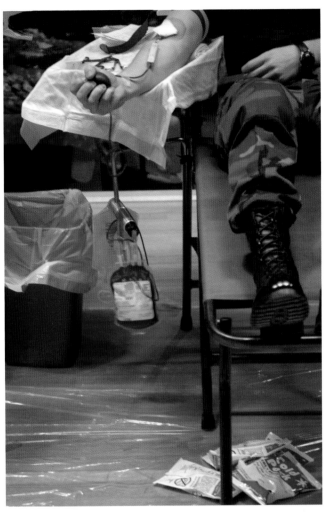

Figure 3. (Above) *Improvised patient information communication written directly onto a dressing following damage control surgery. The current military process involves simultaneous and coordinated operation, resuscitation, and serial evacuation of casualties through several levels of combat casualty care across continents, making accurate communication exceedingly important.*

Figure 4. (Right) *The walking blood bank can rapidly collect fresh whole blood when other blood products are in short supply. Image courtesy of Defense Imagery Management Operations Center (DIMOC).*

The military CCC process involves the simultaneous and coordinated operation, resuscitation, and serial evacuation of the casualty, via both rotary-wing and fixed-wing aircraft, through several levels of military medical care across continents.

Recent advances in the concept of damage control resuscitation (DCR) have resulted in the transfusion of one unit of plasma for each unit of packed red blood cells in the massive transfusion setting.[28] This novel paradigm of resuscitation is thought to be largely responsible for the substantially decreased mortality from coagulopathy in the most severely injured casualties.[29] Another novel concept developed by the military has been the use of the walking blood bank using fresh whole blood donated by soldiers on site, when large stores of fresh frozen plasma and packed red blood cells are in short supply (Fig. 4).[30]

Damage control resuscitation is a strategy that seeks to prevent or mitigate hypothermia, acidosis, and coagulopathy through combined treatment paradigms. Damage control resuscitation comprises early hemorrhage control, hypotensive resuscitation (permissive hypotension), hemostatic resuscitation (minimization of crystalloid fluids and fixed ratio blood product transfusion), prevention or alleviation of hypothermia (through warming measures), and amelioration of acidosis through judicious use of blood products and hemodynamic resuscitation endpoints.

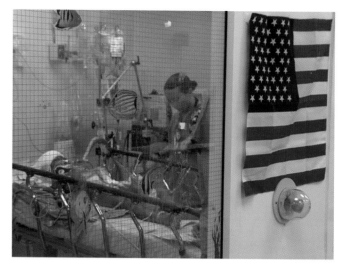

Figure 5. (Top Right) *Intensive care units at Level III facilities are robustly resourced such that care received on the battlefield is akin to care at any Level I trauma center in the US.*

Figure 6. (Bottom Left) *All US and coalition casualties with critical care requirements in the current conflicts in Iraq and Afghanistan are flown out-of-theater to Germany with the assistance of a CCATT. Image courtesy of Donald C. Kowalewski, LTC, MC, USAF.*

Figure 7. (Bottom Right) *The CCATT teams facilitate the rapid evacuation of severely ill patients, which translates into better patient care as well as a significantly decreased forward medical footprint. Image courtesy of Donald C. Kowalewski, LTC, MC, USAF.*

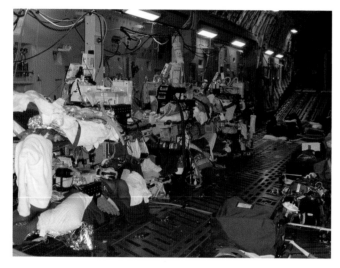 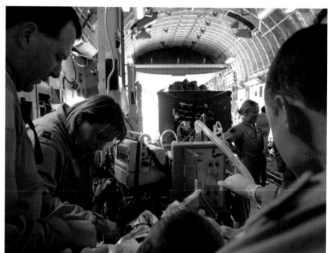

Given the battlefield constraints of multiple-casualty-incidents, the need for rapid turnover of operating rooms, and the limited number of critical care beds, it is more advantageous to resource allocation and utilization to perform damage control procedures early. Intensive care units at Level III facilities are robustly staffed and resourced such that care received on the battlefield of Iraq and Afghanistan is akin to care at any Level I trauma center in the US (Fig. 5). However, operational tempo limits the combat casualty's ability to occupy an ICU bed for an extended length of time.

One of the most substantial advances in recent military medicine, the Critical Care Aeromedical Transport Team (CCATT), has been instrumental in circumventing this problem. These teams provide en-route intensive care to patients requiring evacuation. Most US and coalition casualties spend less than 48 hours in-theater and many times in high-acuity cases, less than 24 hours (Figs. 6 and 7).[31,32,33] With such advanced surgical and critical care capacity, it is feasible to care for the high-acuity patient requiring damage control surgery within the combat theater during the acute surgical, postoperative intensive care stabilization, reoperation, and evacuation phases. As such, the philosophy of damage control continues to be appealing within the realm of CCC, since encompassed within the contingencies of the modern battlefield are a finite pool of manpower and therapeutic resources, a nonlinear battlefield with a highly mobile force, a multiplicity of casualties, and highly destructive mechanisms of injury.

# Thoracic Injury Damage Control

## *Emergency Thoracotomy*

Thoracic damage control surgery can be stratified into two domains: procedures that occur in the emergency department (ED) and those that take place in the operating room. Thoracic procedures that are undertaken in the ED are reserved for those patients who present in extremis with signs and symptoms suggestive of thoracic injury. Collective reviews in the literature have demonstrated survival rates of 8.8 to 11.1 percent for penetrating injury and 1.4 to 1.6 percent for blunt injury after resuscitative thoracotomy for civilian injury.[34,35] In a related combat-environment setting analysis, 12 of 94 patients undergoing resuscitative thoracotomy for penetrating injuries survived, while none of the seven patients with blunt injury survived. Of note, this military study expanded the indication for resuscitative thoracotomy for patients in extremis with injuries to the abdomen (30 percent) and extremities (22 percent).[36]

> The objectives of a thoracotomy are to: (1) confirm ventilatory support by observing expansion of the left lung; (2) open the pericardium to relieve pericardial tamponade; (3) apply occlusive pressure and clamp the descending aorta to restore central perfusion to the brain and heart; (4) provide direct cardiac compression to circulate blood; and (5) control visible hemorrhage.

The basic conduct of resuscitative thoracotomy includes simultaneous left-sided anterolateral thoracotomy with establishment of an airway and ventilatory support, chest tube placement in the contralateral chest cavity, large-bore intravenous access, and initiation of a massive transfusion protocol with a 1:1 ratio of fresh frozen plasma to packed red blood cells or the use of fresh whole blood. The thoracotomy is initiated with an expeditious and generous left anterolateral chest incision in the fifth intercostal space (i.e., below the nipple at the inframammary fold) carried down to the chest wall sharply (Fig. 8). At this point, one blade of a pair of heavy Mayo scissors is inserted into the pleural space on the cephalad edge of the sixth rib, and with a pushing stroke the intercostal musculature is opened both posteriorly and anteriorly to the sternal edge. Care must be taken to incise along the curvature of the ribs to avoid accidentally transecting ribs. This will minimize injury to the intercostal neurovascular bundle and avoid creating sharp bone margins capable of creating iatrogenic injury to careproviders. A rib-spreading retractor is placed within the thoracotomy incision with the handle positioned downward toward the bed and opened to expose the left thoracic cavity. Once the thoracic cavity has been exposed, the objectives of the procedure are to: (1) confirm ventilatory support by observing expansion of the left lung; (2) open the pericardium anterior to the phrenic nerve to relieve pericardial tamponade; (3) apply occlusive pressure and clamp the descending aorta to restore central perfusion to the brain and heart; (4) provide direct cardiac compression to circulate blood; and (5) control visible hemorrhage. Although most careproviders perform cardiac compressions by holding the heart between their hands (mostly fingers due to space constraints), compressions are generally more efficient with placement of the palm of one hand on the posterior heart and pressing upward towards the sternum (Fig. 9).

The pericardium is grasped with DeBakey forceps anterior to the phrenic nerve, and the pericardial sac is opened completely with Metzenbaum scissors in a craniocaudal direction so as not to injure the phrenic nerve. Once the pericardium is incised, the tamponade is relieved and the heart can be delivered into the left chest. If obvious ongoing hemorrhage from the heart is noted, it is initially controlled with digital pressure. The descending aorta can either be compressed manually against the spine or clamped

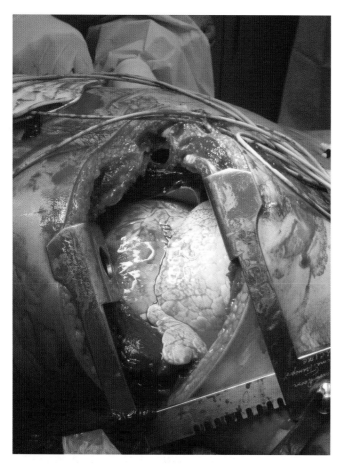

with a vascular clamp. Lifting the lung anteriorly helps to visualize the posterior mediastinum and facilitates direct access to the aorta. Once the posterior mediastinum is visualized, the parietal pleura is incised, and the opening extended bluntly anteriorly as well as posteriorly along the spine to allow insertion of a large vascular clamp across the aorta. Direct visualization is also useful so that the clamp is not inadvertently placed on the esophagus or below the level of an aortic injury, thereby exacerbating hemorrhage. Adjunctive measures to attain visualization and vascular control include a surgical assistant compressing the lung anteriorly, temporarily disconnecting the patient from positive-

Figure 8. (Left) *Emergency thoracotomy is reserved for patients presenting in extremis with signs and symptoms suggestive of thoracic injury. Image courtesy of J. Christian Fox, MD, University of California, Irvine.*

Figure 9. (Below) *Although many careproviders perform cardiac compressions by holding the heart between their hands, compressions may be more efficient by placing the palm of one hand on the posterior heart and pressing upward towards the sternum. Image courtesy of J. Christian Fox, MD, University of California, Irvine.*

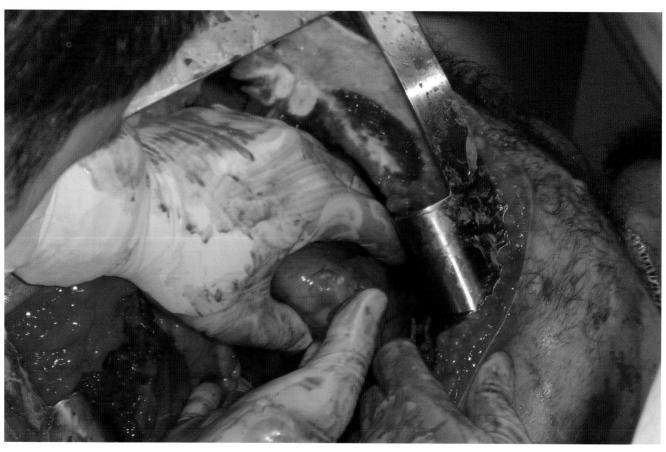

pressure ventilation, or performing a right mainstem bronchus intubation if the patient's cardiopulmonary status can tolerate single-lung ventilation. The inferior pulmonary ligament must be released from the diaphragm via sharp dissection to allow full exposure of the mediastinal structures.

Hemorrhage from penetrating cardiac wounds can often initially be controlled through digital pressure or occlusion. Atrial hemorrhage can also be temporized with a tangential vascular clamp and subsequently undergo a simple 3-0 Prolene™ running suture repair. If digital pressure is not sufficient to control ventricular bleeding, hemorrhage can be temporized with Foley catheter or Fogarty balloon tamponade, suture repair, or stapling (which is quick and effective for small lacerations).[37,38,39,40] If a Foley catheter is used, it is important to completely flush the catheter with crystalloid solution to avoid subsequent air embolism upon introduction of the catheter into the injured heart. While controlling hemorrhage through suture repair of the ventricles, it is paramount to spare the coronary arteries (i.e., avoid accidentally ligating them). This can be performed by tying pledgeted suture bolsters on opposing sides of the coronary artery at-risk using vertical mattress sutures, while at the same time approximating the cardiac wound (Fig. 10).

> If digital pressure or occlusion is not sufficient to control ventricular bleeding, hemorrhage can be temporized with Foley catheter or Fogarty balloon tamponade, suture repair, or stapling.

Control of hemorrhage from major thoracic vascular structures can be obtained by clamping or compressing affected vessels under direct visualization. In the circumstance where additional exposure to the right heart or right hemithorax is required, a left-sided anterolateral thoracotomy can be converted into a clamshell thoracotomy. This is done by extending the incision through the right fifth intercostal space after transecting the sternum with either a Gigli saw, Lebsche knife, heavy bone cutter, or electric sternal saw (Fig. 11). This incision provides the best exposure to the entire anterior and superior mediastinum and both pleural spaces by extending the incision to right chest above the nipple in a gentle S-shaped configuration. Vascular control of the internal mammary arteries following thoracotomy is important to prevent further blood loss and can be obtained by clamping or suture ligation.

Once a cardiac rhythm has been restored and bleeding temporarily controlled, the patient is expeditiously taken to the operating room. Such patients are at significant risk for the lethal triad of coagulopathy, acidosis, and hypothermia, so efforts to prevent and treat these conditions must be made during the resuscitative process. Once in the operating room, the patient is prepped and draped. Cardiac wounds can now be definitively repaired. When suturing ventricular cardiac wounds, it is important to use pledgets fashioned from Teflon® strips or pericardium to prevent suture shearing through the myocardium upon tying. Coronary vascular injuries occurring in combat typically require ligation, as coronary revascularization requires a cardiac bypass technician, bypass pump, and cardiac surgeon.

> When suturing ventricular cardiac wounds, it is important to use pledgets fashioned from Teflon® strips or pericardium to prevent suture shearing through the myocardium upon tying. Additionally, it is paramount to avoid ligation of the coronary arteries when performing suture repair of the heart.

### Intrathoracic Vascular Injury

Vascular injuries to the thorax (aorta and proximal arterial and venous branch vessels) are treated with basic

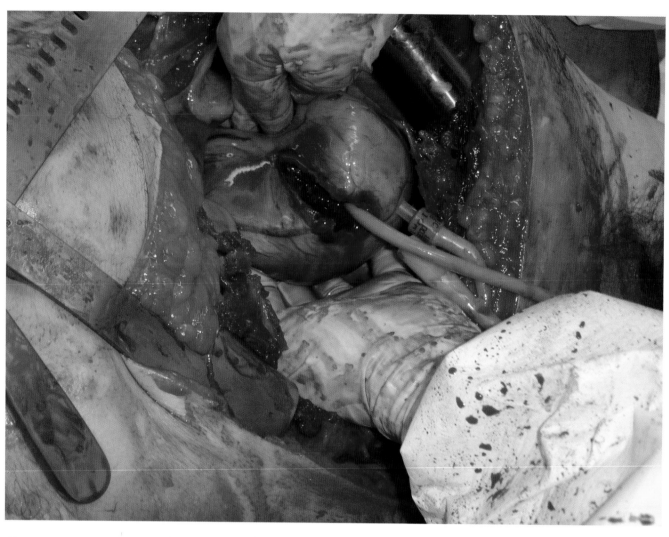

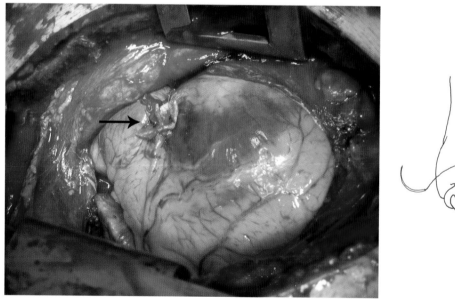

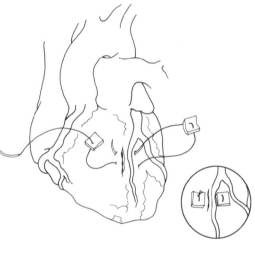

Figure 10. *Bleeding from penetrating trauma to the heart may be temporized with digital pressure (occlusion), Foley catheter or Fogarty balloon tamponade, suture repair, or stapling. When suturing or stapling, it is vital to avoid occlusion of a coronary artery. Images courtesy of J. Christian Fox, MD, University of California, Irvine and the Borden Institute, Office of The Surgeon General, Washington, DC.*

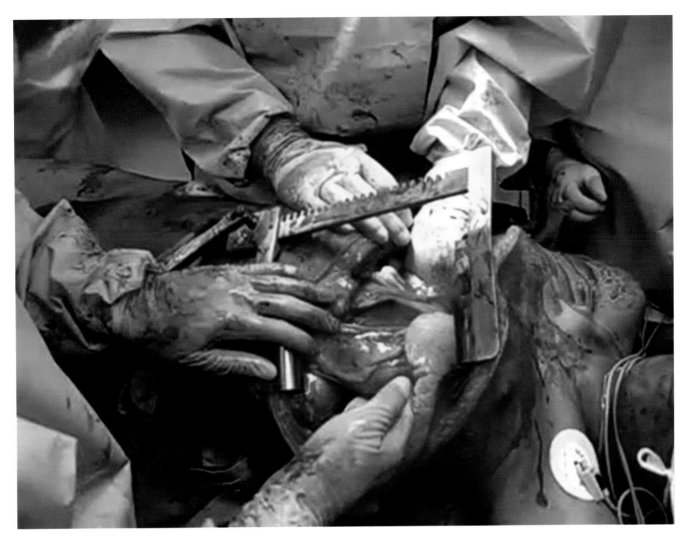

Figure 11. *If additional exposure to the right heart or right hemithorax is required, a left-sided anterolateral thoracotomy can be converted into a clamshell thoracotomy. Image courtesy of J. Christian Fox, MD, University of California, Irvine.*

proximal and distal vascular control and reconstitution of flow principles. Injuries to the aorta require repair. Lateral aortorrhaphy or primary tension-free repair are preferable, although in the authors' experience, in extreme circumstances the aorta can be transiently shunted with a large-bore chest tube tied into position above and below the injury site with large suture or umbilical tape.

Control of the descending thoracic aorta is easily obtainable through a left-sided anterolateral thoracotomy. Exposure of the proximal left subclavian and proximal left common carotid artery is limited from a true left-sided anterolateral thoracotomy and would be better obtained via a more traditional posterolateral thoracotomy. A "book" or "trapdoor" incision would provide better exposure of a long segment of the left common carotid and left subclavian artery. This surgical approach is seldom used due to lack of familiarity, as well as complications related to stretch on the brachial plexus and upper posterior costal junctions, resulting in neurologic and upper back pain syndromes.[41] It should be only used when control and repair are absolutely necessary. A better approach to specifically control subclavian artery hemorrhage would be an anterolateral thoracotomy via a third intercostal space incision combined with a separate infraclavicular incision for definitive repair.[42] Visualization of the subclavian artery and vein, particularly more distally, can be facilitated by resection of the clavicle.

Injuries to the aortic arch vessels and definitive repairs usually require a median sternotomy. As a general principle, dissection into mediastinal hematomas can be disorienting, so it is often useful to open the pericardium and trace vessels upward. The left innominate vein can be divided in order to identify the innominate artery, and the dissection can then continue cephalad. Due to relatively large vessel caliber, the best management method for injuries to thoracic outlet arteries is usually bypass using a synthetic conduit. However, in a damage control scenario, this may not be possible. In extreme circumstances, most aortic arch arteries can be singly ligated since the vigorous collateral flow of the cervical and thoracoacromial region will usually sustain acceptable perfusion. Ligation of cervical vessels carries the risk of stroke, and subclavian and innominate artery ligations carry the risk of limb ischemia. Except for the superior vena cava, injuries to the thoracic venous system can be repaired with lateral venorrhaphy or ligated. Injuries to the superior vena cava should be repaired.

> In extreme circumstances, most aortic arch arteries can be singly ligated since the collateral flow of the cervical and thoracoacromial region will usually sustain acceptable perfusion.

## Pulmonary and Tracheobronchial Injuries

Pulmonary and tracheobronchial damage control procedures are performed to control hemorrhage or air leak. With respect to pulmonary injury, the three main damage control procedures are: (1) nonanatomic pulmonary resection; (2) pulmonary tractotomy; and (3) pneumonectomy (Figs. 12 and 13). Nonanatomic resections using a GIA™ or TA™ stapler are generally preferred for peripheral injuries with ongoing hemorrhage or air leak. The advantage of the nonanatomic resection over anatomic resection is the reduction in time associated with not having to develop formal lobar surgical planes. However, if deeper bleeding persists after pneumorrhaphy or nonanatomic pulmonary resection, this must be addressed with further exposure and repair or ligation. When this occurs or when there is profuse hemorrhage from deeper within

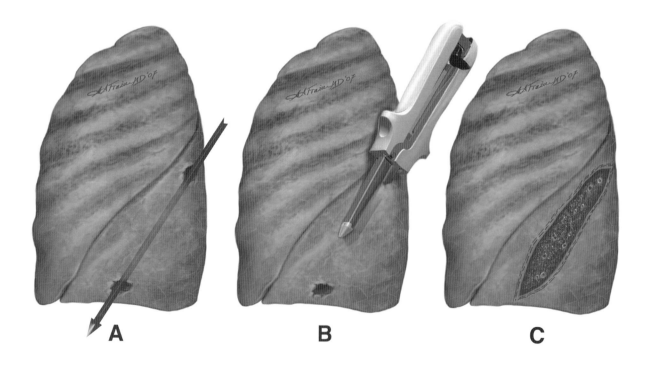

Figure 12. *Illustration of pulmonary tractotomy. Image courtesy of the Borden Institute, Office of The Surgeon General, Washington, DC. Illustrator: Aletta Frazier, MD.*

the lung parenchyma from penetrating injury, a pulmonary tractotomy can be performed. This procedure involves placing two long vascular clamps through the pulmonary wound tract, clamping them, and incising between the two. The lung edges can then be stapled with a TA™ stapler. Alternatively, a GIA™ stapler can be advanced through the tract and fired, creating a linear passage to the source of hemorrhage. The focus of hemorrhage will lie at the base of the tract and can be sutured with 4-0 or 5-0 vascular suture.

> Pulmonary and tracheobronchial damage control procedures that are performed to control hemorrhage or air leak may include: (1) nonanatomic pulmonary resection; (2) pulmonary tractotomy; and (3) pneumonectomy.

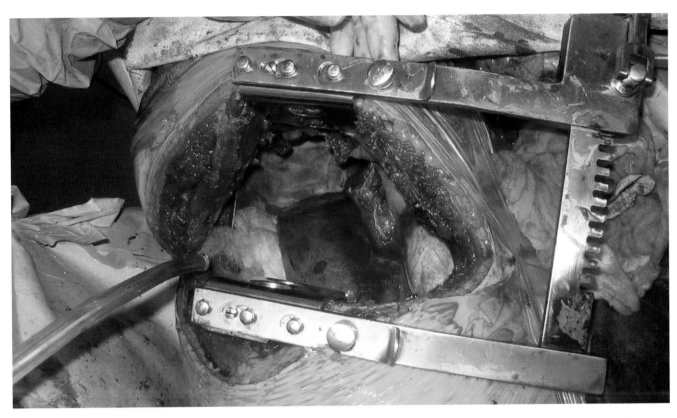

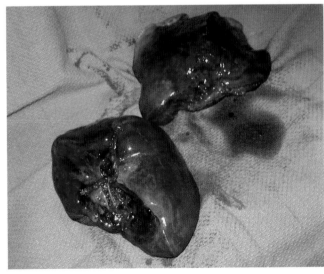

Figure 13. (Above) *Patient with penetrating right chest injury from a mortar round. A posterolateral thoracotomy was perfomed, demonstrating intact lower lobe and stapled upper and middle lobe structures.* (Right) *Resected right upper and middle lobes of the lung. Images courtesy of the Borden Institute, Office of The Surgeon General, Washington, DC.*

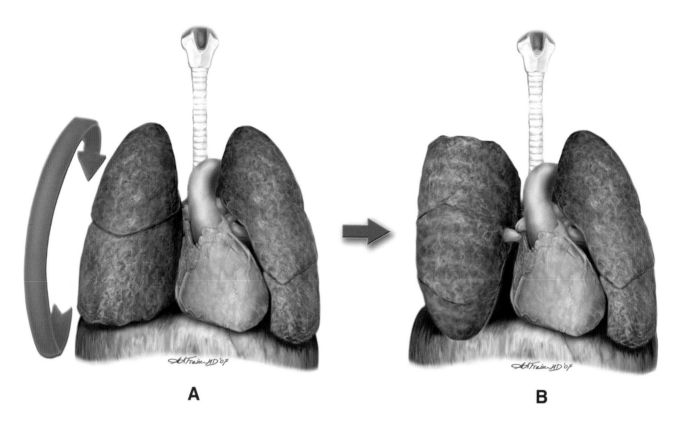

**A**  **B**

Figure 14. *Hilar clamping or "hilar twist." Image courtesy of the Borden Institute, Office of The Surgeon General, Washington, DC. Illustrator: Aletta Frazier, MD.*

In patients with global or hilar parenchymal lung injury, pneumonectomy is an option of last resort. There is a stepwise increase in mortality with more extensive lung resections that is independent of injury severity.[43] The mortality of trauma patients undergoing pneumonectomy is over 50 percent.[43,44,45] Large air leaks from the bronchial tree or major pulmonary hemorrhage can temporarily be controlled by incising the inferior pulmonary ligament and clamping the pulmonary hilum, or by twisting the lung 180 degrees around its hilar axis (Figs. 14 and 15).[46] Should pneumonectomy or hilar clamping be necessary, the hilum of the lung should be clamped slowly. This will give the other lung a chance to accommodate, and volume resuscitation should be minimized to avoid acute right heart failure, which inevitably occurs. Ligation of hilar vascular and bronchial structures should be performed by isolation, stapling, or suture ligation and buttressed with pleural or other easily mobile soft-tissue such as intercostal muscle.

## *Esophageal Injury*

The incidence of esophageal injuries is low, and injuries are most often the result of penetrating trauma.[47] The cervical esophagus represents the most common site of injury. Injuries involving less than 50 percent of the circumference of the esophagus can be closed in layers after debridement. Esophageal repairs need to be buttressed with pleural or intercostal muscles due to the tenuous nature of these types of repairs. If the injury encompasses more than 50 percent of the circumference of the esophagus, or the patient remains physiologically compromised, the esophageal injury is locally resected and the esophagus is stapled in discontinuity. The proximal esophagus should be drained via nasogastric tube. Consideration should be given to concurrently performing gastric decompression (i.e., gastrostomy tube) and feeding jejunostomy; however, both could be performed during definitive repair. The hemithorax must be widely drained with

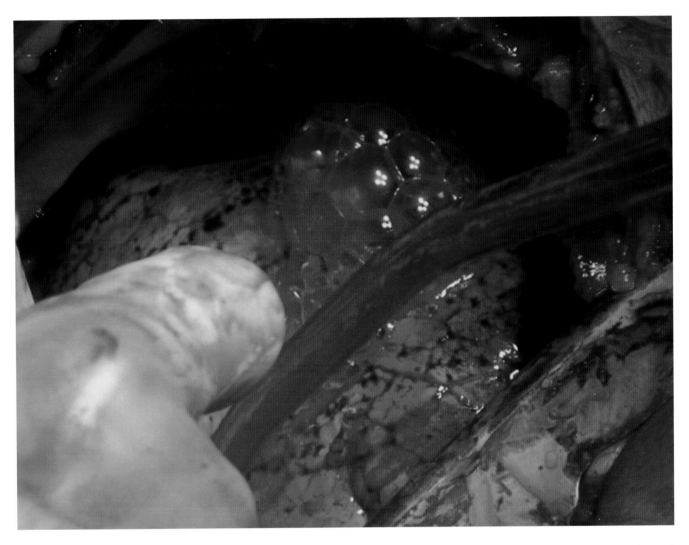

Figure 15. *A patient with penetrating injuries to the right chest. This image demonstrates the right lung after it has been mobilized and twisted around the hilum to achieve hemorrhage control. Image courtesy of the Borden Institute, Office of The Surgeon General, Washington, DC.*

a large-bore (32 French or larger) chest tube. Subsequently, definitive restitution of continuity or cervical esophagostomy can be performed once the patient has stabilized.[48,49]

> The incidence of esophageal injuries is low. Esophageal injuries are most often the result of penetrating trauma, and the cervical esophagus represents the most common site of injury.

## Neck Injury Damage Control

Vascular injury is noted in 20 percent of cases of penetrating neck trauma, and exsanguinating hemorrhage is the primary cause of death.[50] The neck is traditionally divided into three zones to aid decision making and management (Fig. 16). A more detailed discussion of damage control surgery in the neck is provided in the Maxillofacial and Neck Trauma chapter.

Zone II neck injuries with hard signs of vascular injury require immediate exploration (Fig. 17). These hard

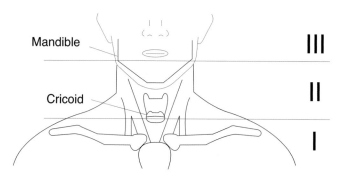

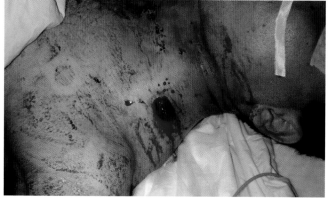

Figure 16. *The neck is commonly divided into three anatomic zones for purposes of initial assessment and management.*

Figure 17. *Penetrating neck trauma with expanding hematoma mandating immediate surgical exploration. Image courtesy of David B. Powers, DMD, MD, COL, US Air Force.*

signs include uncontrollable hemorrhage, rapidly expanding hematoma, pulsatile hemorrhage, palpable thrill or audible bruit, or signs of neurovascular compromise (Table 1).[51,52] As a general principle, the groin and upper thigh should be prepped to allow for saphenous vein interposition graft harvesting prior to vascular exploration. A standard neck incision is made from the mastoid to the sternal notch on the anterior border of the sternocleidomastoid muscle. The facial vein should be identified and ligated and the internal jugular vein retracted posteriorly using a self-retaining retractor. Injuries to the internal jugular vein can be repaired with lateral venorraphy or ligated (Fig. 18). After repairing vascular injuries in this zone, one must have a high index of suspicion and assess for esophageal and tracheal injuries.

| Hard Signs Mandating Immediate Exploration of the Neck |
| --- |
| • Uncontrollable hemorrhage |
| • Rapidly expanding hematoma |
| • Pulsatile hemorrhage |
| • Palpable thrill or audible bruit |
| • Focal neurologic compromise |
| • Absent or decreased pulses in the neck or arms |

Table 1. *Hard signs mandating immediate exploration of the neck.*

> After repairing vascular injuries in Zone II, one must have a high index of suspicion and assess for esophageal and tracheal injuries.

The common carotid artery can be explored from the thoracic inlet to the base of the skull. Suspected proximal (Zone I) carotid injury requires partial sternotomy for proximal vascular control. Injuries to the common or internal carotid arteries may be repaired using lateral arteriorrhaphy, patch angioplasty, end-to-end anastomosis, or bypass.[53] If the patient is in extremis, the common or internal carotid vessels could be ligated. This approach leads to dismal outcomes, with stroke rates exceeding 20 percent and mortality approaching 50 percent.[54] Recent studies suggest patients fare better when the internal carotid artery is repaired rather than ligated.[53] Therefore, it is advisable to repair the injury as long as the patient remains

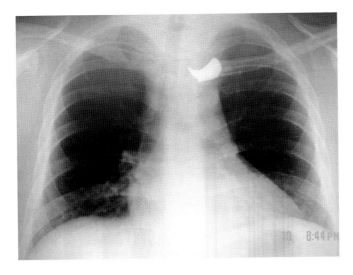

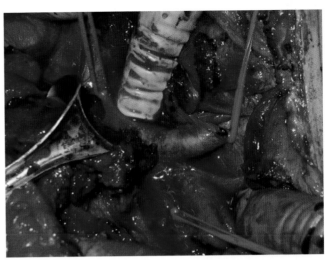

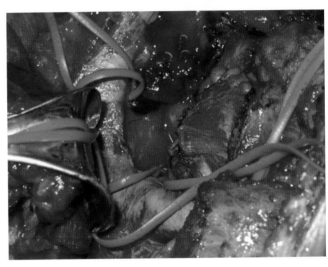

Figure 18. *Penetrating neck injury (initial point of entry was anatomic-right side of neck; Zone II). (Top Left) Preoperative radiograph demonstrates a fragment from a 40-millimeter grenade overlying the left sternoclavicular joint. (Top Right) Upon median sternotomy and exploration, the fragment was noted in the innominate vein, digital pressure was applied, and vascular control was obtained. (Bottom Right) A venorrhaphy was performed. After repairing vascular injuries in this zone, one must have a high index of suspicion and assess for esophageal and tracheal injuries. Images courtesy of the Borden Institute, Office of The Surgeon General, Washington DC.*

clinically stable. An alternative approach to ligation would be placement of a temporary shunt between the two ends tied in place with 2-0 silk suture.

In the case of a distal (Zone III) internal carotid artery injury that is too high for reconstruction, ligation is appropriate if the distal end can be ligated. In the case of a distal carotid lesion that is within the skull base, a size 3 Fogarty embolectomy catheter can be inserted into the distal end of the internal carotid artery, placing two clips just below the balloon to keep it expanded and cutting the shunt to leave the balloon in the internal carotid artery to tamponade it and allowing it to thrombose.[53] Lastly, injuries to the external carotid artery may be repaired using standard techniques or ligated. Transposition of the external carotid artery to the internal carotid artery is particularly useful when the internal carotid artery cannot be primarily repaired. This technique is used as an alternate to ligation.[55]

> Transposition of the external carotid artery to the internal carotid artery is particularly useful when the internal carotid artery cannot be primarily repaired.

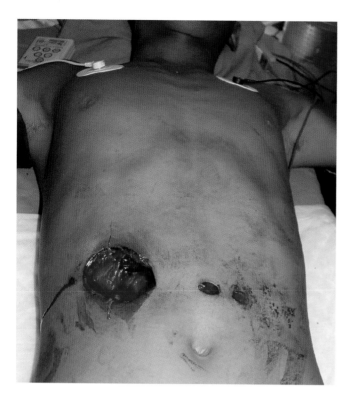

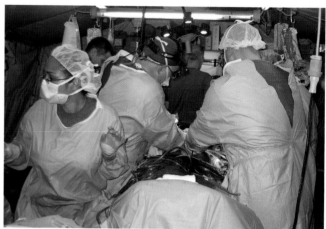

Figure 19. (Left) *Abdominal damage control surgery is indicated for abdominal injury with severe physiologic derangement. This patient was injured by an M16 round. Image courtesy of the Borden Institute, Office of The Surgeon General, Washington, DC.*

Figure 20. (Below) *Resource constraints in a battlefield environment (e.g., mass-casualty-incident) may mandate an abbreviated operation. Image courtesy of Harold Bohman, MD, CAPT, MC, US Navy.*

# Abdominal Injury Damage Control

The battlefield environment presents two discrete conditions in which damage control abdominal surgery is indicated: first and foremost is abdominal injury with severe physiologic derangement and second are the resource constraints of the austere environment. Examples of the former include casualties with penetrating abdominal injury with shock, high-velocity gunshot or abdominal penetrating injury from a secondary blast injury mechanism, or multisystem trauma with major abdominal injury (Fig. 19). An example of the latter is a mass-casualty-incident; each casualty presents with discrete surgical requirements that temporarily overwhelm the capacity of the system. This necessitates performing abbreviated operations (i.e., not definitive repairs) to accommodate all patients in an expedient manner (Fig. 20). In a recent military analysis, the presence of shock and penetrating torso injury was an independent risk factor for the requirement for damage control resuscitation and expedited operative intervention.[29,56]

## *Damage Control Laparotomy*

Early anticipation of the necessity for damage control resuscitation and surgery improves outcomes in this severely injured population.

Adequate patient preparation is essential. Once in the operating room, the patient is placed in the supine position and prepped from chest to groin. A generous midline incision is made and carried down through the midline fascia. Once the peritoneum is opened, the aorta may be manually compressed at the hiatus of the diaphragm if severe arterial hemorrhage is noted, and intraperitoneal blood can be quickly evacuated. This can be rapidly accomplished by pressing the sides of the abdomen together, expressing most of the blood and clot out onto the drapes, and subsequently packing any areas of ongoing hemorrhage. If control of hemorrhage is adequate, time is given to the anesthesiologist to restore intravascular volume in response to any decrease in blood pressure caused by releasing the peritoneal tamponade.

In patients with persistent hemorrhage from abdominal great vessel injury not amenable to packing, priority is given to inflow and outflow control of the injured vessel. Temporary aortic control can be gained at the diaphragmatic hiatus by posterior compression with a Richardson retractor or clamping of the aorta, which can be accessed through the gastrohepatic ligament. Likewise, control of the aorta can be obtained through the left chest via left-sided anterolateral thoracotomy if more proximal control is necessary. Once aortic inflow is controlled, exposure is the key to abdominal vascular control. The entire abdominal aorta and the common iliac vessels can be visualized through a left medial visceral rotation. Conversely, a right medial visceral rotation with a Catell-Braasch maneuver will allow visualization of the infrarenal inferior vena cava and the aorta up to the level of the superior mesenteric artery axis (Fig. 21). Adding a Kocher maneuver will expose the inferior vena cava to the subhepatic level as well as fully mobilize the duodenum and head of the pancreas.

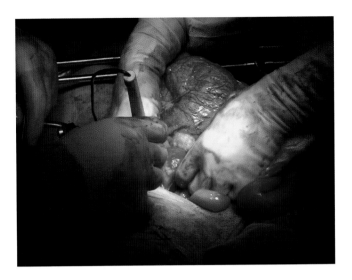

Figure 21. *A right medial visceral rotation with a Catell-Braasch maneuver will allow visualization of the infrarenal inferior vena cava and the aorta up to the level of the superior mesenteric artery axis.*

> In patients with persistent hemorrhage from abdominal great vessel injury not amenable to packing, priority is given to inflow and outflow control of the injured vessel.

Once the injury is identified, a damage control therapeutic plan can be better developed. With injuries to the suprarenal aorta, lateral arteriorrhaphy should be strongly considered since protracted clamping of the aorta at this level during repair will result in visceral ischemia and exacerbation of physiologic anomalies.[57] For an infrarenal aortic injury, an attempt should be made at local repair, and at this point aortic clamping should be reassessed and either removed or repositioned to the most distal portion of the aorta. If not feasible, an interposition tube graft is a better option than patch angioplasty. It should be remembered that in young adults, the aorta is quite small and rarely will accommodate a graft larger than 16 millimeters (mm). Repair in young or thin patients should be buttressed with omentum due to the thin retroperitoneum. In dire circumstances, a temporary chest tube shunt can be considered. The iliac arteries can likewise be shunted in the damage control setting. In select circumstances, the surgeon may need to transect the overlying right common iliac artery to expose and control an injury to the confluence of the common iliac veins for hemorrhage control.

> With injuries to the suprarenal aorta, lateral arteriorrhaphy should be strongly considered since protracted clamping of the aorta at this level during repair will result in visceral ischemia, and exacerbation of physiologic anomalies. For an infrarenal aortic injury, an attempt should be made at local repair.

## Retrohepatic Hematoma

A retrohepatic hematoma controlled with packing should not be explored. If vigorous hemorrhage is emanating from the posterior aspect of the liver, a Pringle maneuver should be performed to control hepatic arterioportal vascular inflow. If this maneuver controls the hemorrhage, then the hemorrhagic source is intrahepatic. If this maneuver does not control the hemorrhage, then there is a high likelihood that the patient has a retrohepatic vena cava injury.[58] Upon identifying a retrohepatic vena cava injury that is not amenable to tamponade by packing, an immediate decision needs to be made to approach the injury via total hepatic vascular isolation. Anesthesia must be forewarned that the isolation procedure will restrict preload from the lower half of the body so large-bore upper central venous access is mandatory. The hepatic arterioportal inflow occlusion is maintained. Then, control of the inferior vena cava above the renal veins is developed.[59] At this point, control of the suprahepatic inferior vena cava is obtained in order to minimize manipulation of the retrohepatic hematoma. This can be done most easily by gaining control within the pericardium. Pericardial access can be developed through the diaphragm or via median sternotomy and pericardiotomy.

> A retrohepatic hematoma controlled with packing should not be explored.

An alternate approach to the suprahepatic inferior vena cava would be to extend the abdominal incision via a right thoracoabdominal incision, which would also offer better exposure to the right and superior portions of the liver. In either approach, it is important to mobilize the right triangular ligament of the liver first. Once the injury is identified, it can be repaired using monofilament suture. Penetrating injuries with suspicion of injury to the subhepatic inferior vena cava require exploration. These juxtarenal caval injuries also require repair. If hemorrhage stops with repair of the anterior hole, it is not necessary and even may be counterproductive to expose the posterior wall of the vena cava looking for a posterior hole in the damage control setting. Infrarenal inferior vena cava injuries can be ligated if patient acuity dictates. Infrarenal inferior vena cava ligation is fairly well tolerated in younger patients.[60] However, ligation of the suprarenal inferior vena cava is usually associated with renal failure and massive lower extremity edema.[61,62]

> Infrarenal inferior vena cava injuries can be ligated if patient acuity dictates. However, ligation of the suprarenal inferior vena cava is usually associated with renal failure and massive lower extremity edema.

## Perihepatic Vascular Injury

Perihepatic vascular injuries require special consideration. Once again, packing is the damage control mainstay, provided it controls hemorrhage. Hepatic artery ligation may be useful in controlling hemorrhage if packing is not successful.[63,64] The supraduodenal portal vein may be ligated for damage control. When both the portal vein and hepatic artery are damaged, at least one of the vessels must be salvaged.

## Hepatic Parenchymal Injury

Bleeding from within the hepatic parenchyma can often be controlled initially with manual compression, with placement of hands on either side of the major laceration(s) and pressing together. This will allow the anesthesia team to restore intravascular volume via blood component transfusions before proceeding. The decision at this point should be whether packing (superiorly, anteriorly, and posteriorly) is adequate to maintain hemostasis.

Adjunctive measures like topical hemostatic agents (e.g., fibrin sealants) in conjunction with packing may be useful with large hepatic lacerations. Topical hemostatic agents may not be readily accessible and are often time-consuming to prepare. Direct suturing is one of the oldest techniques to control deep parenchymal bleeding using large blunt-tipped 0-chromic sutures.[65] The sutures may be placed in a continuous or mattress configuration. Suturing should be limited to lacerations less than three centimeters in size to prevent blind suturing leading to significant bile duct injuries.[66,67] More complex lacerations often involve larger hepatic artery or portal branch vessels, which usually do not respond to packing. Gentle finger fracturing may be used to identify specific bleeding vessels and facilitate ligation.[68] One must be careful not to create excessive additional parenchymal bleeding using this finger-fracturing technique.

> Bleeding from within the hepatic parenchyma can often be initially controlled with manual compression. Suturing should be limited to lacerations less than three centimeters in size, as blind suturing may lead to significant bile duct injuries.

Omental packing has been successfully used for tamponading dead spaces with live-tissue, as well as for achieving hemostasis following hepatic hemorrhage. The omentum is first mobilized from the transverse mesocolon in the avascular plane and then off the greater curvature of the stomach. In general, this technique is superior to most direct techniques of hemorrhage control.[68,69] In civilian study populations, severe and complex liver lacerations treated with formal hepatic resections are associated with low mortality and liver-related morbidity.[70] The authors in these studies achieved 9 percent liver-related mortality and 17.8 percent liver-related morbidity with senior surgeon support (often a surgeon specifically from the liver service). A similar level of surgical expertise (i.e., liver specialists) is not available in a combat theater, hence such surgical interventions are generally avoided in a deployed setting.

## Pancreatic and Duodenal Injuries

The surgical management of duodenal and pancreatic (particular head region) injuries can be challenging and complex. Pancreatic injuries (other than distal injuries) should be treated with hemorrhage control, modest debridement of devitalized tissue, and wide closed-suction drainage.[71,72] Placement of a feeding jejunostomy tube, assessment for pancreatic ductal continuity, and further definitive care should be performed at the next rearward level-of-care. Pancreatic injuries distal to the superior mesenteric artery can be managed with distal pancreatectomy and closed-suction drainage.[73]

> Pancreatic injuries (other than distal injuries) should be treated with hemorrhage control, modest debridement of devitalized tissue, and wide closed-suction drainage. Pancreatic injuries distal to the superior mesenteric artery can be managed with distal pancreatectomy and closed-suction drainage.

Duodenal injuries can be primarily repaired when there is no risk of lumenal compromise.[71] The duodenum should be debrided and closed transversely if the injury involves less than 50 percent of the circumference of the duodenal wall (Fig. 22). If tissue destruction is extensive, the repair will necessitate pyloric exclusion with triple-tube placement: gastrostomy tube, retrograde jejunostomy (to decompress the duodenum), and antegrade feeding jejunostomy.[74] With complete duodenal transection, it would be best to perform closure of the proximal and distal duodenum with definitive repair at the next rearward level-of-care with either Roux-en-Y jejunostomy or duodenojejunostomy.[75] In uncommon cases of destructive combined injuries to the duodenum and pancreatic head, a pancreaticoduodenectomy (Whipple procedure) is a surgical option.[72] This should only be performed by experienced personnel in well-resourced facilities.

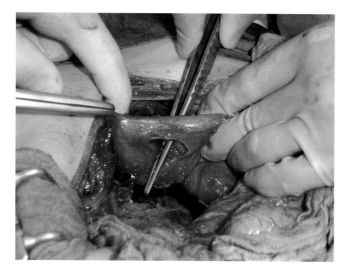

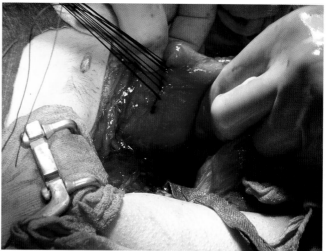

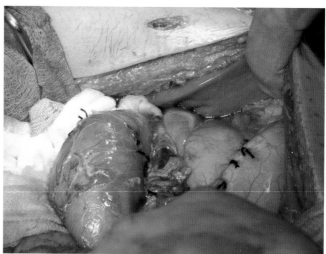

Figure 22. *Duodenal injuries can be primarily repaired when there is no risk of lumenal compromise.* (Top Left) *Kocher maneuver demonstrating through-and-through injury to the duodenum.* (Top Right) *Repair of injury with two-layer closure.* (Bottom Right) *Closed duodenum. Images courtesy of the Borden Institute, Office of The Surgeon General, Washington, DC.*

> A pancreaticoduodenectomy should not be performed in an austere environment. In a damage control surgery setting, destructive injury to the pancreatic head should be treated with drainage.

## Renal Injury

Renal injuries will often respond to compressive tamponade in the damage control setting provided that Gerota's fascia has not been violated. Nonexpanding hematomas within Gerota's fascia need not be explored during a damage control celiotomy. Subsequent management can be determined after the patient is stable.[76,77]

> Although the dictum for renal vascular injuries has been proximal and distal control prior to opening Gerota's fascia, vascular control of the renal hilum has been shown to have no impact on nephrectomy rates, transfusion requirements, or blood loss.

Absolute indications for renal exploration during damage control laparotomy include hemodynamic instability, expanding pulsatile renal hematoma, suspected renal pedicle avulsion, and ureteropelvic junction disruption (Figs. 23 and 24).[76,77] Although the dictum for renal vascular injuries has been proximal and distal control prior to opening Gerota's fascia, vascular control of the renal hilum has been shown to have

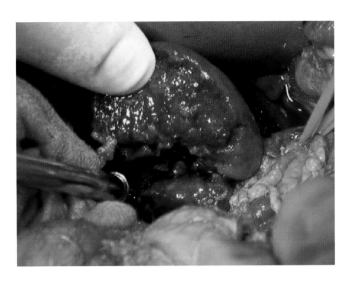

Figure 23. (Top Right) *Penetrating renal injury. A nephrectomy should be performed following complex renal injuries in an unstable patient. Image courtesy of the Borden Institute, Office of The Surgeon General, Washington, DC.*

Figure 24. (Middle) *A renal injury may be locally debrided and closed if operative conditions allow or* (Bottom) *excised in the course of partial nephrectomy. Images courtesy of the Borden Institute, Office of The Surgeon General, Washington, DC. Illustrator: Jessica Shull.*

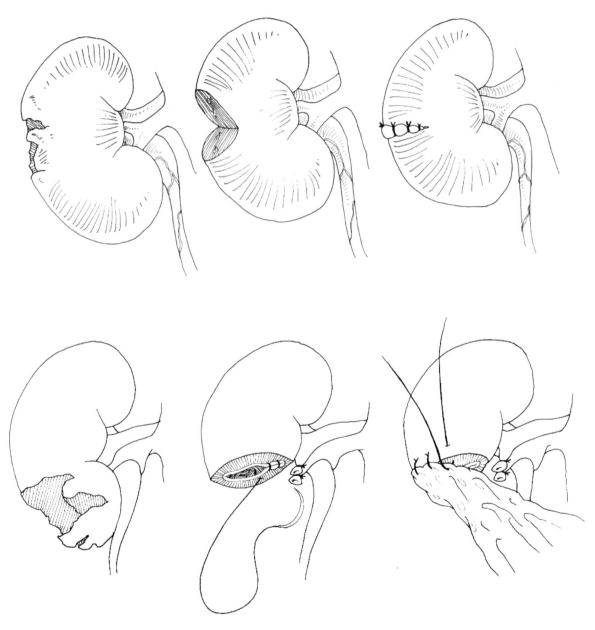

no impact on nephrectomy rates, transfusion requirements, or blood loss.[78] In fact, operative time may be increased with such vascular control techniques. Based on this study and the fact that most surgeons are not experienced in renal hilum isolation, it is recommended to forego renal hilar vascular control prior to entering Gerota's fascia. With complex injuries and/or an unstable patient, a nephrectomy should be performed rather than attempting repair. If nephrectomy is considered, the presence of a contralateral kidney should be confirmed.

> A nephrectomy should be performed following complex renal injuries in an unstable patient, rather than attempting repair.

## Ureteral Injury

Ureteral injuries are uncommon and account for only 1 to 3 percent of penetrating urologic trauma.[79,80,81] They are often overlooked when not appropriately considered and are more likely to be associated with retroperitoneal hematoma and injuries of the fixed portions of the colon, duodenum, and spleen.[82,83,84] Management of ureteral injuries depend on location, severity of injury, and hemodynamic stability of the patient.

Primary ureteral repair is not recommended in patients who present in shock or in those with severe colonic injury requiring colostomy.[83] Ureteral repair in these patients necessitates exteriorization of the ureter via tube or cutaneous ureterostomy, ureteral ligation and nephrostomy, or even ligation and primary nephrectomy.[83] Short proximal and midureteral injuries in hemodynamically stable patients are best managed by end-to-end spatulated anastomosis over a stent. Longer segment injuries may require ureteral exteriorization or ligation with nephrostomy (Fig. 25).[82]

> Short ureteral injuries may be managed by anastomosis over a stent, while longer ureteral injuries may require cutaneous ureterostomy with stent placement or ureteral ligation with tube nephrostomy.

Distal ureteral injuries are best managed by ureteroneocystostomy. This is performed by a transverse cystotomy, which elongates the bladder to the location and fixation of the bladder to the psoas fascia. Both maneuvers facilitate the construction of a tension-free anastomosis.[82] Some have advocated against ureteral reimplantation following distal ureteral injuries associated with rectal injuries due to concerns about wound dehiscence.[82,83] Successful ureteroneocystostomy following distal ureteral injuries complicated by rectal injuries has been reported.[85] Meticulous debridement of all necrotic tissues, urinary and fecal diversion, tension-free wound closure with well-vascularized tissue, and adequate drainage and separation of injured sites with well-vascularized tissue (such as omentum) are integral to reducing the incidence of fistulae formation following combined ureteral and rectal injuries.[85]

## Splenic Injury

Severely injured combat casualties undergoing damage control surgery with active hemorrhage from the spleen should undergo immediate splenectomy (Fig. 26). Observational management or packing of the spleen following injury is not feasible in most injured US service members. Such patients rapidly undergo aeromedical evacuation and are cared for by multiple careproviders as they are moved to more rearward facilities for definitive care. These factors make observational (nonoperative) management of significant splenic injuries impractical. This approach differs significantly from civilian trauma care where

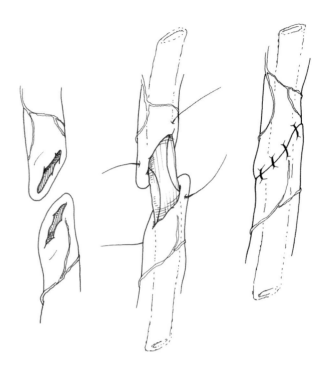

Figure 25. *Ureteral injuries:* (Top Right) *Short proximal and midureteral injuries in hemodynamically stable patients are best managed by end-to-end spatulated anastomosis over a stent. Longer segment injuries may require ureteral exteriorization or ligation with nephrostomy.* (Bottom Left and Bottom Right) *Distal ureteral injuries are best managed by ureteroneocystostomy. This is performed by a cystotomy, which elongates the bladder to the location and fixation of the bladder to the psoas fascia. Images courtesy of the Borden Institute, Office of The Surgeon General, Washington, DC. Illustrator: Jessica Shull.*

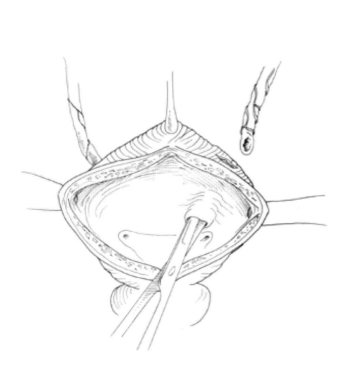

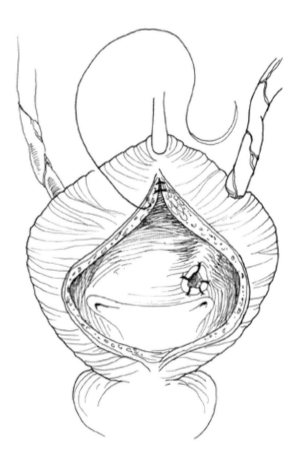

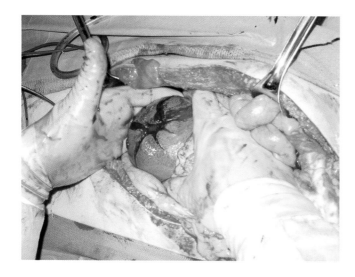

Figure 26. *Splenic laceration due to gunshot wound (GSW). Severely injured combat casualties with active hemorrhage from the spleen should undergo immediate splenectomy. Images courtesy of the Borden Institute, Office of The Surgeon General, Washington, DC.*

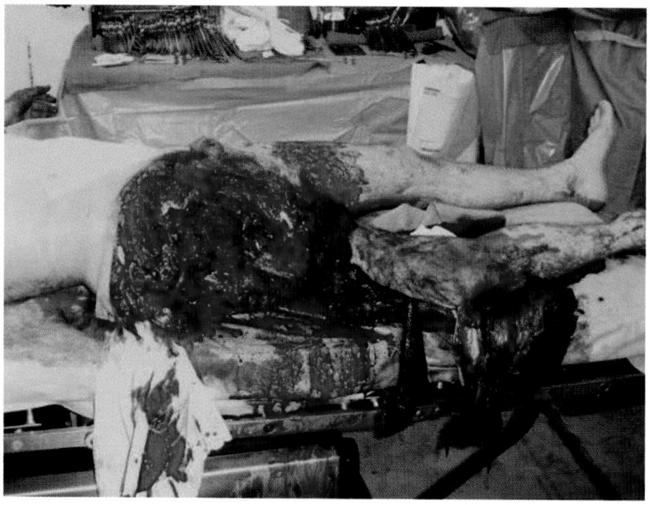

Figure 27. *Large abdominal soft-tissue and retroperitoneal wounds, seen with explosion-related injuries, will have difficult to control hemorrhage. Image courtesy of David Burris, MD, COL, MC, US Army.*

nonoperative management of blunt splenic injury is the treatment of choice for a hemodynamically stable patient, regardless of grade of injury.[86] Angiographic embolization is a useful adjunct in the nonoperative management of a hemodynamically stable patient with continued bleeding from a splenic injury.[87] Unfortunately, this interventional technology is not readily available in Level III facilities in Iraq and Afghanistan.

> Severely injured combat casualties undergoing damage control surgery with active hemorrhage from the spleen should undergo immediate splenectomy.

## Large Soft-Tissue and Retroperitoneal Wounds

Large abdominal soft-tissue and retroperitoneal wounds are not uncommon in the combat environment, particularly with explosion-related injuries (Fig. 27). These wounds present the vexing challenge of controlling a large area of soft-tissue hemorrhage in an often coagulopathic casualty. Temporizing hemorrhage control can be achieved with the combination of topical hemostatic agents such as SURGICEL® NU-KNIT® (Ethicon, Inc.) or GELFOAM® tightly compressed into the wound with laparotomy pads.[88]

## *Intestinal (Enteric) Injuries*

Once control of hemorrhage is obtained, attention is turned to control of contamination. In the damage control laparotomy, all enteric injuries that cannot be repaired by simple suture repair are resected locally, or en bloc if multiple injuries in close proximity are noted (Fig. 28). The bowel is then stapled with a GIA™ stapler and left in discontinuity. No attempt should be made to do a primary enteric anastomosis in the damage control setting.[89] Likewise, enteric diversion should be postponed and not performed during the initial damage control procedure.[90] Abdominal wounds associated with colonic injuries (particularly left-sided) need to be monitored closely, and serial local debridement should be strongly considered since these injuries are often complicated by infections.

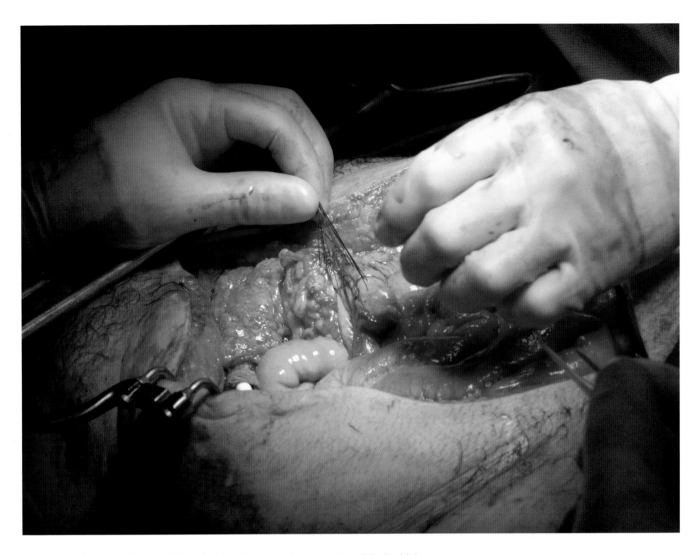

Figure 28. *Suture repair of small bowel perforations following penetrating abdominal injury.*

During damage control laparotomy, all enteric injuries that cannot be repaired by simple suture repair should be resected locally, or en bloc if multiple injuries in close proximity are noted. Primary enteric anastomosis should not be attempted during the initial damage control laparotomy.

## Rectal Injury

Injuries to the rectum should be defined as either intraperitoneal or extraperitoneal. Intraperitoneal rectal injuries follow the same concepts outlined previously with enteric injuries. However, extraperitoneal rectal injuries should be treated with end colostomy or loop colostomy. If the rectal defect is not readily identifiable for closure, one should not perform extensive dissection and mobilization of the rectum. Although civilian data suggest that presacral drains and distal stump washout are of limited benefit, military doctrine remains to place presacral drains and consider a distal washout for massive injuries.[91,92,93]

Extraperitoneal rectal injuries should be treated with end colostomy or loop colostomy.

## Abdominal Wall Closure

Once hemorrhage is controlled and the contamination contained, the abdomen is covered with a sterile dressing and a negative-pressure suction device applied. The open abdomen accommodates abdominal visceral swelling, which is a consequence of reperfusion injury, and minimizes the risk of postoperative abdominal compartment syndrome (Fig. 29).[94,95,96,97] Abdominal compartment syndrome (intraabdominal hypertension) is a potentially lethal disorder caused by conditions that elevate intraabdominal pressure to the point of impairing end-organ function. Excessive fluid resuscitation, reperfusion injury, burn injury, abdominal cavity packing, and intraperitoneal hemorrhage are examples of factors that can lead to abdominal compartment syndrome in the combat casualty.[98,99]

> The fascia is left open following damage control surgery, and the abdomen is temporarily sealed with a sterile dressing and negative-pressure suction device. Skin closure may lead to abdominal compartment syndrome.

The physiologic effects of abdominal compartment syndrome affect many organs.[99,100,101,102] Clinical manifestations result from diminished preload (decreased venous return) and elevated systemic vascular resistance leading to a decrease in end-organ perfusion. Patients will also exhibit evidence of respiratory insufficiency due to diminished lung volumes (due to impeded diaphragmatic excursion). Patients undergoing mechanical ventilation will exhibit high peak airway pressures and decreased urine output caused by falling renal perfusion pressures, despite adequate volume resuscitation. Elevated intracranial pressures and adverse effects on cerebral perfusion pressures have also been linked to abdominal compartment syndrome in patients with severe head injuries. [99,102]

Abdominal compartment syndrome was noted in 33 percent of patients in one case series of patients undergoing a damage control surgery in a civilian setting.[97] The diagnosis of abdominal compartment syndrome is made by indirectly assessing intraabdominal pressures via Foley catheter bladder pressure measurements. A partially filled bladder is very compliant and has been used as an accurate method to assess surrounding intraperitoneal pressures.[98] Abdominal compartment syndrome has been defined by

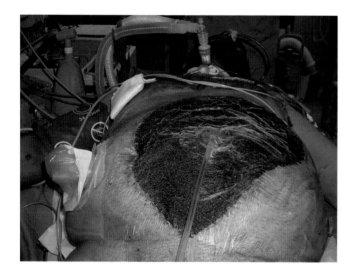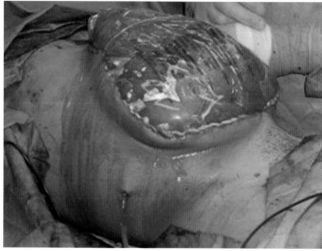

Figure 29. *Temporary abdominal wall closure. Leaving the abdominal wall open accommodates abdominal visceral swelling and minimizes the risk of postoperative abdominal compartment syndrome. (Left) A sterile dressing with negative-pressure suction device. (Right) A sterile three-liter crystalloid solution bag used for closure. Right-sided image courtesy of the Borden Institute, Office of The Surgeon General, Washington, DC.*

intraabdominal pressures greater than 20 mm Hg, abdominal perfusion pressure less than 60 mm Hg (mean arterial pressure minus intraabdominal pressure), and single or multisystem organ failure.[98,100,103] It is important to remember that an abdominal compartment syndrome can develop even with an open abdomen, and it is imperative that serial evaluation for this contingency occurs with revision of the closure if necessary. The exact intraabdominal pressure that warrants an intervention remains unclear. There appears to be consensus agreement that intraabdominal pressures greater than 30 mm Hg require an intervention.[98,99,100,104] Decompressive laparotomy, or an alternative intervention (e.g., loosening of abdominal dressings), to relieve intraabdominal pressures in patients with an open abdomen is indicated when abdominal compartment syndrome is suspected. If left untreated, abdominal compartment syndrome can lead to death.

# Peripheral Vascular Injury Damage Control

The concept of successful damage control surgery for peripheral vascular injury had not been fully realized until the recent implementation of temporary vascular shunts in Afghanistan and Iraq.[105,106] During World War I, German surgeons reported repair of over 100 arterial injuries and pioneered autogenous reconstruction of injured vessels.[105] However, the proclivity for mass casualties, significant soft-tissue injury, and protracted transport times made routine vascular reconstruction impractical, and subsequently, ligation of vessels became standard practice.[105,106,107] DeBakey reported 2,471 arterial injuries treated by ligation in World War II with a 49 percent amputation rate.[108] With these dismal results, the standard of practice became definitive arterial repair in the Korean War with a dramatic reduction in amputation rate to 13 percent.[109] Similar successes were documented during the Vietnam conflict.[105,106,107] Therefore, leading up to the conflicts in Afghanistan and Iraq, damage control with ligation was abandoned in favor of definitive vascular repair with greatly improved results.

## *Arterial Injury and Temporary Vascular Shunts*

Improvements in the paradigm of casualty resuscitation during Operation Enduring Freedom (OEF) and Operation Iraqi Freedom (OIF) have provided greater opportunities for deployed surgeons to successfully perform vascular repair after injury on the battlefield. The use of temporary vascular shunts allowed the extension of this damage control paradigm to the treatment of peripheral vascular injuries. In one report, 57 percent of casualties with peripheral arterial injuries had shunts placed at forward surgical facilities, and 86 percent of these shunts were patent when the patient arrived at the Combat Support Hospital (CSH). In two separate analyses of data from the Joint Trauma Theater Registry (JTTR), damage control resuscitation and damage control surgery techniques applied in the context of vascular injury using temporary shunts allowed for delayed prolonged complex limb revascularizations with limb salvage rates of 95 percent.[110,111] Clouse and Sohn independently demonstrated similar in-theater acute limb salvage rates for revascularization of 92 to 95 percent.[112,113] The successful use of temporary vascular shunts allows for ongoing patient resuscitation and transport to definitive care with a perfused extremity.[114]

> Temporary vascular shunts are an effective tool in the management of extremity vascular injury and allow for ongoing patient resuscitation and extremity perfusion during transport to definitive care.

An important difference between combat and civilian practice is the role of arteriographic study to rule out vascular injury for proximity wounds. Civilian practice has evolved to expectant management of wounds in proximity to critical blood vessels if there are no hard signs of vascular injury. Studies have demonstrated no increase of vascular lesions requiring surgical therapy under these circumstances.[115,116,117] However, the high-energy nature of combat wounds led military investigators to reevaluate this management paradigm in combat casualties (Fig. 30). In a study of 99 patients who underwent angiography after evacuation for wound proximity, 47 percent had vascular abnormalities noted on angiography. Two-thirds of this group had a normal physical examination. Importantly, 52 percent of the patients with an abnormal arteriogram required operative intervention.[118] In an analysis of combat-related penetrating neck trauma by Fox et al., 30 percent of patients undergoing computerized tomographic angiography had occult injury and 50 percent of these required interventional or surgical management.[119]

## Role of Temporary Vascular Shunts in Afghanistan and Iraq

Experience from nearly a decade of war in Afghanistan and Iraq suggests that temporary vascular shunts are a feasible and effective tool in the management of extremity vascular injury.[114,120,121,122] The use of temporary vascular shunts is particularly germane in modern combat where the rate of vascular injury (5 to 7 percent) is much higher than reported in previous wars.[112,120] The increased use of body armor and other force protection measures as well as tourniquets may increase the survivability of wounds that were deadly in previous wars.[123] As such, injured service members who in the past may have succumbed to torso wounds or exsanguination from extremity injuries now survive to have vascular injuries recorded and treated.[120]

In this context, temporary vascular shunts are part of a management triad of: (1) vascular injury exploration; (2) thrombectomy and restoration of flow; and (3) fasciotomy. Following injury exploration, vascular shunts are inserted in both ends (proximal and distal) of the disrupted vessel to bridge and provide flow distal to the defect, and maintain limb viability (Fig. 31). Shunts can typically be placed in an expeditious manner and require less time and technical expertise than formal vascular repair. Data from the Balad Vascular

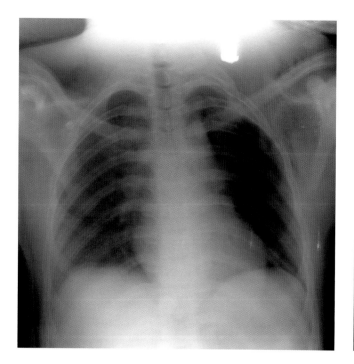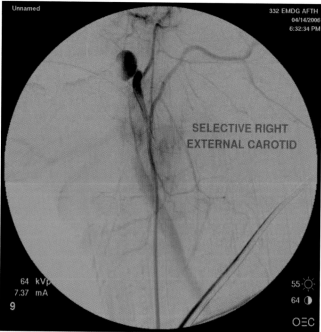

Figure 30. *Proximity wounds.* (Left) *Due to the greater energy imparted by military ballistic projectiles, injury in proximity to critical blood vessels, particularly in the cervical region, should be evaluated by angiography to mitigate the risk of occult vascular injury.* (Right) *The subsequent carotid angiogram revealed a vascular injury requiring coil repair. Images courtesy of David B. Powers, DMD, MD, COL, US Air Force.*

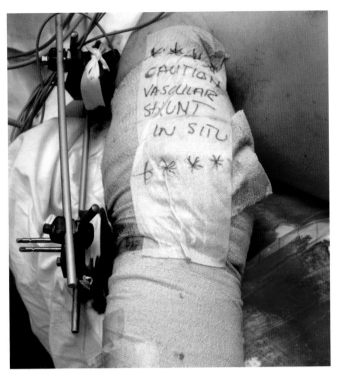

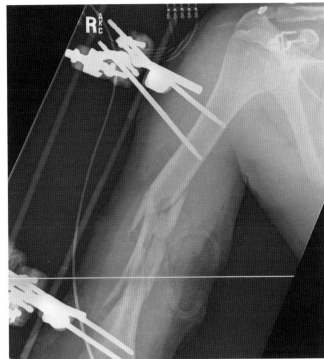

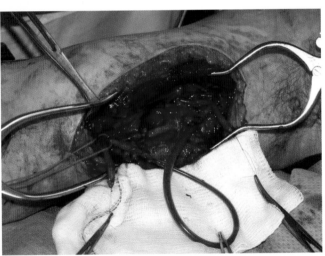

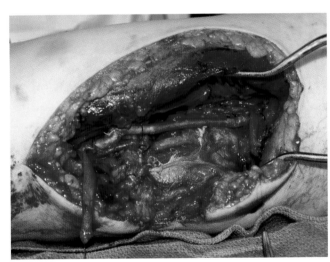

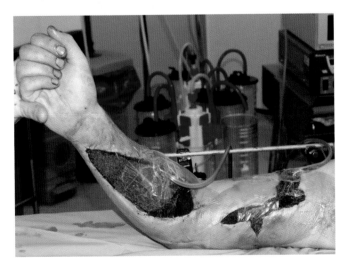

Figure 31. *Vascular repair:* (Top Left) *Level III facility care of a casualty with a GSW to the right upper arm with an open comminuted humeral fracture and transected right brachial artery and median nerve. The casualty was initially treated at a Level II facility and underwent vascular injury exploration, placement of a Javid™ temporary vascular shunt in the right brachial artery, and forearm fasciotomy. An external fixator was applied.* (Top Right) *A radiograph obtained at the Level III ED five hours following injury reveals the presence of an indwelling shunt.* (Center Left) *A patent shunt with excellent Doppler signal was noted during surgical exploration.* (Center Right) *The shunt was removed and an interposition vein graft repair of the brachial artery was performed.* (Bottom Left) *A negative-pressure suction device was applied and the patient was transported to a Level IV facility.*

Registry reveals that a majority of temporary vascular shunts are placed during Level II damage control surgical care, prior to the medical evacuation of casualties to Level III facilities.[112,114] A review of in-theater evacuation data reveals an average time from loading on a helicopter to arrival at a Level III facility of 46 minutes.[120]

> Temporary vascular shunts are part of a management triad of: (1) vascular injury exploration; (2) thrombectomy and restoration of flow; and (3) fasciotomy.

Once placed, shunts maintain perfusion to the extremity (distal to the site of injury) during medical evacuation (MEDEVAC) or treatment of other life-threatening torso or head injuries. In this sense, shunts are amenable to use in forward surgical units where damage control or abbreviated operations (less than one hour) are the goal.[114,121,122] The alternative to initiating the previously mentioned management triad is deferring vascular injury treatment during MEDEVAC and/or management of other injuries. If restoration of flow to the extremity is delayed in these instances, warm-ischemia time compounds increasing neuromuscular damage and decreases the likelihood of limb recovery and salvage.

Data from a large-animal model of hind-limb ischemia and reperfusion demonstrated that early restoration of flow using temporary vascular shunts reduced circulating markers of injury and resulted in improved flow in the injured extremity.[124] Specifically, this study showed that restoration of flow following one hour of ischemia resulted in an 18-hour reperfusion profile that was the same as controls (i.e., no ischemia). In contrast, restoration of extremity flow with a temporary vascular shunt after three to six hours resulted in reperfusion profiles that were incrementally adverse. The conclusion of this study was that early (one hour) versus delayed (greater than three hours) restoration of flow was associated with measurably improved responses.[124] The presence of shock or other soft-tissue or bony injury may even further reduce this ischemic threshold to less than three hours, after which recovery of the limb should not be expected. Results from these large-animal experiments inform surgeons that the critical warm-ischemia time for an extremity in the combat setting (i.e., with hemorrhage and soft-tissue injury) is likely less than three hours and may be as short as one hour.

> Results from large-animal experiments suggest that the critical warm-ischemia time for an extremity in a combat setting (i.e., with hemorrhage and soft-tissue injury) is likely less than three hours and may be as short as one hour.

Early reports from Iraq indicated that shunts were being used effectively at forward Level II facilities.[114,121,122] Specifically, Javid™, Argyl™, and Sundt™ shunts have been extensively used. Shunts remained in place during MEDEVAC to higher levels of in-theater care where they were then removed and definitive reconstruction performed.[114,121,122] During times of high casualty rates in Iraq, shunts were used in up to 50 percent of femoral/popliteal injuries, a frequency that is similar to that currently encountered in Afghanistan by the author (TR).[125]

## Complications

Early temporary vascular shunt-related complications have been rare, and shunt patency, when placed in larger, more proximal arteries of the extremities, approaches 90 percent at four to six hours.[114,121,122] Data from the JTTR, Balad Vascular Registry, and the Walter Reed Vascular Registry demonstrate that use of temporary vascular shunts as an adjunct in damage control surgery did not result in worse outcomes. In fact, the use of shunts extended the window of opportunity for limb salvage in the most severely injured limbs. However, demonstration of definitive benefit was not shown.[126] Late complications associated with revascularization do occur and include thrombosis, infection, and compartment syndrome.[110,127] Interestingly, the factor most significantly associated with post-revascularization morbidity was the use of prosthetic graft implants. Unlike the results of civilian vascular injury, when a prosthetic graft was used with combat vascular injuries, the incidence of graft loss was 80 percent.[110,120,127] Hence, a primary goal of vascular surgeons at Level III facilities is to ensure no temporary vascular shunt or prosthetic conduit be sent out of theater. Definitive repair of vascular injuries with primary or autologous vein repair is a priority.

> Vascular surgeons at Level III facilities should perform definitive repair of vascular injuries that have been previously treated with a temporary vascular shunt or prosthetic conduit prior to transport to a Level IV or Level V facility.

Reperfusion injury often results in extremity compartment syndrome following restoration of perfusion to injured limbs. Hence, prophylactic fasciotomy following definitive vascular repair of an injured limb is recommended.[128] Prophylactic fasciotomy should also be considered (especially if prolonged medical evacuation times are anticipated) concurrent with the placement of temporary vascular shunts, for similar reasons.

Recent increased operational activity in the Afghanistan Theater has provided the opportunity to assess the effectiveness of temporary vascular shunts in an environment with unique casualty evacuation (CASEVAC) and MEDEVAC characteristics. In contrast to OIF, CASEVAC and MEDEVAC in Afghanistan are challenged by mountain passes, which hinder direct rotary-wing transport in many cases. Additionally, the multinational nature of combat casualty care in OEF results in instances of intratheater transport of injured casualties to nation-specific air hubs for preparation for transcontinental air evacuation (AIREVAC). These realities have given rise to a form of MEDEVAC which includes intratheater use of fixed-wing casualty movement referred to as tactical evacuation (TACEVAC). In this setting, vascular injury management has been challenged by instances of longer times between injury and definitive vascular repair. The generally longer TACEVAC times in OEF have given rise to observations by the author (TR) of longer indwell times of temporary shunts (up to 12 to 24 hours) without complication. Although not tested because of rapid and consistent MEDEVAC during OIF, these observations are consistent with experiments demonstrating up to 24-hour patency of shunts without the use of heparin.[124,129] In the author's (TR) experience, the use of temporary vascular shunts in Afghanistan is nearly uniform in extremity vascular injuries, and complications remain uncommon. As in Iraq, even if temporary vascular shunts occlude or clot, it does not preclude removal of the shunt and restoration of flow with formal vascular repair at Level III facilities.

## Conclusions

In aggregate, this data, combined with a decade's experience in OEF/OIF, lead to the conclusions that early restoration of flow (within one hour) using temporary vascular shunts is advantageous. Specifically, when formal vascular repair is not possible, shunts should be used as part of the management triad of: (1) extremity vascular injury exploration; (2) thrombectomy and restoration of flow; and (3) fasciotomy. The application of this management triad should occur as soon as feasible after injury, in the context of tactical considerations and other concomitant life-threatening head and torso injuries. Whether this triad is undertaken at a Level II or III facility is a matter of semantics and is more dependent upon the time from injury to point of surgical care. Temporary vascular shunts are part of the management triad of injury exploration, restoration of flow, and fasciotomy. Ideally, their use reduces warm-ischemia time and extends the window of opportunity for limb salvage. Experienced vascular surgeons, cardiothoracic surgeons, or trauma surgeons are usually only located at Level III facilities. Vascular injuries sustained in the combat environment must undergo arterial reconstruction with autogenous material at Level III facilities, since prosthetic grafts have a much higher rate of infection.

## Venous Injury

In the context of battlefield venous injury, ligation is a safe and effective option. Venous ligation is an expedient solution that allows the surgeon to address other injuries in critically ill patients. A review of the management of 103 venous injuries from the Global War on Terror indicates ligation (63 percent) is more common then repair (37 percent).[130] All patients, regardless of management, developed postoperative edema. While thrombosis of the repair was demonstrated in 16 percent of the repaired veins, there was no acute limb loss or venous graft failure associated with venous ligation.[130] Pulmonary embolus developed in three cases, one in a patient with open repair, and two in cases managed with ligation. Long-term outcomes and follow-up data are needed to determine what the best approach to management should be.

> Ligation is a safe and effective option for combat-related venous injury.

## Proximity to Great Vessel Injury

Contrary to civilian trauma literature recommendations, penetrating extremity injury in proximity to critical blood vessels, particularly in the cervical region, should be evaluated by angiography to mitigate the risk of occult vascular injury due to the greater energy imparted by military ballistic projectiles.[119] It is important to know the patient's total trauma burden and physiology when deciding how to manage that patient's vascular injury. The treatment of vascular injuries in combat casualties can be a challenging endeavor in a resource-limited environment. Optimal care depends upon technical expertise on the part of the operating surgeon and solid judgment regarding when to perform temporizing maneuvers versus definitive repairs. Surgeons at all Level II and III facilities need to be intimately familiar with the use of vascular shunts as a means to stabilize a critically wounded casualty and then move them along the continuum of care.

> Penetrating extremity injury in proximity to critical blood vessels, particularly in the cervical region, should be evaluated by angiography to identify occult vascular injury.

## Extremity Tourniquets

Control of life-threatening hemorrhage following extremity injury has been greatly improved through the field application of the extremity tourniquet.[131,132] Patients requiring damage control procedures for presumed extremity vascular hemorrhage should have the prehospital tourniquet prepped into the operative field or replaced by a sterile tourniquet in the operating room (Fig. 32). Basic vascular surgery principles of proximal and distal control are employed to access extremity vessel injury (Fig. 33). The majority of injuries in patients with penetrating extremity trauma can be explored directly with no need for preoperative arteriography. However, in patients with diffuse or multiple extremity injuries associated with vascular compromise, arteriography is often useful if the patient's physiologic status will tolerate the procedure.[118,133]

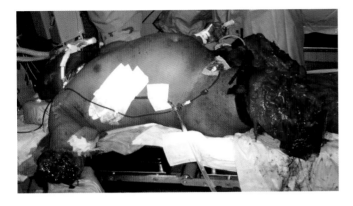

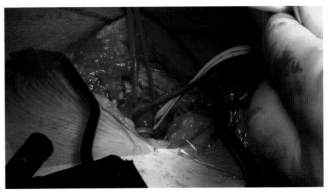

Figure 32. *Control of life-threatening hemorrhage following extremity injury has been greatly improved through the field application of the extremity tourniquet. Image courtesy of Joint Combat Trauma Management Course, 2007.*

Figure 33. *Basic vascular surgical principles of proximal and distal vessel control are a cornerstone of extremity injury management.*

## Upper Extremity Arterial Injury

The axillary artery can be exposed through an infraclavicular incision from midclavicle to the deltopectoral groove through the clavipectoral fascia. The brachial artery is accessed by incising the medial aspect of the upper arm between biceps and triceps. When gaining control of the brachial vessel, care should be taken to avoid injury to the basilic vein and median nerve. An S-shaped incision is required if the incision crosses antecubital fossa. If the vascular injury is below the profunda brachii, the patient will usually tolerate ligation. The radial and ulnar arteries can generally be singly ligated.[134] However, an Allen test is required to assess the vascular integrity of the hand prior to vessel ligation.

## Femoral Vasculature Injury

In the lower extremity, the femoral artery can be accessed proximally via a standard femoral cutdown. For superficial femoral arteries, acute occlusion in young healthy patients without established collateral flow is not well-tolerated.[135] In the damage control setting, the superficial femoral vessels are easily shunted by standard shunting techniques. This vessel can be definitively repaired or an autogenous interposition graft placed once the patient has been adequately resuscitated. The majority of venous injuries can be ligated, especially if the patient is in extremis.[130] After performing a deep venous ligation in the lower extremity, it is incumbent upon the surgeon to be aware of the subsequent lower extremity venous hypertension and risk for the development of a lower extremity compartment syndrome. As such, liberal use of four compartment fasciotomies through extended incisions should be considered.

## Popliteal and Tibial Vasculature Injuries

The popliteal artery behind the knee requires an extended medial approach, dividing tendinous muscular attachments of the hamstring complex and the soleus. Again, depending upon the acuity of the patient and available resources, the therapeutic options include shunting, repair, or bypass. If the popliteal vein is injured, it should be repaired if the patient's condition allows. This will reduce subsequent lower extremity venous hypertension and the risk for compartment syndrome. Tibial arteries are uniformly ligated in the damage control paradigm.[136]

# Pelvic Injury Damage Control

## *Background*

Pelvic fracture is a marker of severe injury and is classically associated with a substantial rate of morbidity and mortality. Although pelvic fractures account for only 3 percent of all acute fractures, mortality in this patient population varies from 10 to 50 percent depending upon fracture pattern.[137,138,139] Morbidity and mortality in this patient population are multifactorial and often associated with concomitant injury to the brain, thorax, and abdomen since the force imparted to fracture the pelvis is also imparted to other regions of the body.[137,138,139] Pelvic fractures can be associated with considerable hemorrhage, especially when the posterior elements of the pelvis are significantly disrupted.[137,138,139] The resultant pelvic hemorrhage can be both arterial and venous and may emanate from the major vasculature or its truncal branches, the presacral venous plexus, the

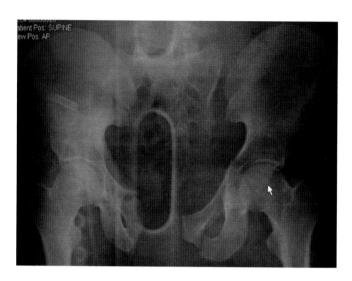

Figure 34. *Pelvic fractures can be associated with considerable hemorrhage, especially when the posterior elements of the pelvis are significantly disrupted as depicted in this radiograph.*

soft-tissue, or the large bulk of open cancellous bone in the region (Fig. 34). Survival of patients with pelvic fracture is optimized by prompt diagnosis of the pelvic fracture, vigorous resuscitation, pelvic stabilization, and definitive control of hemorrhage.[137,138,139]

> Pelvic fractures can be associated with considerable hemorrhage, especially when the posterior elements of the pelvis are significantly disrupted.

The effective management of pelvic fractures and associated hemorrhage, especially in the deployed military environment, requires multidisciplinary cooperation of the emergency physician, trauma surgeon, and the orthopedic surgeon. While the use of interventional angiographic embolization has dramatically improved outcomes in the civilian management of severe pelvic fracture hemorrhage, interventional radiology is not typically available on the battlefield. To date, this has meant that damage control maneuvers such as pelvic wrapping and external fixation have become the primary means for temporizing hemorrhage control. Unfortunately, these maneuvers cannot reliably control pelvic arterial hemorrhage. The relatively recent adoption of extraperitoneal pelvic packing through the space of Retzius has offered a potentially effective damage control procedure for pelvic fracture-associated hemorrhage that may temporarily arrest or abrogate hemorrhage, to allow transport to a facility capable of angiographic embolization.[140]

> Extraperitoneal pelvic packing through the space of Retzius is a potentially effective damage control procedure for pelvic fracture-associated hemorrhage. It may temporize bleeding until angiographic embolization can be performed.

## Physical Examination

Pelvic fracture should be suspected in all patients with appropriate mechanisms of injury. Evidence of systemic hypoperfusion in combination with a pelvic fracture suggests fracture-associated hemorrhage and requires prompt resuscitative and therapeutic interventions.[139] The objectives of the pelvis examination are to estimate the likelihood of fracture, assess pelvic ring stability, and identify injuries to the adjacent structures. The examination begins with visual inspection of the pelvis for signs of injury. Look for abrasions, contusions, and lacerations. The presence of progressive flank, scrotal, perineal ecchymosis, or edema suggests pelvic injury with significant bleeding. Destot's sign is a hematoma above the inguinal ligament. Grey-Turner's sign is a flank ecchymosis secondary to retroperitoneal hemorrhage. Wounds in the pelvic area should be assessed carefully to exclude an open pelvic fracture. Lacerations involving the perineum, vagina, rectum, or scrotum are highly suggestive of an open pelvic fracture. Failure to thoroughly examine the gluteal cleft, buttock fold, rectum, and vagina for open wounds may lead to missed injuries. All patients with pelvic fractures should undergo a rectal exam with special attention to the rectal tone, the presence of rectal bleeding, and the position of the prostate. Diminished rectal tone could result from a pelvic fracture with accompanying lumbosacral nerve plexus injury. Gross blood or stool that tests guaiac-positive could represent a possible open pelvic fracture.[141] A high-riding or free-floating prostate suggests membranous prostatic urethral injury.[142] In patients with a concomitant pelvic hematoma, the outline of the prostate may be indistinct to palpation despite a normal position. A positive Earle's sign is the presence of a bony prominence, palpable hematoma, or tender fracture line on rectal exam. The genitourinary system should be carefully examined. Scrotal swelling or ecchymosis and the presence of bleeding from the urethral meatus are signs of urethral disruption (Fig. 35). A vaginal examination should be performed in female patients to assess for palpable fractures, vaginal lacerations, and blood within the vaginal vault. Pelvic fractures in association with vaginal or rectal lacerations are considered open fractures.[143]

Examination of the lower extremities begins with visual inspection. Discrepancies in leg length, gross rotational deformities, or asymmetry of the hips should be noted. In the absence of a lower extremity fracture, these findings suggest a pelvic fracture or hip dislocation. A patient with a posterior hip dislocation will have a shortened extremity held in an internally rotated position. Range of motion at each hip should be assessed. A study by Ham et al. found that the inability to actively flex the hip was the maneuver most reliably predictive of a pelvic fracture. It had a 90 percent sensitivity and 95 percent specificity for detecting a pelvic fracture.[144] The stability of the pelvis may be assessed by applying lateral-to-medial compression and anterior-posterior compression over the anterior-superior iliac crests. Many clinicians advocate foregoing any forceful manipulation of a potentially injured pelvis for fear of dislodging clots from injured vessels and precipitating renewed pelvic hemorrhage. Neurologic examination should be thorough, as many patients have significant neurological disability, especially when the pelvic fracture extends into or through the sacral foramina. Particular attention should be paid to the lumbar (L5) and sacral (S1) nerve roots to detect an injury to the lumbosacral nerve plexus or its nerve roots. The L5 nerve root may be tested by assessing dorsiflexion of the great toe against resistance and sensation over the dorsum of the foot. The S1 nerve root is tested by evaluating plantar flexion of the great toe against resistance, sensation along the lateral aspect of the foot, and the Achilles tendon reflex.

## Radiographic Evaluation

Contingent upon resources, radiographic evaluation should be performed to allow the surgeon to determine the morphology of the pelvic fracture.

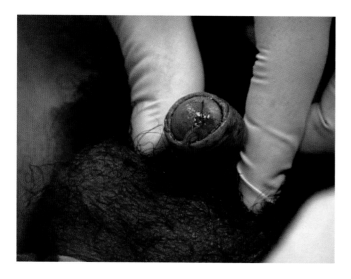 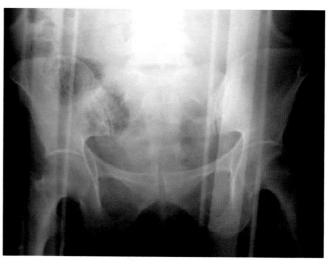

Figure 35. *The presence of urethral meatal bleeding and scrotal swelling or ecchymosis are signs of potential urethral disruption.*

Figure 36. *An anteroposterior (AP) plain radiograph of the pelvis will identify the vast majority of significant pelvic fractures.*

## Plain Radiography

An anteroposterior (AP) plain radiograph of the pelvis will identify the vast majority of pelvic fractures (Fig. 36). It allows for early identification of serious pelvic injuries that may be a source of blood loss. It may also detect proximal femur fractures and hip dislocations. When the patient is in a supine position, the AP pelvis radiograph actually provides an oblique view of the pelvic brim. This is because the pelvis lies 45 to 60 degrees oblique to the long axis of the skeleton. Many acetabular fractures are not visible on the AP pelvic radiographs. Plain radiography is not as accurate as computed tomography (CT) imaging for evaluation of pelvic fractures.[145,146] When compared with CT imaging, plain films missed 57 percent of acetabular rim fractures, 50 percent of femoral head fractures, 40 percent of intraarticular fragments, 34 percent of vertical shear fractures, and 29 percent of sacroiliac diastasis injuries.[147]

## Computed Tomography Imaging

Computed tomography imaging is extremely valuable in the diagnosis and characterization of pelvic injuries. Computed tomography may be utilized to identify or exclude a pelvic injury in equivocal cases or to further delineate a known pelvic fracture. When compared with plain pelvis radiographs, CT is more sensitive in the detection of pelvic fractures and allows better characterization of the fractures and adjacent soft-tissues.[146] The primary advantage of CT imaging is the ability to simultaneously screen for associated injuries (e.g., visceral injuries). In most trauma victims, the bony pelvis is scanned as part of a combined abdomen and pelvis CT study. If a fracture is detected, further imaging with thinner axial sections may be obtained of the area of interest. An important aspect of CT imaging is the use of reformatted images. Multiplanar reconstruction is the reformatting of data to produce images along the sagittal and coronal planes. Inlet and tangential views may be created, eliminating the need for additional plain films. In addition to multiplanar reconstruction, three-dimensional images may also be constructed using three-dimensional image rendering software. Three-dimensional spiral CT images may detect subtle fractures (specifically those in the axial plane), demonstrate spatial relationships of fracture fragments, and guide management (Fig. 37).

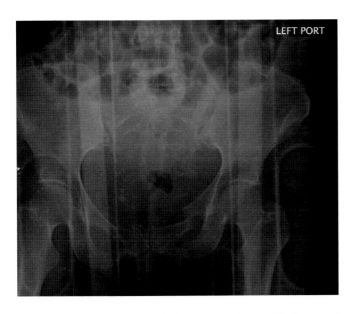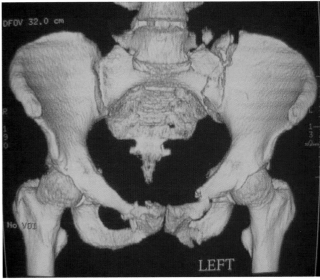

Figure 37. *Three-dimensional CT images may detect subtle fractures, demonstrate spatial relationships of fracture fragments, and guide management. Images courtesy of Swaminatha V. Mahadevan, MD, Stanford University.*

## Angiography

The use of intravenous contrast allows simultaneous evaluation of both osseous and vascular structures. Contrast-enhanced CT imaging can demonstrate active arterial bleeding. This is usually from branches of the internal iliac artery or internal pudendal artery. Nonarterial bleeding may also be detected. These hematomas typically originate from disruption of the posterior pelvic veins or the surfaces of fractured bones. The gold standard test for detecting arterial bleeding associated with pelvic fractures is traditional angiography (Fig. 38). Spiral CT angiography of the pelvis has been shown to be moderately sensitive (84 percent) and specific (85 percent) for the detection of acute pelvic bleeding in trauma.[148] Standard angiography has the important advantage of serving as an excellent diagnostic and therapeutic modality (e.g., embolization).[149,150,151]

## *Acute Management*

The acute management of the patient with pelvic fracture and hemorrhage involves three basic tenets: (1) stabilization of the pelvis; (2) control of pelvic hemorrhage; and (3) identification and control of extrapelvic hemorrhage sources. Pelvic stabilization limits radial expansion of the pelvis and protects against increases in pelvic volume and additional hemorrhage. It is hypothesized that stabilization affects hemostasis via tamponade and clot maintenance.[137,152] Emergent stabilization of the pelvis is almost exclusively temporizing in nature, from the point of view of fracture fixation and serves as a bridge to later definitive internal fixation once the patient is physiologically stable. Potential stabilizing methods include the pelvic sheet sling, pelvic binder, and external fixation (Fig. 39).[153,154]

> The acute management of the patient with pelvic fracture(s) and hemorrhage involves three tenets: (1) stabilization of the pelvis; (2) control of pelvic hemorrhage; and (3) identification and control of extrapelvic hemorrhage sources.

When placing the sheet sling, the boundaries of the wrap should be the anterior-superior iliac spine (cephalad) and the greater trochanter (caudad). After wrapping the pelvis, twist the wrap in front and clip

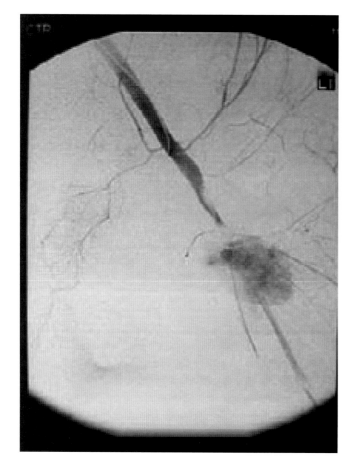 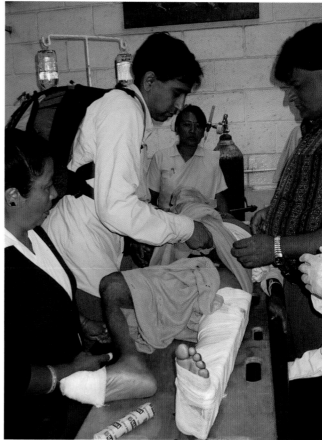

Figure 38. *The gold standard test for detecting arterial bleeding associated with pelvic fractures is traditional angiography.*

Figure 39. *Pelvic stability may be improved with application of a pelvic binder or bed sheet around the patient's hips. Image courtesy of Swaminatha V. Mahadevan, MD, Stanford University.*

or tie the wrap back to itself to maintain the stabilization.[155] The pelvic binder is a useful adjunct in the battlefield environment because it is light, adaptable to any body size, and easy to apply.

External fixation can be applied within minutes by an orthopedic surgeon or a specially trained general surgeon in more remote environments. When the external fixator is placed, crossmembers should be placed, with thought given to potential future therapeutic adjuncts (Fig. 40). A substantial percentage of pelvic hemorrhage is venous and can be controlled through efforts to effect pelvic ring stabilization in conjunction with blood resuscitation to replace volume loss.[153,156] This ongoing resuscitation often requires upwards of 10 units of packed red blood cells and additional blood component therapy to accomplish, and the patient must be cared for in the ICU. In general, pelvic hemorrhage is not approached operatively via celiotomy. The primary reason is that once the hematoma has been released into the peritoneal cavity and tamponade-effect lost, bleeding will increase. It is difficult, if not impossible, to locate and ligate the bleeding vessels. Furthermore, packing the pelvis once the retroperitoneal hematoma has been disrupted into the peritoneal cavity is not effective since there is nothing to pack against. This scenario often results in exsanguination.

Early pelvic stabilization can control hemorrhage and reduce mortality. Potential stabilizing methods for pelvic fractures include the pelvic sheet sling, pelvic binder, and external fixation.

Recent evidence from the civilian literature suggests that an alternative preperitoneal approach and packing

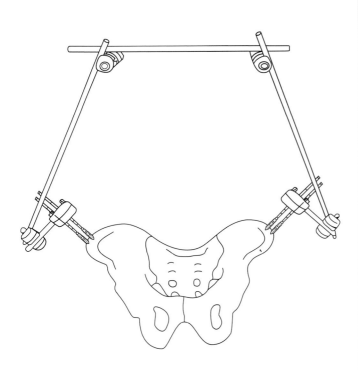

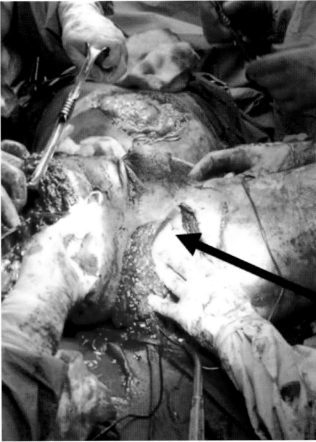

Figure 40. *Early pelvic stabilization can control hemorrhage and reduce mortality. External fixator placement in the iliac crests is often used to stabilize the pelvis. Image courtesy of the Borden Institute, Office of The Surgeon General, Washington, DC.*

Figure 41. *Open pelvic fractures require hemorrhage control, aggressive debridement, and fecal diversion if significant perineal soft-tissue or anorectal disruption exists. Image courtesy of Leopoldo C. Cancio, MD, FACS, COL, MC, US Army.*

of the pelvis through the space of Retzius may be more effective. Such an approach controlled pelvic bleeding and significantly reduced blood product transfusions and mortality in a selected high-risk group of patients.[157,158] Preperitoneal and pelvic packing may prove to be an important intervention in the austere deployed environment where resources and therapeutic options are limited. In this scenario, if a patient does not respond to initial resuscitation, they are taken to the operating room where an initial small laparotomy incision is made above the umbilicus. If the source of hemorrhage is in the abdomen, the incision is extended. On the other hand, if there is a large pelvic retroperitoneal hematoma, a separate lower midline incision is made to enter the extraperitoneal space of Retzius. The pelvic hematoma is evacuated, the bladder displaced, and packs are placed on both sides of the bladder deep into the pelvis. If an unstable pelvic fracture is present, it is necessary to apply a pelvic fixator to provide something to pack against. The patient can then be resuscitated and transported to a rearward facility with angiographic embolization capabilities. Interventional angiography (e.g., embolization) is often only available at Level IV and V care facilities.

## Open Pelvic Fractures

Open pelvic fractures present a unique management challenge to the surgeon (Fig. 41). The same basic management principles apply with some notable additions. Efforts must be made to directly control or tamponade external hemorrhage. Soft-tissue injury must be vigorously debrided. Fecal diversion must be strongly considered in patients with significant perineal soft-tissue or anorectal injuries, though this may be done at subsequent reoperation.[143,159] As with all combat wounds, the early administration (ideally within three hours of injury) of broad-spectrum prophylactic antibiotics is recommended.[160] Exclusive of associated injury, the prognosis of patients with pelvic fractures is directly correlated with severity of injury and prompt institution of therapeutic strategies for temporizing pelvic stabilization and hemorrhage control. Morbidity and mortality of open pelvic fractures are higher than their closed counterparts.[159] This is secondary to difficulty controlling external pelvic hemorrhage and sepsis associated with soft-tissue and enteric injuries.[143,159]

Management of open pelvic fractures includes hemorrhage control, aggressive debridement of soft-tissues, pelvic stabilization, and fecal diversion through a colostomy.

### Bladder and Urethral Injuries

The incidence of genitourinary injuries associated with pelvic fractures is reported to be as high as 25 percent and includes bladder injuries, urethral injuries, and combined injuries.[141,142] The posterior urethra is firmly attached to the pubis (in males), making it prone to injuries with anterior pelvic ring fractures. Urethral injury associated with pelvic fractures is much less common in females due to the female urethra's short length, mobility, and lack of attachments to the pelvis.[161] The bladder is most commonly injured in association with pubic ramus fractures. Injuries to the vagina or rectum may occur in association with pelvic fractures. Most result from the penetration of a bone fragment but may also occur with pubic symphysis diastasis.

Genitourinary tract injuries should be assumed in all patients with pelvic fractures until proven otherwise.

All pelvic fractures should be assumed to have accompanying genitourinary tract injuries until proven otherwise.[141,142] A retrograde urethrogram may diagnose urethral injuries in patients who have characteristic physical exam findings (Fig. 42). These include blood at the urethral meatus, a high-riding prostate, scrotal

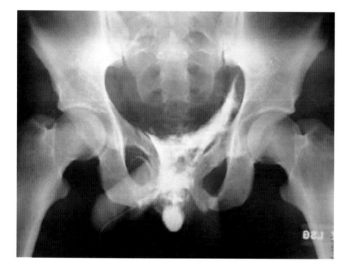

Figure 42. *Retrograde urethrogram demonstrating proximal urethral injury and extraperitoneal extravasation of contrast.*

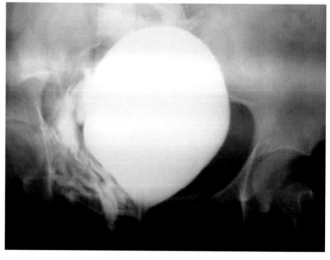

Figure 43. *Retrograde cystogram demonstrating extravasation of contrast from an injured bladder.*

hematoma, an inability to urinate, or difficulty with insertion of a urinary catheter.[141,142] Physical signs may be absent in some patients with urethral injuries. A retrograde cystogram may help to identify bladder ruptures, which often occur in association with pelvic ring injuries (Fig. 43). Evidence of gross hematuria is an indication for performing a retrograde cystogram. The cystogram may be performed using plain radiography or with CT imaging. The latter is often more convenient and provides more accurate imaging.

## Management of Bladder Injuries

Bladder injuries are categorized as intraperitoneal or extraperitoneal. Intraperitoneal injuries are repaired surgically in two-layer fashion with absorbable suture and transurethral catheter drainage. Previous standards included the use of a large-bore suprapubic catheter either alone or in combination with transurethral catheter, but this is no longer recommended due to greater association with complications regardless of degree of bladder injury. In addition, the previous average duration of indwelling suprapubic catheters was 42 days, which with modern treatment standards is now reduced to only 13 days duration of transurethral catheter insertion.[162,163] These advances along with primary bladder repair approaches have improved outcomes.[162,163]

The mainstay treatment of extraperitoneal bladder injuries remains nonoperative management with transurethral catheter drainage for 10 to 14 days with follow-up cystogram prior to removal.[164,165,166] Relative contraindications to nonoperative management of extraperitoneal bladder injuries include bone fragments projecting into the bladder, open pelvic fractures, and bladder injuries associated with rectal perforations.[167]

## Management of Urethral Injuries

Urethral injury in civilian settings is secondary to blunt trauma, occurring in 10 percent of pelvic fractures.[141] However, in combat situations, urethral injury may be associated with pelvic fractures or penetrating gunshot or fragment wounds (Fig. 44). Diagnosis and extent of injury are assessed by retrograde urethrogram. Options for management for partial or complete disruption both include delayed operative reconstruction or primary stenting of injury with a urethral catheter. Either approach appears to have similar complications, impotency rates, and incontinence rates.[168,169,170,171,172] Consequently, in most cases, bladder drainage, either via retrograde urethral catheter or suprapubic catheter alone, is adequate.

> If urethral injury is clinically suspected, urethral integrity can be confirmed by a retrograde urethrogram. Alternatively, a Foley catheter can be gently passed into the urethra. If minimal resistance is encountered the catheter is fully advanced into the bladder and the cuff inflated. If there is difficulty passing the catheter, no further attempts should be made, and a suprapubic tube cystostomy should be performed.

Delayed operative reconstruction requires expertise, which may not be available for host nationals. In these instances, immediate realignment may offer the best chance to reestablish continuity. In the author's experience (AM), based on reports of successful realignment using antegrade cystoscopy, if retrograde urethral catheter placement is unsuccessful, consideration should be given to antegrade urethral catheter placement, particularly if the patient is undergoing laparotomy.[173,174,175] This procedure is performed by opening the dome of the bladder and passing a Foley catheter antegrade into the urethra. A sterile large-bore Foley catheter is sutured to the antegrade catheter and pulled retrograde into the bladder. The bladder is closed in standard two-layer fashion, and the retrograde urethral catheter can be secured to the foreskin

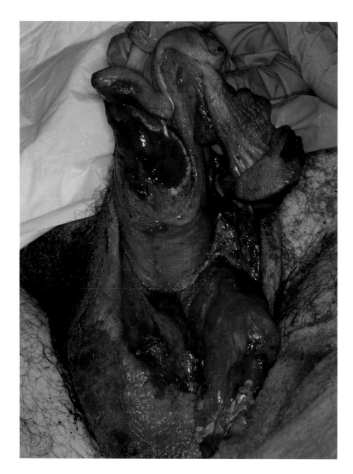

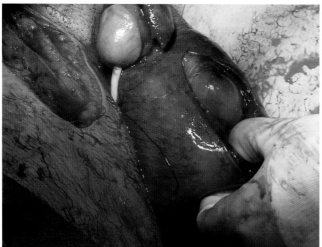

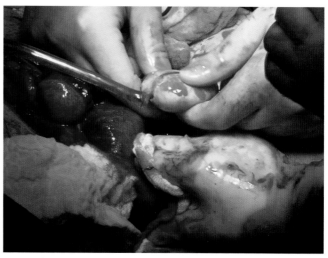

Figure 44. (Left) *External genital trauma. There is significant injury to the glans penis and the transected corpus cavernosum is evident. The proximal urethral opening is visible at the base of the wound. A left-sided orchiectomy was performed while the right testicle was repaired.*

Figure 45. (Bottom Left) *Penetrating scrotal injuries require exploration to examine the testicles and spermatic cords for injury.*

Figure 46. (Bottom Right) *Orchiectomy should not be performed unless the testicle is irreparably damaged or its vascular supply is destroyed.*

of the penis to reduce unintentional removal. The catheter should remain in place for a minimum of three weeks with retrograde urethrogram prior to permanent removal of the catheter to ensure continuity is reestablished.

## Genitalia Injuries

The management of combat wounds to the penis, scrotum, testes, and spermatic cord comprises hemorrhage control, debridement, and early penile repair to prevent deformity.[82] Disruption of Buck's fascia in penile injuries requires suture repair to prevent bleeding and long-term penile deformity.

The management of combat wounds to the penis, scrotum, testes, and spermatic cord comprises hemorrhage control, debridement, and early repair to prevent subsequent complications.

The scrotum is very vascular, and extensive scrotal debridement is unnecessary.[82] Penetrating scrotal injuries require exploration to examine the testes for injury and minimize the risk of hematoma formation (Fig. 45). Management of testicular injuries should be directed toward conservation of tissue with debridement of herniated parenchymal tissue and closure of the tunica albuginea with mattress sutures.[176,177] Orchiectomy should not be performed unless the testicle is irreparably damaged or its vascular supply is destroyed.[178] The testicle should be replaced in the scrotum, which can be closed primarily within eight hours of injury or closed over a Penrose drain, if longer delays to operative care occur (Fig. 46). If scrotal closure is not possible due to extensive tissue loss, the testicle should be placed in available subcutaneous tissue (e.g., thigh soft-tissue).

## Damage Control Summary

Damage control surgery is defined as the rapid initial control of hemorrhage and contamination with packing and temporary closure, followed by resuscitation in the ICU, and subsequent reexploration and definitive repair once normal physiology has been restored. Patients requiring damage control procedures are a higher acuity patient population in whom temporizing procedures to control hemorrhage and contamination improve survival. Damage control techniques are both feasible and effective on the battlefield. This damage control paradigm challenges surgeons in resource-constrained combat environments to have a low threshold to perform damage control procedures in order to mitigate the deleterious consequences of the challenging lethal triad of hypothermia, coagulopathy, and acidosis.

# References

1. Helling TS, McNabney WK. The role of amputation in the management of battlefield casualties: a history of two millennia. J Trauma 2000;49(5):930-939.

2. Larrey DJ. Memoires de chirurgicales militaire et campagnes. Paris; 1812.

3. US War Department. The war of the rebellion: a compilation of the official records of the Union and Confederate Armies. Washington, DC: US Government Printing Office 1880-1901;19(1.27):106-117.

4. Brewer LA III. The contributions of the Second Auxiliary Surgical Group to military surgery during World War II with special reference to thoracic surgery. Ann Surg 1983;197(3):318-326.

5. Jones EL, Peters AF, Gasior RM. Early management of battle casualties in Vietnam. An analysis of 1,011 consecutive cases treated at a mobile army surgical hospital. Arch Surg 1968;97(1):1-15.

6. Stone HH, Strom PR, Mullins RJ. Management of the major coagulopathy with onset during laparotomy. Ann Surg 1983;197(5):532-535.

7. Rotondo MF, Schwab CW, McGonigal MD, et al. 'Damage control': an approach for improved survival in exsanguinating penetrating abdominal injury. J Trauma 1993;35(3):375-382.

8. Hirshberg A, Mattox KL. Planned reoperation for severe trauma. Ann Surg 1995;222(1):3-8.

9. Moore EE, Thomas G. Orr Memorial Lecture. Staged laparotomy for the hypothermia, acidosis and coagulopathy syndrome. Am J Surg 1996;172(5):405-410.

10. Cue JI, Cryer HG, Miller FB, et al. Packing and planned reexploration for hepatic and retroperitoneal hemorrhage: critical refinements of a useful technique. J Trauma 1990;30(8):1007-1011; discussion 1011-1013.

11. Hildebrand F, Giannoudis P, Kretteck C, et al. Damage control: extremities. Injury 2004;35(7):678-689.

12. Giannoudis PV, Pape HC. Damage control orthopaedics in unstable pelvic ring injuries. Injury 2004;35(7):671-677.

13. Rosenfeld JV. Damage control neurosurgery. Injury 2004;35(7):655-660.

14. Reilly PM, Rotondo MF, Carpenter JP, et al. Temporary vascular continuity during damage control: intraluminal shunting for proximal superior mesenteric artery injury. J Trauma 1995;39(4):757-760.

15. Rotondo MF, Zonies DH. The damage control sequence and underlying logic. Surg Clin North Am 1997;77(4):761-777.

16. Feliciano DV, Mattox KL, Burch JM, et al. Packing for control of hepatic hemorrhage. J Trauma 1986;26(8):738-743.

17. Cogbill TH, Moore EE, Jurkovich GJ, et al. Severe hepatic trauma: a multi-center experience with 1,335 liver injuries. J Trauma 1988;28(10):1433-1438.

18. Beal SL. Fatal hepatic hemorrhage: an unresolved problem in the management of complex liver injuries. J Trauma 1990;30(2):163-169.

19. Burch JM, Ortiz VB, Richardson RJ, et al. Abbreviated laparotomy and planned reoperation for critically injured patients. Ann Surg 1992;215(5):476-483; discussion 483-484.

20. Morris JA Jr, Eddy VA, Blinman TA, et al. The staged celiotomy for trauma. Issues in unpacking and reconstruction. Ann Surg 1993;217(5):576-584; discussion 584-586.

21. Hirshberg A, Wall MJ Jr, Mattox KL. Planned reoperation for trauma: a two year experience with 124 consecutive patients. J Trauma 1994;37(3):365-369.

22. Garrison J, Richardson JD, Hilakos AS, et al. Predicting the need to pack early for severe intra-abdominal hemorrhage. J Trauma 1996;40(6):923-927; discussion 927-929.

23. Blackbourne LH. Combat damage control surgery. Crit Care Med 2008;36(7 Suppl):S304-310.

24. Chambers LW, Rhee P, Baker BC, et al. Initial experience of the US Marine Corps forward resuscitative surgical system during Operation Iraqi Freedom. Arch Surg 2005;140(1):26-32.

25. Beekley AC, Watts DM. Combat trauma experience with the United States Army 102nd Forward Surgical Team in Afghanistan. Am J Surg 2004;187(5):652-654.

26. Patel TH, Wenner KA, Price SA, et al. A U.S. Army Forward Surgical Team's experience in Operation Iraqi Freedom. J Trauma 2004;57(2):201-207.

27. Place RJ, Rush RM, Arrington ED. Forward surgical team (FST) workload in a special operations environment: the 250th FST in Operation Enduring Freedom. Curr Surg 2003;60(4):418-422.

28. Borgman MA, Spinella PC, Perkins JG, et al. The ratio of blood products tranfused affects mortality in patients receiving massive transfusions at a combat support hospital. J Trauma 2007;63(4):805-813.

29. Spinella PC, Perkins JG, Grathwohl KW, et al. Effect of plasma and red blood cell transfusions on survival in patients with combat related traumatic injuries. J Trauma 2008;64(2 Suppl):S69-77; discussion S77-78.

30. Spinella PC, Perkins JG, Grathwohl KW, et al. 31st CSH Research Working Group. Fresh whole blood transfusions in coalition military, foreign national, and enemy combatant patients during Operation Iraqi Freedom at a U.S. combat support hospital. World J Surg 2008;32(1):2-6. Epub 2007.

31. Beninati W, Meyer MT, Carter TE. The critical care air transport program. Crit Care Med 2008;36(7 Suppl):S370-376.

32. Bridges E, Evers K. Wartime critical care air transport. Mil Med 2009;174(4):370-375.

33. Rice DH, Kotti G, Beninati W. Clinical review: critical care transport and austere critical care. Crit Care 2008;12(2):207.

34. Working Group, Ad Hoc Subcommittee on Outcomes, American College of Surgeons. Committee on Trauma. Practice management guidelines for emergency department thoracotomy. J Am Coll Surg 2001;193(3):303-309.

35. Rhee PM, Acosta J, Bridgeman A, et al. Survival after emergency department thoracotomy: review of published data from the past 25 years. J Am Coll Surg 2000;190(3):288–298.

36. Edens JW, Beekley AC, Chung KK, et al. Longterm outcomes after combat casualty emergency department thoracotomy. J Am Coll Surg 2009;209(2):188-197.

37. Macho JR, Markison RE, Schecter WP. Cardiac stapling in the management of penetrating injuries of the heart: rapid control of hemorrhage and decreased risk of personal contamination. J Trauma 1993;34(5):711-715; discussion 715-716.

38. Evans BJ, Hornick P. Use of skin stapler for penetrating cardiac injury. Ann R Coll Surg Eng 2006;88(4):413-414.

39. Bowman MR, King RM. Comparison of staples and sutures for cardiorrhaphy in traumatic puncture wounds of the heart. J Emerg Med 1996;14(5):615-618.

40. Wilson SM, Au FC. In extremis use of a Foley catheter in a cardiac stab wound. J Trauma 1986;26(4):400-402.

41. Moore EE, Mattox KL, Feliciano DV. Indication for thoracotomy. In: Moore EE, Mattox KL, Feliciano DV, editors. Trauma manual. 4th ed. McGraw-Hill; 2003. p. 161-169.

42. Moore EE, Mattox KL, Feliciano DV. Injury to the thoracic great vessels. In: Moore EE, Mattox KL, Feliciano DV, editors. Trauma manual. 4th ed. McGraw-Hill; 2003. p. 202-213.

43. Martin MJ, McDonald JM, Mullenix PS, et al. Operative management and outcomes of traumatic lung resection. J Am Coll Surg 2006;203(3):336-344. Epub 2006.

44. Richardson JD. Outcome of tracheobronchial injuries: a long-term perspective. J Trauma 2004;56(1):30-36.

45. Bowling R, Mavroudis C, Richardson JD, et al. Emergency pneumonectomy for penetrating and blunt trauma. Am Surg 1985;51(3):136-139.

46. Wilson A, Wall MJ Jr, Maxson R, et al. The pulmonary hilum twist as a thoracic damage control procedure. Am J Surg 2003;186(1):49-52.

47. Bryant AS, Cerfolio RJ. Esophageal trauma. Thorac Surg Clin 2007;17(1):63-72.

48. Phelan HA, Patterson SG, Hassan MO, et al. Thoracic damage-control operation: principles, techniques, and definitive repair. J Am Coll Surg 2006;203(6):933-941.

49. Rotondo MF, Bard MR. Damage control surgery for thoracic injuries. Injury 2004;35(7):649-654.

50. US Department of Defense (US DoD). Face and Neck Injuries. In: Emergency War Surgery, Third United States Revision. Washington, DC: Department of the Army, Office of the Surgeon General, Borden Institute; 2004. p. 13.1-13.20.

51. Demetriades D, Theodorou D, Cornwell E, et al. Evaluation of penetrating injuries of the neck: prospective study of 223 patients. World J Surg 1997;21(1):41-47; discussion 47-48.

52. Brywczynski JJ, Barrett TW, Lyon JA, et al. Management of penetrating neck injury in the emergency department: a structured literature review. Emerg Med J 2008;25(11):711-715.

53. Ivatury RR, Stoner MC. Penetrating cervical vascular injuries. In: Rich NM, Mattox KL, Hirschberg A, editors. Vascular trauma. 2nd ed. Philadelphia, PA: Elsevier-Saunders; 2004. p. 223-240.

54. du Toit DF, van Schalkwyk GD, Wadee SA, et al. Neurologic outcome after penetrating extracranial arterial trauma. J Vasc Surg 2003;38(2):257-262.

55. Moore WS. Vascular surgery: a comprehensive review. 6th ed. Phildelphia, PA: Elsevier-Saunders; 2002. p. 684-686.

56. McLaughlin DF, Niles SE, Salinas J, et al. A predictive model for massive tranfusion in combat casualty patients. J Trauma 2008;64(2 Suppl):S57-63; discussion S63.

57. Karmy-Jones RC, Salerno C. Thoracic vascular trauma. In: Zelenock GB, Huber TS, Messina LM, editors. Mastery of vascular and endovascular surgery. Philadelphia, PA: Lippincott Williams & Wilkins; 2006. p. 629-635.

58. Feliciano DV, Pachter JL. Hepatic trauma revisited. Curr Probl Surg 1989;26(7):453-524.

59. Buckman RF, Pathak AS, Badellino MM, et al. Injuries to the inferior vena cava. Surg Clin North Am 2001;81(6):1431-1437.

60. Dente CJ, Feliciano DV. Abdominal vascular injury. In: Moore EE, Mattox KL, Feliciano DV, editors. Trauma manual. 6th ed. McGraw-Hill; 2008. p. 746-747.

61. Votanopoulos KI, Welsh FJ, Mattox KL. Suprarenal inferior vena cava ligation: a rare survivor. J

Trauma 2009;67(6):E179-180.

62. Ivy ME, Possenti P, Atweh N, et al. Ligation of the suprarenal vena cava after a gunshot wound. J Trauma 1998;45(3):630-632.

63. Mays ET, Conti S, Fallahzadeh H, et al. Hepatic artery ligation. Surgery 1979;86(4):536-543.

64. Mays ET. Options in treating trauma to the liver. Surg Annu 1980;12:103-121.

65. Trunkey DD, Shires GT, McClelland R. Management of liver trauma in 811 consecutive patients. Ann Surg 1974;179(5):722-728.

66. Moore EE. Edgar J. Poth Lecture. Critical decisions in the management of hepatic trauma. Am J Surg 1984;148(6):712-716.

67. Feliciano DV, Mattox KL, Jordan GL Jr, et al. Management of 1000 consecutive cases of hepatic trauma (1979-1984). Ann Surg 1986;204(4):438-445.

68. Pachter HL, Spencer FC, Hofstetter SR, et al. Significant trends in the treatment of hepatic trauma. Experience with 411 injuries. Ann Surg 1992;215(5):492-500; discussion 500-502.

69. Fabian TC, Stone HH. Arrest of severe liver hemorrhage by an omental pack. South Med J 1980;73(11):1487-1490.

70. Polanco P, Leon S, Pineda J, et al. Hepatic resection in the management of complex injury to the liver. J Trauma 2008;65(6):1264-1269; discussion 1269-1270.

71. Asensio JA, Petrone P, Roldán G, et al. Pancreatic and duodenal injuries. complex and lethal. Scand J Surg 2002;91(1):81-86.

72. Bokhari F, Phelan H, Holevar M, et al. EAST guidelines for the diagnosis and management of pancreatic trauma. Eastern Association for the Surgery of Trauma (EAST) 2009 [cited 2010 May 26]. Available from: URL: http://www.east.org/tpg/pancreas.pdf.

73. Degiannis E, Levy RD, Potokar T, et al. Distal pancreatectomy for gunshot injuries of the distal pancreas. Br J Surg 1995;82(9):1240-1242.

74. Degiannis E, Boffard K. Duodenal injuries. Br J Surg 2000;87(11):1473-1479.

75. Jansen M, Du Toit DF, Warren BL. Duodenal injuries: surgical management adapted to circumstances. Injury 2002;33(7):611-615.

76. Voelzke BB, McAninch JW. The current management of renal injuries. Am Surg 2008;74(8):667-678.

77. Master VA, McAninch JW. Operative management of renal injuries: parenchymal and vascular. Urol Clin North Am 2006;33(1):21-31, v-vi.

78. Gonzalez RP, Falimirski M, Holevar MR, et al. Surgical management of renal trauma: is vascular control necessary? J Trauma 1999;47(6):1039-1042; discussion 1042-1044.

79. Brandes SB, McAninch JW. Reconstructive surgery for trauma of the upper urinary tract. Urol Clin North Am 1999;26(1):183-199.

80. Holden S, Hicks CC, O'Brien DP, et al. Gunshot wounds of the ureter: a 15-year review of 63 consecutive cases. J Urol 1976;116(5):562-564.

81. Walker JA. Injuries of the ureter due to external violence. J Urol 1969;102(4):410-413.

82. US Department of Defense (US DoD). Genitourinary Tract Injuries. In: Emergency War Surgery, Third United States Revision. Washington, DC: Department of the Army, Office of the Surgeon General, Borden Institute; 2004. p. 18.1-18.13.

83. Velmahos GC, Degiannis E, Wells M, et al. Penetrating ureteral injuries: the impact of associated injuries on management. Am Surg 1996;62(6):461-468.

84. Perez-Brayfield MR, Keane TE, Krishnan A, et al. Gunshot wounds to the ureter: a 40-year experience at Grady Memorial Hospital. J Urol 2001;166(1):119-121.

85. Franko ER, Ivatury RR, Schwalb DM. Combined penetrating rectal and genitourinary injuries: a challenge in management. J Trauma 1993;34(3):347-353.

86. Alonso M, Brathwaite C, Garcia V, et al. Practice management guidelines for the nonoperative management of blunt injury to the liver and spleen. Eastern Association for the Surgery of Trauma (EAST), 2003 [cited 2010 May 26]. Available from: URL: http://www.east.org/tpg/livspleen.pdf.

87. Wei B, Hemmila MR, Arbabi S, et al. Angioembolization reduces operative intervention for blunt splenic injury. J Trauma 2008;64(6):1472-1477.

88. Achneck HE, Sileshi B, Jamiolkowski RM, et al. A comprehensive review of topical hemostatic agents: efficacy and recommendations for use. Ann Surg 2010;251(2):217-228.

89. Vertrees A, Wakefield M, Pickett C, et al. Outcomes of primary repair and primary anastomosis in war-related colon injuries. J Trauma 2009;66(5):1286-1291; discussion 1291-1293.

90. Vertrees A, Greer L, Pickett C, et al. Modern management of complex open abdominal wounds of war: a 5-year experience. J Am Coll Surg 2008;207(6):801-809.

91. Burch JM, Feliciano DV, Mattox KL. Colostomy and drainage for civilian rectal injuries: is that all? Ann Surg 1989;209(5):600-610; discussion 610-611.

92. Gonzalez RP, Falimirski ME, Holevar MR. The role of presacral drainage in the management of penetrating rectal injuries. J Trauma 1998;45(4):656-661.

93. Steele SR, Wolcott KE, Mullenix SP, et al. Colon and rectal injuries during Operation Iraqi Freedom: are there any changing trends in management or outcome? Dis Colon Rectum 2007;50(6):870-877.

94. Sugrue M, D'Amours SK, Joshipura M. Damage control surgery and the abdomen. Injury 2004;35(7):642-648.

95. US Department of Defense (US DoD). Abdominal Injuries. In: Emergency War Surgery, Third United States Revision. Washington, DC: Department of the Army, Office of the Surgeon General, Borden Institute; 2004. p. 17.1-17.16.

96. Thal E, Eastridge B, Milhoan R. Operative exposure of abdominal injuries and closure of the abdomen. In: Wilmore, D editor. ACS Surgery. WebMD; 2002.

97. Offner PJ, de Souza AL, Moore EE, et al. Avoidance of abdominal compartment syndrome in damage-control laparotomy after trauma. Arch Surg 2001;136(6):676-681.

98. Harrahill M. Intra-abdominal pressure monitoring. J Emerg Nurs 1998;24(5):465-466.

99. Lozen Y. Intraabdominal hypertension and abdominal compartment syndrome in trauma: pathophysiology and interventions. AACN Clin Issues 1999;10(1):104-112.

100. Schein M, Wittmann DH, Aprahamian CC, et al. The abdominal compartment syndrome: the physiological and clinical consequences of elevated intra-abdominal pressure. J Am Coll Surg 1995;180(6):745-753.

101. Saggi BH, Sugerman HJ, Ivatury RR, et al. Abdominal compartment syndrome. J Trauma 1998;45(3):597-609.

102. Ivatury RR, Diebel L, Porter JM, et al. Intra-abdominal hypertension and the abdominal compartment syndrome. Surg Clin North Am 1997;77(4):783-800.

103. Meldrum DR, Moore FA, Moore EE, et al. Prospective characterization and selective management of the abdominal compartment syndrome. Am J Surg 1997;174(6):667-672.

104. Mayberry JC, Goldman RK, Mullins RJ, et al. Surveyed opinion of American trauma surgeons on the prevention of the abdominal compartment syndrome. J Trauma 1999;47(3):509-513.

105. Rich NM, Rhee P. An historical tour of vascular injury management: from its inception to the new millennium. Surg Clin North Am 2001;81(6):1199-1215.

106. Rich N. Military surgery: "bullets and blood vessels." Surg Clin North Am 1978;58(5):995-1003.

107. Rich NM. Vascular trauma. Surg Clin North Am 1973;53(6):1367-1392.

108. DeBakey ME, Simeone FA. Battle injuries of the arteries in World War II: an analysis of 2,471 cases. Ann Surg 1946;123(4):534-579.

109. Hughes CW. The primary repair of wounds of major arteries; an analysis of experience in Korea in 1953. Ann Surg 1955;141(3):297-303.

110. Fox CJ, Gillespie DL, Cox ED, et al. Damage control resuscitation for vascular surgery in a combat support hospital. J Trauma 2008;65(1):1-9.

111. Fox CJ, Gillespie DL, Cox ED, et al. The effectiveness of a damage control resuscitation strategy for vascular injury in a combat support hospital: results of a case control study. J Trauma 2008;64(2 Suppl):S99-106; discussion S106-107.

112. Clouse WD, Rasmussen TE, Peck MA, et al. In-theater management of vascular injury: 2 years of the Balad Vascular Registry. J Am Coll Surg 2007;204(4):625-632.

113. Sohn VY, Arthurs ZM, Herbert GS, et al. Demographics, treatment, and early outcomes in penetrating vascular combat trauma. Arch Surg 2008;143(8):783-787.

114. Rasmussen TE, Clouse WD, Jenkins DH, et al. The use of temporary vascular shunts as a damage control adjunct in the management of wartime vascular injury. J Trauma 2006;61(1):8-12; discussion 12-15.

115. Dennis JW, Frykberg ER, Crump JM, et al. New perspectives on the management of penetrating trauma in proximity to major limb arteries. J Vasc Surg 1990;11(1):84-92; discussion 92-93.

116. Frykberg ER, Crump JM, Vines FS, et al. A reassessment of the role of arteriography in penetrating proximity extremity trauma: a prospective study. J Trauma 1989;29(8):1041-1050; discussion 1050-1052.

117. Francis H III, Thal ER, Weigelt JA, et al. Vascular proximity: is it a valid indication for arteriography in asymptomatic patients? J Trauma 1991;31(4):512-514.

118. Johnson ON III, Fox CJ, White P, et al. Physical exam and occult post-traumatic vascular lesions: implications for the evaluation and management of arterial injuries in modern warfare in the endovascular era. J Cardiovasc Surg (Torino) 2007;48(5):581-586.

119. Fox CJ, Gillespie DL, Weber MA, et al. Delayed evaluation of combat-related penetrating neck trauma. J Vasc Surg 2006;44(1):86-93.

120. Rasmussen TE, Clouse WD, Jenkins DH, et al. Echelons of care and the management of wartime vascular injury: a report from the 332nd EMDG/Air Force Theater Hospital, Balad Air Base, Iraq. Perspect Vasc Surg Endovasc Ther 2006;18(2):91-99.

121. Chambers LW, Green DJ, Sample K, et al. Tactical surgical intervention with temporary shunting of peripheral vascular trauma sustained during Operation Iraqi Freedom: one unit's experience. J Trauma 2006;61(4):824–830.

122. Taller J, Kamdar JP, Greene JA, et al. Temporary vascular shunts as initial treatment of proximal extremity vascular injuries during combat operations: the new standard of care at Echelon II facilities? J Trauma 2008;65(3):595-603.

123. Zouris JM, Walker GJ, Dye J, et al. Wounding patterns for U.S. Marines and sailors during Operation Iraqi Freedom, major combat phase. Mil Med 2006;171(3):246-252.

124. Gifford SM, Eliason JL, Clouse WD, et al. Early versus delayed restoration of flow with a temporary vascular shunt reduces circulating markers of injury in a porcine model. J Trauma 2009;67(2):259-265.

125. Woodward EB, Clouse WD, Eliason JL, et al. Penetrating femoropopliteal injury during modern warfare: experience of the Balad Vascular Registry. J Vasc Surg 2008;47(6):1259-1264; discussion 1264-1265.

126. Gifford SM, Aidinian G, Clouse WD, et al. Effect of temporary shunting on extremity vascular injury: an outcome analysis from the Global War on Terror vascular injury initiative. J Vasc Surg 2009;50(3):549-555.

127. Fox CJ, Gillespie DL, O'Donnell SD, et al. Contemporary management of wartime vascular trauma. J Vasc Surg 2005;41(4):638-644.

128. US Department of Defense (US DoD). Vascular Injuries. In: Emergency War Surgery, Third United States Revision. Washington, DC: Department of the Army, Office of the Surgeon General, Borden Institute; 2004. p. 27.1-27.9.

129. Dawson DL, Putnam AT, Light JT, et al. Temporary arterial shunts to maintain limb perfusion after arterial injury: an animal study. J Trauma 1999;47(1):64-71.

130. Quan RW, Gillespie DL, Stuart RP, et al. The effect of vein repair on the risk of venous thromboembolic events: a review of more than 100 traumatic military venous injuries. J Vasc Surg 2008;47(3):571-577.

131. Kragh JF Jr, Walters TJ, Baer DG, et al. Survival with emergency tourniquet use to stop bleeding in major limb trauma. Ann Surg 2009;249(1):1-7.

132. Kragh JF Jr, Walters TJ, Baer DG, et al. Practical use of emergency tourniquets to stop bleeding in major limb trauma. J Trauma 2008;64(2 Suppl):S38-49; discussion S49-50.

133. Perry MO. Vascular trauma. Adv Surg 1995;28:59-70.

134. Thal ER. Vascular injuries of the extremities. In: Rutherford RB, editor. Vascular surgery. 4th ed. Philadelphia, PA: WB Saunders; 1995. p. 713-735.

135. Perry MO, Bongard F. Vascular trauma. In: Moore WS. Vascular surgery a comprehensive review. 6th Ed. WB Saunders; 2002. p. 648-666.

136. Joint Theater Trauma System (JTTS) Clinical Practice Guideline. Vascular injury. 2008 Nov 07 [cited 2010 May 26]. Available from: URL: http://www.usaisr.amedd.army.mil/cpgs.html.

137. Dalal SA, Burgess AR, Siegel JH, et al. Pelvic fracture in multiple trauma: classification by mechanism is key to pattern of organ injury, resuscitative requirements and outcome. J Trauma 1989;29(7):981-1000; discussion 1000-1002.

138. Burgess AR, Eastridge BJ, Young JW, et al. Pelvic ring disruptions: effective classification system and treatment protocols. J Trauma 1990;30(7):848-856.

139. Eastridge BJ, Starr A, Minei JP, et al. The importance of fracture pattern in guiding therapeutic decision-making in patients with hemorrhagic shock and pelvic ring disruptions. J Trauma 2002;53(3):446-450; discussion 450-451.

140. Papakostidis C, Giannoudis PV. Pelvic ring injuries with haemodynamic instability: efficacy of pelvic packing, a systematic review. Injury 2009;40(Suppl 4):S53-61.

141. Brandes S, Borrelli J Jr. Pelvic fracture and associated urologic injuries. World J Surg 2001;25(12):1578-1587.

142. Lowe MA, Mason JT, Luna GK, et al. Risk factors for urethral injuries in men with traumatic pelvic fractures. J Urol 1988;140(3):506-507.

143. Faringer PD, Mullins RJ, Feliciano PD, et al. Selective fecal diversion in complex open pelvic fractures from blunt trauma. Arch Surg 1994;129(9):958-963; discussion 963-964.

144. Ham SJ, van Walsum AD, Vierhout PA. Predictive value of the hip flexion test for fractures of the pelvis. Injury 1996;27(8):543-544.

145. Resnik CS, Stackhouse DJ, Shanmuganathan K, et al. Diagnosis of pelvic fractures in patients with acute pelvic trauma: efficacy of plain radiographs. AJR Am J Roentgenol 1992;158(1):109-112.

146. Falchi M, Rollandi GA. CT of pelvic fractures. Eur J Radiol 2004;50(1):96-105.

147. Theumann NH, Verdon JP, Mouhsine E, et al. Traumatic injuries: imaging of pelvic fractures. Eur Radiol 2002;12(6):1312-1330.

148. Cerva DS Jr, Mirvis SE, Shanmuganathan K, et al. Detection of bleeding in patients with major pelvic fractures: value of contrast-enhanced CT. AJR Am J Roentgenol 1996;166(1):131-135.

149. Velmahos GC, Chahwan S, Hanks SE, et al. Angiographic embolization of bilateral internal iliac arteries to control life-threatening hemorrhage after blunt trauma to the pelvis. Am Surg 2000;66(9):858-862.

150. Velmahos GC, Toutouzas KG, Vassiliu P, et al. A prospective study on the safety and efficacy of angiographic embolization for pelvic and visceral injuries. J Trauma 2002;53(2):303-308.

151. Agolini SF, Shah K, Jaffe J, et al. Arterial embolization is a rapid and effective technique for controlling pelvic fracture hemorrhage. J Trauma 1997;43(3):395-399.

152. Bottlang M, Simpson T, Sigg J, et al. Noninvasive reduction of open-book pelvic fractures by circumferential compression. J Orthop Trauma 2002;16(6):367-373.

153. Rommens PM, Hofmann, A, Hessmann MH. Management of acute hemorrhage in pelvic trauma: an overview. Eur J Trauma Emerg Surg 2010;2:91-99.

154. Eastridge BJ. Butt binder. J Trauma 2007;62(6 Suppl):S32.

155. Simpson T, Krieg JC, Heuer F, et al. Stabilization of pelvic ring disruptions with a circumferential sheet. J Trauma 2002;52(1):158-161.

156. Tucker MC, Nork SE, Simonian PT, et al. Simple anterior pelvic external fixation. J Trauma 2000;49(6):989-994.

157. Cothren CC, Osborn PM, Moore EE, et al. Preperitonal pelvic packing for hemodynamically unstable pelvic fractures: a paradigm shift. J Trauma 2007;62(4):834-839; discussion 839-842.

158. Osborn PM, Smith WR, Moore EE, et al. Direct retroperitoneal pelvic packing versus pelvic angiography: a comparison of two management protocols for haemodynamically unstable pelvic fractures. Injury 2009;40(1):54-60. Epub 2008.

159. Grotz MR, Allami MK, Harwood P, et al. Open pelvic fractures: epidemiology, current concepts of management and outcome. Injury 2005;36(1):1-13.

160. Gerhardt RT, Matthews JM, Sullivan SG. The effect of systemic antibiotic prophylaxis and wound irrigation on penetrating combat wounds in a return-to-duty population. Prehosp Emerg Care 2009;13(4):500-504.

161. Venn SN, Greenwell TJ, Mundy AR. Pelvic fracture injuries of the female urethra. BJU International 1999;83(6):626-630.

162. Thomae KR, Kilambi NK, Poole GV. Method of urinary diversion in nonurethral traumatic bladder injuries: retrospective analysis of 70 cases. Am Surg 1998;64(1):77-80.

163. Volpe MA, Pachter EM, Scalea TM, et al. Is there a difference in outcome when treating traumatic intraperitoneal bladder rupture with or without a suprapubic tube? J Urol 1999;161(4):1103-1105.

164. Corriere JN Jr, Sandler CM. Management of the ruptured bladder: seven years of experience with 111 cases. J Trauma 1986;26(9):830-833.

165. Cass AS, Luxenberg M. Features of 164 bladder ruptures. J Urol 1987;138(4):743-745.

166. Corriere JN Jr, Sandler CM. Mechanisms of injury, patterns of extravasation and management of extraperitoneal bladder rupture due to blunt trauma. J Urol 1988;139(1):43-44.

167. Cass AS, Luxenberg M. Management of extraperitoneal ruptures of bladder caused by external trauma. Urology 1989;33(3):179-183.

168. Morehouse DD, Mackinnon KJ. Management of prostatomembranous urethral disruption: 13-year experience. J Urol 1980;123(2):173-174.

169. Follis HW, Koch MO, McDougal WS. Immediate management of prostatomembranous urethral disruptions. J Urol 1992;147(5):1259-1262.

170. Herschorn S, Thijssen A, Radomski SB. The value of immediate or early catheterization of the traumatized posterior urethra. J Urol 1992;148(5):1428-1431.

171. Kotkin L, Koch MO. Impotence and incontinence after immediate realignment of posterior urethral trauma: result of injury or management? J Urol 1996;155(5):1600-1603.

172. Elliott DS, Barrett DM. Long-term followup and evaluation of primary realignment of posterior urethral disruptions. J Urol 1997;157(3):814-816.

173. Koraitim MM. Pelvic fracture urethral injuries: evaluation of various methods of management. J Urol 1996;156(4):1288-1291.

174. Moudoni, SM, Patard JJ, Manunta A, et al. Early endoscopic realignment of post-traumatic posterior urethral disruption. Urology 2001;57(4):628-632.

175. Chapple C, Barbagli G, Jordan G, et al. Consensus statement on urethral trauma. BJU Int 2004;93(9):1195-1202.

176. Brandes SB, Buckman RF, Chelsky MJ, et al. External genitalia gunshot wounds: a ten-year experience with fifty-six cases. J Trauma 1995;39(2):266-271; discussion 271-272.

177. Cline KJ, Mata JA, Venable DD, et al. Penetrating trauma to the male external genitalia. J Trauma 1998;44(3):492-494.

178. Yap SA, DeLair SM, Ellison LM. Novel technique for testicular salvage after combat-related genitourinary injury. Urology 2006;68(4):890.e11-12.

# MAXILLOFACIAL AND NECK TRAUMA

*Chapter 6*

**Contributing Authors**
Robert G. Hale, DDS, COL, US Army
David K. Hayes, MD, COL, US Army
George Orloff, MD
Kyle Peterson, DO, CDR, US Navy
David B. Powers, DMD, MD, COL, US Air Force
Swaminatha Mahadevan, MD

All figures and tables included in this chapter have been used with permission from Pelagique, LLC, the UCLA Center for International Medicine, and/or the authors, unless otherwise noted.

Use of imagery from the Defense Imagery Management Operations Center (DIMOC) does not imply or constitute Department of Defense (DOD) endorsement of this company, its products, or services.

**Disclaimer**
The opinions and views expressed herein belong solely to those of the authors. They are not nor should they be implied as being endorsed by the United States Uniformed Services University of the Health Sciences, Department of the Army, Department of the Navy, Department of the Air Force, Department of Defense, or any other branch of the federal government.

# Table of Contents

# Introduction

This chapter will review maxillofacial and neck injuries combat casualty care (CCC) providers will likely encounter at Level II and III care facilities. The chapter is intended to convey lessons learned in Operation Enduring Freedom (OEF) and Operation Iraqi Freedom (OIF). Pertinent anatomy, injury patterns, treatment of battle injuries, and differences between civilian trauma management in the United States (US) versus CCC are presented. The generalist CCC provider will be presented with the information required to assess and stabilize maxillofacial and neck injuries. Special consideration is given to airway management since significant trauma to the maxillofacial and neck areas greatly influences airway management (Fig. 1). Evidence-based recommendations to prevent and manage infections of combat-related injuries of the head and neck are provided. Additionally, information is provided to prepare the specialist CCC provider, deployed for the first time, to both stabilize and definitively manage (typically in host nation patients) maxillofacial and neck battle injuries.

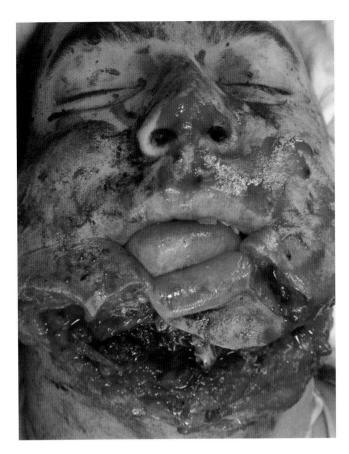

Figure 1. *The first consideration in this casualty with significant head and neck trauma is securing the airway. Image courtesy of Tamer Goksel, DDS, MD, COL, US Army.*

## Overview

The combat theater will produce varying combinations of blunt and penetrating injuries to the head and neck. Blunt trauma can result from motor vehicle accidents, blast injury (tertiary effect), falls, heavy equipment injuries, sport injuries, and altercations. Many of these blunt trauma injury mechanisms are similar to those experienced in the US. The majority of these blunt trauma-related maxillofacial injuries are closed fractures and lacerations. Management of these injuries involves: (1) airway management, (2) prevention of disability from central nervous system injuries, and (3) systematic reconstruction of facial structures (Figs. 2 and 3).

Combat (gunshot wounds and blast injuries) often results in penetrating maxillofacial and neck injuries. Penetrating trauma results in a combination of complex lacerations, open fractures, and wounds complicated by tissue avulsions and burns (Fig. 4).[1] There is an increased frequency of maxillofacial injuries in OEF/OIF compared to previous American wars in the past century. The incidence of head and neck region injuries in World War II and the Korean War was 21 percent, in the Vietnam War it was 16 percent, and in OEF/OIF is 30 percent.[2] Recent advances in body armor and cranial vault protection have led to the increase in the percentage of head and neck casualties that survive initial injuries (Fig. 5).[3] The high incidence of blast injuries caused by improvised explosive devices (IEDs) is likely an additional factor contributing to the higher frequency of head and neck injuries in OEF/OIF.[4]

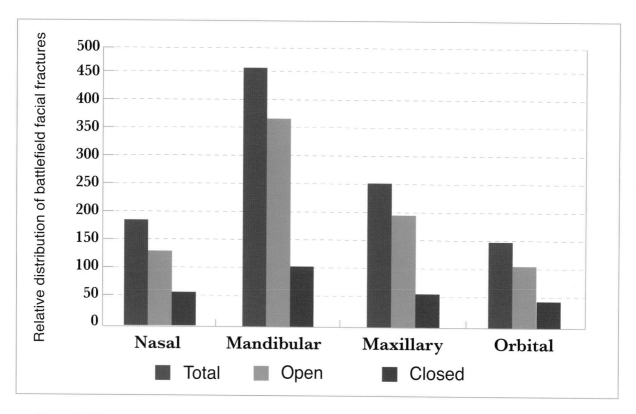

Figure 2. *Relative distribution of battlefield facial fractures. Most battlefield injury facial fractures are open. Data source: Joint Theater Trauma Registry (unpublished).*

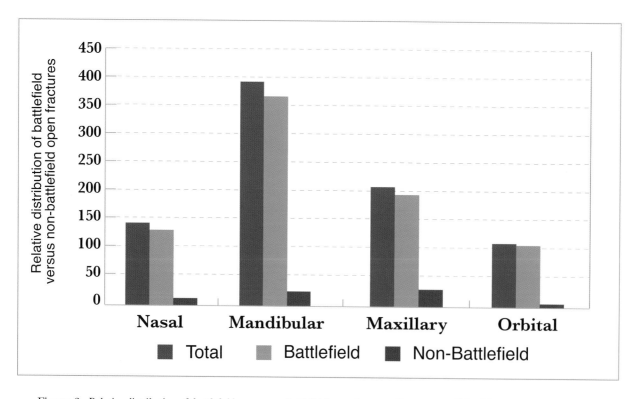

Figure 3. *Relative distribution of battlefield versus non-battlefield open fractures. Data source: Joint Theater Trauma Registry (unpublished).*

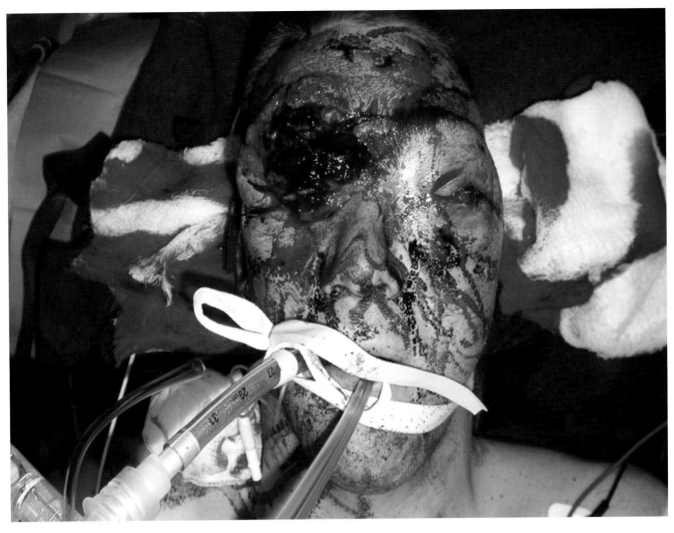

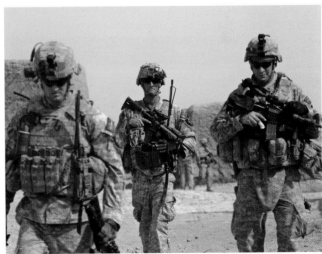

Figure 4. (Above) *Explosive blast trauma can result in a combination of complex facial lacerations, open fractures, tissue avulsion, and burns. Image courtesy of Tamer Goksel, DDS, MD, COL, US Army.*

Figure 5. (Right) *Recent advances in body armor and cranial vault protection have led to an increase in the percentage of head and neck casualties that survive initial injuries. Defense Imagery Management Operations Center (DIMOC).*

Combat injuries often cause complex penetrating maxillofacial and neck wounds, including lacerations, open fractures, tissue avulsions, and burns.

Lew et al. analyzed the Joint Theatre Trauma Registry (JTTR) database to describe the type, distribution, and mechanism of injury of maxillofacial injuries experienced by US service members in OEF/OIF (Tables 1, 2 and 3).[1] The JTTR is a military healthcare database, started at the beginning of military operations in Afghanistan (October 19, 2001), of all US military service members injured and treated at any medical facility throughout the evacuation system and spanning all military services at all levels of care.[5] During the six-year study period there were 7,770 injured service members entered into the JTTR. Approximately 26 percent of injured service members (2,014/7,770) had maxillofacial injuries.[1] There were 4,783 maxillofacial injuries among the 2,014 injured service members (average 2.4 injuries per service member with range of 1 to 8). The majority of patients were male (98 percent) and the average age was 26-years-old, with a range of 18 to 57 years of age. The relative distribution of maxillofacial injuries stratified by branch of military service was 72 percent (Army), 24 percent (Marines), 2 percent (Navy), and 1 percent (Air Force).

| Body Region | Body Surface Area (Percent) | WWII | Korea | Vietnam | OEF/OIF |
|---|---|---|---|---|---|
| Head/Neck | 12 | 21 | 21.4 | 16.0 | 30.0 |
| Thorax | 16 | 13 | 10 | 13.4 | 5.9 |
| Abdomen | 11 | 8 | 8.4 | 9.4 | 9.4 |
| Extremities | 61 | 58 | 60.2 | 61.1 | 54.5 |

Table 1. *Percent distribution of wounds by body region. Adapted from Lew, 2010.*[1]

| Craniomaxillofacial Wound Types | Number | Percent |
|---|---|---|
| Total Soft-Tissue | 2788 | 58 |
| Complicated Penetrating Soft-Tissue | 660 | 14 |
| Simple Penetrating Soft-Tissue | 2128 | 44 |
| Fractures | 1280 | 27 |
| Abrasions | 231 | 5 |
| Dental | 204 | 4 |
| Contusions | 111 | 2 |
| Dislocations | 6 | <1 |
| Skull | 15 | <1 |
| Unknown | 148 | 3 |

Table 2. *Characterization of craniofacial injuries sustained in battle by US service members in OEF and OIF. Adapted from Lew, 2010.*[1]

| Mechanism of Injury | Number of Injuries | Percent |
|---|---|---|
| Explosive | 4061 | 84 |
| IED | 3228 | 67 |
| Grenade/Rocket-propelled grenade (RPG) | 428 | 9 |
| Mortar | 263 | 5 |
| Landmine | 142 | 3 |
| Bomb | 26 | <1 |
| Gunshot Wound | 400 | 8 |
| Motor Vehicle Accident | 77 | 2 |
| Other / Not Documented | 81 | 2 |
| Fragment / Shrapnel | 43 | 1 |
| Helicopter / Plane Crash | 40 | 1 |
| Miscellaneous | 55 | 1 |

Table 3. *Mechanism of injury of combat-related craniomaxillofacial injuries in OEF and OIF. Adapted from Lew, 2010.*[1]

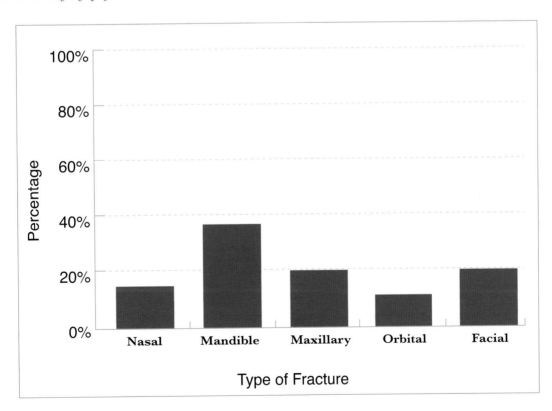

Figure 6. *Distribution of combat facial fractures in OEF and OIF. Adapted from Lew, 2010.*[1]

Based on analysis of the JTTR, the majority of maxillofacial combat injuries were penetrating soft-tissue injuries and fractures. A majority of the fractures were open. The primary mechanism of injury to the maxillofacial region was explosive devices.

The majority of maxillofacial combat injuries were penetrating soft-tissue injuries (58 percent) and fractures (27 percent). A majority of the fractures (76 percent) were open. Amongst the facial fractures, the mandible (36 percent) most frequently involved bone, followed by the maxilla and zygoma (19 percent), nasal bone (14 percent), and orbital wall (11 percent). The remaining fractures (20 percent) were not otherwise specified facial fractures (Fig. 6).[1] The primary mechanism of injury to the maxillofacial region was explosive devices (84 to 88 percent); this injury mechanism is much higher than previous wars.[1,2] Improvised explosive device wounds are the consequence of high-energy projectiles and are characterized by tissues grossly contaminated with dirt, rocks, plastic, glass, animal or human remains, and other materials.[6] Gunshot wounds (GSWs) accounted for just 8 percent of maxillofacial combat injuries. Burns traditionally account for 5 percent of all evacuated combat casualties. Explosions were the primary cause of combat burns (86 percent), which involved the face in 77 percent of cases.[7]

## Lessons Learned - Maxillofacial Injuries

Maxillofacial battle injuries are present in 26 percent of casualties evacuated from Combat Support Hospitals (CSHs).[1] These highly visible injuries, although bloody, are rarely the sole cause of shock. Death resulting from airway loss following maxillofacial injury is the primary concern. Establishing a secure airway is paramount for casualties with severe head and neck injuries. Direct laryngoscopy with endotracheal intubation and surgical cricothyroidotomy are commonly used techniques to secure an airway in combat casualties.

Although they are often bloody, maxillofacial injuries are rarely the source of shock. The critical, immediate life-threat following maxillofacial injury is airway compromise due to oropharyngeal bleeding, swelling, and loss of mandibular structural integrity.

During direct laryngoscopy, exposure of the glottis is highly dependent on displacement of the tongue with a laryngoscope blade against an intact mandibular arch. Once mandibular body integrity is disrupted by fracture or avulsion, anterior displacement of the tongue is easier, but blood, soft-tissue swelling, and debris may continue to obscure the glottis. A maneuver to consider if the glottis is obscured despite aggressive suctioning is to push air through the glottis by compressing the chest; bubbles will localize the glottis for intubation. If this fails, and bag-valve-mask ventilation is not feasible, the CCC provider needs to perform an immediate cricothyroidotomy.

Once the casualty has a secured airway, in the authors' experience, direct pressure and aggressive packing of open bleeding wounds or bleeding nasal and oropharyngeal cavities will control all but the most catastrophic hemorrhages (Figs. 7 and 8). Flail mandible fractures may compromise a patient's airway and, if left untreated, cause considerable pain and morbidity. Early tracheotomy and external pin fixation to stabilize mandible fractures prior to air evacuation should be considered. An orthopedic pin fixator, such as the Hoffman® II device, works well to obtain gross alignment and fixation of the fractured mandible (Fig. 9).

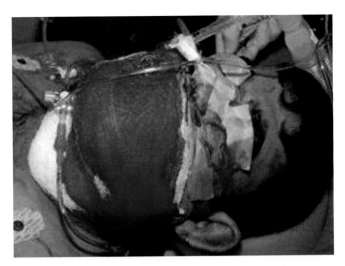

Figure 7. (Left) *With the airway secure, a compression dressing has been applied to control bleeding in the oropharyngeal cavity.*

Figure 8. (Below) *A casualty with explosive blast-related penetrating fragmentation wounds to the torso and head. Note the secured airway and compression dressings applied to the head and face. Image courtesy of Kurt W. Grathwohl, MD, COL, MC, US Army.*

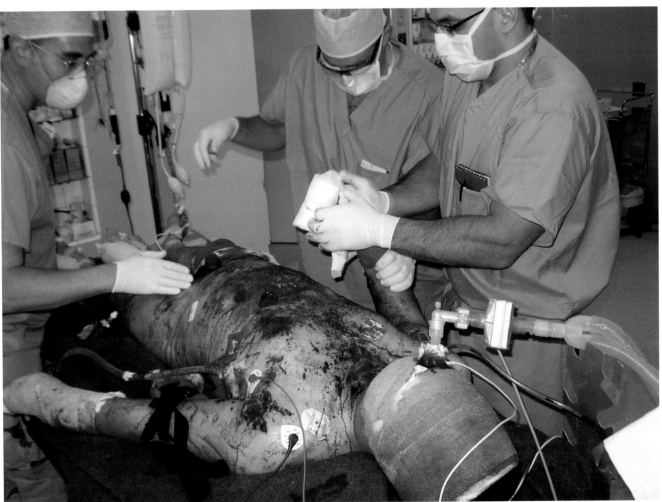

For uncontrolled hemorrhage from open wounds and nasal or oropharyngeal cavities, the airway should be secured and the wounds or cavities aggressively packed.

Head and neck wounds should be copiously irrigated, wound contaminants should be removed, and clearly nonviable tissue fragments should be debrided. Judicious initial debridement of facial wounds will provide the face surgeon with a subsequent opportunity to assess viability of critical structures. Facial

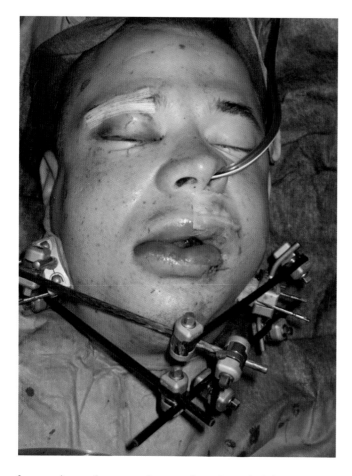

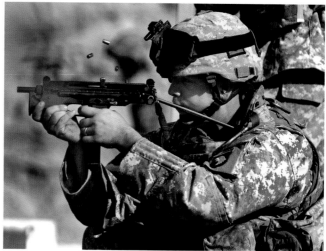

Figure 9. (Left) *An orthopedic pin fixator, such as the Hoffman® II device, works well to obtain gross alignment and fixation of a fractured mandible prior to transport. Image courtesy of Tamer Goksel, DDS, MD, COL, US Army.*

Figure 10. (Below) *The maxillofacial region corresponds to head structures not protected by a Kevlar® helmet. Image courtesy of Defense Imagery Management Operations Center (DIMOC).*

lacerations that can be explored and debrided effectively should be closed primarily unless underlying fractures are present.[8] Facial fractures are frequently accessed through existing lacerations. Packing the wound open (temporarily), rather than closing the wound, will prevent open facial fractures from being overlooked in later evacuation phases. Wound packing should be changed at least every 24 hours. Definitive facial fracture repair can be delayed up to two weeks without significantly affecting the outcome in most cases.[8]

> With the exception of fractures that significantly alter normal dental occlusion or compromise the airway, definitive facial fracture repair can be delayed up to two weeks.

# Information for the Generalist - Maxillofacial Injuries

Improvised explosive devices cause a majority of injuries in OEF/OIF.[2] The face of combat casualties is particularly vulnerable to explosive injuries. Explosions cause a high incidence of ocular injuries, facial fractures, and complex soft-tissue wounds and burns.[1,7] The critical, immediate problem following maxillofacial injury is airway compromise due to oropharyngeal bleeding, swelling, and loss of mandibular structural integrity. Initial treatment of oromaxillofacial injury involves securing the patient's airway and controlling bleeding, while simultaneously protecting the brain, cervical spine, and eyes from further injury. Once the airway is stabilized, efforts can be focused upon hemorrhage control and treatment of additional injuries identified in the secondary survey.

Maxillofacial anatomy comprises the bony and soft-tissue structures anterior and inferior to the base of the skull, from the ears forward and from the brow down to the chin. This region corresponds to head structures not protected by a Kevlar® helmet (Fig. 10). The tongue is attached to the forward projecting mandible, which supports the patency of the upper airway. Beneath the skin, critical structures at risk from penetrating trauma are the parotid glands, parotid ducts, and major facial nerve branches. Unrecognized injuries to these structures may result in high morbidity.[9]

The midface is the area between the eyebrows and base of the nose. The midface contains pneumatized (air-filled) paranasal sinuses. The bones encasing the sinus cavities are thin and lined by mucosa. Projectiles can easily perforate and traverse the midface and lead to subsequent infections. Globe injuries, vascular injuries, and intracranial penetration are critical associated injuries following penetrating trauma to the midface.[10,11]

The lower face is the area from the base of the nose to the chin, including the tooth-bearing parts of the maxilla and the entire mandible. The lower face skeleton is composed of thick cortical bone and dense dental structures. The tongue, surrounded by these hard structures, is at risk for severe injury leading to airway obstruction when high-speed projectiles fragment surrounding structures and produce secondary projectiles.

## *Airway Control and Breathing Support*

Airway management is arguably the single most important skill taught to and possessed by emergency careproviders. Effective airway management in the combat casualty often makes the difference between life and death and takes initial precedence over most other clinical considerations.

There are fundamental differences in the management of casualties arriving to treatment facilities with blunt trauma to the face versus penetrating injury. Patients with isolated blunt force trauma to the face and neck typically undergo standard spinal immobilization measures (e.g., in-line traction) during initial airway management (when the tactical setting allows). Combat casualties with penetrating injuries to the face and neck often pose significant airway visualization challenges (Fig. 11). The primary priority in such patients (at immediate risk for airway obstruction) is securing a stable airway. This often results in more liberal initial manipulation of the head and neck to enable lifesaving airway interventions. Fortunately, studies performed in civilian and combat settings suggest that most patients with normal neurological motor exams following isolated penetrating trauma to the neck will not have a mechanically destabilized spinal column.[12,13] Of note, blast injury management is complicated by the fact that combined blunt force and penetrating injuries to the face and neck often occur.

> Studies performed in civilian and combat settings suggest that following isolated penetrating trauma to the neck, most patients with normal neurological motor exams will not have a mechanically destabilized spinal column.

### Airway and Breathing Assessment

The initial casualty assessment determines whether the airway is open and protected and if breathing is present and adequate. This is achieved through inspection, auscultation, and palpation (look, listen, and feel). Start by observing the patient for objective signs of airway compromise. Note the presence

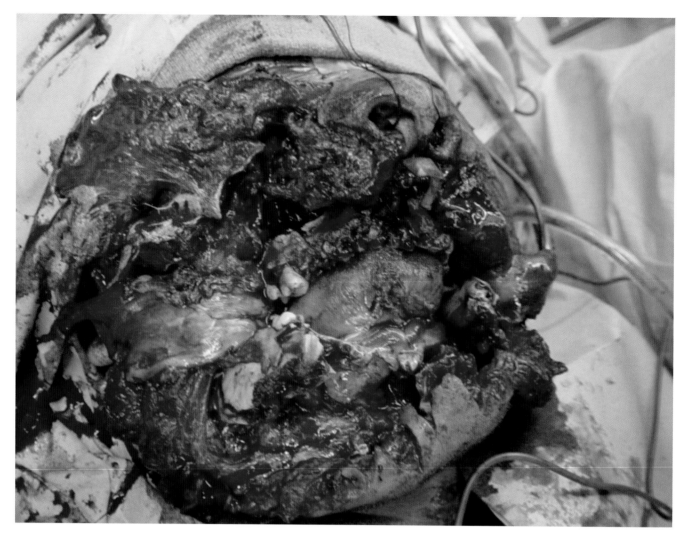

Figure 11. *Penetrating trauma to the maxillofacial region can make visualization of the airway extremely challenging. Image courtesy of Tamer Goksel, DDS, MD, COL, US Army.*

or absence and quality of speech. A normal voice suggests that the airway is adequate for the moment. Gurgling is a consequence of obstruction of the upper airway by liquids, such as blood or vomit, pooling in the oral cavity or hypopharynx. Snoring usually indicates partial airway obstruction at the pharyngeal level, while hoarseness suggests a laryngeal process. Snoring is classically due to obstruction of the upper airway by the tongue. This can occur due to loss of muscle tone secondary to loss of consciousness or as a result of loss of structural integrity of the mandible, as is seen in explosive or ballistic trauma. Stridor, a high-pitched sound, may be associated with partial airway obstruction at the level of the larynx (inspiratory stridor) or at the level of the trachea (expiratory stridor). Wheezing is usually secondary to narrowing of the lower airways. This can result from exacerbation of preexisting disease (e.g., reactive airway disease) or due to compression of the airway by soft-tissue edema, a foreign object, or an expanding hematoma. Aphonia in the conscious patient is an extremely worrisome sign. A patient who is too short of breath to speak is in grave danger of impending respiratory compromise.

Feel for air movement at the mouth and nose. Open the mouth and inspect the upper airway, taking care not to extend or rotate the neck. Look for and remove any vomitus, blood, or other foreign bodies. Identify swelling of the tongue or uvula, any sites of bleeding, or any other visible abnormalities of the oropharynx. The gentle use of a tongue blade may facilitate this task. The patient's ability to spontaneously swallow and handle secretions indicates airway protective mechanisms are intact. In the unconscious patient, the absence of a gag reflex has traditionally been equated to a loss of protective airway reflexes.

The midface and mandible should be inspected and palpated for structural integrity. Injuries to these structures may lead to distortion and loss of airway patency. Mandible fractures can lead to a loss of structural support and subsequent airway obstruction. Patients with these injuries may refuse to lie down in an attempt to maintain airway patency. The anterior neck should be carefully inspected for penetrating wounds. Asymmetry or swelling (i.e., from a vascular injury) of the neck may herald impending airway compromise. The detection of crepitus upon palpation of the neck suggests injury to the airway or a communicating pneumomediastinum. Auscultation should demonstrate clear and equal breath sounds. Diminished breath sounds may result from respiratory splinting causing atelectasis, pneumothorax, hemothorax, or pleural effusion. Wheezing and dyspnea imply lower airway obstruction. Patient agitation may represent hypoxia. Obtundation suggests hypercarbia. Cyanosis indicates hypoxemia. Hypoxia represents low oxygen at the cellular level, whereas hypoxemia is low oxygen solely with reference to arterial blood. In essence, each relates to low oxygen levels. Note the patient's respiratory rate and pattern.

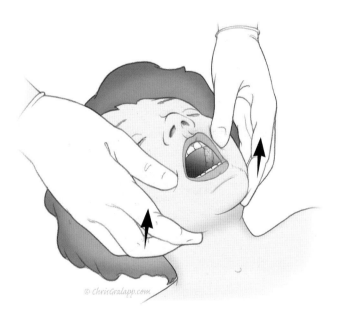
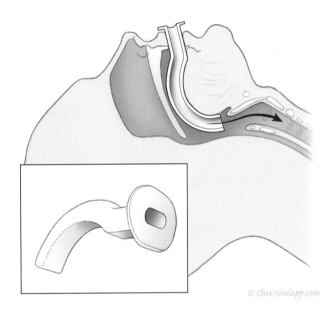

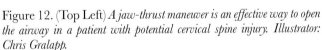

Figure 12. (Top Left) *A jaw-thrust maneuver is an effective way to open the airway in a patient with potential cervical spine injury. Illustrator: Chris Gralapp.*

Figure 13. (Top Right) *The oropharyngeal airway is a C-shaped device designed to hold the tongue off the posterior pharyngeal wall while providing an air channel through the mouth. Illustrator: Chris Gralapp.*

Figure 14. (Bottom Right) *Example of oropharyngeal airway (top) and nasopharyngeal airway (below).*

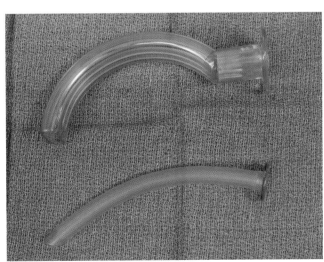

Bradypnea or tachypnea may be a sign of respiratory compromise. Respiratory muscle fatigue may result in the recruitment of accessory muscles of respiration. This is clinically manifested as suprasternal, supraclavicular, or intercostal muscle retractions. Look for a symmetrical rise and fall of the chest. Significant chest trauma may result in paradoxical or discordant chest wall movement (e.g., flail chest).

## Initial Airway Control

Ensuring airway patency is essential for adequate oxygenation and ventilation and is the first priority in airway control. The conscious patient uses the musculature of his/her upper airway and protective reflexes to maintain a patent airway and protect against aspiration of foreign substances (e.g., vomitus). In the severely ill or unconscious trauma patient, protective airway mechanisms may be impaired or lost, predisposing the patient to aspiration of secretions, blood, and gastric contents.

Opening the airway is the first step in airway management. Upper airway obstruction in the unconscious

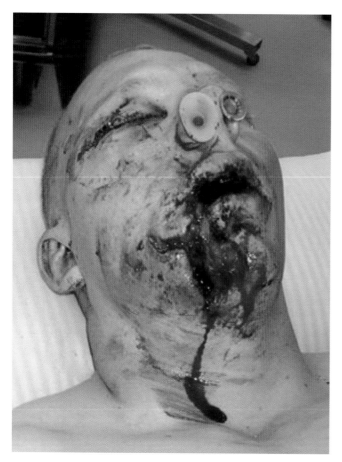

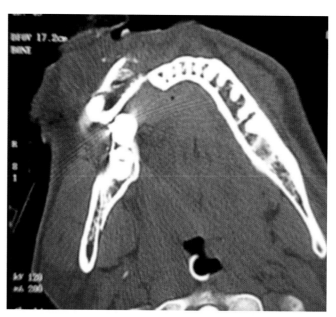

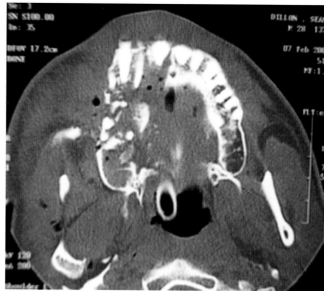

Figure 15. (Top Left) *Nasopharyngeal airways inserted in a combat casualty. A nasopharyngeal airway can establish a temporary, nonsurgical airway in a spontaneously breathing patient. (Top Right, Bottom Right) Though it does not provide definitive airway protection, these CT images clearly demonstrate the effectiveness of the nasopharyngeal airway as an adjunct in maintaining airway patency.*

patient is most commonly the result of posterior displacement of the tongue and epiglottis. Simple bedside maneuvers can remove this occlusion and reestablish airway patency and airflow. Carefully remove a casualty's helmet or any headgear while maintaining manual in-line stabilization of the cervical spine. The chin-lift with head-tilt maneuver is a simple, effective technique for opening the airway but should be avoided in any patient with a potentially unstable cervical spine. The jaw thrust without head-tilt maneuver can be performed while maintaining cervical spine alignment (Fig. 12). Between 2 to 4 percent of patients with facial fractures from blunt trauma (in civilian studies) have concomitant cervical spinal fractures, and approximately 10 to 12 percent have cervical ligamentous injury.[14,15] Although these techniques work well, they require the continuous involvement of several careproviders to maintain airway patency and cervical spine alignment.

> Although effective in opening the airway, the chin-lift with head-tilt maneuver should be avoided in any patient with a potential cervical spine injury.

### Oral and Nasal Airways

Oral and nasal adjunctive airway aids can establish a nonsurgical airway in a spontaneously breathing patient (Fig. 13). Though an oropharyngeal or nasopharyngeal airway may help establish a temporary airway, they do not provide definitive airway protection (e.g., protect against aspiration of vomitus).

> Nasal airways should not be placed in the setting of midface craniofacial injuries, as they can inadvertently be introduced into the cranial vault in cases of concomitant midface and skull base fractures.

The oropharyngeal airway is a C-shaped device designed to hold the tongue off the posterior pharyngeal wall while providing an air channel and suction conduit through the mouth (Fig. 14). An oropharyngeal airway is most effective in patients who are spontaneously breathing and lack a gag or cough reflex. The use of an oropharyngeal airway in a patient with a gag or cough reflex is contraindicated as it may stimulate vomiting or laryngospasm. Oral airways can cause complications; when used in conscious or semiconscious casualties, they may stimulate vomiting, laryngospasm, or patient agitation. Hence, inappropriate use of oral airways may worsen airway problems (e.g., potentially exacerbate cervical spinal injuries). They are also useful in assisting bag-valve-mask ventilation efforts in patients with respiratory failure. The oropharyngeal airway comes in various sizes to accommodate children to large adults. Proper oropharyngeal airway size is estimated by placing the oropharyngeal airway flange at the corner of the mouth. The distal tip of the airway should then reach the angle of the jaw.

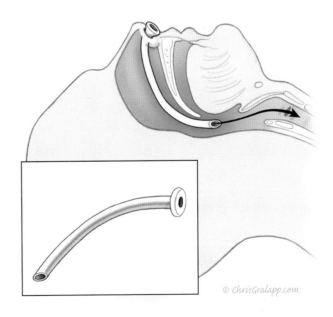

Figure 16. *The nasopharyngeal airway is an uncuffed curved tube made of soft rubber or plastic that provides a conduit for airflow between the nares and pharynx. Nasal airways should not be used in the setting of midface craniofacial injuries. Illustrator: Chris Gralapp.*

The nasopharyngeal airway is an uncuffed, curved tube made of soft rubber or plastic that provides a conduit for airflow between the nares and pharynx (Fig. 15). Nasopharyngeal airways are commonly used in intoxicated or semiconscious patients who do not tolerate an oropharyngeal airway. They are also effective when trauma, trismus (i.e., clenched teeth), or another obstacle (i.e., wiring of the teeth) preclude the placement of an oropharyngeal airway. Proper nasopharyngeal airway length is determined by measuring the distance from the tip of the nose to the tragus of the ear. Nasal airways may induce bleeding from the nose. Nasal airways should not be placed in the setting of midface craniofacial injuries, as they potentially can be introduced into the cranial vault in cases of concomitant midface and skull base fractures (Fig. 16).[16]

## Cervical Spine Protection and Control

All patients with significant blunt trauma to the head or face are at risk for cervical spine injury. The amount of force required to fracture the facial bones ranges from 275 to 1800 pounds per square inch, and careful consideration for unstable cervical spinal injury must be maintained throughout the process of securing the airway.[17] Inadvertent movement of the neck of a patient with an unstable cervical spine injury can lead to permanent neurologic disability or death. Accordingly, many combat casualties are transported to the CSH with spinal immobilization.

An effective approach to airway management in patients with possible cervical spine injuries is rapid sequence intubation with in-line spinal immobilization. Pharmacologically paralyzing the patient reduces the risk of the patient moving during intubation attempts, improves airway visualization, and facilitates subsequent endotracheal intubation. A second individual maintaining immobilization of the head and neck in the neutral position throughout the procedure prevents inadvertent movement of the cervical spine by the laryngoscopist (Fig. 17). Careproviders need to ensure the patient can be effectively bag-valve-mask ventilated or that an alternative rescue airway intervention is planned (e.g., surgical airway) prior to pharmacologically paralyzing the patient, in the event endotracheal intubation is not possible.

As previously noted, combat casualties with penetrating injuries to the face and neck often pose significant

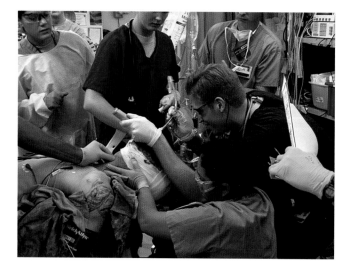

Figure 17. *In-line cervical spine immobilization in a casualty with penetrating maxillofacial injury.*

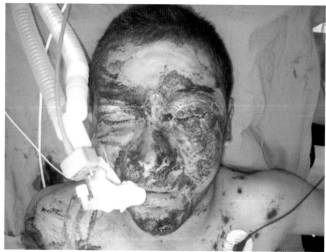

Figure 18. *A combat casualty with a definitive airway. A secured endotracheal tube is positioned in the trachea with its cuff inflated, attached to an oxygen-rich ventilation device.*

airway visualization challenges, which often result in more liberal manipulation of the head and neck to enable lifesaving airway interventions. Studies suggest that most patients with normal neurological motor exams following penetrating trauma to the neck will not have a mechanically destabilized spinal column.[12,13]

## Definitive Airway Control and Breathing Support

A definitive airway ensures airway patency and protection. It requires an endotracheal tube (ETT) or tracheostomy tube in the trachea with the cuff inflated, secured in place, and attached to an oxygen-rich ventilation device (Fig. 18). Failure to secure a definitive airway in a timely manner can have adverse consequences for the combat casualty. The decision to intubate a combat casualty is often complicated and may depend on a variety of clinical factors. There are several fundamental reasons for securing a definitive airway in such patients. These include: (1) failure of ventilation or oxygenation; (2) inability to maintain or protect an airway; (3) potential for deterioration based on the patient's clinical presentation; and (4) facilitation of patient management (e.g., combative head injury patient who needs a neuroimaging or aeromedical evacuation). At this stage, intubation should be attempted with one of the following modalities:

- Standard oral or nasal endotracheal intubation
    - Adjuncts include the GlideScope®, Light Wand® or fiberoptic scope
    - Extreme caution should be used with nasal endotracheal intubation in patients with known midface fractures due to potential violation of the anterior cranial vault.
- Laryngeal mask airway (LMA™)
- Esophageal tracheal Combitube®

The benefit of endotracheal intubation or a Combitube® is that the casualty can be transported with either of these devices after they are properly secured. Should an LMA™ be used and patient transport remains an issue, the patient should be considered to only have a temporary airway since the LMA™ does not actually enter the trachea and dislodgement or movement is a potential complication. In addition, the LMA™ has limitations associated with decreased ability to ventilate at increased airway pressures, contraindications in penetrating upper airway trauma or central airway obstruction with foreign body, and potential aspiration risks.[18] In a Level III or higher care facility where immediate patient movement is not a tactical concern, the LMA™ serves as an appropriate adjunct to facilitate ventilation prior to performing endotracheal intubation or a surgical airway.

> Extreme caution should be used with nasal endotracheal intubation in patients with known midface fractures due to potential violation of the anterior cranial vault.

### Preparation for Endotracheal Intubation

Careful preparation prior to attempting endotracheal intubation is essential to achieving success. This point cannot be emphasized enough. Careproviders need to ensure adequate suction, oxygen flow, airway equipment, pharmacologic agents, and monitoring equipment are present. This includes airway adjuncts and alternative airway devices, including a cricothyroidotomy tray in case initial methods are unsuccessful. Suction systems should be tested and readily available at the bedside for removal of blood, vomitus, and foreign bodies. A high-flow oxygen mask and bag-valve-mask ventilation device should be ready for use. Ideally, patients should be preoxygenated with 100 percent high-flow oxygen to enable several attempts at intubation without the need for bag-valve-mask ventilation (which causes gastric distention and increases the risk of passive regurgitation of gastric contents). At least two functioning laryngoscope handles and appropriately sized and shaped laryngoscope blades should be obtained. The anticipated blade of choice should be clicked into position to ensure that the light functions properly. An ETT should be chosen based on the patient's anatomy and one smaller size should be prepared as well. The average adult male will require a 7.5- or 8.0-millimeter (internal diameter) ETT, the average adult female requires a 7.0- or 7.5-millimeter ETT. In children, the ETT size may be estimated by the formula: ETT size = 4 + (age in years /4). The ETT cuff should be inflated to test for an air leak. A stylet should be inserted within the ETT to shape it into a configuration that will facilitate insertion into the airway. Care must be taken to ensure that the tip of the stylet does not protrude from the end of the ETT or through the small distal side port (Murphy's eye). The patient should have at least one intravenous (IV) catheter inserted, and patency of the line should be verified and ensured. The specific rapid sequence intubation medications, proper dosing, and sequence of administration should be determined. These pharmacological agents should be drawn up and syringes labeled. Cardiac monitoring, blood pressure monitoring, and pulse oximetry are mandatory for all patients. If available, an end-tidal $CO_2$ monitor should be readied as well.

---

In children, the ETT size may be estimated by the formula: ETT size = 4 + (age in years /4).

---

## Endotracheal Intubation Technique

With the laryngoscope in the left hand (assuming a right-hand-dominant laryngoscopist), the mouth is gently opened with the right hand. The laryngoscope is gently inserted into the right side of the patient's mouth, and the tongue is displaced to the left (Fig. 19). The curved (Macintosh) blade is slid into the vallecula and the straight (Miller) blade is positioned below the epiglottis (Fig. 20). The handle is pushed along the axis of the handle at a 45-degree angle to the patient's body. Avoid the tendency to leverage (i.e., crowbar) the laryngoscope blade against the teeth, as this may fracture the teeth.

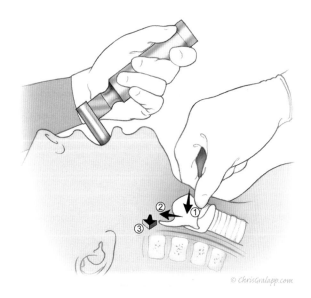

Figure 19. *Insertion of laryngoscope and application of cricoid pressure during intubation. Illustrator: Chris Gralapp.*

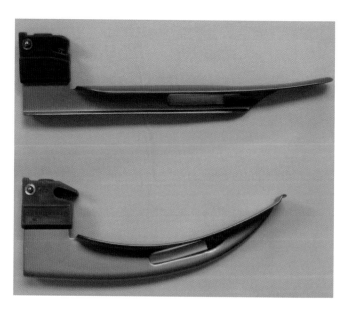

Figure 20. *The straight (Miller) blade is positioned below the epiglottis whereas the curved (Macintosh) blade is placed in the vallecula during endotracheal intubation.*

With a clear view of the glottis, the right hand gently inserts the ETT until the cuff is about two to three centimeters past the vocal cords. Blind intubation (i.e., passing the ETT without visualization of the vocal cords) increases the likelihood of esophageal intubation. In the average-size adult male, the 23-centimeter mark of the ETT will be located at the corner of the mouth (21 centimeters in women). Once the ETT is in place, the stylet should be removed and the cuff inflated until there is no audible air leak with bag ventilation. The ETT cuff pressure should be kept below 25 cm $H_2O$ pressure. This will minimize the risk of tracheal mucosal injury attributable to excessive cuff pressures.[19] Adequate preoxygenation should allow the laryngoscopist multiple attempts at intubation before arterial oxygen desaturation occurs. A dedicated team member should be focused on the patient's cardiac rhythm, blood pressure, and oxygen saturation during laryngoscopy and should alert the endoscopist to any abnormalities.

Endotracheal tube cuff pressure should be kept below 25 cm $H_2O$ to minimize the risk of tracheal mucosal injury.

After any unsuccessful attempt, always recheck the patient's position, and make the necessary adjustments. It is important to attempt to improve your chance of successfully intubating the patient with each successive attempt. This is often done by changing the size or type of laryngoscope blade, repositioning the patient, or by utilizing additional techniques (e.g., fiberoptic intubation).

### Rapid Sequence Intubation

Rapid sequence intubation is a series of defined steps intended to allow for rapid endotracheal intubation of a patient with minimal bag-valve-mask ventilation. Given that most patients requiring emergent intubation have not fasted and may have full stomachs, bag-valve-mask ventilation may inadvertently lead to gastric distention and passive regurgitation and increase the risk of aspiration. To perform rapid sequence intubation and avoid this complication, the patient is first preoxygenated to provide adequate blood oxygentation despite a period of apnea without interposed assisted ventilation. This is followed by the sequential administration of an induction agent and a rapidly acting neuromuscular blocking agent to induce a state of unconsciousness and paralysis, respectively. An assistant should apply Sellick's maneuver (cricoid pressure), just as the patient is noted to lose consciousness (Fig. 19). This application of firm pressure to the cricoid cartilage is intended to compress the esophagus (although recent studies suggest the postcricoid hypopharynx is the site of compression) and prevent passive regurgitation of gastric contents.[20] Sellick's maneuver should be maintained until the ETT has been placed, its position verified, and the cuff inflated. Cricoid pressure can occasionally hinder airway visualization; hence, pressure should be reduced to facilitate vocal cord visualization as indicated.[21] Sellick's maneuver should be discontinued in patients who are actively vomiting (versus passive regurgitation). Esophageal compression in a patient who is actively vomiting risks esophageal rupture.

### Awake Endotracheal Intubation

Performing oral intubation on a patient who is awake is an intervention that will require liberal topical airway anesthesia and patient sedation prior to inspection or intubation of the patient's airway. This approach allows for the preservation of the patient's airway reflexes and spontaneous breathing while the laryngoscopist takes a quick look at the glottis, vocal cords, and internal airway anatomy. The classic scenario for employing such a technique is the patient with distorted upper airway anatomy (Fig. 16). Under these circumstances, intubation by rapid sequence intubation is often unsuccessful. Subsequent bag-valve-mask ventilation may be ineffective due to loss of normal architecture and inability to create an adequate mask-to-mouth seal (e.g., displaced mandible fractures and soft-tissue loss) or can cause air to dissect into the tissue planes of the neck (e.g., following penetrating oropharyngeal injuries), further distorting airway anatomy. Disadvantages of oral intubation of a patient who is awake include oversedation, discomfort and stress, deleterious effects in patients with cardiac disorders, or increased intracranial pressure. Fiberoptic laryngoscopy assessment of the airway (when available) and subsequent ETT placement are alternatives and very valuable methods of performing an awake oral intubation.

## Crash Endotracheal Intubation

A crash intubation is the immediate endotracheal intubation of a patient without the use of any medications. It is indicated in patients with respiratory arrest, agonal respirations, or deep unresponsiveness. The advantages of this approach often include technical ease and rapidity. Disadvantages include the potential for increased intracranial pressure from the stress of intubation as well as emesis and aspiration.

## Confirmation of Endotracheal Tube Placement

As inadvertent intubation of the esophagus can occur during airway management, proper positioning of the ETT within the trachea needs to be confirmed after every intubation. Failure to recognize an esophageal intubation can result in patient death. Methods used to detect ETT placement include clinical assessment, pulse oximetry, end-tidal carbon dioxide ($ETCO_2$) detection, suction bulb or syringe aspiration techniques, and ultrasonography.[22] Chest radiography can be used to assess ETT position but does not confirm ETT placement within the trachea. Since the esophagus lies directly behind the trachea, an ETT placed incorrectly in the esophagus may appear to be within the trachea on an anterior-posterior chest radiograph.

---

Failure to recognize an esophageal intubation can result in patient death. Clinical observations, end-tidal $CO_2$ colorimetry, and continuous noninvasive pulse oximetry can be used to help confirm appropriate positioning of the ETT within the trachea.

---

Classically, a combination of clinical observations has been used to confirm correct ETT placement. These include (1) direct visualization of the ETT passing through the vocal cords during intubation; (2) auscultation of clear and equal breath sounds over both lung fields; (3) absence of breath sounds when auscultating over the epigastrium; (4) observation of symmetrical chest rise during ventilation; and (5) observation of condensation (fogging) of the ETT during ventilation. Though these clinical findings should be assessed in every intubated patient, they are subject to failure as the sole means for confirming ETT placement.

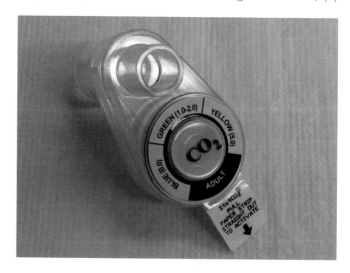

Figure 21. *A colorimetric end-tidal $CO_2$ detector can be placed between the ETT and bag following intubation, with a (depending on brand) blue- or purple-to-yellow color change indicating a correctly placed ETT.*

Continuous noninvasive pulse oximetry should be standard for every patient being intubated. A drop in oxygen saturation following intubation is suggestive of an esophageal intubation. However, this drop may be delayed for several minutes if the patient was adequately preoxygenated. In certain patients (i.e., hypotensive), oxygen saturation measurements may be unreliable or difficult to detect. Detection and measurement of exhaled carbon dioxide is a highly reliable method for detecting proper placement of the ETT within the trachea.[23] A colorimetric end-tidal $CO_2$ detector is a small disposable device that connects between the bag and the ETT. When the device detects end-tidal volume $CO_2$, its colorimetric indicator (depending on brand) changes from blue or purple to yellow (Fig. 21). The absence of this color change usually indicates the tube is incorrectly placed in the esophagus. An important exception is that the colorimetric indicator will remain purple even with correct ETT placement within the trachea in patients with prolonged cardiac arrest. These patients are not circulating carbon dioxide to their pulmonary circulation and into their airways. The recovery prognosis for such patients is dismal.[23]

Aspiration devices may also be used for confirmation of ETT placement and work based on the principle that the trachea is a rigid air-filled structure, whereas the esophagus is soft-walled.[22] Attempts to draw air through an ETT placed in the esophagus will meet resistance from collapse of the esophageal wall around the distal ETT, whereas air will freely flow when drawn through an ETT in the trachea. Two commonly used aspiration appliances are a bulb suction device and a large-volume syringe.

## Surgical Airway Management

Despite active bleeding and gaping facial wounds, the fastest and most direct technique to establish a definitive airway is often direct laryngoscopy and oral endotracheal intubation. If direct laryngoscopy fails, a cricothyroidotomy is an expedient technique to establish a definitive airway. Even in the hands of experienced careproviders, alternative surgical airways (e.g., tracheotomy) require a formal surgical setting, proper patient positioning, surgical assistance, and good lighting. The degree of skill required to surgically create such alternative airways coupled with the required resources conspire to make such surgical interventions challenging for generalists providing CCC.

> If attempts at direct laryngoscopy and endotracheal intubation fail, a cricothyroidotomy is an expedient technique to establish a definitive airway.

### *Cricothyroidotomy*

Surgical airway management entails the creation of an opening into the trachea to provide oxygenation and ventilation. Proficiency with surgical airway techniques can mean the difference between life and death. Should difficulty arise in obtaining a secure airway via endotracheal intubation (and bag-valve-mask ventilation is not feasible), there should be no hesitation to proceed directly to a surgical cricothyroidotomy. In an emergency, a surgical cricothyroidotomy is preferred to a tracheotomy, as the distance from the skin to the cricothyroid membrane in most adults is approximately 10 millimeters (mm), compared to the average distance from the skin to the trachea being approximately 20 to 30 mm.[24] In addition, at the level of the second and third tracheal rings, the potential exists for violating the highly vascular thyroid isthmus. The resultant hemorrhage can complicate visualization of the trachea.

> A cricothyroidotomy is preferred to a tracheotomy as an emergency surgical airway.

A cricothyroidotomy creates an immediate surgical opening through the cricothyroid membrane to allow the placement of an ETT or cuffed tracheostomy tube. The primary indication for a cricothyroidotomy is the immediate need for an airway when oral endotracheal intubation is not achievable and bag-valve-

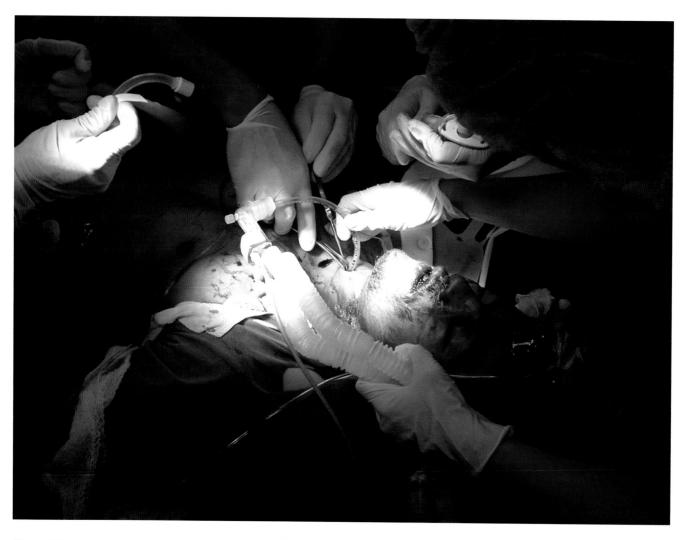

Figure 22. *A cricothyroidotomy creates an immediate surgical opening through the cricothyroid membrane to allow the placement of an ETT or cuffed tracheostomy tube. It requires decisive action and a coordinated team effort.*

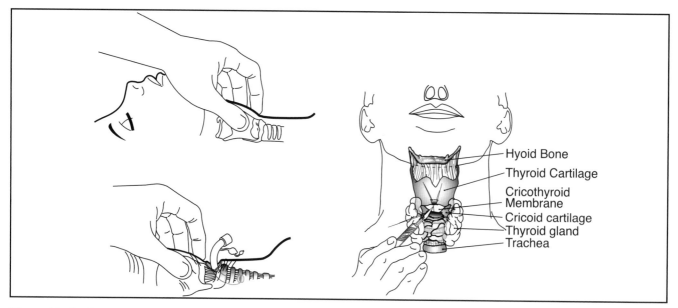

Hyoid Bone
Thyroid Cartilage
Cricothyroid Membrane
Cricoid cartilage
Thyroid gland
Trachea

Figure 23. *Landmarks for cricothyroidotomy. Image courtesy of the Borden Institute, Office of The Surgeon General, Washington, DC. Illustrator: Bruce Maston.*

## STEPS OF SURGICAL CRICOTHYROIDOTOMY

1. Identify the cricothyroid membrane, which is positioned between the cricoid ring and thyroid cartilage

2. Prepare and sterilize the skin widely to allow for increased visualization of the operative field

3. Anesthetize the site if time or circumstances allow

4. Grasp and secure the thyroid cartilage with your nondominant hand, placing digits one and three along the outer contour of the thyroid cartilage, and use your second digit to identify the cricothyroid membrane

5. Make a one- to two-centimeter vertical skin incision* placed just inferior to the thyroid cartilage past the level of cricothyroid membrane through the following structures:
   a. Skin
   b. Subcutaneous tissues
   c. Cervical fascia
   * The author prefers vertical incisions, as the potential is decreased for injuring the anterior jugular veins or superior thyroid arteries that lay lateral to the cricothyroid membrane[25]

6. Bluntly dissect the tissues to expose the cricothyroid membrane

7. Make a horizontal incision through the lower half of the cricothyroid membrane and pass a tracheal hook under the inferior surface of the thyroid cartilage and retract upward with the tracheal hook

8. Open the membrane with dilator forceps or the back of a scalpel handle

9. Insert a lubricated, small-cuffed endotracheal tube (6.0 to 7.0 mm internal diameter tube works well in adults) until you see the balloon of the tube disappear below the level of the membrane

10. Confirm tracheal intubation:
    a. End-tidal $CO_2$ colorimetry
    b. Chest rise
    c. Bilateral breath sounds

11. Secure the endotracheal tube with sutures to the skin

Table 4. *Steps of surgical cricothyroidotomy.*

mask ventilation is not feasible (Figs. 22 and 23). A classic example is the patient with severe facial trauma in whom conventional airway management might be extremely complicated or impossible (Fig. 11). The steps of surgical cricothyroidotomy are outlined in Table 4.

A CCC provider inexperienced in performing cricothyroidotomy should not attempt a smaller stab incision of only the cricothyroid membrane in an emergency situation unless the patient has a thin soft-tissue profile with readily apparent thyroid and cricoid cartilages. The characteristic thick, muscular neck of many US service members makes correct performance of an isolated stab incision into the cricothyroid membrane extremely difficult.

Contraindications to cricothyroidotomy include: (1) the ability to secure an orotracheal intubation; and (2) complete tracheal transection with retraction of distal trachea into the mediastinum. Relative contraindications include the presence of injuries or infections of the larynx and children under the age of 12 years. In children of this age, poorly defined anatomic landmarks and an extremely small cricothyroid membrane make the procedure difficult, if not impossible to perform. These age-based guidelines are variable. If a younger child is large for his or her age and has well-developed anatomy, the procedure may be successful. A surgical tracheotomy is the preferred method for airway stabilization in children under the age of 12, if conditions allow. Complications of cricothyroidotomy include incorrect location of tube placement, hemorrhage (and tube obstruction), tracheal or laryngeal injury, infection, pneumomediastinum, subglottic stenosis, and voice change.[26,27]

### Percutaneous Transtracheal Ventilation (Needle Cricothyroidotomy)

An important (particularly in young children) surgical airway procedure is needle cricothyroidotomy with percutaneous transtracheal ventilation (PTTV) (Fig. 24). Percutaneous transtracheal ventilation involves inserting a 14-gauge transtracheal catheter into the cricothyroid membrane with the catheter connected to a ventilation system; lungs are insufflated with 15 liters per minute oxygen flow, one second on and four seconds off.[28,29] Advantages of this technique include its simplicity, safety, and speed. There is typically less bleeding when compared with cricothyroidotomy, and age is not a contraindication, making it a valuable airway management adjunct in children younger than age 12. During PTTV, the upper airway must be free of obstruction to allow for complete exhalation; otherwise, the patient is at risk for barotrauma from air stacking. All patients receiving PTTV should have oral and nasal airways placed. Unlike cricothyroidotomy, PTTV does not provide airway protection. Therefore, it should be thought of as a temporizing measure until a definitive airway can be established.

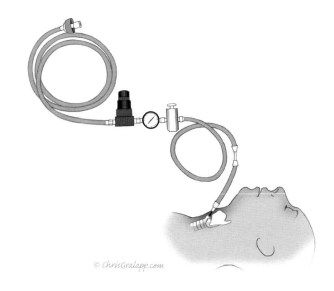

Figure 24. *Percutaneous transtracheal ventilation (PTTV). Illustrator: Chris Gralapp.*

### The Difficult Airway

A recurring difficult-to-manage scenario in OEF/OIF is a casualty with avulsion of the lower face. Despite injury severity, such casualties often present conscious, sitting up in an air-hungry position, and drooling a combination of saliva and blood. Attempts to place these patients in a supine position is resisted by the patient because the airway becomes immediately impaired. In addition, such patients are not easy to bag-valve-mask ventilate, as creating a tight mask seal is impeded by missing anatomy and active bleeding. The inability to bag-valve-mask ventilate a patient is a contraindication to administering a muscle paralytic medication (rapid sequence induction).

There are several approaches to such a scenario. One approach involves the use of a nonparalytic medication such as ketamine (1 to 2 milligrams [mg] per kilogram intravenous bolus infusion) and an antisialogogue like atropine (0.01 mg per kilogram) to facilitate direct laryngoscopy. This often provides the endoscopist with the ability to visualize the vocal cords and perform intubation or gain confidence that intubation is achievable if a paralytic medication is subsequently administered. A surgical cricothyroidotomy is another airway intervention that can be performed under ketamine anesthesia (1 to 2 mg per kilogram intravenous bolus infusion), which preserves a patient's ability to maintain airway tonicity and respiratory drive. Alternatively, if equipment and trained careproviders are available, fiberoptic laryngoscopy can be attempted. However, fiberoptic laryngoscopy efforts are often unsuccessful due to active bleeding obscuring airway visualization or the unavailability of instruments and trained personnel.

An additional approach involves preoxygenating such patients with 100 percent high-flow oxygen for several minutes and then initiating rapid sequence induction while the patient is still sitting upright. Once the patient is unconscious and supine, direct laryngoscopy is immediately attempted. Exposure of the glottis is highly dependent on displacement of the tongue with a laryngoscope blade against an intact mandibular arch. Once mandibular body integrity is disrupted by fracture or avulsion, anterior displacement of the tongue is easier; but blood, soft-tissue swelling, and debris may continue to obscure the glottis. To aid exposure of the glottis in these situations, traction on a suture passed through the tip of the tongue can assist in opening the airway for intubation. If the glottis is still obscured despite aggressive suctioning, pressing on the chest to push air through the glottis may produce bubbles that will help localize the glottis for intubation. If this fails, a surgical cricothyroidotomy is rapidly performed.

> When mandibular body integrity is disrupted, traction on a suture passed through the tip of the tongue can assist in exposure of the glottis and in opening the airway for intubation.

## Initial Management Considerations

Once a definitive airway is established, active bleeding is controlled with nasal packs, oropharyngeal packs, and pressure dressings that are applied by wrapping the head with Kerlix™ gauze. The goal is to at least slow blood loss to a level that can be replaced by blood products and allow the patient to be fully assessed and stabilized before transfer to the operating room. Patients with suspected ocular globe injuries should not have compression dressings applied, pending exclusion of globe rupture. After primary survey and stabilization of other injuries, secondary survey of severely injured maxillofacial structures is performed along with appropriate imaging.

Computed tomography (CT) imaging of the maxillofacial region and cervical spine (to screen for spinal injury) is often required prior to maxillofacial reconstruction. The sequence of treatment steps includes fracture management and soft-tissue repair. In the combat theater, time and resource-consuming maxillofacial reconstruction is avoided in casualties eligible for evacuation. The administration of an initial course of broad-spectrum prophylactic antibiotics should be considered following head and neck combat-related injuries (especially open fractures). A comprehensive review of the literature fails to support prophylactic antibiotic coverage beyond 24 hours of initial surgical intervention.[8] Hence, perioperative antibiotics should be terminated 24 hours after primary repair of maxillofacial wounds.

### Mandible Fractures

Definitive management of maxillofacial fractures is best deferred to face specialists. A Barton bandage is an effective measure a generalist may use to stabilize a flail mandible fracture. This temporizing measure incorporates an extension of the head wrap bandage under the chin to stabilize the mandible against the

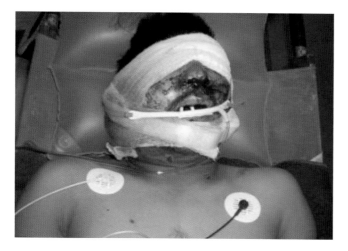

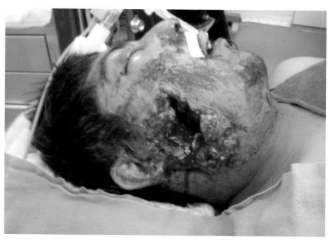

Figure 25. *Casualty arrives at a Field Hospital with a pressure dressing in place. An AK-47 bullet entrance wound is adjacent to the nose (anatomical left side of patient).*

Figure 26. *Rapid sequence induction is immediately performed with oral endotracheal intubation. Note exit wound on anatomical right side of face.*

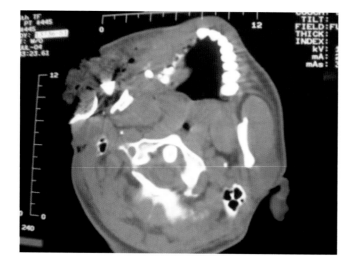

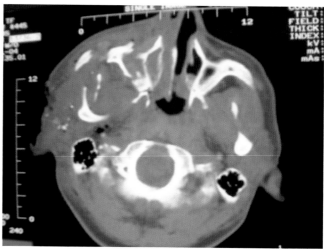

Figures 27 and 28. *Two axial CT images demonstrating the bullet's path from the base of the nose (anatomical left side of face) traversing the face and causing fragmented dentition and extensive soft-tissue injury to the anatomical right side of the face.*

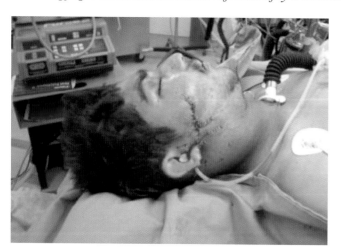

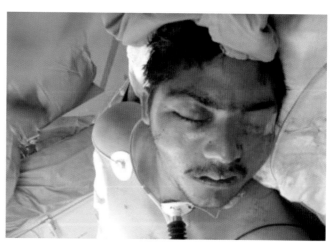

Figures 29 and 30. *Definitive care on this nontransferable host nation casualty occurred in one step. This included tracheotomy, debridement of hopelessly comminuted fragments and debris, fracture repair with open reduction and internal fixation, and parotidectomy and facial nerve repair with greater auricular nerve graft to the upper division, followed by oral and skin flaps for closure.*

maxilla to control pain. This intervention should be delayed until the airway is secured or deemed safe and uncompromised (Figs. 25 to 30). Application of dental wires and arch bar techniques requires dental expertise; these techniques can effectively stabilize fractures and control pain (Fig. 31). Wiring the teeth together, however, compromises the airway and should be avoided in most cases of severe maxillofacial trauma treated in-theater. Elastic intermaxillary fixation with lightly applied rubber band ligatures is an excellent substitute to wire fixation for the ambulatory patient.

> Wiring the teeth together compromises the airway and should be avoided in most cases of severe maxillofacial trauma treated in-theater.

## Dental Injury

Teeth avulsed on the battlefield should be discarded. Even under the most ideal conditions of immediate root canal therapy and dental fixation, reimplanted teeth activate a chronic inflammatory response that causes irreversible root resorption. An exception is if the avulsion time for an anterior maxillary root is less than 30 minutes, and dental expertise is readily available for reimplantation as a temporizing measure to preserve alveolar bone until a dental implant is placed.[30] Likewise, dentoalveolar fragments suspended in the airway from a scant soft-tissue pedicle should be removed to prevent aspiration of loose dentition. Lost dentoalveolar structures can be replaced by tissue grafting techniques and dental implants once the casualty is evacuated to the US.

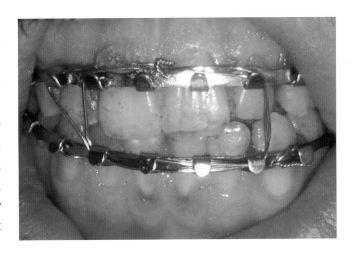

Figure 31. *Intermaxillary fixation is used judiciously in the combat theater and only on ambulatory patients with no airway compromise. Elastic bands between the dental arches instead of wire ligatures are highly recommended for transport. Image courtesy of the Borden Institute, Office of The Surgeon General, Washington, DC.*

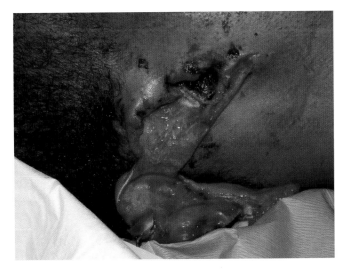

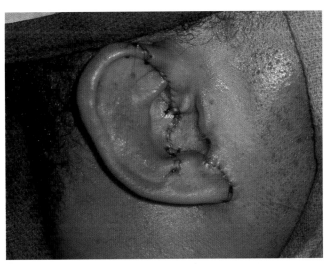

Figure 32. *Near complete avulsion of the ear.* (Left) *Prior to surgical intervention, note small soft-tissue pedicle.* (Right) *Following repair, venous congestion threatens tissue survival. Medical leeches can be beneficial in such cases.*

Teeth avulsed on the battlefield should be discarded. The primary exception is an anterior maxillary tooth with an avulsion time of less than 30 minutes.

Facial Injury

Facial features such as the ears, nose, and lips are at risk for avulsion on the battlefield. Following complete avulsion, very little can be done to reattach the body part without immediate microvascular surgical resources. Partially avulsed structures should be assessed by a face specialist before debridement. Even a small soft-tissue pedicle can perfuse an ear or nose, and the consequence of failure is no worse than not trying at all. Venous congestion of reattached tissue can be treated with leeches (Fig. 32).[31,32,33] Access to leeches for such interventions is limited in OEF/OIF. In the authors' experience, the resourcefulness of host nationals (e.g., obtaining leeches from a nearby riverbank) should be not be underestimated.

Even a small soft-tissue pedicle can perfuse a partially avulsed ear or nose, and the consequence of failure is no worse than not trying at all.

*Parotid and Facial Nerve Injuries*

Penetrating injuries to the face can disrupt the parotid capsule, sever parotid ducts, and injure major branches of the facial nerve. Careful evaluation and inspection are necessary to rule out these injuries prior to wound closure because significant morbidity occurs when these injuries go unrecognized.[34] A reference line dropped vertically from the lateral canthus helps identify the parotid duct as posterior to the line, just below the nasal base, and lying over the masseter (Figs. 33 and 34). If there is any doubt regarding parotid duct integrity, the laceration should be cleaned, packed open, dressed wet-to-dry, and referred for treatment by a specialist. The same reference line is used to establish reparability of

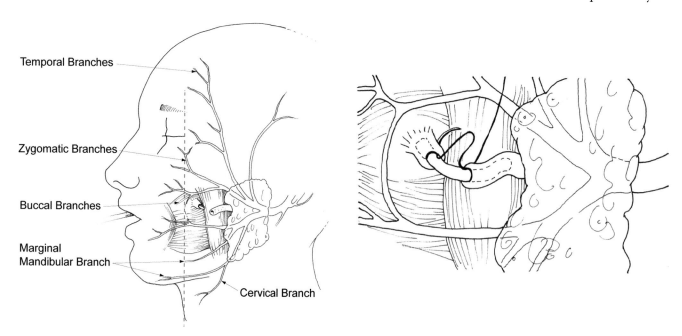

Figure 33. *Branches of the facial nerve and a parotid duct injury. Parotid duct injuries and severed facial nerve branches posterior to a vertical line drawn down from the lateral canthus of the eye should be cleaned, packed open, and referred for treatment by a specialist. Image courtesy of the Borden Institute, Office of The Surgeon General, Washington, DC.*

Figure 34. *Repair of the parotid duct should be completed by a face specialist. Image courtesy of the Borden Institute, Office of The Surgeon General, Washington, DC.*

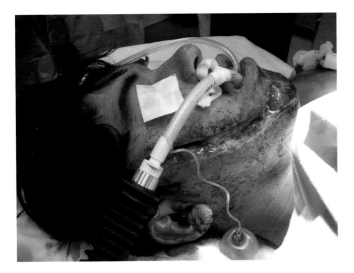
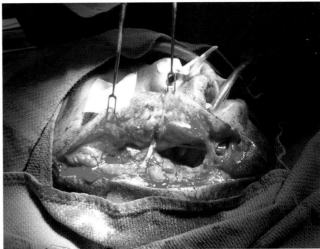
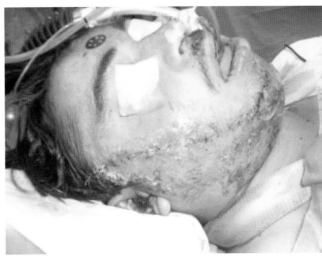

Figure 35. *Through-and-through cheek laceration.* (Top Left) *Penetrating injuries to the face can disrupt the parotid capsule, sever parotid ducts, and injure major branches of the facial nerve.* (Top Right) *Parotid duct and branches of marginal mandibular nerve were identified and repaired, followed by watertight closure of the mucosa and* (Bottom Right) *repair of deep layers and dermis.*

facial nerve branches. Wounds posterior to this reference line are packed open for specialist care if nerve dysfunction is clinically evident. Parotid capsule disruption requires special closure, pressure bandages, and possibly botulinum (toxin) injections (Fig. 35). These injections minimize saliva secretion as the wound heals and are intended to prevent cutaneous fistula formation.

> Parotid duct injuries and severed facial nerve branches posterior to a vertical line drawn down from the lateral canthus of the eye should be cleaned, packed open, and referred for treatment by a specialist.

### Facial Lacerations

Facial lacerations are anesthetized by subcutaneous injection of 1 percent lidocaine with epinephrine through the wound edges (the addition of 0.25 percent bupivacaine will add hours of postoperative pain relief), followed by careful cleansing and inspection of the wound. After hemostasis is achieved, deep lacerations are closed in layers with absorbable 4-0 polyglycolic interrupted sutures starting with the deep subcutaneous layer, then the dermis to approximate the wound edges. Finally, 4-0 to 6-0 (depending on exact location) nylon skin sutures are used to create a tension-free closure of the skin. Petroleum gel coverage of the wound maintains a physiologic environment for favorable healing. Facial sutures should be removed within three to five days to prevent track scars, and adhesive skin closure interventions (e.g., Steri-Strips™ or cyanoacrylate tissue glue) are applied for an additional two weeks.

Facial lacerations that can be explored and debrided effectively should be closed primarily unless underlying fractures are present.[8] In the authors' experience, simple lacerations can be packed open and closed in a delayed fashion (up to four days later) without significant cosmetic compromise, whereas complex lacerations should be definitively treated within two days to achieve the best possible repair. Macerated or abraded facial soft-tissue should be cleaned and covered with petroleum gel (ophthalmic petroleum gel if wounds are near eyes). Closing facial wounds with advanced flaps should be deferred (when possible) until arrival at Level IV and V facilities.

> Facial lacerations that can be explored and debrided effectively should be closed primarily unless underlying fractures are present.

## Information for the Specialist - Maxillofacial Injuries

### Overview

According to a study of a six-year period of battle injuries recorded in the JTTR, penetrating trauma is the mechanism of injury in 92 percent of US service members evacuated from theater with maxillofacial injuries.[1] Face burns occur in 77 percent of service members evacuated from theater with combat-related burns.[7] Maxillofacial blast injury is characterized in the JTTR database as a combination of complex lacerations and open comminuted fractures, complicated by avulsions and burns.[1] This is in sharp contrast to maxillofacial injuries encountered in the civilian setting, which are predominately caused by blunt trauma. While most injured US service members are stabilized for evacuation to a Level IV or V medical facility for definitive care, the deployed surgeon will be expected to provide definitive care to injured host

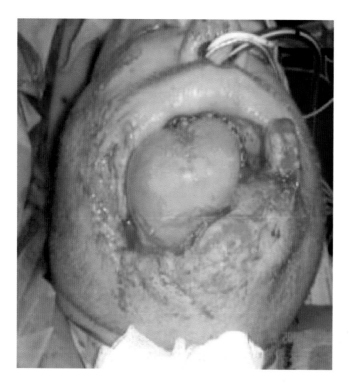 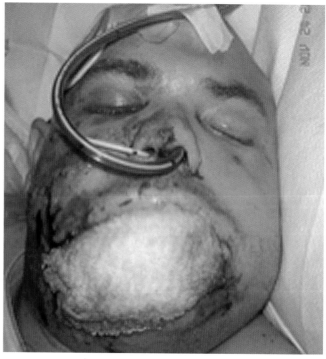

Figure 36. *Casualties with complex facial wounds that can be transferred to higher levels of care should have their wounds cleaned, stabilized, and packed wet-to-dry.*

nation patients, security forces, and detainees. This is especially true in Afghanistan, where transfer to local surgical facilities is rarely possible. Since severe blast injury is uncommon in the US, the nature of injuries the deployed face surgeon will likely encounter will be outside his/her usual scope of practice. This section will help bridge this experience gap for the newly deployed face surgeon by addressing penetrating maxillofacial battle injuries.

> As severe blast injury is uncommon in the US, the nature of injuries the deployed face surgeon will encounter will likely be outside his/her usual scope of practice.

## Initial Management

The high incidence of airway compromise following severe maxillofacial trauma requires immediate interventions to stabilize and secure a patient's airway. Endotracheal intubation (when feasible) and surgical cricothyroidotomy are well established first-line interventions for securing a casualty's airway. Face specialists may also need to reduce fractured and displaced facial bones that are encroaching on a patient's airway. Severe hemorrhage from fractured bony segments may necessitate immediate surgery to ligate injured vessels or reduce fragments to control hemorrhage (covered later in this chapter).

Once the airway is secured and active bleeding controlled with application of pressure bandages, damage control resuscitation and, when indicated, damage control surgery are immediate priorities. Initial maxillofacial fracture stabilization and soft-tissue repair can be delayed for several days until the casualty is deemed stable from the trauma surgeon's perspective (Fig. 36).

## Maxillofacial Wound Care

"The maxillofacial region is anatomically complex with skin and mucosa lining structures that support the upper airway, deglutition apparatus, and specialized sensory organs of sight, smell, hearing, taste, and touch."[8] Although the integrity of the mucosal lining is often disrupted by penetrating maxillofacial battle injuries, the rich blood supply allows for early primary closure after appropriate debridement.[8] The risk of cavitation necrosis to the head and neck following gunshot wounds is low. This is because the head and neck lack large muscle masses, the investing tissues are highly vascular, and the potential space for disruption is limited in depth prior to encountering the hard tissues of the mandible.[8]

> Primary closure of penetrating maxillofacial injuries may be performed following judicious wound debridement.

Maxillofacial wounds suffered in combat will often require serial debridement and irrigation to remove gross debris and foreign bodies. Such interventions can be scheduled in coordination with the multiple trips to the operating room casualties undergo during damage control surgery for concurrent injuries. The surgeon should consider early lateral canthotomies for maxillofacial wounds complicated by burns involving the periorbita to prevent orbital compartment syndrome and loss of vision (Fig. 37). Tracheotomy should also be considered at this early phase. Frost sutures (intermarginal sutures placed between the eyelids to protect the cornea) and bolster dressings will help protect against corneal injury and ectropion formation (Fig. 38).

Application of arch bars and external pin fixation (Hoffman® II orthopedic devices) are expedient

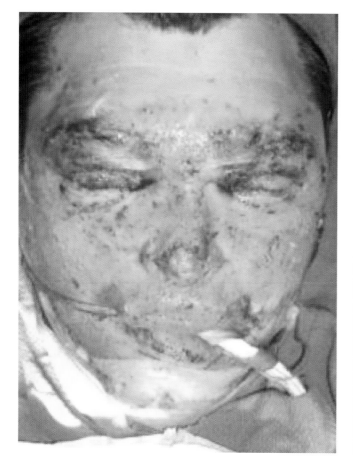

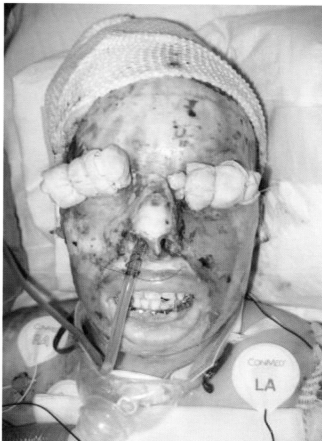

Figure 37. *Second-degree face burns involving the periorbita. Lateral canthotomies are performed to prevent orbital compartment syndrome. Using tape or Velcro® straps to secure the endotracheal tube interferes with wound healing and risks accidental extubation. A better technique is to wire the tube to the lower teeth.*

Figure 38. *Bolster dressings and Frost sutures will help prevent ectropion in the acute phase of burn recovery. Likewise, a plastic lip retractor will help prevent microstomia.*

techniques to stabilize flail mandible fractures (Fig. 39). Nasal packs should be removed at three days. Facial pressure dressings should be removed and replaced, wet-to-dry, daily. Standard ear-nose-throat (ENT) textbooks routinely recommend prophylactic antibiotic administration while the nose is packed to prevent complications associated with *Staphylococcus aureus* dissemination.[35]

## Infection Prevention and Management

Infection prevention and management are integral components of all phases of CCC. In 2007, the US Army Surgeon General commissioned a group of researchers to review the literature and publish evidence-based recommendations for the prevention and treatment of combat-related infections.[36] A team consisting of an infectious disease specialist, a head and neck surgeon, an ophthalmologist, and an oral and maxillofacial surgeon focused on infections of maxillofacial and neck combat-related injuries.[8]

### War Wounds

War wounds are traditionally considered contaminated. Animal studies have demonstrated that animals become rapidly colonized with bacteria found in the immediate environment in which projectile-related wounding occurs.[37] The integrity of the mucosal lining (especially the oral cavity) is an important factor

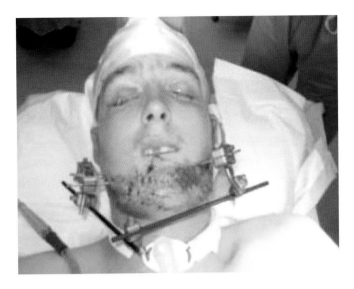

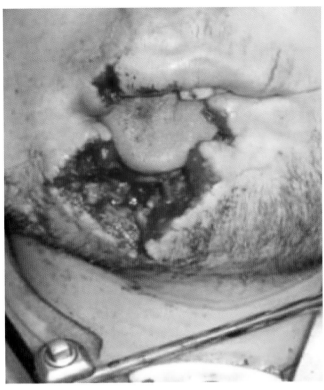

Figure 39. *Flail mandible.* (Above) *Avulsed dentate mandible was stabilized with a wrist external pin fixator and the lower lip wound temporarily closed.* (Right) *Once sutures were released at a Level V facility, the preexisting two-thirds avulsion of the lower lip, chin, and oral vestibule become apparent.*

following injuries to the maxillofacial region. Wounds characterized by disruption of the integrity of the mucosal lining within the oral cavity are prone to infection by bacteria found within saliva. Despite these characteristics, the rich vascular supply of the face (among other factors) does allow for early primary wound closure of face wounds following wound irrigation and debridement.[8]

Early definitive treatment with debridement, irrigation, early repair of soft- and hard-tissues, and early administration of broad-spectrum prophylactic antibiotics are interventions that decrease war infections.[8,38,39,40] All war wounds to the head and neck should be treated with 24 hours of prophylactic antibiotic therapy. There is no evidence to indicate that longer courses of antibiotics are of any benefit, provided war wounds are repaired in less than 12 hours, and prophylactic antibiotics are administered within six hours of initial head and neck injury.[41,42,43] Third-generation cephalosporin antibiotics provide adequate perioperative prophylaxis for maxillofacial, head, and neck injury surgical interventions.[44] Current US Army recommendations are that maxillofacial war injuries not repaired in less than or equal to 12 hours, or without prophylactic antibiotics greater than or equal to six hours following injury, have a high risk of infection and require a treatment course of 10 to 14 days of antibiotics.[15] Combat casualty care data supporting these recommendations are limited. However, similar recommendations are widely published in civilian oral and maxillofacial textbooks.[39,40] High-risk maxillofacial wound characteristics include those with comminuted fractures or avulsed mandible defects, wounds with compromised blood supply, wounds closed under tension, and tissue flap or skin graft closures. Such wounds may benefit from a more prolonged course of prophylactic antibiotic therapy.[8]

Early definitive treatment with debridement, irrigation, repair of soft- and hard-tissues, administration of broad-spectrum prophylactic antibiotics, minimal introduction of foreign surgical material during initial surgery, and coverage of bone with tension-free closure are all interventions that decrease war infections.

## Epidemiology of Wound Infection

Infection rates following war-related maxillofacial injuries are outlined in Table 5. The actual pathogens that cause infections following war-related maxillofacial injury are poorly characterized.[45,46] Civilian studies in non-trauma patient populations have found that the cause of infection was polymicrobial in 88 to 96 percent of patients who develop infections following head and neck surgery.[47,48] Aerobic organisms were found in 54 to 91 percent of infections and anaerobic organisms were found in 54 to 74 percent of infections.[47,48] The specific pathogens cultured in the aforementioned studies were highly variable and included *Staphylococcus aureus*, *Pseudomonas aeruginosa*, *Klebsiella* species, *Escherichia coli*, *Proteus mirabilis*, *Bacteroides fragilis*, *Peptococcus*, *Fusobacterium* species, *Peptostreptococcus*, and fungi (among others). Osteomyelitis is a notable infectious complication in several civilian gunshot wound injury studies.[49,50,51] Inadequate wound exploration, debridement, foreign body removal, and closure of pharyngoesophageal injuries were cited as reasons for developing osteomyelitis.

| WAR-RELATED MAXILLOFACIAL INJURY INFECTION RATES |
| --- |
| Vietnam: 7 percent rate of infection[52] |
| Iran-Iraq War: 11 percent rate of infection[53] |
| Balkan conflict: 19 percent rate of infection[54] |

Table 5. *War-related maxillofacial injury infection rates.*

## Prevention of Infection: Surgical Management

Early repair of soft- and hard-tissues following irrigation, conservative wound debridement, early administration of broad-spectrum prophylactic antibiotics, minimal introduction of foreign surgical material during initial surgery, and coverage of bone with tension-free closure have been cited as interventions that decrease war infections.[39,40,55,56,57] The inner mucosal lining of maxillofacial structures should be maximally preserved during debridement efforts. Avulsion defects of the mandible are best treated by early stabilization of existing bone fragments, primary soft-tissue closure, wound drainage, repeated debridements, and delayed bone reconstruction (e.g., eight weeks following injury).[8] Bone grafting of mandibular injuries is best deferred to Level IV and V care facilities and performed in a delayed fashion. Bone grafting of mandibular defects is best performed on infection-free and well-perfused wound beds.[58,59] Further studies are required to determine whether rigid internal fixation of maxillofacial war wounds (as is often practiced in the course of host national care in OEF/OIF) has favorable outcomes (e.g., decreasing wound infection rates).

> Avulsion defects of the mandible are best treated by early stabilization of existing bone fragments, primary soft-tissue closure, wound drainage, repeated debridements, and delayed bone reconstruction.

## Diagnosis of Infection

Signs of a head and neck infection include erythema, edema, warmth, lymphadenopathy, drainage, or fluctuance at the wound site. Patients may complain of fever, increased pain at the site of injury, malaise, fevers, or difficulty tolerating oral intake. Laboratory testing may reveal evidence of inflammation (e.g., elevated white blood cell count). Radiographic imaging such as ultrasonography and CT or magnetic resonance imaging (MRI) can be used to help define the infection. Radionuclide scanning and MRI can be used to screen for evidence of early osteomyelitis. Of note, the ferromagnetic characteristics of embedded projectiles need to be assessed prior to MRI. Plain radiograph findings of osteomyelitis occur late in the disease course, following significant destruction of cortical bone.[60]

### Management of Infection

The following interventions are helpful in treating wound infections: (1) incision and drainage of accumulated purulent collections; (2) debridement of foreign bodies or necrotic material; (3) stabilization of fracture fragments; and (4) broad-spectrum antibiotic therapy.[45,54] There are no definitive studies in war settings to determine optimal choice or duration of antibiotic therapy for established infections. Standard expert-based recommendations include a 10 to 14 day course (or two to three days following wound closure and no evidence of infection) of broad-spectrum antibiotic therapy.[36] Osteomyelitis typically requires a minimum of six weeks of antibiotic therapy.[8] Ampicillin/sulbactam, clindamycin and a quinolone, and piperacillin/tazobactam have all been described as reasonable first-line agents for treatment of established infections of the head and neck in war settings.[8] Complications of wound infections of the head and neck include delayed healing, scarring/deformity, sinus tracts, nonunion of bone fragments, ocular infections, osteomyelitis, venous and cerebral sinus thrombosis, and necrotizing fasciitis.[40,45,50,51]

> Although no definitive studies exist, standard recommendations for treatment of established combat wound infections include 10 to 14 days of broad-spectrum antibiotic therapy.[36]

### Definitive Management

Over the past 25 years, the development of modern craniomaxillofacial surgical principles and techniques has resulted in dramatic improvements in facial fracture surgery. However, these principles and techniques are primarily based on the experience of civilian patients with blunt trauma. The preponderance of penetrating maxillofacial battle injuries (complicated by tissue avulsions and burns) caused by explosive devices in OEF/OIF has increased treatment requirements, including the application of microvascular composite tissue transfer, a technology driven by oncologic surgery. Even the combination of these technologies falls short of reconstructing the face to a natural form and function, because transferred tissues lack both the delicate contours and features of the face and neuromuscular integration.

Research in regenerative medicine and composite tissue allotransplantation over the next five to 10 years holds promise to improve reconstruction results for severely wounded service members. For now, the deployed face surgeon needs to stabilize US casualties with severe maxillofacial wounds for transfer to Level IV and V facilities for definitive care. Face specialists need to apply time-honored techniques to close severe facial wounds on casualties not eligible for evacuation, which, in the experience of the authors, make up the largest surgical patient load. Basic principles are reviewed in this section with emphasis placed on management of unique wounds the face specialist will most likely encounter in the combat zone versus within the US. Unless otherwise noted, the following recommendations are based on the training and experience of the authors.

> Severe maxillofacial wounds in US casualties should be stabilized and transferred to Level IV and V facilities for definitive care.

## Evaluation and Treatment Planning

Beyond the primary and secondary surveys and initial resuscitation of a combat casualty, maxillofacial examination begins with an overall inspection of the face for asymmetry, contusions, swellings, and lacerations. Palpate the entire facial skeleton for areas of irregularity or instability. The canthal attachments should be tested for stability, especially in cases of midface trauma. The nose should be palpated and inspected for signs of fracture. Mandibular range of motion should be assessed and jaw joints palpated. Evaluate for malocclusion, signs of dental trauma, intraoral lacerations, through-and-through lacerations, embedded debris, disruption of salivary ducts, and cranial nerve dysfunction. Evaluation of visual acuity, inspection of the anterior and posterior chambers, pupillary reflexes, and extraocular movements may be difficult to perform on the traumatized patient, and ophthalmology consultation is desirable. A detailed discussion of the ocular exam is provided in the Ocular Trauma chapter.

## Radiographic Imaging

Three-dimensional reconstruction of CT scans is the imaging procedure of choice for facial injuries. Computed tomography scans can be extended to the cervical spine and cranium to define trauma to these areas. Panoramic tomography (Panorex) provides additional information on the dentition of an ambulatory patient should this modality be available in the deployed setting. Preinjury photographs and identification cards are also helpful during the evaluation phase.

## Fracture Stabilization

After thorough maxillofacial evaluation and specialty consultations, a list of injuries is developed in order to plan definitive treatment. Clinical judgment is a critical factor in determining the indication, scope, and timing of surgery. As noted earlier, if the severely injured casualty can be evacuated to a higher level of care, the focus should then be on stabilizing the maxillofacial wounds for transfer. Often two to three days of damage control surgery in-theater will allow the face specialist the opportunity to secure a definitive surgical airway, serially debride and irrigate wounds and remove foreign material and necrotic tissue, address grossly unstable fractures, and apply wound dressings.

A small bone (Hoffman® II) or specific craniomaxillofacial external pin fixation device is an expedient technique to temporarily stabilize flail mandible fractures. Arch bars and bridle wires for intra-arch stabilization are also helpful, but wire intermaxillary fixation should be avoided (Figs. 40 and 41). Wiring the teeth together compromises the airway and should be avoided in most cases of severe maxillofacial trauma treated in-theater. Elastic intermaxillary fixation with lightly applied rubber band ligatures is an excellent substitute to wire fixation for the ambulatory patient.

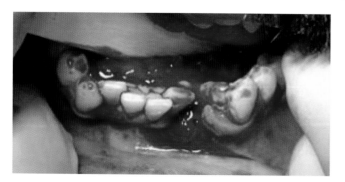 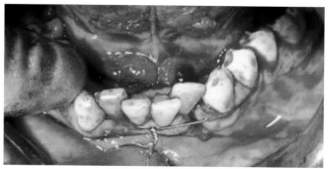

Figure 40. *Bridle wires may be used for intra-arch stabilization.*

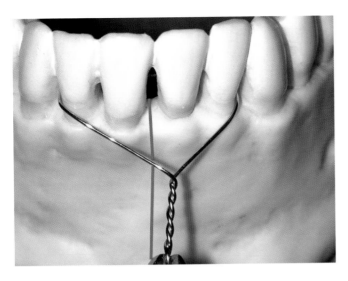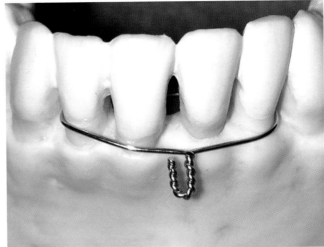

Figure 41. *Bridle wire placement (red line denotes fracture line).*

For transferable patients, a small bone (Hoffman® II) or specific craniomaxillofacial external pin fixation device is an expedient technique to temporarily stabilize flail mandible fractures. Wiring the teeth together compromises the airway and should be avoided in most all cases of severe maxillofacial trauma treated in-theater.

## Definitive Repair

Definitive treatment of the nontransferable casualty requires preoperative analysis of incisions to expose the skeleton for fracture mobilization and reduction, methods of bony fixation, need for primary bone grafting, and repair of soft-tissues. The presence of tissue avulsions and burns obviously complicates planning. In those situations, wound closure may require local and regional flaps or, in the case of burns, stabilization of fractures through external pin fixation and interdental fixation techniques. Incisions may involve the use of existing lacerations, scalp incisions, periorbital incisions, cervical incisions, and incisions in the oral cavity (Fig. 42). Rigid internal fixation is desirable, but if the soft-tissue envelope is compromised, external pin and/or dental fixation may be required. Airway management, both during and after the operation, should be collaboratively performed with input from the anesthesiologist and trauma surgeon. Oral or nasal intubations are airway options, but if access to the surgical field or associated injuries (e.g., unstable cervical spine or basilar skull fractures) prevents their use, an elective tracheotomy should be considered.

### Informed Consent

Even in the combat theater, informed consent for an elective operation is a feature of comprehensive care. If the patient is not able to make an informed consent, review the potential risks with the patient's family. The concerned parties should be aware that despite your best efforts, preinjury appearance will unlikely be achieved. The possibility of revision or staged surgeries to achieve the best results cannot be realistically determined or promised in the combat theater. The consent process with the potential for loss of vision, intracranial injury, and even death, although rare, needs to be accepted and documented.

### Timing of Surgery

It is prudent to delay surgery on unstable patients with intracranial injuries. Once intracranial injuries

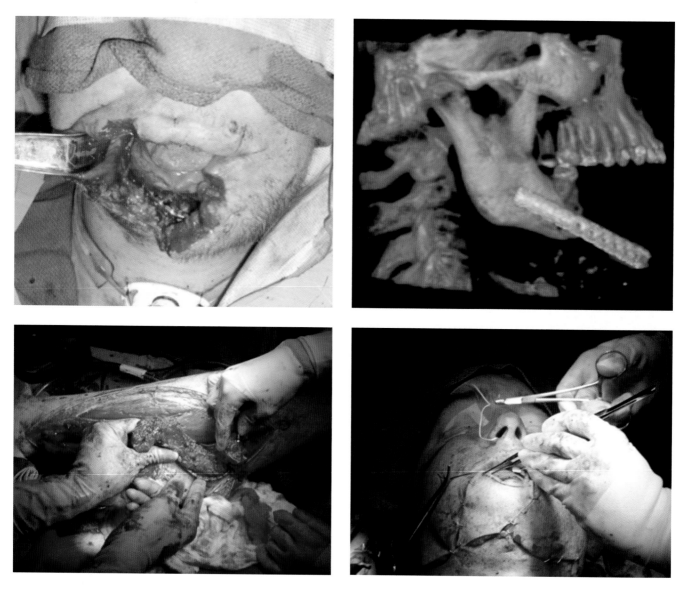

Figure 42. (Top Left) *Improvised explosive device injury to lower face resulting in lower lip and chin avulsion and avulsion of entire dentate mandible.* (Top Right) *Three-dimensional CT imaging is the modality of choice for facial injuries.* (Bottom Left) *A fibular microvascular flap is grafted and restores soft-tissue and bone continuity.* (Bottom Right) *The flap will remain insensate, adynamic, different in color and texture, and hairless.*

stabilize, early repair of facial fractures in these patients should be considered with input from neurosurgical consultants. It is difficult to predict when an unconscious patient will neurologically improve. If maxillofacial surgery is delayed beyond two to three weeks, subsequent attempts at repair are exceedingly difficult, if not impossible, because of soft-tissue envelope contracture and fibrous unions.[61]

It is prudent to delay facial reconstruction in unstable patients with intracranial injuries. However, delayed maxillofacial repair is more difficult after two to three weeks due to soft-tissue envelope contracture and fibrous unions.

### Surgical Principles

The overall plan to treat hard- and soft-tissue injuries to the maxillofacial region is to reconstruct facial fractures before definitively closing the soft-tissue wounds. The goal of fracture repair is to reconstruct preinjury facial projection, proportions, and form and function, and to support subsequent soft-tissue

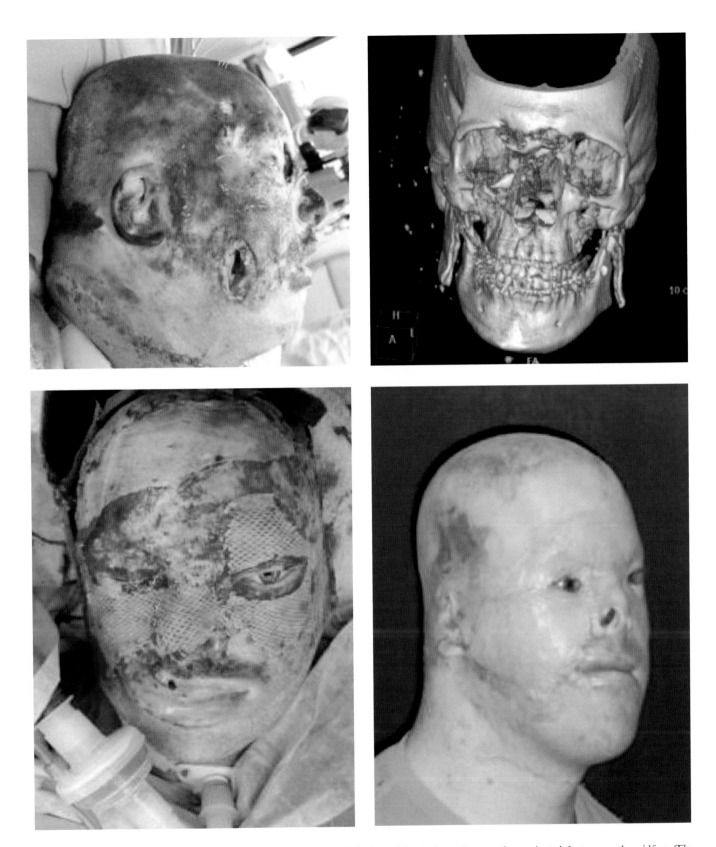

Figure 43. (Top Left and Top Right) *An explosive device caused third- and fourth-degree burns and comminuted fractures to the midface. The mandible fracture was reconstructed primarily through cervical incisions. Burn closure took precedence over midface bony reconstruction.* (Bottom Left) *After one to two weeks, the burns on the face will demarcate tissue requiring debridement. The resultant soft-tissue bed is dressed until healthy enough to receive split-thickness skin grafts.* (Bottom Right) *Multiple secondary procedures are expected in cases of burns and soft-tissue avulsion.*

reconstruction. The soft-tissue wounds can then be redraped over a rigid and correct facial framework. In cases of severe facial burns and avulsions, soft-tissue care often precedes definitive fracture care, and extensive revisions are expected (Fig. 43).

> The goal of facial fracture repair is to restore preinjury facial projection, proportions, and form and function, and to support subsequent soft-tissue reconstruction.

## Facial Soft-Tissue Injuries

Penetrating trauma on the battlefield tends to injure both hard- and soft-tissues. This section will initially address soft-tissue injuries, but composite tissue injuries are discussed later by region (upper face, midface, and lower face) because penetrating battle injuries are manifested differently in those regions. Blunt trauma injury patterns and treatment to the maxillofacial area will not be discussed in detail since it is expected that the deployed face specialist is competent in this injury pattern (commonly seen in the US civilian setting). The deployed face surgeon should ensure access to reference sources that cover maxillofacial trauma, orbital trauma, soft-tissue management, and pedicle and rotational flap management. Beyond book references, the deployed face surgeon should develop online communication with rear echelon experts in their respective fields. This online connection, more than any collection of books, will give the face specialist access to expert consultation and provide a forum to discuss difficult management decisions.

Penetrating trauma to the face causes a variety of soft-tissue defects. This section will outline facial wound closure and surgery to reconstruct the lips and nose, features that remain extremely challenging to reconstruct. Ear avulsions are seen with combat injuries. The face surgeon may have the opportunity to salvage avulsed ear cartilage in a postauricular skin pouch. The avulsed ear is prepared by removing or dermabrading the skin but leaving perichondrium intact over the cartilage. In general, cheek defects from penetrating trauma are closed by wide undermining of wound edges, or development of a rhomboid or cervicofacial flap. Buccal, tongue, or floor of mouth flaps will close the mucosal lining of most full-thickness cheek defects. Severed parotid ducts should be cannulated and repaired primarily. Repair of at least the severed temporal nerve or upper division of the facial nerve is critical to restore the protective function of the eyelid.

As a general rule, lip defects with less than 33 percent vermillion-lip-length loss can be closed primarily by modifying the defect to a "V" or "M" and advancing the skin-muscle flaps.[62] The blood supply to even macerated facial skin and mucosa is surprisingly robust, and no tissue should be discarded until defect closure is carefully planned. Defects measuring 33 to 67 percent of vermillion-lip-length can be closed with staged lip switch flaps, such as Abbe-Estlander flaps.[62,63] Larger lip defects can be treated by dissection of perioral skin-muscle flaps and advancing flaps circumferentially to provide orbicularis oris function using classic procedures of Karapandzic and Giles.[63] All of these flaps cause microstomia, but lip function is preserved. Loss of over 67 percent of vermillion-lip-length will require lateral sliding cheek flaps or nasolabial flaps to close the wound, along with buccal mucosa advancement or pedicle ventral tongue flaps to replace the vermillion.[62] Total lip avulsion in a nontransferable patient will require multiple staged tissue transfers (i.e., temporoparietal or cervicofacial flaps). Staged flap reconstruction is necessary to reconstruct commissure defects. Patients, families, and command need to make the commitment for host nation patients to return for staged procedures.

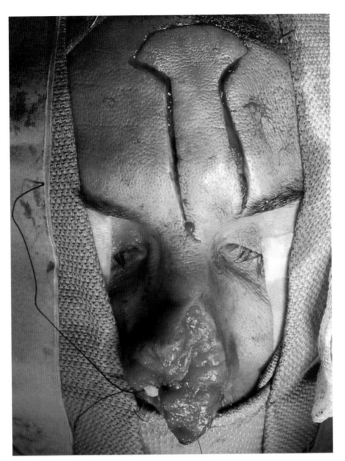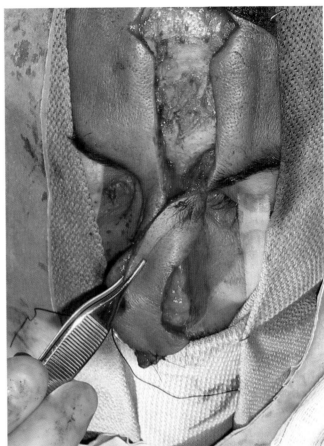

Figure 44. *Gunshot wound to the nose in a host nation male.* (Left) *A median forehead flap was fashioned.* (Right) *Rotation of the flap onto the defect.* *Image courtesy of the Borden Institute, Office of The Surgeon General, Washington, DC.*

> As a general rule, lip defects with less than 33 percent vermillion-lip-length loss can be closed primarily by modifying the defect to a "V" or "M" and advancing the skin-muscle flaps.

Staged forehead flaps based on supraorbital, supratrochlear, infratrochlear, and superficial temporal vessels are robust flaps useful for immediate reconstruction of the avulsed nose (Fig. 44). Full-thickness nasal avulsion with loss of mucosal lining can lead to synechiae and chronic nasal airway obstruction unless the lining is replaced. The author (**RGH**) prefers a separate broad-based pericranial flap to replace intranasal lining.[64] Loss of septal support is reconstructed with a cantilever cranial bone graft. Melolabial flaps are useful to reconstruct alar defects.

Facial Burns

The immediate concern for significant facial burns (second- and third-degree) is to evaluate the patient for airway burns and secure the airway accordingly. After irrigating the wounds, sterile dry dressings should be applied to wounds. The choice of topical burn dressings and when to apply them are often based on provider preference, available supplies, and transport times between successive medical facilities. Providers in the field should simply cover burns with a clean, dry dressing and avoid applying any topical ointments, including burn creams, to the wounds.[65]

This approach eliminates the need for careproviders to later have to remove creams when patients present at the next facility in the evacuation chain. The use of silver-impregnated dressing such as Silverlon®, Acticoat®, or SilverSeal® as the initial dressing is an alternative option. These materials are easy to apply, provide topical antimicrobial protection, and do not impede the subsequent wound evaluation and care. A more detailed discussion of burn management is found in the Acute Burn Care chapter.

Oral ETTs are best secured by keeping tape and straps off the face and affixing the tube to several lower anterior teeth. Significant burn involvement of the periorbita puts the patient at risk for orbital compartment syndrome, which is prophylactically treated by lateral canthotomies (discussed in detail in the Ocular Trauma chapter). Corneal protection and ectropion prevention are achieved by bolstering eyelids together or performing a Frost suture. Intercommissure lip distance is maintained by a plastic oral prosthesis for perioral burns. Sepsis is not risked by delaying face debridement until burn margins fully demarcate, typically by seven to 10 days. Debridement of deep second- and third-degree burns is followed by dressing changes until the wound bed is ready for closure with skin grafts. Split-thickness skin grafts are used in areas where contracture will minimally harm function (i.e., contracture can be tolerated). Full-thickness skin grafts are preferred in areas such as the perioral region and lower eyelid. Use sutures, Xeroform™ bolsters, and face dressings to secure grafts on the face.

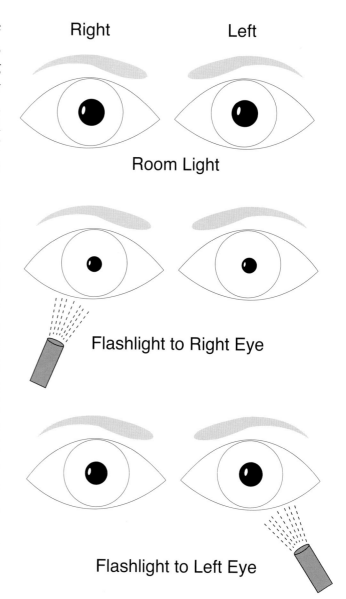

Figure 45. *Swinging flashlight test reveals an afferent pupillary defect in the left eye (anatomical left).*

## Upper and Midface Injuries

### *Ocular Assessment*

Management of maxillofacial blast injuries requires the face surgeon to diagnose and treat conditions that threaten vision following trauma or surgery. This is a difficult but important task, especially when treating foreign-speaking, uncooperative, sedated, or obtunded patients. In these situations, an objective clinical method to assess for an afferent pupillary defect (Marcus Gunn pupil) indicates optic nerve dysfunction is helpful (Fig. 45). A field expedient test is the swinging flashlight test. The test is performed in a dark room by methodically swinging a flashlight from one eye to the other. An abnormal exam that indicates optic nerve dysfunction-related vision loss will demonstrate that both pupils will dilate symmetrically when

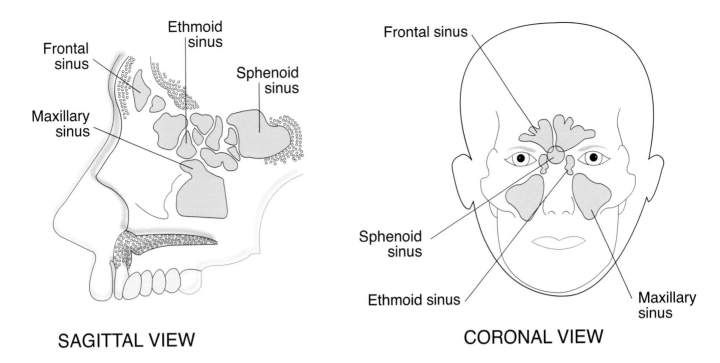

Frontal sinus

Ethmoid sinus

Sphenoid sinus

Maxillary sinus

**SAGITTAL VIEW**

Frontal sinus

Sphenoid sinus

Ethmoid sinus

Maxillary sinus

**CORONAL VIEW**

Figure 46. *Schematic of facial sinuses.*

the light is directed into the affected eye, and both pupils will constrict symmetrically when the light is directed into the normal eye.

### Frontal Sinus Fractures

The frontal sinus is a paranasal cavity lined by mucosa located between the anterior cranial fossa and the naso-orbito-ethmoidal (NOE) region of the frontal bone. Sinus drainage is through ducts located in the anterosuperior part of the anterior ethmoid complex into the middle meatus. Thin bone separates this sinus from the cranium, which puts the brain at risk from penetrating trauma. Additionally, injury to the frontonasal ducts prevents drainage of mucosal secretions, which can lead to intracranial complications (Fig. 46).[66] Frontal sinus and NOE fractures that extend intracranially can cause a cerebrospinal fluid leak manifested as rhinorrhea (Fig. 47). Significantly displaced posterior wall fractures are usually associated with torn dura.[67] An indication for surgery is the presence of a foreign body in the frontal sinus. Bloody nasal drainage can be field tested at bedside for cerebrospinal fluid by placing the fluid on a linen sheet. Cerebrospinal fluid diffuses faster than blood and creates a clear halo around a bloodstain.[68] Of note, this test is not very accurate and maintaining a high index of suspicion for these injuries is prudent irrespective of test results. The definitive laboratory diagnosis for the presence of cerebrospinal fluid is beta-2 transferrin, which is not routinely available in the combat theater.[69,70,71]

> Frontal sinus and NOE fractures that extend intracranially can cause a cerebrospinal fluid leak manifested as rhinorrhea.

The frontal sinus can be approached through an existing skin laceration, but a coronal incision provides the best exposure. The sinus should be explored, irrigated, and all foreign bodies and devitalized tissue removed. If a nasofrontal outflow tract (frontonasal duct) injury is absent, the anterior sinus wall is anatomically reduced and fixated. If significant bone loss is present or if the fragments are comminuted beyond repair, fixated cranial bone grafts are useful to fill the defects. Fractures involving the nasofrontal outflow tract (frontonasal duct) may produce obstruction and infection. Treatment designed to prevent infection involves sinus membrane ablation and frontonasal duct obliteration.[72] This is performed through a frontal bone flap with removal of all mucosa from the sinus with a rotary diamond burr. A pericranial flap elevated from the coronal flap and placed over bone grafts to plug the duct system is useful to isolate the nasal cavity from the cranium.[73] Obliteration of the sinus with fat or muscle-free grafts is frequently recommended in the literature, but the operated sinus can also be left empty for spontaneous osteogenesis.[74,75,76,77]

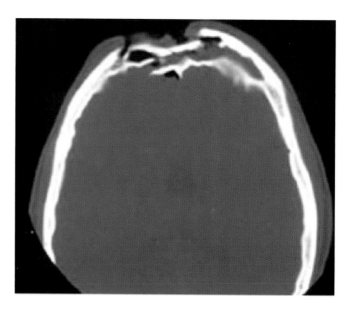

Figure 47. *An axial CT image of a posteriorly displaced frontal sinus fracture. Fracture displacement of the posterior wall of the frontal sinus with cerebrospinal fluid leakage or a foreign body lodged in the frontal sinus is an indication for surgery.*

Significantly displaced frontal bone fractures associated with a cerebrospinal fluid leak require a cranialization procedure in consultation with neurosurgery, if available (Figs. 48 to 55). Cranialization is the removal of the posterior wall of the frontal sinus to repair torn dura and allow anterior displacement of the brain into the prepared sinus cavity. Care must be taken to avoid injury to the dura and superior sagittal sinus during the flap osteotomy. The author (RGH) uses a powered perforator to develop burr holes in the frontotemporal areas, followed by a craniotome with a guarded side-cutting burr to cut and remove two parasagittal frontal bone flaps, leaving a two-centimeter wide bone strut in the midline. The dura over the superior sagittal sinus can then be elevated from the frontal crest and protected during removal of the midline bone strut. This technique adds several minutes to the cranialization procedure but helps avoid tremendous blood loss from violation of the superior sagittal sinus; avoiding neurosurgical complications in a CSH is important because consultation may only be available by Internet. After the posterior wall of the frontal sinus is removed, the dura injury can be repaired. Complete mucosal ablation of the remaining sinus walls is followed by obliteration of the frontonasal ducts. A pericranial flap dissected from the coronal flap can be advanced over the ducts to provide a vascularized brain–nose barrier. It is important to note that performing a cranialization procedure on US service members in a deployed setting without neurosurgical support is not advised. Ideally, such an intervention should be deferred until service members are evacuated to Level IV or V care facilities due to the potential for a catastrophic bleed from the superior sagittal sinus. The face specialist may be forced to perform such an intervention on host nationals, as they typically do not have access to higher levels of care.

### Naso-Orbito-Ethmoid (NOE) Region Fractures

The NOE region is beneath the frontal bone and is located below the floor of the anterior cranial fossa and between the medial orbital walls. Besides involving issues relating to nasofrontal outflow tract drainage described above, fractures and penetrating trauma can also cause displacement of the medial canthal ligaments. Instability of the medial canthal ligaments can be assessed by palpating the medial canthus while applying traction on the lateral canthus (bowstring test). A bimanual exam is performed by inserting an instrument intranasally into the area of the medial canthus while placing the index finger externally on the medial canthus. All displaced or unstable NOE fractures require surgery to reconstruct intercanthal distance and nasal projection.

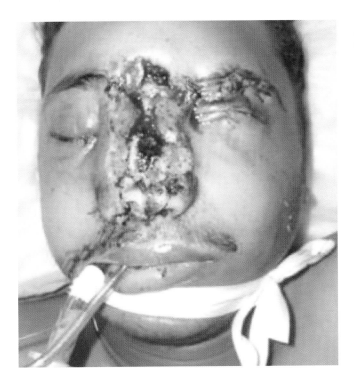

Figure 48. *A 16-year-old Afghan male with an avulsed nose and penetrating injury to the frontal sinus and anterior cranial fossa and left eye from an explosive device. Cranialization of frontal sinus and repair of dura were indicated.*

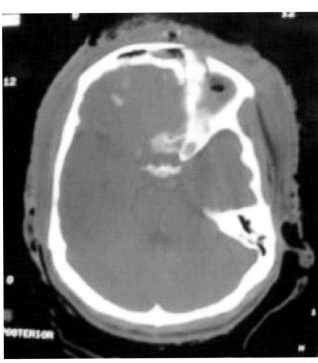

Figure 49. *CT image demonstrating frontal sinus and anterior cranial fossa injury.*

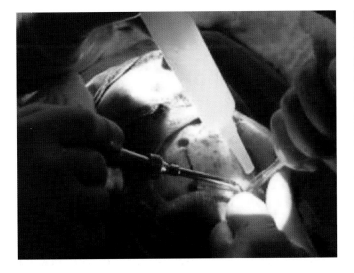

Figure 50. *A guarded craniotome connected the burr holes and the bone flap was carefully elevated to avoid damaging the superior sagittal sinus.*

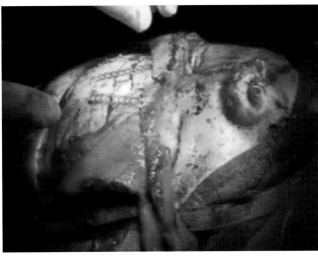

Figure 51. *The frontal flap and fragments are replaced and fixated rigidly.*

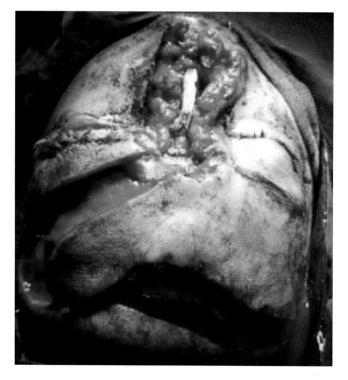

Figure 52. *Skin flap reapproximation.*

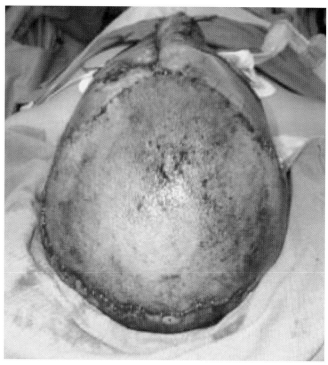

Figure 53. *Occipital view of scalp wound closure.*

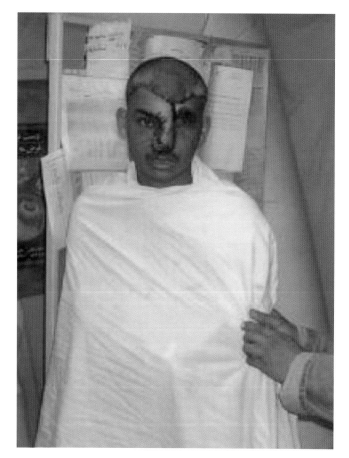

Figure 54. *Patient at one week following injury.*

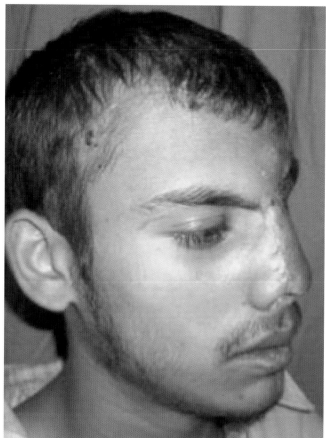

Figure 55. *Patient at three months following injury after flap division and minor revision.*

Type I NOE fractures involve a large bone fragment with the medial canthi attached. This fracture can be reduced and managed by rigidly fixating the fragment to stable bones superiorly and inferiorly. Type II is a comminuted fracture with the medial canthi attached to operable central bone fragments.[78] Type III NOE fractures involve avulsion of the medial canthus from bone. Type II and III fractures are difficult to treat and require wide exposure through multiple incisions or reflection of a coronal flap beyond the level of the nasofrontal junction with placement of transnasal wires to restore intercanthal distance. Reconstruction of comminuted NOE fractures may require a cantilever cranial bone graft to support nasal projection. The cantilever bone graft engages the area between the upper lateral cartilages and fixates superiorly with miniplates and screws.

Battle injuries to the maxilla, zygomas, orbits, and nose make up at least 44 percent of the injuries to the maxillofacial area.[1] The maxilla occupies the mid-aspect of the face between the cranial base and dentition. Three bony struts support the maxilla: the nasomaxillary, the zygomaticomaxillary, and the pterygomaxillary buttresses. The zygoma articulates with the frontal bone, maxilla, temporal bone, and greater wing of the sphenoid bone. The orbital floor extends back 35 to 40 mm from the rim to the posterior wall of the maxillary sinus. Exploding debris easily penetrates the thin walls of the orbits and paranasal sinuses. The fracture pattern from penetrating trauma varies from typical LeFort to comminuted fractures with avulsed bony fragments. Fractures with no displacement require only observation. Blast debris in the sinuses and airway should be removed. If the fracture is displaced, exploration with anatomic reduction and fixation is indicated. The experience and clinical judgment of the surgeon will dictate the exposure and methods of fixation.

> Naso-orbito-ethmoid fractures without displacement require observation only, whereas displaced fractures necessitate exploration with anatomic reduction and fixation.

### Zygoma Fractures

Reconstruction of a significantly displaced zygoma fracture requires multiple exposure sites in areas of fracture: the zygomaticofrontal suture, the infraorbital rim, the zygomaticomaxillary buttress, and occasionally the zygomatic arch. The zygomatic arch is an important consideration in aligning significantly displaced or comminuted zygoma fractures because the arch defines midface width and projection. The zygomatic arch should be reduced and fixated as a relatively straight structure. A maxillary vestibule incision provides exposure of the zygomaticomaxillary buttress and infraorbital area. The choice of lower eyelid incision depends on the surgeon's training and experience, but the transconjunctival incision, with or without a canthotomy, has the least risk for lower lid retraction. The zygomaticofrontal suture is exposed by a separate incision in the lateral aspect of the supratarsal fold of the upper eyelid.

For comminuted or severely displaced zygoma fractures, a coronal incision is performed to reconstruct the facial width and projection by exposing the zygomatic arch. In front of the ear and above the arch, the superficial layer of the deep temporal fascia is identified and then incised to the fatty space (superficial temporal fat pad); dissection is carried out in this layer to the arch to avoid injury to the frontal branch of the facial nerve. The zygomatic arch is reduced and fixated, followed by figure-of-eight wire ligature to the zygomaticofrontal fracture and a microplate to the rim. The fractured zygoma can then be rotated into proper position and fixated at the zygomaticomaxillary buttress after confirming intraorbitally that the zygomaticosphenoid (greater wing) articulation is aligned. Cranial bone grafts should be used in areas of avulsion or severe comminution.

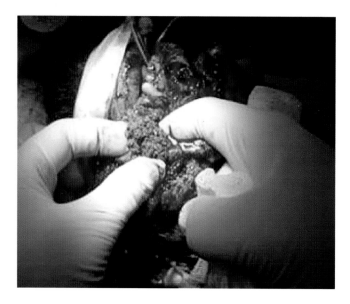 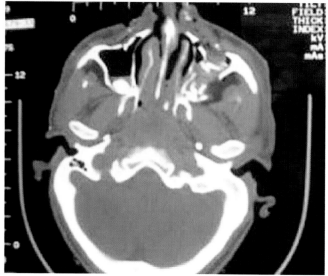

Figure 56. (Left) *A piece of shrapnel removed from a combat casualty suffering penetrating fragmentation injuries to the face.* (Right) *Axial CT image revealing shrapnel that has perforated and comminuted the thin bones of the midface.*

### Orbit Fractures

Orbital floor fractures are reconstructed in the usual fashion by identifying the residual floor ledge of the posterior orbit through a lid incision with dissection beneath periorbita. If available, an endoscope inserted into the maxillary sinus can visualize the posterior ledge and confirm adequacy of reduction and reconstruction. Large floor defects are reconstructed with a variety of materials, but in the combat theater choices are limited. To avoid late complications of infection and extrusion, the author (RGH) prefers cranial bone graft shavings harvested from the temporoparietal area with the pericranium attached. These grafts are harvested using a wide, short, and sharp osteotome angled at a low profile and engaged by a heavy mallet. The resultant bone shaving, slightly curled and attached to pericranium, is placed over floor defects. Several stacked shavings may be necessary to correct orbital volume defects; fixation is not necessary.

### LeFort Fractures

LeFort fractures present with malocclusion, midface instability, nasal bleeding, and periorbital edema. Penetrating trauma of the maxilla above the dentition can cause a LeFort fracture or penetrate the thin bony walls and lodge debris into paranasal sinuses (Fig. 56). Caldwell Luc access may be necessary to remove debris from the sinus followed by nasal antrostomy (endoscopic equipment is not necessarily available in Level III care facilities). LeFort fractures are manipulated through vestibule incisions and reduction performed to reconstruct facial height, projection, and occlusion. Typically, 1.5 to 2.0 mm bone plates are used to fixate the fracture at the nasomaxillary and zygomaticomaxillary buttresses, and bone grafts are placed in defect areas.

## Lower Face Injuries

Penetrating trauma to the lower face by explosive debris can fragment and avulse the thick cortical bones of the mandible and dentoalveolar structures. Fragmentation of the mandible and dentoalveolar structures places the tongue and surrounding areas at risk of laceration with subsequent airway compromise (Fig. 57). Securing a definitive airway is an important consideration for penetrating trauma to the lower face.

The U-shaped mandible has a dentate portion and an articular portion. The dentate portion has a thick, compact, inferior border and a dense dentoalveolar process superiorly. The ascending ramus ends as the condylar process that articulates with the cranium to form the temporomandibular joint. Blood supply to the mandible varies with anatomical area: the ramus, condyles, and symphysis have large muscular attachments to nourish the bone; however the mandibular body receives the majority of blood supply centrally from the inferior alveolar vessels.[79]

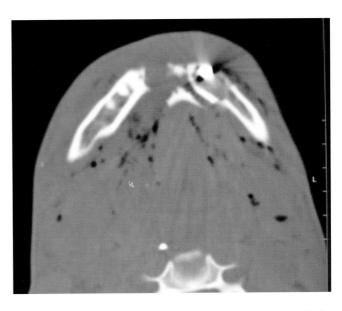

Figure 57. *An axial CT image demonstrating a comminuted mandibular fracture. Fragmentation of the lower face can result in loss of mandibular tongue support and supraglottic edema leading to airway compromise.*

### Evaluation

Evaluation of the lower face begins with inspection and palpation of the face along the inferior border and joints to reveal point tenderness, instability, or step-off deformities. Orally, evaluate for malocclusion and disruptions of the soft-tissue envelope, teeth, and dental arch. Anterior traction on the mandible by grasping the mandibular incisors and chin will often cause pain at the fracture sites. Likewise, pushing inward at the angles of the mandible will also reveal fracture sites. Radiographic evaluation of the mandible is best done with a CT scan.

### Treatment

The goal of mandibular reconstruction is restoration of the lower facial height, chin projection, arch form, and occlusion. The location and condition of the fracture dictates the surgical approach. Nondisplaced fractures without occlusal disturbances are treated with a soft diet. Closed reduction is used when a fracture is displaced with minimal occlusal disturbances. Grossly displaced fractures usually require open reduction with internal or external fixation.

> The goal of mandibular reconstruction is restoration of lower facial height, chin projection, arch form, and occlusion.

Uncorrectable or irreparably comminuted open mandibular fractures should be debrided of small, devitalized fragments. Larger, viable fragments should be reduced and fixated as soon as possible to minimize pain, soft-tissue injury, and risk of infection. Reduction of the fractured mandible is aided by dental knowledge and intraoperative intermaxillary fixation to align major dentoalveolar fragments (Fig. 58). The decision to debride or retain a fragment rests with the surgeon's clinical judgment and experience. Any retained fragment needs to be large enough to be fixated and yet remain attached or covered with an adequate soft-tissue envelope for healing. Keep in mind, the soft-tissue envelope of a severely comminuted mandibular body fracture is not only torn and compromised, but also contaminated by bacteria-laden saliva in a nondependent wound bed. The prudent face surgeon chooses the least risky course of action for the situation. An overly limited debridement puts the polytrauma casualty at risk for complications of mandibular infection, while an overly aggressive debridement adds multiple major future interventions to an already complicated treatment course. Of the two extremes, mandibular

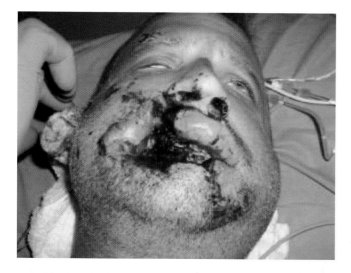

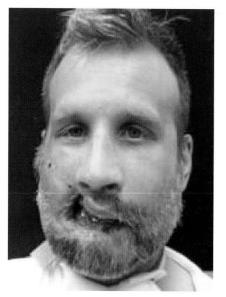

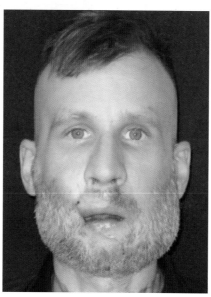

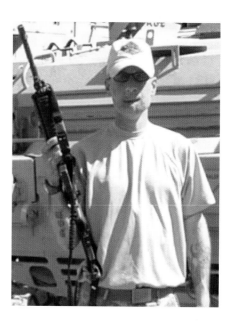

Figure 58. (Top Left) *An explosion caused avulsions of 40 percent of the upper lip and 80 percent of the lower lip in this casualty. Shrapnel perforated through the posterior face to cause a LeFort fracture and comminuted bilateral mandible fractures.* (Bottom Left) *Six weeks after bone reconstruction, a series of soft-tissue procedures attempt lip reconstruction (rhomboid, lateral sliding cheek, buccal mucosa flaps, bilateral cervicofacial flap, and ventral tongue flap) with limited success.* (Bottom Center and Bottom Right) *Reconstruction replaced facial features, but microstomia and lip incompetence persisted. This soldier chose to redeploy to Iraq after lip reconstruction.*

infection will likely delay other surgical services from performing critical and timely procedures, whereas complex mandibular reconstruction for a continuity defect can be electively delayed for months until the casualty is sufficiently recovered from multiple other wounds. Likewise, overly limited debridement of a complicated mandible fracture on host nation patients risks infection with the possibility of not having access to timely or sufficient care. Overly aggressive treatment may leave a mandibular continuity defect unrepaired. The treatment decision in a combat zone is difficult; but, in the case of the US service member, the decision can be deferred to a higher level of care. In the case of the injured host nation patient in the combat zone, decision making should involve the patient, family, and command.

Immediate bone grafting of mandibular body defects is not recommended because the wound bed is compromised by injury, contaminated by saliva, and is essentially a nondependent wound of the floor of the mouth.[80] Late grafting of bone defects requires adequate soft-tissue bed and in cases of avulsion, regional soft-tissue flaps (pectoralis) are often needed to prepare the recipient site. Mandibular body continuity defects greater than six centimeters, especially central, are problematic to reconstruct without the advantage of microvascular surgery to perform osseous free flaps.[81,82,83] Consultation with the host nation patient and family, along with command input, will lessen the burden of decision-making since long-term follow-up by the same face surgeon is unlikely.

## Panfacial Fractures

The two basic approaches to panfacial fractures have traditionally been from bottom-to-top or from top-to-bottom.[84,85] The bottom-to-top approach is based on the premise that the mandible can be anatomically reconstructed to provide an intact relationship for positioning of the maxilla. Facial width reconstruction in this technique is based on correct anatomical reduction of the mandibular body, ramus, and condyles. Positioning of the fractured maxilla to the cranium is then based on seating the condyles into the glenoid fossae, as dictated by intermaxillary fixation, followed by zygoma and frontonasal reconstruction. The bottom-to-top approach is preferred in cases of blunt trauma when mandibular continuity can be assured through anatomic alignment and fixation of large fragments.

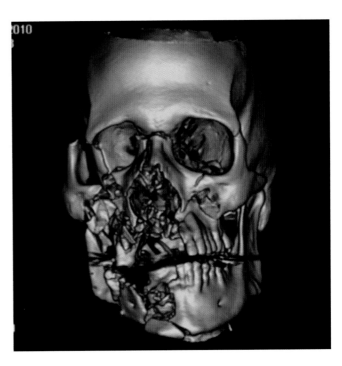

Figure 59. *Complex right orbit, zygoma, maxilla, and mandible fractures due to an IED. Partial avulsion of the maxilla and mandible will challenge the surgeon's ability to symmetrically reconstruct facial width and height. Computer reconstruction of image from a live patient. Stereolithographic resin models and computer imaging are useful reconstruction tools (used at Level V care facilities) when avulsion of key anatomical parts occurs.*

In cases of severe mandibular comminution from a maxillofacial blast injury, anatomical reduction of the mandible may be impossible (Fig. 59). In the top-to-bottom approach, midface projection is defined initially by reconstructing the outer facial frame to include the zygomatic arch, zygoma, and frontal areas. Second, the inner facial frame – including the nasoethmoid complex and infraorbital rims – is reconstructed. Third, the maxilla is repositioned and reconstructed by plating the zygomaticomaxillary and nasomaxillary buttresses. Lastly, temporary intermaxillary fixation followed by open reduction and fixation of the mandible is performed using interdental relationships to dictate mandibular projection. Mandibular continuity defects are reconstructed with reconstruction plates and bone grafted secondarily.

## *Summary*

Management of maxillofacial battle injuries ranges from the simple to the highly complex. Penetrating trauma on the battlefield is the predominant mechanism of maxillofacial injuries. Injuries include multiple complex soft-tissue wounds and open fractures, occasionally complicated by tissue avulsions and burns. Infection of combat-related wounds remains a problem. Broad-spectrum prophylactic antibiotic therapy, administered one hour prior to surgical intervention and continued for a 24-hour period, is recommended. An important consideration to prevent infections is early wound care, early stabilization, preservation of soft-tissue, and early evacuation.

Following patient stabilization, including securing a definitive airway, US service members with severe maxillofacial wounds should undergo conservative wound debridement and be transported to higher levels of care. Difficulty arises in the appropriate planning and execution of definitive repair in host nation civilians, local forces, and detained personnel. In such cases, complex battle injuries are best approached with interventions that have the least risk of postoperative complications but are consistent with predictable and favorable outcomes. Before surgery, it is critical to communicate the operative plan and the possibility of deviation depending on operative findings or postoperative complications. The patient, family, and military command need to be aware of the severity of the injury and the high likelihood that further future reconstructive surgeries and treatment will be needed.

# Penetrating Neck Wounds

## Introduction

Three percent of wounds sustained in OEF and OIF from October 2001 through January 2005 were neck wounds. Seventy-eight percent of wounds were sustained from explosions.[2] The patterns of injury created by high-energy explosive devices (e.g., IEDs), the weapon of choice of insurgents in Iraq and Afghanistan, are more variable, less predictable, and not as well understood as those seen in previous conflicts or at civilian US trauma centers. Several studies are in the data collection phase, but comprehensive data on battle injuries to the neck and outcomes of treatment have not yet been compiled and published. With that understood, historical studies of trauma management remain a useful starting point for making clinical decisions. In particular, the Advanced Trauma Life Support (ATLS) protocols developed by the American College of Surgeons are largely based on civilian trauma experience, but are the basis of a logical approach to trauma casualties that has stood the test of time.[86]

> The patterns of injury created by high-energy explosive devices are more variable, less predictable, and not as well understood as those seen in previous conflicts or at civilian US trauma centers.

During the 50 years prior to the widespread use of IEDs, injury patterns and treatment outcomes following penetrating neck wounds were fairly consistent. In 1963, Stone et al. reported that vascular injuries in the neck accounted for 50 percent of deaths following penetrating neck trauma.[87] Thirty years later, in a multi-institutional review of penetrating neck injuries from 16 US medical centers, McConnell et al. also reported the number one leading cause of death from penetrating neck trauma was exsanguinating hemorrhage.[88] In that study, the following incidence of injury to structures of the neck was reported: larynx and trachea (10 percent), internal jugular vein (9 percent), common and internal carotid arteries (7 percent), subclavian artery (2 percent), external carotid artery (2 percent), and vertebral artery (1 percent). Other relevant observations in the study include: (1) that one-third of initially asymptomatic patients with Zone I neck trauma were ultimately diagnosed with significant Zone I neck injuries; and (2) 25 percent of initially asymptomatic patients with neck Zone III trauma were diagnosed with an arterial injury. Penetrating trauma to Zone II managed by mandatory neck exploration was negative 30 to 50 percent of the time. A major cause of late mortality was missed esophageal injuries because esophageal and pharyngeal injuries were often asymptomatic on presentation. When surgical repair or drainage was performed less than 24 hours after the injury, the survival rate was greater than 90 percent; when performed more than 24 hours after the injury, survival dropped to 65 percent.[88,89]

## Anatomy

It is useful to divide structures of the neck into five major functional groups to ensure a comprehensive assessment is performed and as a map for focusing a secondary survey and surgical approaches (Table 6). Two muscles of the neck serve as key landmarks and their importance must be understood. The platysma defines superficial from deep structures of the neck. If a wound does not penetrate deep to the level of the platysma, it is not classified as a penetrating neck wound. Although the transverse cervical veins, running superficial to the platysma, may be large and can bleed profusely when severed, they are easily controlled with direct pressure and can be managed with simple ligature. The sternocleidomastoid muscle further divides the neck into the anterior triangle and posterior triangle (Fig. 60). Generally speaking, the posterior triangle contains the spine and muscles, whereas the anterior triangle contains the vasculature, nerves, airway, esophagus, and glands.

> If a wound does not penetrate the platysma, it is not classified as a significant penetrating neck wound.

| NECK ANATOMY |
| --- |
| • Airway (pharynx, larynx, trachea, lung) |
| • Major Vessels (carotid arteries, innominate artery, aortic arch vessels, jugular veins, subclavian veins) |
| • Gastrointestinal Tract (pharynx, esophagus) |
| • Nerves (spinal cord, brachial plexus, peripheral nerves, cranial nerves) |
| • Bones (mandibular angles, styloid processes, spine) |

Table 6. *Neck anatomy.*

## Neck Zones

When evaluating penetrating injuries, the neck is commonly divided into three anatomic zones for purposes of initial assessment and management planning (Fig. 61). The utility of this division is based upon two concepts: injury patterns and surgical management approaches. As discussed above, injury patterns from high-energy explosives are variable, lowering the predictive value of observing a penetrating wound in a particular zone. However, the limitations associated with surgical exploration and control of hemorrhage in each zone still make the concept useful. The boundaries and major contents of each zone are reviewed here. The impact of injuries on management planning is discussed by zone in a later section.

Zone I is the horizontal area between the clavicle/suprasternal notch and the cricoid cartilage (including the thoracic inlet). Surgical access to this zone may require thoracotomy or sternotomy, management of vascular injuries here is challenging, and injury mortality is high.[90] The proximal common carotid, vertebral and subclavian arteries, subclavian, innominate and jugular veins, proximal trachea, recurrent laryngeal nerves, esophagus, thoracic duct, lower thyroid and parathyroid glands, and thymus are located in this zone. Zone II is the area between horizontal lines drawn at the level of the cricoid cartilage and the angle of the mandible. Surgical access to this zone is straightforward, via a standard neck exploration incision. Zone II contains the internal and external carotid arteries, jugular veins, pharynx, larynx, esophagus, recurrent laryngeal nerves, spinal cord, trachea, upper thyroid, and parathyroid glands. Zone III lies between the angle of the mandible and the base of the skull. Surgical access to this zone often requires mandibulotomy or maneuvers to anteriorly displace the mandible, and may require craniotomy. Management of vascular injuries here is difficult, and injury mortality is high.[91,92] Zone III contains the extracranial carotid and vertebral arteries, the jugular veins, cranial nerves IX through XII, and the sympathetic nerve trunk.

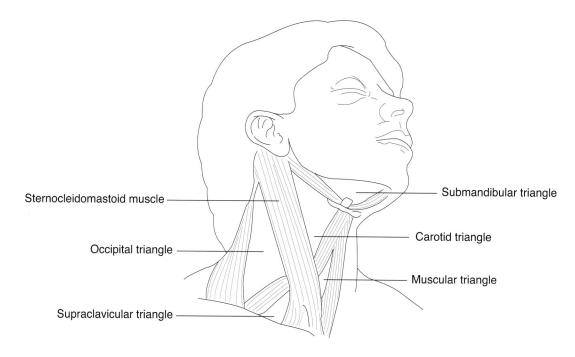

Figure 60. *Triangles of the neck. The sternocleidomastoid muscle divides the neck into the anterior triangle and posterior triangle.*

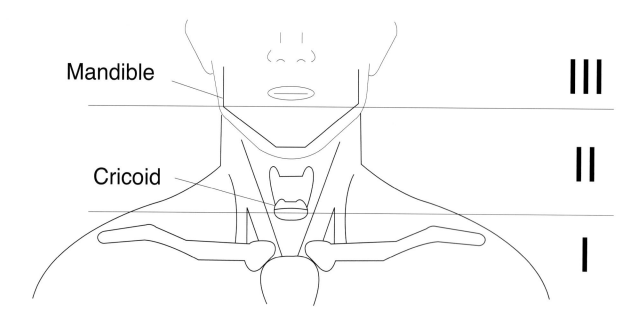

Figure 61. *The neck is commonly divided into three anatomic zones for purposes of initial assessment and management.*

# Information for the Generalist - Neck Wounds

## Initial Assessment and Management

> Casualties with signs of significant neck injury, including active pulsatile hemorrhage, expanding hematoma, bruit, pulse deficit, subcutaneous emphysema, hoarseness, stridor, respiratory distress, or hemiparesis, have indications for immediate operative management and require urgent surgical consultation.[93]

### Airway

The first priority in penetrating neck trauma is to assess and secure the airway, keeping in mind the potential for concomitant cervical spine injury. It may be difficult to fully assess the cervical spine until the airway is controlled, and rigorous spinal precautions should not be maintained at the expense of managing life-threatening airway or vascular injuries. Orotracheal intubation is the initial method of choice for securing the airway under most circumstances in Level III care facilities. Nasal intubation and fiberoptic intubation techniques are technically more difficult, require special equipment, and should be reserved for elective airway management. Use of a LMA™ to ventilate a casualty may serve as a bridge to buy time but is not a secure airway. A pharynx filled with blood or distortion of laryngeal landmarks can make endotracheal intubation difficult, and repeated blind intubation attempts risk enlarging a penetrating injury of the pharynx.

As discussed earlier in the chapter, cricothyroidotomy is the preferred method for establishing an immediate airway if rapid endotracheal intubation is not possible or is contraindicated. In casualties with large penetrating anterior neck wounds that require an urgent airway, consider extending the wound as necessary and intubating through the wound by isolating the trachea between two fingers and completing an incision into the anterior trachea. An emergency tracheotomy is the preferred method of establishing a definitive airway in cases of suspected tracheal disruption. Attempts at endotracheal intubation could convert a partial tracheal disruption into a complete transection, while attempts at a cricothyroidotomy would be futile, as the injured segment lies distal to the incision site.

The airway should be considered at-risk in any casualty that presents with a penetrating neck wound. An unremarkable physical exam in a soldier with well-developed cervical musculature who presents with a small penetrating wound(s) to the neck can be deceiving (Fig. 62). Casualties who appear to have a minor neck wound may still have a significant injury. Stridor, hoarseness or dysphonia, hemoptysis, and subcutaneous air should be specifically looked for and indicate potentially significant injury to deeper structures. Fiberoptic laryngoscopy (when available) is a helpful adjunct for identifying airway injuries.

> In difficult to intubate casualties with large penetrating anterior neck wounds that require an urgent airway, consider extending the wound as necessary and intubating through the wound by isolating the trachea between two fingers and completing an incision into the anterior trachea.

### Bleeding

Do not blindly clamp bleeding vessels in the neck. Most survivable hemorrhage from neck wounds can

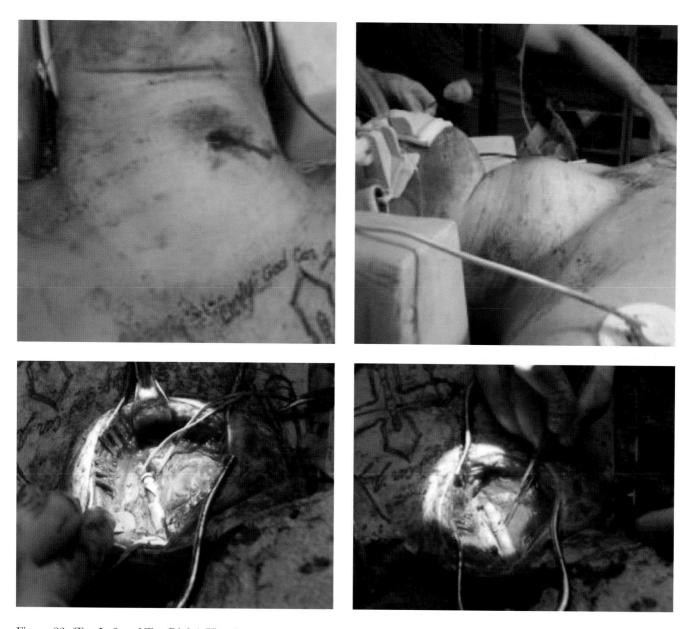

Figure 62. (Top Left and Top Right) *These images illustrate a gunshot wound to the neck with an expanding hematoma. Casualties who appear to have a minor neck wound may still have a significant injury.* (Bottom Left) *Proximal and distal ligature control.* (Bottom Right) *Primary repair of a common carotid injury with saphenous vein graft. Images courtesy of Joel Nichols, MD.*

be controlled with directed pressure above and/or below the wound (compressing a bleeding vessel against the vertebrae), application of pressure directly over the wound, or by packing the wound with gauze. Vaginal tampons inserted into wounds (one- to two-centimeter size bleeding lacerations) caused by shrapnel can be effective at controlling hemorrhage. Pharyngeal packing after an airway has been secured is effective at controlling severe oral bleeding but must be under pressure and may require a full Kerlix™ roll or more to tamponade bleeding. Do not probe open neck wounds. This may lead to clot dislodgement and vigorous bleeding can occur. Injuries that do not penetrate the platysma do not cause significant injuries.[94] If violation of the platysma is uncertain, gently spread wound edges without probing. Stop as soon as platysma violation is recognized and call a surgeon. Suspect subclavian artery or vein injury in casualties with Zone I penetrating neck injuries. Intravenous access should be attained on the side of the body opposite the site of injury or in the lower torso/extremities to avoid potential extravasation of fluids.

> Do not blindly clamp bleeding vessels in the neck. Most survivable hemorrhage from neck wounds can be controlled through application of pressure directly over the wound or by packing the wound with gauze.

## Considerations for the Specialist

### Operative Indications

It is useful to triage patients with penetrating neck injuries as either symptomatic or asymptomatic. Symptomatic injuries require immediate surgical exploration. Evidence of significant injury includes active pulsatile hemorrhage, expanding hematoma, bruit, pulse deficit, hoarseness, stridor, respiratory distress, or hemiparesis. Asymptomatic patients may be observed pending completion of appropriate studies. Choice of studies is guided by the location of the wound and often dictated by availability of resources.

### Role of Imaging

Improvements in imaging technology, particularly computed tomographic angiography (CTA), are changing the management of patients with penetrating injuries of the neck in combat zones. In many Level III CSHs, CTA for examination of the vasculature has become the preferred method of evaluation due to the possibility of retained projectiles and occult injuries to the great vessels of the neck.[95] This reflects civilian trauma center experience. In a five-year retrospective study from 2000 to 2005 evaluating the role of CTA in clinical decision-making in the management of penetrating injuries to the neck, Osborn et al. reported that the use of CTA eliminated the performance of negative neck explorations without increasing adjunctive studies (esophagography, angiography, and various endoscopic procedures). No difference in morbidity or mortality was reported between their two study groups.[96]

### Immediate Hemorrhage Control

In the authors' experience, external carotid artery injuries are easily managed by suture ligation. All veins in the neck can be safely ligated to control hemorrhage. Casualties with large venous injuries should have their wounds covered with tightly adherent dressing (e.g., Vaseline® gauze dressing) and should be placed in the Trendelenburg position if there is any concern about internal jugular vein injury and possible air embolus. If both internal jugular veins are interrupted by the injury, an attempt to repair one is appropriate. Exsanguinating oropharyngeal hemorrhage should be controlled by obtaining an immediate surgical airway (cricothyroidotomy or tracheotomy) followed by packing the pharynx. The casualty is then taken to the operating room, where a wide apron-incision is made from the mastoid tip to the midline of the neck at the cricoid level for definitive exploration. Although studies have shown that it is safe to close uncontaminated penetrating neck wounds primarily within six hours of injury, there is insufficient evidence to make a recommendation regarding primary closure of neck wounds caused by IEDs.[97]

> Exsanguinating oropharyngeal hemorrhage should be controlled by obtaining an immediate surgical airway followed by packing the pharynx.

### Zone I

Zone I injuries are reported to have a mortality rate as high as 12 percent.[90] The bony thorax and clavicle make surgical exploration of the root of the neck challenging. Stable casualties with Zone I injuries should be further evaluated by arteriography, laryngoscopy, and esophagoscopy. Unstable casualties with Zone I injuries require a median sternotomy or left anterior thoracotomy to control hemorrhage. Surgical repair is preferred unless the patient has already developed neurological changes consistent with coma and arteriogram confirms absence of antegrade flow. The decision to explore a Zone I injury should be reserved for surgeons with experience with these approaches.

> Unstable casualties with Zone I injuries require a median sternotomy or left anterior thoracotomy to control hemorrhage.

### Zone II

Management of Zone II injuries continues to be debated. Multiple civilian studies have documented the safety of selective exploration of neck wounds that penetrate the platysma, and the management of casualties without significant symptoms is changing as technology advances. The most recent thorough review published on this subject was performed by Tisherman et al. in 2008.[98] These authors evaluated 112 articles examining the issue of mandatory exploration of all patients with penetrating neck wounds versus selective exploration based on physical examination with or without use of current imaging technologies and summarized their conclusions as clinical practice guidelines. They found strong evidence that selective operative management and mandatory exploration of penetrating injuries to Zone II of the neck have equivalent diagnostic accuracy and recommended selective exploration to minimize unnecessary surgery. They identified multiple studies that showed selective operative management of these injuries by experienced surgeons was safe in both community hospital and trauma center settings, with no difference in morbidity or mortality.[99,100,101] Tisherman et al. cited studies demonstrating CTA can safely reduce the number of negative neck explorations and that CTA or duplex ultrasound can be used in lieu of arteriography to rule out Zone II arterial injury following penetrating trauma to Zone II of the neck.[102,103,104,105] Based on the strength of evidence cited, the authors recommended high-resolution CTA as the initial diagnostic study of choice for Zone II penetrating injury to the neck. They also found evidence that careful serial physical examination, including auscultation of the carotid artery, is greater than 95 percent sensitive for detecting arterial or aerodigestive tract injuries requiring repair, but cautioned that clinicians should have a low threshold for obtaining imaging studies.[106,107]

The review by Tisherman et al. is thorough and timely, but caution must be exercised in extrapolating conclusions drawn from civilian experience to current combat environments.[98] In the authors' experience, the following management practices have been successfully employed in OEF and OIF. Symptomatic casualties (e.g., active pulsatile hemorrhage, audible bruit, rapidly expanding hematoma, airway or neurovascular compromise) with penetrating Zone II neck wounds undergo neck exploration. Asymptomatic casualties with penetrating Zone II neck wounds may be observed with frequent monitoring while being further evaluated for injury to the great vessels, trachea, or aerodigestive tract. Computed tomographic angiography or conventional arteriography, laryngoscopy and esophagoscopy are performed if the wounds are not surgically explored. If CTA or conventional arteriography, laryngoscopy, and esophagoscopy are not available, asymptomatic casualties with penetrating Zone II neck wounds are monitored continuously until transfer to a facility with advanced capabilities, or the wounds are surgically explored.

> Although there is strong evidence that selective operative management and mandatory exploration of penetrating injuries to Zone II of the neck have equivalent diagnostic accuracy, caution must be exercised in extrapolating conclusions drawn from civilian experience to current combat environments.

A low threshold for proceeding to surgical exploration is suggested for casualties with multiple penetrating Zone II neck wounds such as shrapnel injuries from a high-energy explosive device. Further studies of high-energy blast wounds are necessary to determine whether CTA is sufficiently sensitive for detecting injuries that require surgical intervention and whether CTA may be relied upon to guide patient management. Based on the authors' experience, strict observation of casualties with penetrating Zone II neck wounds from blast injuries without concurrent radiographic evaluation of the great vessels, trachea, and esophagus (observation alone) is not recommended (Fig. 63).

### Zone III
Zone III injuries are also associated with a high mortality rate.[91,92] The skull base, styloid process, and

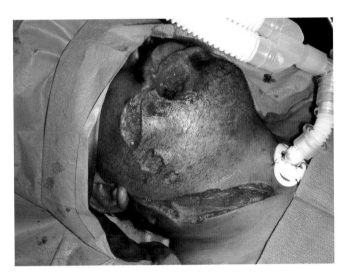

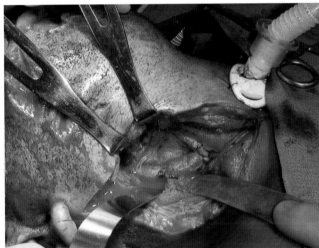

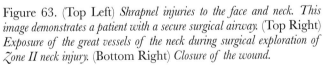

Figure 63. (Top Left) *Shrapnel injuries to the face and neck. This image demonstrates a patient with a secure surgical airway.* (Top Right) *Exposure of the great vessels of the neck during surgical exploration of Zone II neck injury.* (Bottom Right) *Closure of the wound.*

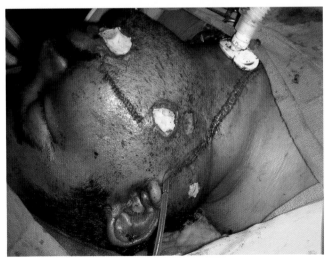

mandible make surgical exposure in this area difficult. The mandible may need to be divided or displaced anteriorly by dividing the stylomandibular ligament. Craniotomy may be required to control a high-carotid injury in this location. Stable casualties with Zone III should be further evaluated by arteriography to exclude carotid/vertebral artery injuries and a Gastrografin® contrast swallow imaging study should be considered if there is any suspicion of esophageal injury.[89, 93,108] When arteriography is not available, frequent intraoral examination should be performed to observe for edema or expanding hematoma within the parapharyngeal or retropharyngeal spaces. Nerves exiting the skull base are in close proximity to the great vessels, thus neurological deficits in a casualty with a Zone III injury are suggestive of injury to the great vessels.[91]

> The decision to explore a Zone III injury should be reserved for surgeons with experience performing these approaches.

Bleeding from the internal carotid artery in Zone III may be controlled by passing a small-diameter (e.g., 4 French size) Fogarty catheter proximal to the injury and inflating the balloon to occlude the lumen. Alternatively, the internal carotid artery may be ligated through an incision parallel to the anterior border of the sternocleidomastoid muscle. If the internal carotid artery is ligated, the distal injury may continue to bleed from collateral circulation through the Circle of Willis and require packing as the artery enters the skull base. Achieving hemorrhage control of penetrating vertebral artery injuries can be very challenging and is associated with high morbidity and mortality rates.[92] The decision to explore a Zone III injury should be reserved for surgeons with experience performing these approaches.

## Esophageal Injury

Esophageal injuries may be clinically silent initially. Signs of esophageal injury include subcutaneous air, crepitus, dysphagia, odynophagia, drooling, and hematemesis. Missed esophageal injuries are the cause of the majority of delayed complications seen with penetrating neck injuries.[89,108] When an esophageal leak progresses to mediastinitis, morbidity and mortality are significant.[89,107,109] Either contrast esophagography or esophagoscopy should be used to rule out an esophageal perforation that requires operative repair. Diagnostic workup should be expeditious as management delayed by more than 24 hours increases morbidity and mortality.[89,108] Early diagnosis may allow primary repair to be performed and generally results in superior outcomes.[109]

> If esophageal injury is suspected, either contrast esophagography or esophagoscopy should be used to rule out an esophageal perforation that requires operative repair. Diagnostic workup should be expeditious as management delayed by more than 24 hours increases morbidity and mortality.

The accuracy of the evaluation for esophageal injury is dependent on the skills of the careproviders and the availability of diagnostic equipment. The sensitivity of esophagography to detect an esophageal injury is 62 percent to 100 percent, and the sensitivity of esophagoscopy is 43 percent to 100 percent.[110,111] In cases in which the cervical spine has not been cleared, flexible endoscopy is helpful in evaluating injuries of the pharynx and esophagus.[112,113] There have been reports of missed perforations near the cricopharyngeus muscle or in the hypopharynx, where flexible endoscopy is less effective because of mucosal redundancy.[114,115,116] Studies utilizing a combination of flexible endoscopy and rigid esophagoscopy to examine the entire cervical and upper thoracic esophagus generally demonstrate the best results. No perforations were missed in those series that used both techniques to evaluate all patients.[117] Gastrografin®

is recommended as a first-line contrast study agent for evaluation of esophageal injury.[118] Barium is used as a second-line agent because barium extravasation radiographically distorts soft-tissue planes for future studies, and it is more toxic to the peritoneal cavity. Care must be exercised to ensure patients do not aspirate Gastrografin®, which can cause significant pulmonary toxicity.[119]

If suspicion of a pharyngeal perforation remains despite an initial negative examination or exploration, the casualty should be kept nil per os (NPO), observed for seven days, and a swallow study should be repeated prior to advancing the diet to clear liquids. Fever, tachycardia, or widening of the mediastinum on serial chest radiographs or CT indicates the need for repeat endoscopy or neck exploration. When an esophageal injury is found early, surgical management should include copious wound irrigation, cautious debridement, a two-layer closure, and adequate drainage.[116] After repair of the mucosal perforation, a muscle flap should be placed over the esophageal suture line for further protection. If an extensive esophageal injury is present, a lateral cervical esophagostomy should be created and definitive repair performed later.[116]

> If an extensive esophageal injury is present, a lateral cervical esophagostomy should be created and definitive repair performed later.

## Laryngotracheal Injury

When a wound involves the larynx or upper trachea, a tracheotomy should be established below the level of the injury. After a definitive airway is established, laryngotracheal injuries are not life-threatening, and definitive management may be delayed while treating more acute injuries. Laryngeal injuries may be evaluated with flexible endoscopy to differentiate between wounds that need only observation (small or shallow lacerations, nondisplaced fractures) and those that require a thyrotomy for open fracture reduction and mucosal approximation. If rigid endoscopy is performed, care must be taken to avoid extending lacerations.

> When a wound involves the larynx or upper trachea, a tracheotomy should be established below the level of the injury. Definitive tracheal repair may be delayed while treating more acute injuries.

Multiple authors recommend repair of laryngeal mucosal lacerations from a penetrating injury as soon as possible and have found an increase in debilitating long-term sequelae, including airway stenosis and poor voice quality associated with delayed repair.[51,120] Danic reported that even extensive laryngotracheal injuries may be safely repaired early.[97] When the inner laryngeal mucosa in an adult patient is badly macerated, a soft laryngeal stent fashioned from a six-centimeter segment of a 7.0 mm ETT, which has been permanently crimped in the middle by clamping it while heated, should be inserted. The crimp should be at the level of the vocal cords and fixed in place with through-and-through 1-0 Prolene® suture secured to the skin of the neck. An appropriately sized ETT should be selected and fashioned accordingly in smaller adults and children. In the authors' experience, tracheal lacerations extending less than 50 percent of the tracheal circumference do not require repair or tracheotomy. Longer lacerations without significant disruption of the tracheal mucosa may be reapproximated with interrupted 5-0 Prolene® sutures spaced two to three millimeters apart, without the need for a tracheotomy. More severe disruptions are initially treated by placing a tracheotomy either below or through the injury.

*Summary*

As with all trauma patients, initial management priorities include airway protection, breathing, and circulatory support. Casualties who present with signs and symptoms of shock and continuous hemorrhage from a neck wound should undergo immediate surgical exploration. After life-threatening injuries are stabilized, a more focused evaluation of the penetrating neck wound is undertaken. Upon wound exploration, if the platysma is not violated, surgical exploration is not indicated. Symptomatic casualties (e.g., active pulsatile hemorrhage, audible bruit, rapidly expanding hematoma, airway, or neurovascular compromise) with penetrating Zone II neck wounds should undergo neck exploration. Asymptomatic casualties with Zone II injuries that penetrate the platysma should be evaluated to rule out significant injury to the great vessels, trachea, or esophagus. The evaluation of stable casualties may be delayed if they are carefully monitored at frequent intervals. Casualties with Zone I and III penetrating injuries and penetrating esophageal and laryngotracheal injuries should be transferred to a Level IV or V facility for definitive management as soon as possible.

# References

1. Lew TA, Walker JA, Wenke JC, et al. Characterization of craniomaxillofacial battle injuries sustained by United States service members in the current conflicts of Iraq and Afghanistan. J Oral Maxillofac Surg 2010;68(1):3-7.

2. Owens BD, Kragh JF Jr, Wenke JC, et al. Combat wounds in Operation Iraqi Freedom and Operation Enduring Freedom. J Trauma 2008;64(2):295-299.

3. Kosashvili Y, Hiss J, Davidovic N, et al. Influence of personal armor on distribution of entry wounds: lessons learned from urban-setting warfare fatalities. J Trauma 2005;58(6):1236-1240.

4. Dobson JE, Newell MJ, Shepherd JP. Trends in maxillofacial injuries in war-time (1914-1986). Br J Oral Maxillofac Surg 1989;27(6):441-450.

5. Eastridge BJ, Jenkins D, Flaherty S, et al. Trauma system development in a theater of war: experiences from Operation Iraqi Freedom and Operation Enduring Freedom. J Trauma 2006;61(6):1366-1372; discussion 1372-1373.

6. Nessen SC, Lounsbury DE, Hetz SP, editors. High-energy facial injuries. In: War Surgery in Afghanistan and Iraq: A Series of Cases, 2003-2007. Washington, DC: Department of the Army, Office of the Surgeon General, Borden Institute, 2008. p. 74-81.

7. Kauvar DS, Wolf SE, Wade CE, et al. Burns sustained in combat explosions in Operation Iraqi and Enduring Freedom (OIF/OEF explosion burns). Burns 2006;32(7):853-857.

8. Petersen K, Hayes DK, Blice JP, et al. Prevention and management of infections associated with combat-related head and neck injuries. J Trauma 2008;64(3 Suppl):S265-276.

9. Akinbami BO. Traumatic diseases of parotid gland and sequelae. Review of literature and case reports. Niger J Clin Pract 2009;12(2):212-215.

10. Cole RD, Browne JD, Phipps CD. Gunshot wounds to the mandible and midface: evaluation, treatment and avoidance of complications. Otolaryngol Head Neck Surg 1994;111(6):739-745.

11. Chen AY, Stewart MG, Raup G. Penetrating injuries to the face. Otolaryngol Head Neck Surg 1996;115(5):464-470.

12. Ramasamy A, Midwinter M, Mahoney P, et al. Learning the lessons from conflict: pre-hospital cervical spine stabilisation following ballistic neck trauma. Injury 2009;40(12):1342-1345.

13. Barkana Y, Stein M, Scope A, et al. Prehospital stabilization of the cervical spine for penetrating injuries of the neck - is it necessary? Injury 2000;31(5):305-309.

14. Ardekian L, Rosen D, Klein Y, et al. Life-threatening complications and irreversible damage following maxillofacial trauma. Injury 1998;29(4):253-256.

15. US Department of Defense (US DoD). Face and Neck Injuries. In: Emergency War Surgery, Third United States Revision. Washington, DC: Department of the Army, Office of the Surgeon General, Borden Institute; 2004. p. 13.1-13.20.

16. Muzzi DA, Losasso TJ, Cucchiara RF. Complication from a nasopharyngeal airway in a patient with a basilar skull fracture. Anesthesiology 1991;74(2):366-368.

17. Fonseca RJ, Walker RV, Betts NJ, et al. Diagnosis and treatment of midface fractures. In: Fonseca RJ, Walker RV, Betts NJ, et al, editors. Oral and maxillofacial trauma vol 2. 1st ed. St Louis, MO: WB Saunders Co; 2005.

18. Pollack CV Jr. The laryngeal mask airway: a comprehensive review for the emergency physician. J Emerg Med 2001;20(1):53-66.

19. Weiss M, Dullenkopf A, Fischer JE, et al. Prospective randomized controlled multi-centre trial of cuffed or uncuffed endotracheal tubes in small children. Br J Anaesth 2009;103(6):867-873.

20. Rice MJ, Mancuso AA, Gibbs C, et al. Cricoid pressure results in compression of the postcricoid hypopharynx: the esophageal position is irrelevant. Anesth Analg 2009;109(5):1546-1552.

21. Ellis DY, Harris T, Zideman D. Cricoid pressure in emergency department rapid sequence tracheal intubations: a risk-benefit analysis. Ann Emerg Med 2007;50(6):653-666.

22. Rudraraju P, Eisen LA. Confirmation of endotracheal tube position: a narrative review. J Intensive Care Med 2009;24(5):283-292.

23. Varon AJ, Morrina J, Civetta JM. Clinical utility of a colorimetric end-tidal $CO_2$ detector in cardiopulmonary resuscitation and emergency intubation. J Clin Monit 1991;7(4):289-293.

24. Feinberg SE, Peterson LJ. The use of cricothyroidostomy in oral and maxillofacial surgery. J Oral Maxillofac Surg 1987;45(10):873-878.

25. Boon JM, Abrahams PH, Meiring JH, et al. Cricothyroidotomy: a clinical anatomy review. Clin Anat 2004;17(6):478-486.

26. Sise MJ, Shackford SR, Cruickshank JC, et al. Cricothyroidotomy for long-term tracheal access. A prospective analysis of morbidity and mortality in 76 patients. Ann Surg 1984;200(1):13-17.

27. Gallo AC, Adams BD. Emergency battlefield cricothyrotomy complicated by tube occlusion. J Emerg Trauma Shock 2009;2(1):54-55.

28. Ravussin P, Bayer-Berger M, Monnier P, et al. Percutaneous transtracheal ventilation for laser

endoscopic procedures in infants and small children with laryngeal obstruction: report of two cases. Can J Anaesth 1987;34(1):83-86.

29. Smith RB, Myers EN, Sherman H. Transtracheal ventilation in paediatric patients; case reports. Br J Anaesth 1974;46(4):313-314.

30. Block MS, Casadaban MC. Implant restoration of external resorption teeth in the esthetic zone. J Oral Maxillofac Surg 2005;63(11):1653-1661.

31. Cho BH, Ahn HB. Microsurgical replantation of a partial ear, with leech therapy. Ann Plast Surg 1999;43(4):427-429.

32. Weinfeld AB, Yuksel E, Boutros S, et al. Clinical and scientific considerations in leech therapy for the management of acute venous congestion: an updated review. Ann Plast Surg 2000;45(2):207-212.

33. Aydin A, Nazik H, Kuvat SV, et al. External decontamination of wild leeches with hypochloric acid. BMC Infect Dis 2004;4:28.

34. Steinberg MJ, Herrera AF. Management of parotid duct injuries. Oral Surg Oral Med Oral Pathol Oral Radiol Endod 2005;99(2):136-141.

35. Bailey BJ. Nasal Fractures. In: Bailey BJ, Johnson JT, Newlands SD, editors. Head & neck surgery–otolaryngology. 4th ed. Philadelphia: Lippincott; 2006. p. 995-1008.

36. Hospenthal DR, Murray CK, Andersen RC, et al. Guidelines for the prevention of infection after combat-related injuries. J Trauma 2008;64(3 Suppl):S211-220.

37. Bellamy R, Zajtchuk R. The management of ballistic wounds of soft tissue. In: Bellamy RF, Zajtchuk R, editors. Textbook of military medicine. Part I: Conventional warfare: ballistic, blast and burn injuries. Vol 3. Washington, DC: U.S. Government Printing Office; 1991. p. 163-220.

38. Chole RA, Yee J. Antibiotic prophylaxis for facial fractures. A prospective, randomized clinical trial. Arch Otolaryngol Head Neck Surg 1987;113(10):1055-1057.

39. Lieblich SE, Topazian RG. Infection in the patient with maxillofacial trauma. In: Fonseca RG, Walker RV, Tetts JN, editors. Oral and maxillofacial trauma. 3rd ed. St Louis, MO: Elsevier Saunders; 2005. p. 1009-1129.

40. Haug R, Assael L. Infection in the maxillofacial trauma patient. In: Topazian R, Goldberg M, Hupp J, editors. Oral and maxillofacial infections. 4th ed. Philadelphia, PA: WB Saunders; 2002. p. 359-380.

41. Johnson JT, Schuller DE, Silver F, et al. Antibiotic prophylaxis in high-risk head and neck surgery: one-day vs. five-day therapy. Otolaryngol Head Neck Surg 1986;95(5):554-557.

42. Abubaker AO, Rollert MK. Postoperative antibiotic prophylaxis in mandibular fractures: a

preliminary randomized, double-blind, and placebo-controlled clinical study. J Oral Maxillofac Surg 2001;59(12):1415-1419.

43. Miles BA, Potter JK, Ellis E III. The efficacy of postoperative antibiotic regimens in the open treatment of mandibular fractures: a prospective randomized trial. J Oral Maxillofac Surg 2006;64(4):576-582.

44. Johnson JT, Yu VL, Myers EN, et al. Efficacy of two third-generation cephalosporins in prophylaxis for head and neck surgery. Arch Otolaryngol 1984;110(4):224-227.

45. Zaytoun GM, Shikhani AH, Salman SD. Head and neck war injuries: 10-year experience at the American University of Beirut Medical Center. Laryngoscope 1986;96(8):899-903.

46. Kwapis BW. Early management of maxillofacial war injuries. J Oral Surg (Chic) 1954;12(4):293-309.

47. Rubin J, Johnson JT, Wagner RL, et al. Bacteriologic analysis of wound infection following major head and neck surgery. Arch Otolaryngol Head Neck Surg 1988;114(9):969-972.

48. Brook I, Hirokawa R. Microbiology of wound infection after head and neck cancer surgery. Ann Otol Rhinol Laryngol 1989;98(5 Pt 1):323-325.

49. Altman MM, Joachims HZ. Osteomyelitis of the cervical spine after neck injuries. Arch Otolaryngol 1972;96(1):72-75.

50. Jones RE, Bucholz RW, Schaefer SD, et al. Cervical osteomyelitis complicating transpharyngeal gunshot wounds to the neck. J Trauma 1979;19(8):630-634.

51. Schaefer SD. The treatment of acute external laryngeal injuries. 'State of the art.' Arch Otolaryngol Head Neck Surg. 1991;117(1):35-39.

52. Tinder LE, Osbon DB, Lilly GE, et al. Maxillofacial injuries sustained in The Vietnam conflict. Mil Med 1969;134(9):668-672.

53. Akhlaghi F, Aframian-Farnad F. Management of maxillofacial injuries in the Iran-Iraq War. J Oral Maxillofac Surg 1997;55(9):927-930.

54. Puzovic D, Konstantinovic VS, Dimitrijevic M. Evaluation of maxillofacial weapon injuries: 15-year experience in Belgrade. J Craniofac Surg 2004;15(4):543–546.

55. Morgan HH, Szmyd L. Maxillofacial war injuries. J Oral Surg 1968;26(11):727-730.

56. Kelly JF, ed. Management of war injuries to the jaws and related structures. Washington, DC: US Government Printing Office;1977;66-67.

57. Osbon DB. Early treatment of soft tissue injuries of the face. J Oral Surg 1969;27(7):480-487.

58. Motamedi MH. Primary management of maxillofacial hard and soft tissue gunshot and shrapnel injuries. J Oral Maxillofac Surg 2003;61(12):1390-1398.

59. Taher AA. Management of weapon injuries to the craniofacial skeleton. J Craniofac Surg 1998;9(4):371-382.

60. Topazian RG. Osteomyelitis of the jaws. In: Topazian RG, Goldberg MH, Hupp JR, editors. Oral and maxillofacial infections. 4th ed. Philadelphia, PA: W.B. Saunders; 2002. p. 214-242.

61. Benzil DL, Robotti E, Dagi TF. Early single-stage repair of complex craniofacial trauma. Neurosurgery 1992;30(2):166-71; discussion 171-172.

62. Renner G. Reconstruction of the lip. In: Baker S, editor. Local flaps in facial reconstruction. 2nd ed. Philadelphia, PA: Mosby; 2007. p. 475-525.

63. Lee P, Mountain R. Lip reconstruction. Curr Opin Otolaryngol Head Neck Surg 2000;8(4):300-304.

64. Potter JK, Ducic Y, Ellis E III. Extended bilaminar forehead flap with cantilevered bone grafts for reconstruction of full-thickness nasal defects. J Oral Maxillofac Surg 2005;63(4):566-570.

65. US Department of Defense (US DoD). Burn Injuries. In: Emergency War Surgery, Third United States Revision. Washington, DC: Department of the Army, Office of the Surgeon General, Borden Institute; 2004. p. 28.1-28.15.

66. Helmy ES, Koh ML, Bays RA: Management of frontal sinus fractures. Review of the literature and clinical update. Oral Surg Oral Med Oral Pathol. 1990;69(2):137-148.

67. Luce EA. Frontal sinus fracture: guidelines to management. Plast Reconstr Surg 1987;80(4):500-510.

68. Dula DJ, Fales W. The 'ring' sign: is it a reliable indicator for cerebrospinal fluid? Ann Emerg Med 1993;22(4):718-720.

69. Rouah E, Rogers BB, Buffone GJ, et al. Transferrin analysis by immunofixation as an aid in the diagnosis of cerebrospinal fluid otorrhea. Arch Pathol Lab Med 1987;111(8):756-757.

70. Zapalac JS, Marple BF, Schwade ND. Skull base cerebrospinal fluid fistulas: a comprehensive diagnostic algorithm. Otolaryngol Head Neck Surg 2002;126(6):669-676.

71. Nandapalan V, Watson ID, Swift AC. Beta-2-transferrin and cerebrospinal fluid rhinorrhoea. Clin Otolaryngol Allied Sci 1996;21(3):259-264.

72. Heckler FR. Discussion of frontal sinus fractures. Guidel Manage Plast Reconstr Surg 1987;80:509-520.

73. Parhiscar A, Har-El G. Frontal sinus obliteration with the pericranial flap. Otolaryngol Head Neck Surg 2001;124(3):304-307.

74. Weber R, Draf W, Keerl R, et al. Osteoplastic frontal sinus surgery with fat obliteration: technique and long-term results using magnetic resonance imaging in 82 operations. Laryngoscope. 2000;110(6):1037-1044.

75. Rohrich RJ, Mickel TJ. Frontal sinus obliteration: In search of the ideal autogenous material. Plast Reconstr Surg 1995;95(3):580-585.

76. Wallis A, Donald PJ. Frontal sinus fractures: a review of 72 cases. Laryngoscope 1988;98(6 Pt 1):593-598.

77. Kay PP. Frontal sinus fractures—to obliterate or not to obliterate. Outlook Plast Surg 1989;9:6-11.

78. Markowitz BL, Manson PN, Sargent L, et al. Management of the medial canthal tendon in nasoethmoid orbital fractures: the importance of the central fragment in classification and treatment. Plast Reconstr Surg 1991;87(5):843-853.

79. Stewart MG. Penetrating face and neck trauma. In: Bailey BJ, Johnson, JT, editors. Head & neck surgery—otolaryngology. 4th ed. Philadelphia: Lippincott, 2006. p. 1013-1026.

80. Clark N, Birely B, Manson PN, et al. High-energy ballistic and avulsive facial injuries: classification, patterns, and an algorithm for primary reconstruction. Plast Reconstr Surg 1996;98(4):583-601.

81. Hidalgo DA. Fibula free flap: a new method of mandible reconstruction. Plast Reconstr Surg 1989;84(1):71-79.

82. Hidalgo DA, Pusic AL. Free-flap mandibular reconstruction: a 10-year follow-up study. Plast Reconstr Surg 2002;110(2):438-449.

83. Cordeiro PG, Disa JJ, Hidalgo DA, et al. Reconstruction of the mandible with osseous free flaps: a 10-year experience with 150 consecutive patients. Plast Reconstr Surg 1999;104(5):1314-1320.

84. Gruss JS, Bubak PJ, Egbert MA. Craniofacial fractures. An algorithm to optimize results. Clin Plast Surg 1992;19(1):195-206.

85. Manson PN, Hoopes JE, Su CT. Structural pillars of the facial skeleton: an approach to the management of Le Fort fractures. Plast Reconstr Surg 1980;66(1):54-62.

86. American College of Surgeons Committee on Trauma. Advanced trauma life support program for doctors. 8th ed. Chicago, IL: American College of Surgeons; 2008.

87. Stone HH, Callahan GS. Soft tissue injuries of the neck. Surg Gynecol Obstet 1963;117:745-752.

88. McConnell DB, Trunkey DD. Management of penetrating trauma to the neck. Adv Surg 1994;27:97-127.

89. Asensio JA, Berne J, Demetriades D, et al. Penetrating esophageal injuries: time interval of safety for preoperative evaluation—how long is safe? J Trauma 1997;43(2):319-324.

90. Rao PM, Bhatti MF, Gaudino J, et al. Penetrating injuries of the neck: criteria for exploration. J Trauma 1983;23(1):47-49.

91. Levine ZT, Wright DC, O'Malley S, et al. Management of zone III missile injuries involving the carotid artery and cranial nerves. Skull Base Surg 2000;10(1):17-27.

92. Liekweg WG Jr, Greenfield LJ. Management of penetrating carotid arterial injury. Ann Surg 1978;188(5):587-592.

93. Carducci B, Lowe RA, Dalsey W. Penetrating neck trauma: consensus and controversies. Ann Emerg Med 1986;15(2):208-215.

94. Prgomet D, Danic D, Milicic D, et al. Management of war-related neck injuries during the war in Croatia, 1991–1992. Eur Arch Otorhinolaryngol 1996;253(4-5):294-296.

95. Fox CJ, Gillespie DL, Weber MA, et al. Delayed evaluation of combat-related penetrating neck trauma. J Vasc Surg 2006;44(1):86-93.

96. Osborn TM, Bell RB, Qaisi W, et al. Computed tomographic angiography as an aid to clinical decision making in the selective management of penetrating injuries to the neck: a reduction in the need for operative exploration. J Trauma 2008;64(6):1466-1471.

97. Danic D, Prgomet D, Milicic D, et al. War injuries to the head and neck. Mil Med 1998;163(2):117-119.

98. Tisherman SA, Bokhari F, Collier B, et al. Clinical practice guideline: penetrating zone II neck trauma. J Trauma 2008;64(5);1392-1405.

99. Cabasares HV. Selective surgical management of penetrating neck trauma. 15-year experience in a community hospital. Am Surg 1982;48(7):355-358.

100. Biffl WL, Moore EE, Rehse DH, et al. Selective management of penetrating neck trauma based on cervical level of injury. Am J Surg 1997;174(6):678-682.

101. Golueke PJ, Goldstein AS, Sclafani SJ, et al. Routine versus selective exploration of penetrating neck injuries: a randomized prospective study. J Trauma 1984;24(12):1010-1014.

102. Mazolewski PJ, Curry JD, Browder T, et al. Computed tomographic scan can be used for surgical decision making in zone II penetrating neck injuries. J Trauma 2001;51(2):315-319.

103. Inaba K, Munera F, McKenney M, et al. Prospective evaluation of screening multislice helical computed tomorgraphic angiography in the initial evaluation of penetrating neck injuries. J Trauma 2006;61(1):144-149.

104. Woo K, Magner DP, Wilson MT, et al. CT angiography in penetrating neck trauma reduces the need for operative neck exploration. Am Surg 2005;71(9):754-758.

105. Bell RB, Osborn T, Dierks EJ, et al. Management of penetrating neck injuries: a new paradigm for civilian trauma. J Oral Maxillofac Surg 2007;65(4):691-705.

106. Metzdorff MT, Lowe DK. Operation or observation for penetrating neck wounds? A retrospective analysis. Am J Surg 1984;147(5):646-649.

107. Demetriades D, Charalambides D, Lakhoo M. Physical examination and selective conservative management in patients with penetrating injuries of the neck. Br J Surg 1993;80(12):1534-1536.

108. Asensio JA, Chahwan S, Forno W, et al. Penetrating esophageal injuries: multicenter study of the American Association for the Surgery of Trauma. J Trauma 2001;50(2):289-296.

109. Cheadle W, Richardson JD. Options in management of trauma to the esophagus. Surg Gynecol Obstet 1982;155(3):380-384.

110. Noyes LD, McSwain NE Jr, Markowitz IP. Panendoscopy with arteriography versus mandatory exploration of penetrating wounds of the neck. Ann Surg 1986;204(1):21-31.

111. Wood J, Fabian TC, Mangiante EC. Penetrating neck injuries: recommendations for selective management. J Trauma 1989;29(5):602-605.

112. Arantes V, Campolina C, Valerio SH, et al. Flexible esophagoscopy as a diagnostic tool for traumatic esophageal injuries. J Trauma 2009;66(6):1677-1682.

113. Flowers JL, Graham SM, Ugarte MA, et al. Flexible endoscopy for the diagnosis of esophageal trauma. J Trauma 1996;40(2):261-265; discussion 265-266.

114. Fetterman BL, Shindo ML, Stanley RB Jr, et al. Management of traumatic hypopharyngeal injuries. Laryngoscope 1995;105(1):8-13.

115. Roden DM, Pomerantz RA. Penetrating injuries to the neck: a safe, selective approach to management. Am Surg 1993;59(11):750-753.

116. Shama DM, Odell J. Penetrating neck trauma with tracheal and oesophageal injuries. Br J Surg 1984;71(7):534-536.

117. Weigelt JA, Thal ER, Snyder WH III, et al. Diagnosis of penetrating cervical esophageal injuries. Am J Surg 1987;154(6):619-622.

118. James AE Jr, Montali RJ, Chaffee V, et al. Barium or gastrografin: which contrast media for diagnosis of esophageal tears? Gastroenterology 1975;68(5 Pt 1):1103-1113.

119. Trulzsch DV, Penmetsa A, Karim A, et al. Gastrografin-induced aspiration pneumonia: a lethal complication of computed tomography. South Med J 1992;85(12):1255-1256.

120. Leopold DA. Laryngeal trauma. A historical comparison of treatment methods. Arch Otolaryngol 1983;109(2):106-112.

# OCULAR TRAUMA
## *Chapter 7*

**Contributing Authors**
Raymond I. Cho, MD, LTC, MC, US Army
Eric Savitsky, MD

All figures and tables included in this chapter have been used with permission from Pelagique, LLC, the UCLA Center for International Medicine, and/or the authors, unless otherwise noted.

**Disclaimer**

The opinions and views expressed herein belong solely to those of the authors. They are not nor should they be implied as being endorsed by the United States Uniformed Services University of the Health Sciences, Department of the Army, Department of the Navy, Department of the Air Force, Department of Defense, or any other branch of the federal government.

# Table of Contents

# Introduction

Trauma to the eye and its associated structures accounts for a significant number of combat-related injuries. Despite the fact that the eyes cover less than 1 percent of the total body surface area, the proportion of combat injuries involving ocular structures has exceeded 10 percent in recent conflicts, with an increasing trend over the past century of warfare. Ocular injuries accounted for 2 percent of all combat injuries during the First and Second World Wars, compared to 13 percent during Operation Desert Storm (Fig. 1).[1] Although combat-related ocular injuries in the United States (US) military have decreased somewhat over the past several years due to the widespread implementation of combat eye protection, these injuries remain a significant cause of disability and suffering among wounded combat veterans (Fig. 2).

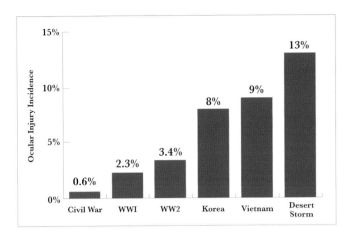

Figure 1. *Ocular injury incidence as a percentage of combat injuries, American Civil War through Operation Desert Storm. Adapted from Wong, 1997.*[1]

Penetrating projectile injuries have had a significant effect on the nature of modern combat ocular trauma, most commonly causing open-globe injuries (55 percent), eyelid injuries (33 percent), orbital fractures (13 percent), orbital foreign bodies (12 percent), corneal/conjunctival foreign bodies (11 percent), and traumatic optic neuropathy/optic nerve avulsion (3 percent).

Many valuable lessons have been learned through the experience of caring for thousands of ocular combat casualties during Operation Enduring Freedom (OEF) and Operation Iraqi Freedom (OIF). As has been noted by combat casualty care (CCC) providers throughout the history of warfare, combat injuries tend to be much more severe and extensive than those seen as a result of civilian trauma. These conflicts have also demonstrated that, in counterterrorism and counterinsurgency operations, blast injuries tend to account for a higher proportion (78 percent) of trauma when compared to conventional battlefields of the past.[2] These penetrating projectile injuries have had a significant effect on the nature of modern combat ocular trauma. There has also been a high incidence (62 percent) of concomitant head, face, and neck trauma in ocular trauma patients.[3] This finding in large part has led to the establishment of integrated multispecialty head and neck surgical teams that have been successfully deployed by the US Army in Iraq. Finally, the large number of host national injuries treated by coalition medical personnel has required a rethinking of many

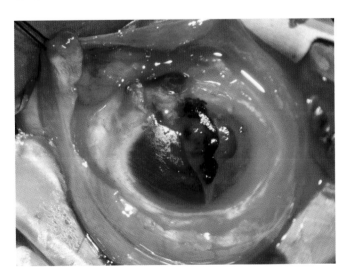

Figure 2. *Open-globe injury with large corneoscleral laceration and uveal prolapse following gunshot wound.*

trauma management patterns that are commonly practiced in the US, but have questionable applicability in resource-limited countries. For example, open-globe repair versus primary enucleation following open-globe injury is addressed later in this chapter.

The most common types of ocular injury requiring specialized ophthalmic care during OIF from 2003 to 2005 were open-globe injuries (55 percent), eyelid injuries (33 percent), orbital fractures (13 percent), orbital foreign bodies (12 percent), corneal/conjunctival foreign bodies (11 percent), and traumatic optic neuropathy/optic nerve avulsion (3 percent) (Table 1).[4] A separate study during OIF from 2005 to 2006 also reported that 20 percent of patients with combat ocular trauma were treated for orbital compartment syndrome.[5] The prevalence of less serious injuries such as corneal abrasion or hyphema has not been recently reported, although during the Vietnam War, hyphemas were seen in 15 percent of ocular combat casualties.[6]

| Injury Type | Percent |
|---|---|
| Open-globe injuries | 55 |
| Eyelid injuries | 33 |
| Orbital fractures | 13 |
| Orbital foreign bodies | 12 |
| Corneal / conjunctival foreign bodies | 11 |
| Traumatic optic neuropathy/optic nerve avulsion | 3 |

Table 1. *Most common types of ocular injury requiring specialized ophthalmic care during OIF 2003 to 2005. Adapted from Thatch, 2008.*[4]

## Levels of Ophthalmic Combat Casualty Care (CCC)

### Levels I and II

The resources available for treating ocular injuries at Level I and II facilities are limited, but certain actions taken at these levels may prove critical to optimizing ultimate outcomes. It is of utmost importance for providers at this level to recognize when an ocular injury is severe enough to warrant evacuation to the next level of care, and this requires an appropriately thorough ophthalmic examination. It is often difficult to examine an injured eye due to the frequent presence of eyelid edema, hemorrhage, tissue damage, or pain. However, it is possible in most cases to open the eyelids long enough to obtain at the very least a cursory glance at the globe and a gross assessment of visual acuity. If necessary, Desmarres retractors, a lid speculum, or even a bent paper clip can be used to carefully retract the eyelids while avoiding pressure on the globe (Fig. 3). A topical anesthetic (e.g., 0.5 percent proparacaine or tetracaine drops) may be used to decrease the discomfort caused by examination. However, excessive manipulation of the eyelids in the presence of a ruptured globe can increase the risk of intraocular content extrusion. The moment the examiner notes findings suggestive of globe rupture, the examination should be terminated and the injured globe should be protected from further manipulation. The specific exam findings suggestive of an open-globe injury are discussed later in this chapter.

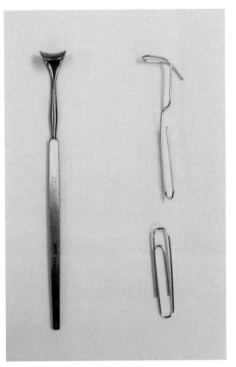

Figure 3. (Right) *Desmarres retractors or a bent paper clip can be used to retract the eyelids during the assessment of the acutely injured eye.*

Figure 4. (Far Right) *Placement of Fox eye shield (right eye) and truncated disposable drinking cup (left eye) for eye protection. The rim of the device rests on the frontal and maxillary bones.*

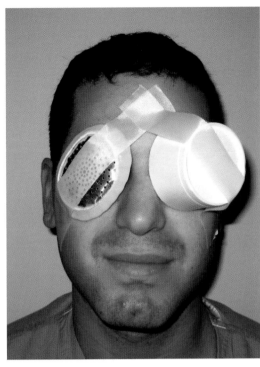

Patients with ocular injuries should undergo as complete an ophthalmic examination as possible. A detailed description of this exam is provided below, although some aspects, such as the slit-lamp exam, are not feasible at this level. At a minimum, visual acuity, pupils, extraocular motility, and visual fields by confrontation should be assessed. Gross examination of the eyelids, conjunctiva, sclera, cornea, and anterior chamber structures may reveal lacerations, anatomic disruption, hemorrhage, or foreign bodies.

---

Combat casualty care providers at Level I and II facilities must perform thorough ophthalmic examinations and recognize when an ocular injury is severe enough to warrant evacuation to the next level of care. If globe rupture is suspected, the eye examination should be terminated and the eye protected from further injury. Foreign bodies protruding from the eye or orbit should be left in place unless they are too large to safely immobilize during evacuation. Patients with severe vision loss, pupillary abnormalities, gross proptosis, or limited ocular motility should be evacuated whenever possible.

---

The most important action medical personnel at Level I or II facilities can perform for a patient with an ocular injury requiring evacuation is to protect the eye from further injury. To this end, Fox eye shields have been recently added as a standard item to the combat medic bag. This eye shield is designed to rest on the bony support of the face and vault over the ocular structures and can be secured with one or more strips of tape spanning the forehead and cheek. In the absence of a Fox eye shield, any item that can effectively perform the same function, such as a specimen cup or truncated disposable drinking cup, can be substituted (Fig. 4). It is important to make the distinction between shielding, as described above, and patching, (i.e., placing a pressure dressing on the eye). Patching of the eye should never be performed by nonophthalmic personnel on a suspected ocular injury. Similarly, the application of solutions or ointments to a suspected open-globe is not recommended. As a rule, foreign bodies protruding from the eye or orbit should be left in place unless they are too large to safely immobilize during evacuation (Figs. 5 and 6).

The decision to evacuate a patient to a Level III facility for ophthalmologic evaluation is not always clear-

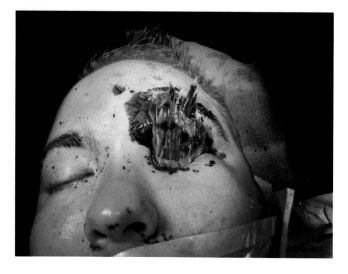

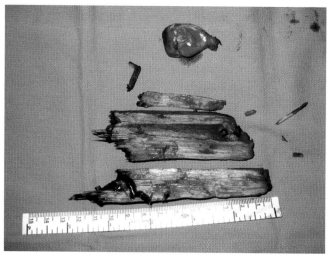

Figure 5. *Left orbit impaled with large wooden plank. The plank had been part of a fence, and the portion embedded in the patient's face had to be broken off in order to facilitate transport from the accident scene.*

Figure 6. *Removed wooden fragments adjacent to the primarily enucleated globe.*

cut and must take into account many nonclinical variables such as operational security, the availability of evacuation assets, and the impact of evacuation on the unit's mission. In general terms, patients with severe vision loss, pupillary abnormalities, gross proptosis, or limited ocular motility should be evacuated whenever possible. More specific indications for evacuation include suspected open-globe injuries, corneal infections, large hyphemas, retinal detachments, full-thickness eyelid lacerations, orbital compartment syndromes, and orbital fractures. As discussed below, suspected orbital compartment syndrome must be immediately treated by the first qualified CCC provider prior to evacuating the patient to the next level of care. This list is by no means all-inclusive, and additional guidelines for evacuation are provided later in this chapter. If telephonic or electronic consultation with an ophthalmologist is available in-theater, it should be utilized in cases where doubt exists about the severity of an ocular injury.

## Level III

Under current doctrine, specialized ophthalmic care is first available in the combat zone at Level III (Fig. 7). As stated above, ophthalmologists at Level III care facilities are typically deployed as part of multidisciplinary head and neck teams that include neurosurgery, otolaryngology, and oral maxillofacial surgery. Facilities and equipment vary, but the bare minimum should include a slit-lamp biomicroscope, Tono-Pen®, indirect ophthalmoscope, and an operating room with a surgical microscope and complete sets of ophthalmic surgical instruments. Surgical loupes can also be very useful, particularly when treating periocular and orbital injuries. Essential supplies include balanced salt solution (BSS), viscoelastics, microsurgical sponges, orbital implants, and other medications and surgical devices unique to ophthalmic surgery. Individual surgeons should ensure that their preferred sutures are available. Some of the more commonly employed sutures include: 8-0, 9-0, and 10-0 nylon; 4-0, 5-0, and 6-0 polyglactin; 5-0 polydiaxanone; 4-0 and 6-0 silk; 6-0 chromic gut or plain gut; and 6-0 polypropylene.

The mission of the Level III ophthalmologist is to provide treatments that are as definitive as possible within the physical and operational constraints of the care facility. Patients who require more specialized surgery, extensive rehabilitation, or are rendered indefinitely combat ineffective will be evacuated to a Level IV facility and beyond. Conversely, if a soldier can be treated in-theater and returned to duty within

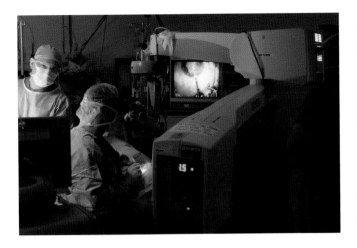

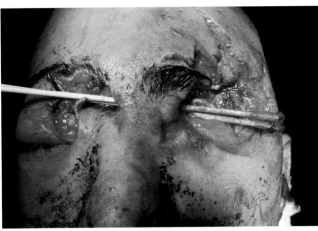

Figure 7. *Ophthalmologic procedure being performed at a Level III facility in Balad AFB, Iraq.*

Figure 8. *Combined ocular and cranial injury caused by gunshot wound. Bullet path is demonstrated by cotton-tipped applicators. The patient underwent decompressive hemicraniectomy, enucleation of the left eye, and left orbital reconstruction.*

a reasonable timeframe, this course of action should be considered. The extent to which host nationals or other noncombatants should be treated is determined by the medical commander.

> The Level III facility-based ophthalmologist should provide treatments that are as definitive as possible within the physical and operational constraints of the facility. For patients requiring evacuation, photographic documentation of pertinent clinical findings is helpful to the receiving careproviders.

For patients requiring evacuation out-of-theater, proper medical record keeping is of great importance in optimizing follow-up and appropriate treatment by Level IV and V careproviders. Photographic documentation of pertinent clinical findings, obtainable through the use of a standard point-and-shoot digital camera, can be particularly helpful to careproviders receiving patients evacuated out-of-theater. Photographs can be taken externally or through the lens of the operating microscope or slit-lamp biomicroscope and electronically transmitted to points of contact at the next level of care.

## Levels IV and V

Definitive and subspecialized ophthalmic care, such as retinal surgery, intraocular foreign body (IOFB) removal, or traumatic cataract extraction, is available at Level IV and V facilities located outside the theater of operations. Detailed discussion of treatment at this level falls beyond the scope of this chapter.

# Evaluation of the Ocular Trauma Patient

## *History*

A detailed ocular history aids in the assessment of injury severity and guides subsequent patient evaluation. In cases of chemical exposure to the eye, treatment should be initiated immediately while history and physical examination are deferred or performed in concert with immediate copious irrigation of the eyes. The ophthalmologic history should establish the premorbid visual acuity. It should also include the patient's use of corrective lenses, ophthalmologic medications, tetanus status, and previous eye surgery.[7,8,9] Patients with a history of prior ocular surgery are at risk for corneal or scleral rupture, even with minor trauma.

---

In cases of chemical exposure to the eye, treatment should be initiated immediately while history and physical examination are deferred or performed in concert with immediate copious irrigation of the eyes.

---

In cases of blunt trauma, the mechanism, force, and direction of impact are important in determining the extent of injury. A history of ocular exposure to high-speed projectiles should alert the provider to the possibility of an IOFB.[9] For penetrating injuries, it is important to determine the composition of the potentially retained foreign body. Certain foreign bodies can elicit an intense inflammatory reaction or lead to infection within the globe, while others are well tolerated.[7]

As stated in the introduction to this chapter, combat ocular injuries are often found in conjunction with head, face, and neck injuries (Fig. 8). For example, during OIF from 2005 to 2006, 33 percent of patients with cranial trauma had a concomitant open-globe injury.[5] It is therefore important for CCC providers to maintain a high level of suspicion for the presence of ocular injuries when trauma to the head, face, or neck is recognized. This is particularly true for unconscious patients in whom it is not possible to ascertain the presence of ocular pain, decreased vision, or limited motility.

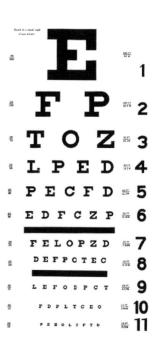

Figure 9. *A Snellen eye chart read at 20 feet, or a near card viewed at 14 inches, should be used to assess visual acuity.*

## Visual Acuity

Visual acuity is the vital sign of the eye and its measurement is the first step in all ophthalmologic exams. Visual acuity must be measured in all responsive patients with ocular trauma, as it is a critical factor in establishing diagnosis, guiding treatment, and predicting visual outcome in these patients.[10]

Visual acuity should be determined independently in each eye using a Snellen eye chart at 20 feet or a near card viewed at 14 inches (Fig. 9). The best-corrected visual acuity should be obtained using the patient's spectacle correction or a pinhole test. Binocular acuity testing is not useful in the trauma setting. Topical anesthetics may facilitate visual acuity testing in patients with acute eye pain and blepharospasm.

---

Visual acuity is the vital sign of the eye, and its measurement is the first step in all ophthalmologic exams.

---

If an eye chart is unavailable, any form of typed print such as a magazine or packaging from medical supplies may be used. If a patient is unable to visualize typed print, visual acuity should be recorded as counting fingers at a specified distance, hand motion, light perception, or no light perception.

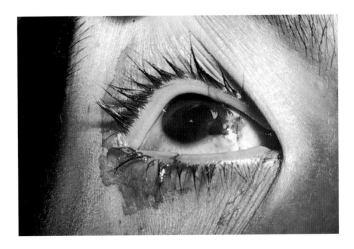

Figure 10. *Teardrop-shaped pupil with the apex of the teardrop pointing to rupture site. Image courtesy of Swaminatha V. Mahadevan, MD, Stanford University.*

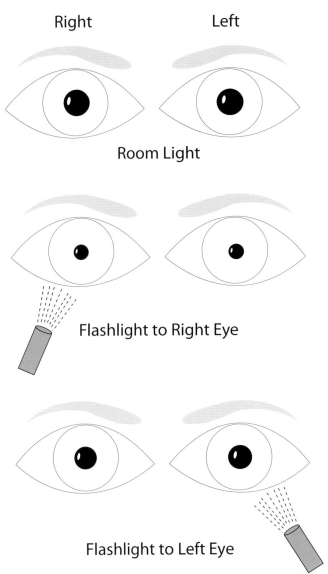

Figure 11. *Afferent pupillary defect. The swinging flashlight test reveals an afferent pupillary defect in the left eye.*

## Pupil Examination

The pupil should be examined, noting size, shape, symmetry, and reaction to light. Pupil size is recorded in millimeters (mm). Blunt trauma may cause pupillary irregularities or traumatic mydriasis (i.e., dilated pupil). A teardrop-shaped pupil is suggestive of globe rupture, with the apex of the teardrop pointing to the rupture site (Fig. 10). Each pupil should be assessed for direct and consensual response to light stimulation (i.e., pupillary light reflex). Patients should be screened for the presence of an afferent pupillary defect (APD), also known as the Marcus-Gunn pupil, using the swinging flashlight test (Fig. 11). This test is based upon the assumption that fellow eyes with normal optic nerve function have equal consensual constriction to light. When optic nerve function (the afferent visual pathway) is compromised on one side, the pupil on the involved side will still constrict when light is shined into the fellow normal eye. However, when the light is swung to the abnormal eye, the pupil will be observed to dilate from its once-constricted state, due to the decreased input to the Edinger-Westphal nucleus.

An afferent pupillary defect should alert the examiner to the presence of optic nerve pathology or severe retinal injury.

## Ocular Motility

The corneal light reflex should be at the same relative position on each cornea and the patient should be able to move his or her eyes in all directions of gaze (supraduction, infraduction, adduction, and abduction). Limited extraocular motility may indicate orbital fractures, cranial nerve injury, extraocular muscle injury or entrapment, or restriction of globe motility from intraorbital edema or blood.

It is important to distinguish whether patients complaining of diplopia are experiencing monocular versus binocular diplopia. Diplopia that persists when the uninjured eye is covered (i.e., monocular diplopia) suggests an abnormality in the ocular media, such as corneal irregularity, lens abnormality, or iridodialysis. Diplopia that resolves with occluding either eye (i.e., binocular diplopia) is indicative of a defect in coordinated eye movement.

> It is important to distinguish whether patients complaining of diplopia are experiencing monocular versus binocular diplopia.

## *Visual Field Testing*

Visual field testing can detect disorders affecting the retina, optic nerve, anterior and posterior visual pathways, and visual cortex. Patients with visual complaints irrespective of visual acuity should always be screened for visual field defects. Confrontational visual fields are measured one eye at a time and can be assessed by comparing the patient's responses to the examiner's own field with the opposite eye closed (assuming that the examiner has normal visual fields). At a normal conversational distance, any target (e.g., fingers or cotton-tipped applicators) can be presented at the periphery of the visual field equidistant between the examiner and patient. Care must be taken to ensure that the unexamined eye of the patient is completely covered.

## *Intraocular Pressure Measurement*

Intraocular pressure (IOP) may be measured using an applanation tonometer, Tono-Pen®, or Schiotz tonometer (Fig. 12). However, these devices are not usually available at Level I or II facilities. Topical anesthesia (e.g., 0.5 percent proparacaine or tetracaine) is necessary to enable their use in conscious patients. Normal IOP ranges between 10 and 21 mm Hg. Elevated IOP can result from numerous traumatic conditions, including hyphema, angle closure, retrobulbar hemorrhage, or carotid-cavernous fistula. Decreased IOP can result from open-globe injury, uveitis, cyclodialysis (separation of the ciliary body from the sclera), or retinal detachment.[11]

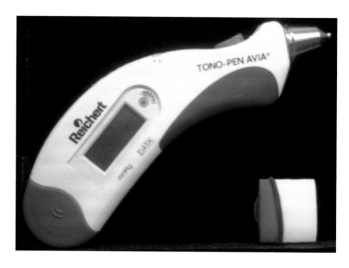

Figure 12. *The Tono-Pen® is a portable device that can be used by ophthalmic and nonophthalmic personnel to accurately measure intraocular pressure.*

> If an open-globe injury is suspected, IOP measurements should be deferred to prevent further eye injury.

## *External Ocular Examination*

The eyelids and periocular region should be inspected, taking note of asymmetry, edema, ecchymosis, lacerations, foreign bodies, or abnormal eyelid position. Ptosis (drooping of the upper eyelid) is common

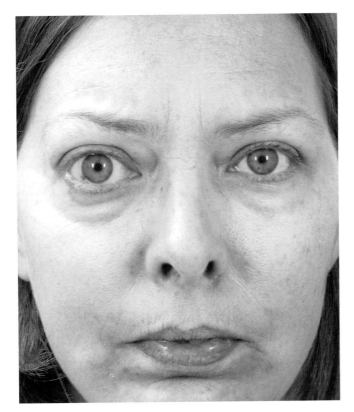

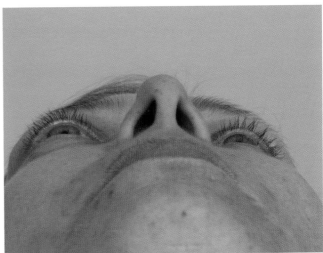

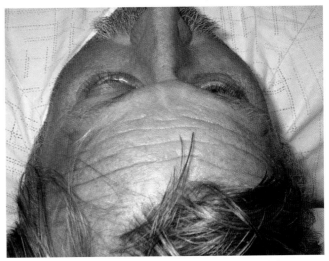

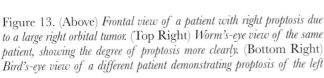

Figure 13. (Above) *Frontal view of a patient with right proptosis due to a large right orbital tumor.* (Top Right) *Worm's-eye view of the same patient, showing the degree of proptosis more clearly.* (Bottom Right) *Bird's-eye view of a different patient demonstrating proptosis of the left eye.*

in trauma settings and is typically the result of edema, but other potential causes include third nerve palsy, levator muscle injury, or a traumatic Horner's syndrome (miosis, ptosis, anhidrosis). Medial eyelid lacerations should raise the suspicion of canalicular injury. The presence of fatty tissue within a lid laceration indicates violation of the orbital septum, raising the suspicion for orbital injury or foreign body. The presence of proptosis (protruding eyeball) should be noted, and may be indicative of a retrobulbar hemorrhage or other pathology such as infection, inflammation, or tumor. Looking at the orbits from above (bird's-eye view) or below (worm's-eye view) can assist in determining the degree of proptosis (Fig. 13). The orbital rims should be palpated and bony step-offs or tenderness noted. Periorbital subcutaneous emphysema is highly suggestive of a fracture involving the orbital floor or medial orbital wall (Figs. 14 and 15). A detailed discussion of examination for the presence of orbital fractures is presented in the Maxillofacial and Neck Trauma chapter.

## Anterior Segment Examination

Gross inspection and slit-lamp examination can detect injuries of the anterior segment including the conjunctiva, sclera, cornea, iris, and lens. The conjunctiva and the sclera should be examined for injection, bleeding, lacerations, chemosis (i.e., conjunctival edema), exposed tissues (e.g., darkly pigmented uveal tissues), and foreign bodies. The presence of hemorrhagic chemosis is suggestive of open-globe injury

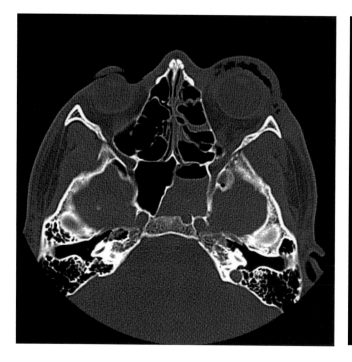

Figure 14. *Axial computed tomography image of a patient with subcutaneous emphysema in the left upper eyelid resulting from an orbital floor fracture.*

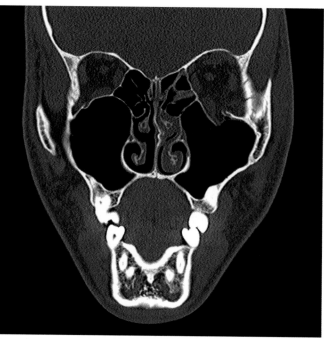

Figure 15. *Coronal computed tomography image of the same patient demonstrating the orbital floor fracture.*

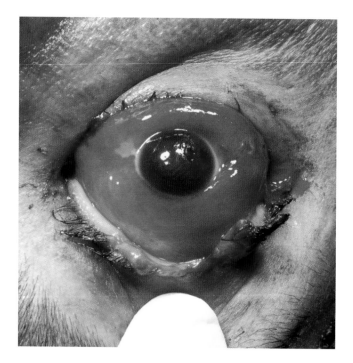

Figure 16. *Presence of hemorrhagic chemosis suggesting open-globe injury.*

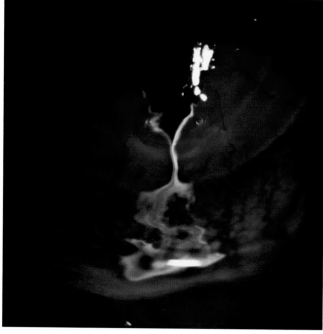

Figure 17. *Positive Seidel's sign identifying aqueous humor leakage. Image courtesy of the University of Michigan Kellogg Eye Center.*

(Fig. 16). The cornea should be examined for lack of clarity, surface irregularities, and foreign bodies. Fluorescein staining of the cornea may assist with the diagnosis of corneal epithelial defects. Removal of contact lenses prior to the application of fluorescein will prevent permanent staining of the contact lens.

(Note: in accordance with DA PAM 40-506, chapter 4-13.c, the US Army prohibits the wearing of contact lenses in field and combat environments.)

> The presence of hemorrhagic chemosis is suggestive of open-globe injury.

In cases of suspected corneal perforation, a Seidel test can identify aqueous humor leakage (Fig. 17). A Seidel test is performed by applying a moistened fluorescein strip directly to the area in question, creating a puddle of dark orange concentrated fluorescein. Leaking aqueous humor will dilute the fluorescein and create a stream that fluoresces bright yellow-green under cobalt blue light. While a positive Seidel test is pathognomonic for corneal perforation, a negative test does not necessarily rule it out, as some corneal wounds can be self-sealing.

> In cases of suspected corneal perforation, a Seidel test can identify aqueous humor leakage. While a positive Seidel test is pathognomonic for corneal perforation, a negative test does not necessarily rule it out, as some corneal wounds can be self-sealing.

The irides are inspected for color, defects, and irregularities in shape. The crystalline lens is not normally visible on gross inspection, and is best examined with a slit-lamp. Traumatic subluxation of the lens often manifests as a dark crescent moon in the center of the pupil. Gross examination of the anterior chamber may reveal an excessively shallow or deep anterior chamber (in comparison with the opposite eye), suggestive of open-globe injury or lens dislocation. Normally, the anterior chamber is optically clear, but gross inspection may reveal red blood cells (i.e., hyphema) or purulent exudate (i.e., hypopyon). Cell and flare, which are signs of anterior chamber inflammation, can usually only be seen through a slit-lamp biomicroscope. The magnified view of the oblique slit beam reveals individual white blood cells or proteinaceous debris, which resemble dust particles or smoke within a movie projector beam.[8]

## Posterior Segment Examination

The vitreous, retina, and optic disc can be visualized through a careful fundoscopic exam. The fundoscopic exam should begin by documenting the status of the red reflex. An abnormal red reflex suggests corneal edema, cataract, vitreous hemorrhage, or a large retinal detachment. Any opacity that disturbs the transmission of light (e.g., foreign body, corneal laceration, or lens injury) will show up as a dark shadow against the red reflex.

> An abnormal red reflex suggests corneal edema, cataract, vitreous hemorrhage, or a large retinal detachment.

A complete fundoscopic examination may be facilitated by pharmacologic dilation of the pupils with topical mydriatics (e.g., phenylephrine) and cycloplegics (e.g., tropicamide). Prior to inducing pharmacologic dilation, patients should have a complete pupillary exam and be screened for contraindications to dilation such as significant head trauma or a history of angle-closure glaucoma. All patients with possible posterior segment injuries should be referred to an ophthalmologist for a complete 360-degree retinal examination.

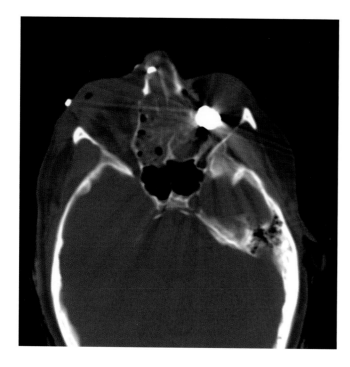

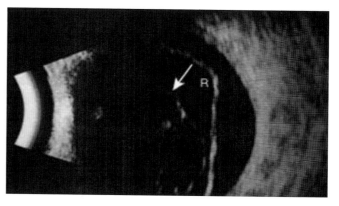

Figure 18. (Left) *Axial computed tomography image of a patient with a left intraorbital foreign body resulting from an improvised explosive device (IED) blast. The metallic foreign body traveled through the right orbit and both ethmoid and nasal sinuses before coming to rest in the medial left orbit adjacent to the optic nerve. It was successfully removed through a transcaruncular medial orbitotomy.*

Figure 19. (Top Right) *B-scan ultrasound image showing retinal detachment (R). The vitreous cavity is black and the curved surface of the posterior sclera (white) is seen on the right side of the image. Image courtesy of Mitchell Goff, MD.*

## Ocular Imaging Techniques

Plain film radiography, computed tomography (CT), ultrasound, and magnetic resonance imaging (MRI) have all been used in the evaluation of ocular trauma. Computed tomography has largely replaced conventional plain film radiography for the evaluation of ocular trauma. It is particularly useful in the evaluation of orbital fractures, intraocular and orbital foreign bodies, globe rupture, and retrobulbar hemorrhage.[12,13] However, radiolucent foreign bodies such as glass, plastic, or wood may be difficult to detect on CT or plain film.[14] Standard CT examination should include both axial and direct coronal imaging, although direct coronals are often not obtainable in trauma patients who are unconscious or under cervical spine precautions. Contrast administration is not necessary. Thin cuts (e.g., 1 mm) can be obtained for specific indications, such as localizing foreign bodies, viewing the optic canal, or for coronal reconstruction when direct coronals cannot be obtained (Fig. 18). If CT is unavailable, conventional plain films may be used to screen for metallic foreign bodies or evaluate for orbital fractures and sinus injury.

> Within the first 24 to 72 hours following injury, the most valuable imaging modality for the evaluation of ocular trauma is CT scanning, which is widely available at Level III facilities.

When ocular examination is obscured by opaque media (e.g., intraocular hemorrhage), B-scan ultrasound may provide detailed intraocular anatomic information.[15] Ultrasound may detect the presence of an IOFB, retinal detachment, choroidal hemorrhage, vitreous hemorrhage, and orbital hemorrhage (Fig. 19).[13,16] Because the transducer applies pressure to the globe, ultrasound testing should be avoided in cases of suspected globe violation.

Within the first 24 to 72 hours following injury, the most valuable imaging modality for the evaluation of ocular trauma is CT imaging, which is widely available at Level III facilities. B-scan ultrasound can be useful in select cases, but its availability at Level III is variable. Magnetic resonance imaging is not particularly useful in the setting of acute ocular trauma, and is not generally available prior to Level IV.

## Closed Globe Injuries

### *Corneal Abrasion*

In most cases, corneal abrasions (traumatic corneal epithelial defects) can be safely managed by nonophthalmic providers. The cause of the abrasion is usually traumatic and the onset of symptoms (pain, foreign body sensation, photophobia, and blurred vision) is immediate. The defect can be visualized with the aid of fluorescein, which stains exposed epithelial basement membrane and fluoresces bright yellow-green when viewed under a Wood's lamp or cobalt blue light (Fig. 20). In most cases, the recommended treatment is a prophylactic topical antibiotic (erythromycin, bacitracin ophthalmic ointment, or polymyxin B sulfate and trimethoprim [Polytrim®] ophthalmic solution) instilled four times a day. Patching is generally discouraged, but sunglasses can provide symptomatic relief. The dispensing of topical anesthetics to any patient for any reason is contraindicated, as they can lead to neurotrophic keratopathy and persistent epithelial defects.[17] Depending on the size of the defect, most corneal abrasions heal spontaneously within a few days. Special care must be taken in contact lens wearers or when the presence of an embedded corneal foreign body or corneal infection (e.g., corneal ulcer) is suspected. Since slit-lamp biomicroscopy, which is not available at Level I or II facilities, is necessary to evaluate and treat these conditions, such cases should be referred to an eye care professional (optometrist or ophthalmologist) when operationally feasible.

> In most cases, non-ophthalmic providers can safely manage corneal abrasions using a prophylactic topical antibiotic. If a superficial foreign body is embedded within or on the surface of the cornea, care must be taken to rule out corneal perforation.

### *Corneal Foreign Bodies*

Combat casualties will often present with superficial foreign bodies embedded within or on the surface

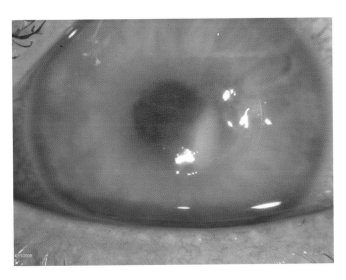

Figure 20. *Corneal ulcer. Note the opaque white inflammatory infiltrate and overlying epithelial defect. Image courtesy of the University of Michigan Kellogg Eye Center.*

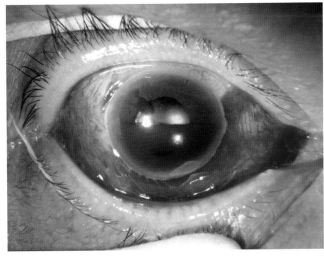

Figure 21. *This hyphema demonstrates extensive blood in the anterior chamber.*

of the cornea. Without the aid of a slit-lamp, it may be difficult to determine whether the foreign body has perforated the cornea, which is only 0.5 to 0.9 mm in thickness.[18] In cases where the foreign body is thought to be superficial, the first-line treatment should be irrigation of the eye with sterile saline or eye wash solution. If irrigation is unsuccessful, instrument removal of the foreign body should be performed by an eye care professional. However, if circumstances prevent this from occurring, only experienced nonopthalmic personnel should attempt removal of corneal foreign bodies, using slit-lamp or loupe magnification, and exercising extreme caution. Seidel testing should be performed following foreign body removal and topical antibiotics should be administered until the epitheleal defect has healed. Metallic foreign bodies can leave a rust ring in the cornea, which should be removed by an ophthalmologist, ideally within several days of the injury.

## *Hyphema*

Hyphema is defined as the presence of blood in the anterior chamber, and is usually caused by blunt trauma, unless it is associated with an open-globe injury. The source of bleeding is usually from tears in the iris or ciliary body, and irregular mydriasis or iridodialysis (separation of the iris root) is often an associated finding. In sufficient quantity, the blood is grossly visible as it layers across the bottom of the anterior chamber (Fig. 21). Visual acuity can be affected, depending on the size of the hyphema, and pain and photophobia are often present as the result of coexisting injuries, such as traumatic iritis.

Most hyphemas resolve spontaneously and their treatment is usually nonoperative, consisting of observation, eye protection, and bed rest with head elevation. However, complications sometimes arise that require medical or surgical intervention. The greatest risk of vision loss from isolated hyphemas occurs with rebleeding, which usually occurs two to five days after injury. Permanent vision loss can result from hyphema-related complications, which include glaucoma, corneal bloodstaining, and ischemic optic neuropathy. Patients with sickle trait or disease are at particular risk for these complications, and all hyphema patients of African descent should undergo sickle screening if their status is unknown.

---

Most hyphemas resolve spontaneously and their treatment is usually nonoperative, consisting of observation, eye protection, and bed rest with head elevation. Small hyphemas (occupying less than one-third of the anterior chamber) with normal vision and IOP can potentially be monitored for resolution at Level I or II facilities. Patients experiencing vision loss, increased IOP, or larger hyphemas (involving one-third or more of the anterior chamber) should be evacuated to a Level III facility for ophthalmologic management.

---

Small hyphemas (occupying less than one-third of the anterior chamber) with normal vision and IOP can potentially be monitored for resolution at Level I or II facilities, but eventual evaluation by an ophthalmologist is advisable. Patients with vision loss, increased IOP, or larger hyphemas (involving one-third or more of the anterior chamber) should be evacuated to a Level III facility for ophthalmologic management. Medical treatment includes topical steroids, cycloplegics, and IOP-lowering agents when necessary. Aminocaproic acid has been used to prevent rebleeding in select cases, but its marginal benefits must be weighed against the potential risks of clotting and stroke. Anterior chamber paracentesis with washout is indicated in cases with persistent IOP elevation despite maximal medical therapy, and a lower threshold for surgery is maintained for patients with sickle disease.

## Traumatic Iritis

Blunt eye trauma can lead to irritation of the iris and ciliary body, inciting an inflammatory reaction within the anterior chamber known as traumatic iritis or iridocyclitis. Symptoms include deep eye pain, photophobia, and blurred vision. These symptoms may be delayed for 24 to 48 hours following the injury. Evaluation of these patients should include a complete slit-lamp exam, fundoscopic exam, and documentation of IOP. The key physical exam finding is a mild to severe anterior chamber reaction (cells and flare), which, as mentioned previously, can be best appreciated with an oblique slit beam through the slit-lamp biomicroscope. Additional findings include perilimbal injection (i.e., ciliary flush), photophobia, consensual photophobia (i.e., pain in the affected eye when light is shone in the opposite eye), and occasionally decreased vision. Other clues to the diagnosis include pain that does not improve with topical anesthetics and pain with accommodation.[19,20] Treatment regimens can include cycloplegic drops, topical steroids, or topical nonsteroidal antiinflammatory agents (NSAIDs). Isolated traumatic iritis is self-limited and carries a good prognosis, and in the absence of findings suggesting coexisting ocular injuries may be managed at Level I or II facilities. If symptoms worsen or fail to resolve within one week, ophthalmologic evaluation is indicated.

> In the absence of findings suggesting coexisting ocular injuries, isolated traumatic iritis is self-limited, carries a good prognosis, and may be managed at Level I or II facilities.

## Lens Subluxation / Dislocation

Patients with lens subluxation or dislocation can present with a history of ocular trauma, distorted vision, monocular diplopia, and pain. Critical findings include a displaced lens on direct ophthalmoscopy, phacodonesis (i.e., quivering of the lens), and iridodonesis (i.e., quivering of the iris). Additional findings include cataract, acute pupillary block glaucoma, and acquired myopia. Partial disruption of the zonular fibers that support the lens will result in subluxation. A subluxed lens can still remain partially visible within the pupillary aperture. Complete disruption of the zonular fibers results in lens dislocation, where the lens may no longer be visible through the pupillary aperture.

> All patients with lens subluxations or dislocations warrant immediate ophthalmologic consultation.

A potential vision-threatening complication of lens dislocation is acute pupillary-block glaucoma.[21] This results from the dislocated lens preventing the aqueous from flowing from the posterior chamber through the pupil into the anterior chamber, which pushes the iris forward and closes the anterior chamber angle where the aqueous exits the eye. Traumatic cataract, another complication, may follow even the most trivial injury to the lens, and can be removed electively at Level IV or V facilities.[21]

## Vitreous Hemorrhage

Vitreous hemorrhage may occur from a variety of mechanisms including iris injuries, ciliary body trauma, vitreous detachment, retinal vessel injury, and choroidal rupture.[22] Patients with vitreous hemorrhage can present with varying degrees of vision loss, ranging from hazy vision with cobwebs or floaters to bare light perception vision.

Visualizing blood within the vitreous cavity with direct or indirect ophthalmoscopy confirms the diagnosis of vitreous hemorrhage. It is important to document IOP measurements in these patients, as they are at risk for acute glaucoma. The treatment of vitreous hemorrhage involves bed rest (with head of bed elevation), a protective eye shield, and analgesics (avoiding aspirin and nonsteroidal antiinflammatory drugs). All vitreous hemorrhages, traumatic or otherwise, should be assumed to be secondary to retinal injury and referred for immediate ophthalmologic evaluation.

## Retinal / Choroidal Injuries

Ocular trauma may result in a variety of retinal injuries including retinal breaks, retinal detachments, choroidal hemorrhage, and choroidal rupture.[23] Patients with retinal injuries may present with a recent or remote history of ocular trauma. Symptoms include floaters, photopsias (flashes of light), a curtain or shadow over the visual field, and varying degrees of vision loss. Peripheral retinal breaks may initially be asymptomatic only to later lead to retinal detachment. Detailed dilated fundoscopic examination by an ophthalmologist is necessary to diagnose most retinal injuries.

Commotio retinae (Berlin's edema) is a retinal injury resulting from a contrecoup mechanism of injury.[24] The injury is characterized by a transient whitening of the deep sensory retina following ocular trauma, which is visible on direct or indirect ophthalmoscopy. Patients present with variable degrees of vision loss, which is more severe with macular involvement. While there is no specific treatment for commotio retinae, most cases are self-limited and they rarely result in permanent vision loss.

> Patients with retinal injuries may present with a recent or remote history of ocular trauma. Symptoms include floaters, photopsias (flashes of light), a curtain or shadow over the visual field, and varying degrees of vision loss. Careproviders should be able to identify patients with signs or symptoms consistent with retinal injury and refer them for appropriate ophthalmologic consultation.

Combat casualty careproviders must maintain a high suspicion for retinal injuries in all patients with significant ocular trauma. The visual morbidity from delayed treatment of these injuries is high. Definitive diagnosis of these injuries is well beyond the scope of most physicians. Thus, providers should be able to identify patients with signs or symptoms consistent with retinal injury and refer them for appropriate ophthalmologic consultation. In some cases, specialized treatment must be performed within 24 to 72 hours of injury to optimize visual outcomes.[25]

# Open-Globe Injuries

## Overview

An open-globe injury is defined as any full-thickness violation of the cornea or sclera. While the distinction is largely semantic, a laceration generally implies direct violation by a sharp object, while rupture is usually used to describe the forceful splitting of the eye wall induced by blunt trauma. Foreign body penetration denotes the entry of an object without exiting the involved structure, while perforation indicates the complete through-and-through passage of the object.

Signs and symptoms of open-globe injury include loss of vision, hemorrhagic chemosis, anterior chamber asymmetry, intraocular hemorrhage (hyphema or vitreous hemorrhage), uveal prolapse, hypotony (IOP less than 5 mm Hg), positive Seidel test, and visible protrusion of a foreign body from the globe (Figs.

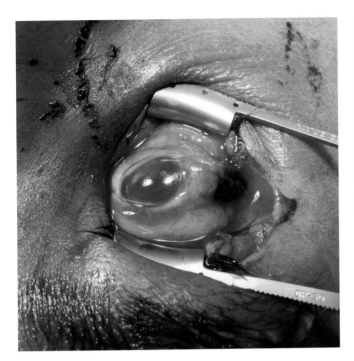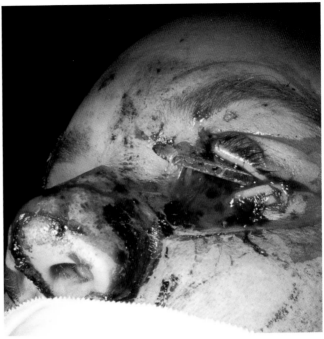

Figure 22. *Signs of open-globe injury:* (Left) *Uveal prolapse and misshapened globe.* (Right) *Protruding intraocular foreign body.*

16, 17, and 22). On CT scan, IOFB or air are diagnostic of open-globe injury, and globe deformation, intraocular hemorrhage, and lens disruption are highly suggestive (Fig. 23).

The prognosis for open-globe injury is highly variable and dependent on the severity of the injury. According to the Ocular Trauma Score, out of all the prognostic indicators for visual outcome, poor initial visual acuity (light perception or worse) is the most important negative predictor.[26] This is followed by globe rupture, endophthalmitis, perforating injury, retinal detachment, and afferent pupillary defect. The prognostic applicability of the Ocular Trauma Score to combat injuries was nicely validated by a study from OEF and OIF.[27] Corneoscleral laceration length and posterior extension more than five mm past the limbus are also negative predictors for globe survival. Barr reported an enucleation rate of 68 percent for globes with corneoscleral lacerations over 13 mm in length in contrast to only 4 percent with lacerations less than nine mm.[28]

An open-globe is defined as any full-thickness violation of the cornea or sclera. Signs and symptoms of open-globe injury include loss of vision, hemorrhagic chemosis, anterior chamber asymmetry, intraocular hemorrhage (hyphema or vitreous hemorrhage), uveal prolapse, hypotony (IOP less than five mm Hg), positive Seidel test, and visible protrusion of a foreign body from the globe. Casualties with open-globe injuries should undergo eye shielding and be evacuated to a Level III facility.

## Initial Management of Open-Globe Injuries

Patients with signs and symptoms consistent with open-globe injury require emergent evacuation to a Level III facility for ophthalmologic evaluation. As described above, the eye should be protected with a Fox shield and the patient's tetanus status updated as needed. In anticipation of possible surgery, the patient's last meal should be recorded and they should receive nothing by mouth until they have been evaluated by an ophthalmologist. Pain, nausea, and anxiety should be treated if present, as excessive blepharospasm or valsalva can increase IOP and exacerbate open-globe injuries.

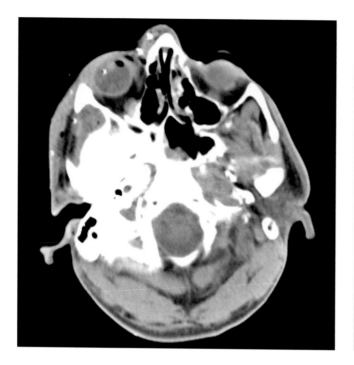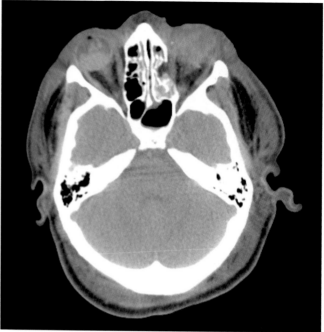

Figure 23. *CT scan findings in open-globe injury:* (Left) *Intraocular foreign body and air.* (Right) *Vitreous hemorrhage and lens disruption, right eye. Deformed and poorly defined globe, left eye.*

## Open-Globe Injury Repair

The Level III ophthalmologist is responsible for the definitive treatment of open-globe injuries in the vast majority of cases. Even for the most experienced ophthalmologist, the diagnosis of open-globe injury is not always clear-cut, and the decision to take the patient to the operating room can be difficult. However, if any doubt exists, a low threshold for surgical exploration should be maintained. General anesthesia is required, as retrobulbar injection is clearly contraindicated. It has been suggested that the use of depolarizing paralytic agents is contraindicated in open-globe injuries due to the risk of increased IOP, but this has never been clearly demonstrated to be a problem.[29] Intraoperative findings dictate the extent of the exploration, but one can never be faulted for performing a 360-degree peritomy in order to directly visualize the entire scleral surface. Conjunctival traction sutures (e.g., 4-0 silk) placed at the oblique quadrants can improve surgical exposure dramatically (Fig. 24). Scleral lacerations often originate at or extend beneath the extraocular muscle insertions, and in these instances it is helpful to detach the muscle at its insertion in order to fully visualize and repair the defect. Double-armed 6-0 polyglactin sutures preplaced through the tendon can facilitate retraction and exposure of the field, as well as reattachment of the muscle to the globe at the end of the case.

The overarching principle in the treatment of open-globe injury is to restore the physical integrity of the globe wall. Every attempt should be made to reposit prolapsed intraocular structures prior to wound approximation. The exception to this rule is the crystalline lens, which should be removed if it is prolapsed into the anterior segment or out of the globe. Viscoelastics are quite useful in preventing incarceration of intraocular tissue in the wound during repair. Typically, 10-0 nylon suture is used in the cornea, 9-0 nylon at the limbus, and 8-0 nylon in the sclera. If the limbus is involved, it is generally the first structure to be sutured, being the most critical and easily recognizable anatomic landmark. Basic wound closure principles must be strictly observed, particularly in the cornea. These include: (1) vertical entry and exit

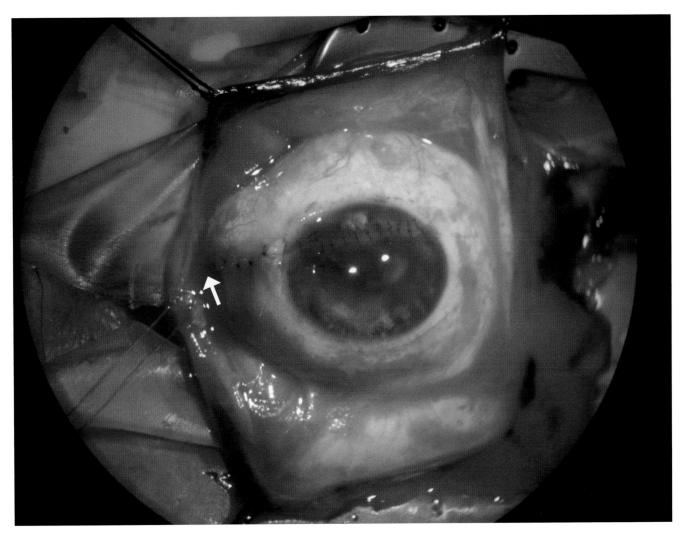

Figure 24. *Corneoscleral laceration repair, right eye. The scleral portion of the laceration extends posteriorly beneath the insertion of the medial rectus muscle, which has been tagged with a double-armed 6-0 polyglactin suture and detached. Note conjunctival traction sutures.*

of the needle point with respect to the corneal surface; (2) 90 percent-stromal-thickness suture passes; (3) exact matching of suture depth and width on each side of the wound; (4) orientation of each suture orthogonal to the wound axis; (5) proper and even spacing of interrupted sutures (space between each suture slightly less than the suture length); and (6) tying of sutures under proper tension (approximation, not strangulation). The use of the adjustable slipknot can greatly aid in achieving the last goal. All corneal suture knots should be buried and directed away from the visual axis if possible.

Occasionally, a watertight closure cannot be achieved with sutures alone, such as in corneal lacerations with a stellate pattern or tissue maceration. In these cases, cyanoacrylate glue can be very useful. Prior to applying the glue, any residual corneal epithelium should be removed from the surface to which the glue will be applied. Nylon 10-0 sutures can then be placed in a criss-crossing or grid pattern to create a scaffold across the defect. The glue is drawn up from the ampule in a tuberculin syringe and sparingly applied to the defect through a small-gauge needle. A completely dry wound surface is necessary for adherence of the glue, but this may be difficult to maintain in the presence of an aqueous leak. Viscoelastic, preferably a cohesive type, can be injected directly beneath the laceration to prevent the egress of fluid. A bandage contact lens should be placed after the glue is applied, and can subsequently be removed once the plug

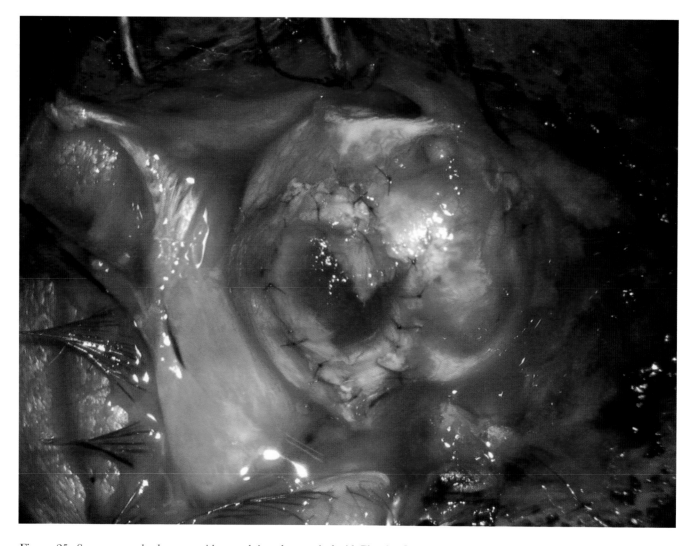

Figure 25. *Severe corneoscleral rupture with corneal tissue loss repaired with Tutoplast® patch graft.*

spontaneously detaches, usually within two to four weeks. Another option for the closure of wounds with damaged or missing tissue is the use of allografts or xenografts, such as acellular dermis or processed pericardium, which can be cut to the size and shape of the defect and sewn into place as a patch graft (Fig. 25).

> The overarching principle in the treatment of open-globe injury is to restore the physical integrity of the globe wall. Every attempt should be made to reposit prolapsed intraocular structures prior to wound approximation.

In some cases, intraocular pathology may be addressed during primary globe repair if technically feasible. Foreign bodies in the anterior chamber or within easy reach of the anterior segment can often be safely removed. Disrupted lens material or prolapsed vitreous may also be removed at the discretion of the surgeon. However, as stated above, the primary goal of open-globe repair is to simply close the defect and allow the eye an opportunity for further rehabilitation in the future. Procedures that add surgical time or increase risk to the globe, such as posterior segment foreign body removal, retinal detachment repair, or intraocular lens implantation are not advisable under these circumstances.

Intraocular air may be found either clinically or radiographically in some penetrating globe injuries. While not a major treatment concern, the presence of air may potentially impact the patient's ability to safely undergo aeromedical evacuation, due to the expansion of gas within the globe at high altitude. However, this concern is mitigated by several factors: (1) the rise in IOP at altitude is dependent on the volume of air present within the globe, and studies indicate that eyes with less than 10 percent gas fill (0.6 milliliters) may safely undergo air travel; (2) the half-life of air in the human eye is only 1.3 days; and (3) most open globes, including those that have just undergone repair, are hypotonus and can accommodate moderate increases in IOP. [30,31,32] With these considerations in mind, it is advisable for the ophthalmologist to remove any air that is easily accessible during the course of open-globe injury repair. However, based upon the information provided above, volumes of retained intraocular air less than 0.6 milliliters (approximately 10 mm in diameter on CT scan) should not prevent aeromedical evacuation of a combat casualty.

> Intraocular air may be found either clinically or radiographically following penetrating globe injuries. The presence of air may potentially impact the patient's ability to safely undergo aeromedical evacuation due to the expansion of gas within the globe at high altitude. Volumes of retained intraocular air less than 0.6 milliliters (approximately 10 mm in diameter on CT scan) should not prevent aeromedical evacuation of a combat casualty.

While definitive evidence proving benefit is lacking, prophylactic administration of systemic antibiotics is widely recommended for open-globe injuries. [33,34] A variety of single- or multiple-agent regimens have been used, including fluoroquinolones, cephalosporins, or beta-lactams. Topical antibiotics are also advisable. However, the use of intravitreal antibiotics on a prophylactic basis in this setting is of questionable value. [34] A study from OEF and OIF reported no cases of endophthalmitis in 79 eyes with retained IOFBs, despite the fact that only three of them received intravitreal antibiotics at the time of primary globe repair. [35]

## Sympathetic Ophthalmia
An uncommon but potentially devastating complication of open-globe injury that can lead to blindness in the fellow eye is sympathetic ophthalmia. Defined as a diffuse bilateral granulomatous uveitis following penetrating globe injury, sympathetic ophthalmia is believed to represent an autoimmune response to the exposure of uveal or retinal antigens previously sequestered within the blood-aqueous or blood-retinal barrier. Incidence reports of sympathetic ophthalmia after wartime open-globe injuries vary widely from 0.02 to 56 percent. [36]

It is widely believed that sympathetic ophthalmia can be prevented by enucleating a severely damaged eye within two weeks of injury, although this time frame is largely based on anectodal data. Evisceration (i.e., removal of the contents of the globe) is generally discouraged in the setting of trauma, due to the potential presence of uveal proteins within the emissary canals of the retained scleral shell. The true risk of developing sympathetic ophthalmia if enucleation is not performed is unknown. Modern estimates of the overall incidence of sympathetic ophthalmia after open-globe injury (including patients who underwent enucleation) range from 0.3 to 1.9 percent. [36]

## Globe Repair versus Enucleation
Repair of severe open-globe injuries should be attempted whenever technically feasible, unless proper follow-up care is doubtful. Deciding between primary globe repair and primary enucleation can sometimes

be extremely difficult. In smaller globe lacerations where preoperative vision is at least light perception, the decision to repair is clear. On the opposite end of the spectrum, when a globe is so severely damaged that repair is not technically possible, enucleation must be performed to prevent sympathetic ophthalmia and socket contracture.[37,38] In the middle of the spectrum, however, the ophthalmologist will encounter cases in which repair is possible, but the ultimate prognosis for vision or globe survival is slim to nonexistent. In such cases, it is generally felt that repair should be attempted whenever technically feasible. The benefits to the patient are multiple: (1) the patient is assured that a reasonable effort was made to try to save the eye; (2) the lack of visual function despite repair is demonstrated to the patient; (3) the patient is included in the decision-making process leading to removal of the eye; and (4) the patient has time to come to terms with the loss of a major sensory organ before enucleation is performed. This guidance is appropriate in cases where the availability of proper follow-up and ophthalmic surgery can be reasonably assured, such as is the case for service members being evacuated to higher levels of care (Level IV and V facilities). However, if a patient in the same clinical situation may not be able to obtain proper follow-up care (e.g., host national in a country with no reliable health care system), primary enucleation may be more advisable for the patient's long-term welfare.

> Repair of severe open-globe injuries should be attempted whenever technically feasible, unless proper follow-up care is doubtful.

## Enucleation

Enucleation, defined as surgical removal of the entire globe, is typically performed under general anesthesia, although a retrobulbar block may be utilized if necessary. A 360-degree peritomy is performed, sparing as much conjunctiva as possible. Tenon's capsule is bluntly dissected from the sclera in the oblique quadrants with curved blunt scissors. The rectus muscles are isolated with muscle hooks, and double armed 5-0 or 6-0 polyglactin sutures can be preplaced before detaching them from the globe at their insertions. The oblique muscles are usually cut and not preserved, although some surgeons advocate attaching one or both of them to the orbital implant or to the rectus muscles (e.g., the superior oblique to the superior rectus and the inferior oblique to the lateral rectus). The globe is then retracted by the muscle stumps, with traction sutures (e.g., 4-0 silk passed through the limbus), or with an enucleation spoon, and the optic nerve is strummed and cut with curved scissors (Fig. 26). The length of the optic nerve segment is not critical, as long as the nerve is severed distal to its entrance into the globe. Clamping or cauterizing the optic nerve prior to cutting it may assist in hemostasis. Once adequate hemostasis is achieved by packing with cold-soaked gauze or other hemostatic materials, orbital implant sizers can be used to determine the appropriate implant size. The implant should provide adequate volume replacement while at the same time rest easily within Tenon's capsule without placing undue tension on the Tenon's closure. For ideal orbital volume replacement, the optimal implant

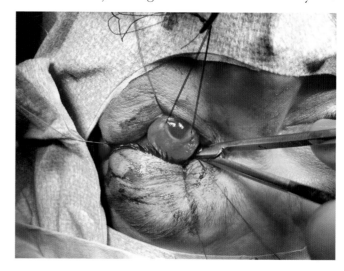

Figure 26. *Enucleation of globe. The four rectus muscles are tagged with 5-0 polyglactin sutures. The globe is retracted with 4-0 silk sutures passed through the limbus as the optic nerve is cut.*

diameter should be approximately two mm less than the axial length of the globe.[39] Given that the average axial length of the adult globe is approximately 24 mm, most orbital implants should be between 20 and 22 mm in diameter, although a smaller size may be used if there is tissue loss or a specific concern for implant extrusion. Care should be taken in the presence of large orbital fractures, which may need to be repaired in order to prevent implant migration into the maxillary or ethmoid sinus. Much debate remains regarding the ideal orbital implant material, and there is insufficient data in the literature to definitively recommend one type over another. Once the implant is placed within Tenon's capsule, the extraocular muscles can be attached to the anterior surface of the implant in order to maximize postoperative motility. Tenon's capsule and conjunctiva are then closed over the implant with absorbable sutures. Separate layered closure of posterior Tenon's capsule (with 4-0 polyglactin) and anterior Tenon's (with 5-0 or 6-0 polyglactin) may decrease the risk of postoperative implant extrusion. A conformer is placed into the socket with antibiotic ointment, and some surgeons perform a temporary suture tarsorrhaphy, which can be left in place for up to three weeks. A pressure patch may also be applied for two to three days to limit postoperative edema. Six to eight weeks of postoperative healing should be allowed before ocular prosthesis fitting is attempted.

## *Intraocular Foreign Body (IOFB)*

By definition, IOFBs are open-globe injuries, and the signs and symptoms are the same as those described at the beginning of this chapter segment. However, the severity of IOFB injuries varies widely, and as one would expect is largely dependent on the size of the offending object. Intraocular foreign bodies should be suspected with blast injury mechanisms, sanding, drilling, grinding, or hammering metal-on-metal. High-velocity metal or glass splinters may enter the eye painlessly. The initial ocular examination may appear deceptively benign, revealing only slight injection or local discomfort (Fig. 27). Visual acuity is typically decreased, but can be normal. Some corneal or scleral perforations can be difficult to detect. Additional findings suggestive of an IOFB include conjunctival chemosis, hyphema, localized cataract, iris injury, pupillary asymmetry, vitreous hemorrhage, decreased IOP, or an aqueous humor leak (as evidenced by a positive Seidel test). CT scanning is helpful in identifying IOFBs in eyes with opaque media. Although small pieces of wood, glass, or plastic may not be seen on CT, the majority of IOFBs can be visualized. The utility of ultrasonography for detecting IOFBs in the setting of open-globe injury is limited by the need to avoid direct pressure to the injured globe.

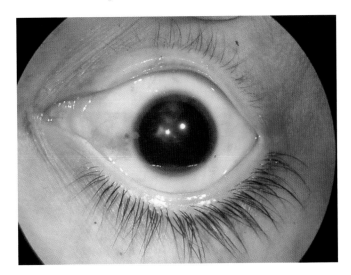 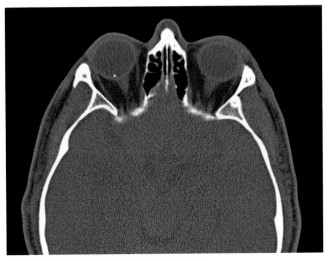

Figure 27. *Penetrating globe injury caused by a rocket-propelled grenade blast fragment.* (Left) *Anterior segment exam appears relatively benign with mild focal corneal edema seen in the inferior cornea.* (Right) *Posterior segment IOFB is visible on CT scan.*

Intraocular foreign bodies are open-globe injuries and should be suspected with blast injury mechanisms, sanding, drilling, grinding, or hammering metal-on-metal. Level III facility-based ophthalmologists should only remove IOFBs that are easily accessible within the anterior segment. Posterior segment foreign bodies should be left for potential future removal by a vitreoretinal specialist at Level IV or V facilities.

Management of IOFBs depends on the foreign body size, composition, and location within the eye.[40,41] The reactivity of IOFBs is highly variable. Wood, vegetable matter, and metals such as iron, copper, and steel typically incite an intense inflammatory reaction when left in the eye, and surgical removal is indicated.[42] On the other hand, inert foreign bodies such as glass, lead, plaster, rubber, silver, and stone, are often left in the eye if they are minimally symptomatic.[43] As stated above, Level III facility-based ophthalmologists should only remove IOFBs that are easily accessible from the anterior segment. Posterior segment foreign bodies should be left for potential future removal by a vitreoretinal specialist at Level IV or V facilities.

# Ocular Adnexal Trauma

## *Eyelid Lacerations*

Lacerations of the eyelid and periocular region are common in combat injuries, and can be seen in isolation or concomitantly with other ocular injuries (Fig. 28). Proper eyelid function is critical to preserving vision and maintaining the health of the ocular surface and cornea. The most important discriminating factor in the management of eyelid lacerations is involvement of the lid margin.[44] This will be manifested as notching or gaping along the lid contour due to violation of the tarsal plate, the dense connective tissue that provides structural support to the eyelid. Orbital fat prolapsing thru an eyelid laceration is indicative of violation of the orbital septum.

Partial-thickness eyelid lacerations that do not involve the lid margin or violate orbital septum can be repaired by careproviders at Level I or II facilities. Absorbable 6-0 or nonabsorbable sutures are generally used, and layered closure is recommended for absorbable sutures. Full-thickness lid lacerations should be repaired at the earliest opportunity by an ophthalmic surgeon at a Level III facility, preferably within 24 to 48 hours of injury. If ocular surface exposure is evident prior to evacuation, a lubricating eye ointment should be instilled until repair of the laceration can be performed.

The principles of lid laceration repair are simple: (1) reapproximation of vital anatomic landmarks, especially the lid margin; (2) preservation of tissues; and (3) avoidance of vertical tension on the lids. While in many other body sites, debridement of devitalized or necrotic-appearing tissue is advocated, such is not the case with the eyelids. Due to their excellent vascular supply, eyelid tissues that appear to be unsalvageable may end up surviving after being anatomically restored. It is also common for lacerated eyelid tissues to roll up or retract, giving the false impression of tissue loss. Careful wound exploration often reveals the presence of tissue previously thought to be missing, making repair or reconstruction much more achievable (Fig. 29).

Partial-thickness eyelid lacerations that do not involve the lid margin or violate orbital septum can be repaired by careproviders at Level I or II facilities. Full-thickness lid lacerations should be repaired by an ophthalmologist or facial plastic surgeon. Canalicular involvement must be ruled out in medial eyelid lacerations.

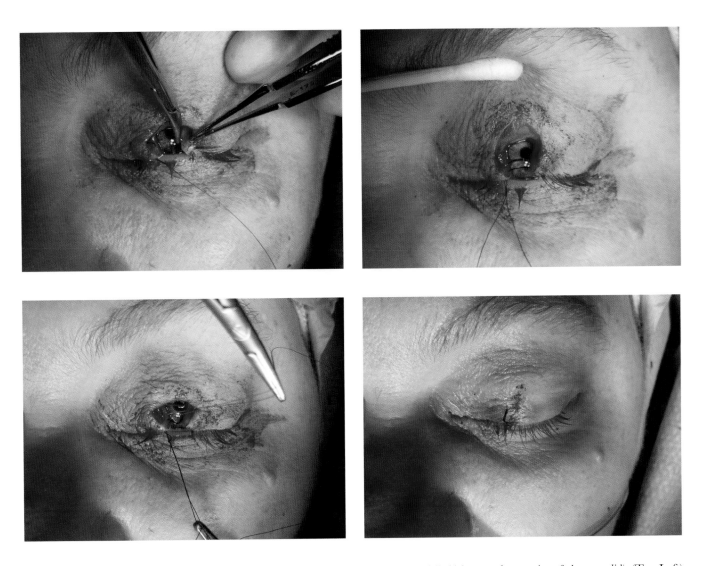

Figure 28. *Stepwise repair of a full-thickness eyelid laceration (demonstrated following a full-thickness wedge resection of the upper lid):* (Top Left) *A 6-0 silk suture is passed through the gray line on both sides of the defect, taking healthy bites of the tarsal plate.* (Top Right) *The same suture is passed in a vertical mattress fashion.* (Bottom Left) *The remainder of the tarsus is repaired with partial thickness passes of 6-0 polyglactin.* (Bottom Right) *The skin is closed with 6-0 fast-absorbing gut sutures. The tails of the margin sutures can be secured with the skin sutures to prevent them from contacting the cornea.*

Repair of full-thickness lid lacerations should begin with approximation of the wound at the lid margin. This is typically performed at the gray line in a vertical mattress fashion with 5-0 or 6-0 silk or polyglactin suture. Additional margin sutures can be placed in similar fashion at the posterior and/or anterior lash lines. To avoid contact with the ocular surface, the suture tails can be cut long and tied down with the tails of the more anterior sutures. Deep absorbable sutures (e.g., 6-0 polyglactin) should also be used to repair the tarsus. The orbicularis and skin can be closed with any of a number of braided or monofilament sutures.

With lacerations involving the medial eyelid, damage to the lacrimal drainage system should be suspected. This can be confirmed by canalicular probing with or without irrigation. Canalicular lacerations should be repaired over a silicone stent (e.g., Crawford tubes), which can either be placed through the entire nasolacrimal duct system, through the upper and lower canaliculi with a pigtail probe, or through the involved canaliculus alone with a monocanalicular stent. The latter option should only be used in proximal

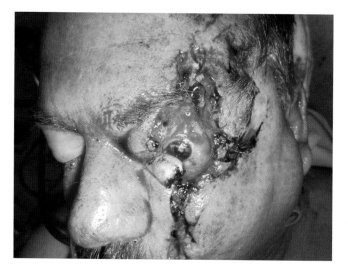 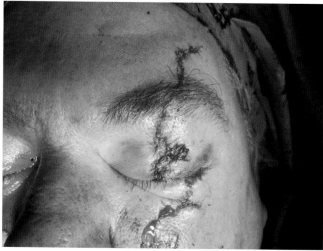

Figure 29. (Left) *Preoperative photograph of a patient who sustained a chainsaw injury to the left globe and orbit. At first glance, a significant amount of tissue appears to be missing, but careful wound exploration revealed minimal tissue loss, and primary repair was successfully accomplished. The globe was repaired prior to eyelid reconstruction.* (Right) *Postoperative photograph.*

canalicular lacerations with a normal punctum. Once the canaliculus is intubated, the pericanalicular tissues are approximated with 7-0 or 8-0 polyglactin suture. It should be remembered that damage to the medial canthal tendon is often seen with canalicular lacerations. Repair of both the posterior and anterior cruri of the medial canthal tendon should be performed as necessary.

Occasionally, lid lacerations will be encountered in association with an open-globe injury or proptotic eye. In these cases, it may be advisable to perform a lateral canthotomy and cantholysis to relieve the pressure on the globe and decrease the tension on the lid repair. If a significant amount of eyelid tissue is lost, reconstruction may be attempted depending on the expertise and comfort level of the ophthalmologist. However, it is acceptable to perform a temporary suture tarsorrhaphy and evacuate the patient to Level IV or V facility, where ophthalmic plastic and reconstructive surgery services are available.

## *Conjunctival Lacerations*

Patients with conjunctival lacerations following ocular trauma may present with eye pain, foreign body sensation, and conjunctival injection or hemorrhage. Physical exam often reveals a conjunctival laceration upon white light examination. The damaged conjunctiva typically folds over on itself at the site of the laceration providing an unobstructed view of exposed white sclera. The damaged region of conjunctiva may fluoresce bright yellow-green following fluorescein staining and cobalt blue light illumination. The presence of a conjunctival laceration should raise the suspicion of potential open-globe injury and/or IOFB, and merits evaluation by an ophthalmologist.

Patients with small conjunctival defects, less than one centimeter (cm), will typically heal without surgical intervention. Patients with conjunctival defects larger than one cm will often need surgical repair, which should be performed by an ophthalmologist.[45] Aftercare involves topical antibiotic administration for up to one week until the affected area has healed.

# Orbital Trauma

## *Retrobulbar Hemorrhage*

Retrobulbar hemorrhage is typically caused by blunt trauma to the orbit, and frequently results in an acute orbital compartment syndrome, a true ocular emergency.[46,47] Another potential cause of orbital compartment syndrome in the setting of trauma is third-spacing of fluid into the orbit following massive fluid resuscitation for burn patients. Signs and symptoms of orbital compartment syndrome include acute vision loss, eye pain, headache, proptosis, resistance to retropulsion, increased IOP (typically over 40 mm Hg), afferent pupillary defect, ophthalmoplegia (loss of extraocular motility), and hemorrhagic chemosis. When orbital compartment syndrome is suspected clinically, lateral canthotomy and inferior cantholysis should be performed immediately. Timing is critical, as experimental studies suggest that permanent vision loss occurs with orbital ischemia lasting greater than 100 minutes.[48] While imaging studies can help to confirm the presence of retrobulbar hemorrhage, the diagnosis of orbital compartment syndrome is clinical, and treatment should not be delayed to obtain a CT scan (Fig. 30).

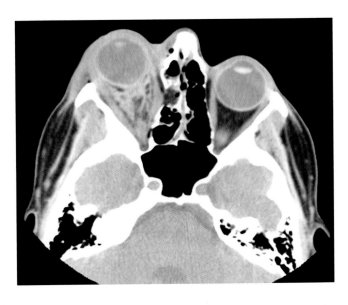

Figure 30. *CT scan appearance of right retrobulbar hemorrhage. Note the loculated pattern of blood within the orbital fat, posterior tenting of the globe from optic nerve traction, and severe proptosis.*

The goal of lateral canthotomy and inferior cantholysis is to convert the orbit from a closed to an open compartment by releasing the attachment of the lower lid to the lateral orbital rim (Fig. 31). Scissors are used to make a horizontal cut from the lateral commissure to the orbital rim, effectively separating the lateral canthal tendon into its superior and inferior portions (lateral canthotomy). The lower lid is then grasped with forceps and pulled away from the rim to place the lateral canthal tendon under tension, and the tendon is "strummed" and cut with scissors (inferior cantholysis). The hand grasping the lid during this maneuver should feel an immediate release when the tendon is cut. Significant drainage of blood from the orbit is not necessary for the procedure to be effective, nor is it expected. However, if the decompressive effect from the inferior cantholysis is insufficient, a superior cantholysis can be performed by releasing the upper lid in the same manner as the lower. The efficacy of the treatment can be assessed soon after the procedure through repeat IOP measurements and visual acuity assessment.

> Retrobulbar hemorrhage is typically caused by blunt trauma to the orbit, and frequently results in an acute orbital compartment syndrome, a true ocular emergency. When orbital compartment syndrome is suspected clinically, lateral canthotomy and inferior cantholysis should be performed immediately. There is no other procedure in all of ophthalmology that can more simply, quickly, and dramatically treat and prevent such devastating vision loss and so profoundly impact a patient's final visual outcome.

If orbital ischemia persists despite complete inferior and superior cantholysis, additional maneuvers may be attempted. Blunt scissors can be placed through the canthotomy incision and used to spread the orbital fat in

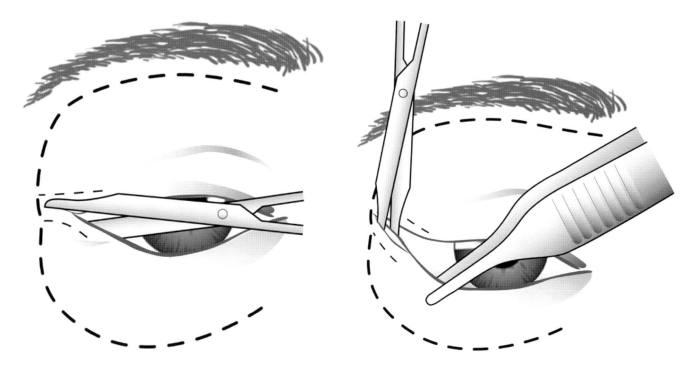

Figure 31. *Lateral canthotomy and inferior cantholysis. Heavy dotted line represents the orbital rim, lighter dotted lines represent the superior and inferior cruri of the lateral canthal tendon. (Left) The lateral canthotomy is created by cutting horizontally from the lateral commissure to the lateral orbital rim. (Right) The lower lid is distracted away from the lateral orbital rim and the inferior crus of the lateral canthal tendon is cut, separating the lower lid from the lateral orbital rim. Image courtesy of Juan D. Nava, Medical Illustrator, Brooke Army Medical Center.*

the inferotemporal quadrant, releasing any pockets of loculated blood within the orbit.[49] If this maneuver fails, the patient may be taken to the operating room for formal orbitotomy and decompression by whatever means necessary. Medical therapy with intraocular-pressure-lowering agents such as osmotics or aqueous suppressants may also be considered.

The value of canthotomy and cantholysis in the setting of orbital compartment syndrome cannot be overstated. There is no other procedure in all of ophthalmology that can more simply, quickly, and dramatically treat and prevent such devastating vision loss and so profoundly impact a patient's final visual outcome. Performed promptly enough, it can literally make the difference between no-light-perception and 20/20 vision. Given the time-critical nature of this condition, ophthalmologists are strongly encouraged to train fellow CCC providers on the indications for and use of this simple technique.

## Orbital Foreign Bodies

Penetrating orbital injury from projectiles or stab injuries can result in retained orbital foreign bodies (Fig. 32). Patients typically present with varying

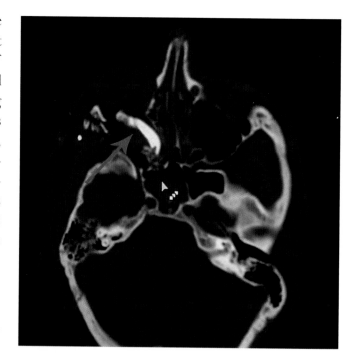

Figure 32. *Orbital foreign body sustained from a blast injury.*

degrees of periocular edema/ecchymosis, proptosis, impaired ocular motility, decreased vision, and pain. Orbital compartment syndrome can also result, and must be managed in the manner described above. As is the case with IOFBs, the composition of the object is important in predicting its long-term tolerability within the orbit and determining the need for removal. Removal of organic foreign bodies is generally recommended, while inorganic foreign bodies can in many cases be observed.[50] Complications of orbital foreign bodies include vision loss, proptosis, diplopia, cellulitis, or a chronic draining fistula. Foreign body removal can be attempted in such cases, although the unique anatomy of the orbit can make this procedure technically difficult, and it should only be performed by an experienced orbital surgeon. The use of intraoperative fluoroscopy has been described as an adjunct to increase the ease of orbital foreign body removal.[51]

### Orbital Fractures

Diagnosis and management of orbital fractures are covered in detail in the Maxillofacial and Neck Trauma chapter.

## Miscellaneous Ocular Injuries

### Chemical Eye Injuries

Chemical exposure of the eye is a true ophthalmologic emergency and may occur with acid or alkali agents. The resulting damage to the eyelids, conjunctiva, cornea, and anterior segment structures may produce permanent visual impairment. In general, alkali burns are more severe than acid burns.[52] Alkali burns cause a liquefactive necrosis, saponifying corneal proteins and initiating corneal collagen destruction. Acid burns cause injury through coagulation necrosis and tend to precipitate corneal proteins, which serve to limit penetration of the acid. Alkali agents are found in more commercially available products than acids, making alkali exposure a relatively more frequent occurrence. Exposure of the eyes to chemical warfare agents is also an ocular emergency. Blistering agents such as mustard gas are particularly toxic to the ocular surface, and the acute management of exposure to these agents mirrors that for standard chemical exposures.

A patient who presents with chemical exposure should undergo immediate copious irrigation of the eye before any time is wasted on additional history and physical examination.[53] In terms of efficacy, no therapeutic difference exists between normal saline, normal saline with bicarbonate, lactated Ringer's solution, or balanced salt solution.[54] Irrigation with a minimum of one liter of irrigating solution is recommended. During irrigation, the lids should be retracted and the stream of irrigating fluid should be directed onto the globe and conjunctival fornices. The fornices should be carefully swabbed to remove any chemical particulate matter. Topical anesthesia will facilitate these maneuvers. Irrigation should continue until the pH of the tear film obtained at the inferior conjunctival fornix is neutral, as measured with litmus paper or the pH indicator of a urine dipstick.[55] Waiting several minutes after completion of irrigation will allow for pH equilibration. No attempt should be made to neutralize chemicals with either acids or alkalis. The immediate irrigation of metallic sodium, metallic potassium, or yellow or white phosphorous has the theoretic potential to initiate further chemical injury. Despite this concern, authorities still recommend copious irrigation of eyes exposed to these chemicals.[53]

Chemical injury to the eye is a true ophthalmologic emergency and may occur with acid or alkali agents. A patient who presents following chemical exposure should undergo immediate copious irrigation of the eye before any time is wasted on additional history and physical examination.

The severity of a chemical eye injury is related to the type of chemical, surface area of contact, duration of chemical contact, and depth of chemical penetration. If an epithelial defect is highly suspected but none is found on initial staining with fluorescein, the procedure should be repeated, as sloughing of the corneal basement membrane may result in delayed fluorescein uptake. The ultimate prognosis depends on the loss of corneal clarity and degree of limbal ischemia, graded on a scale of I to IV. Patients with mild injuries (grade I) may be treated with a cycloplegic (avoiding mydriatics such as phenylephrine due to their vasoconstrictor effects), a topical antibiotic (e.g., erythromycin), and oral pain medication. These patients should be seen by an ophthalmologist daily until healing is documented, after which they may return to duty in the absence of visually significant complications. Patients with moderate to severe injuries (grades II to IV) warrant emergent ophthalmologic assessment and evacuation out-of-theater. Subsequent treatment will focus on lysis of adhesions, minimizing infection potential, and treatment of iritis and elevated IOP. Long-term complications of chemical injuries include corneal scarring and neovascularization, adhesions of the lids to the globe (symblepharon), glaucoma, cataracts, and retinal necrosis.

## *Traumatic Optic Neuropathy*

Traumatic optic neuropathy (i.e., injury to the optic nerve) may occur with blunt or penetrating ocular trauma. It is often associated with a blow to the eyebrow or forehead, the force of which can be transmitted through the orbital roof to the optic canal. Patients with traumatic optic neuropathy typically note an immediate and profound loss of vision and present with an afferent papillary defect.[56] The optic disc usually appears normal upon initial fundoscopic examination, as optic disc pallor can take several weeks to develop following the injury. The underlying etiology of nerve injury may be nerve compression, transection, or ischemic injury.[57] The diagnosis of traumatic optic neuropathy is typically made only after other causes of vision loss are excluded by an ophthalmologist. Computed tomography imaging often shows associated orbital fractures, but radiographically evident optic canal fractures are much less common.[58] Therapeutic options for traumatic optic neuropathy include high-dose corticosteroids or surgical decompression of the optic nerve if impingement is suspected. However, controversy remains over the efficacy of these treatments. The International Optic Nerve Trauma Study, the most extensive prospective study of traumatic optic neuropathy to date, showed no definitive benefit from either steroids or surgery, and both of these modalities can pose significant potential risks to the multisystem trauma patient.[59] The decision to treat should be individualized for each patient, taking into account their ocular status, mechanism of injury, presence of fracture on CT scan, and comorbid conditions.

Traumatic optic neuropathy may occur following blunt or penetrating ocular trauma. Patients with traumatic optic neuropathy typically note an immediate and profound loss of vision and present with an afferent papillary defect.

# Summary

The basic principles of ocular trauma management in combat do not differ significantly from those followed in the civilian sector. Recent developments during OEF and OIF in casualty evacuation and combat trauma systems have facilitated the delivery of ocular trauma care which replicates the standards of care maintained in civilian trauma system. However, the overall severity and complexity of these injuries are generally much greater in combat, calling for the utmost skill and dedication from military ophthalmologists and other combat health support personnel. Combat casualty care providers at Level I and II facilities must be able to recognize ocular injuries that require further evacuation and take appropriate steps to protect the eye during transport. Ophthalmologists at Level III facilities must be prepared to make difficult clinical decisions and perform technically challenging surgery within the physical and operational constraints of the theater level hospital. Every attempt should be made to repair open-globe injuries, except for severely ruptured globes in patients for whom proper access to further ophthalmologic care is doubtful. Given the frequent association of ocular injuries with head, face, and neck injuries, ophthalmologists should expect to work in close conjunction with surgeons in other specialties, particularly neurosurgery, otolaryngology, oral maxillofacial surgery, and facial plastic surgery.

# Case Studies

## *Case 1*

A 26-year-old male enlisted soldier arrived intubated at a Level III hospital after sustaining a blast injury to his head and face from an IED. Examination of his right eye revealed a large perilimbal scleral laceration with uveal prolapse and a large complex laceration to his right upper eyelid and brow (Fig. 33). His left eye was markedly proptotic and resistant to retropulsion, with marked upper eyelid edema and ecchymosis, a mid-dilated non-reactive pupil, and inferior hemorrhagic chemosis (Fig. 34). Based

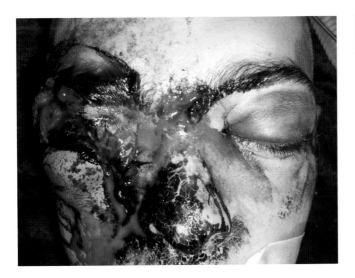

Figure 33. *Preoperative photograph of a combat casualty following blast injury to the head and face from an IED.*

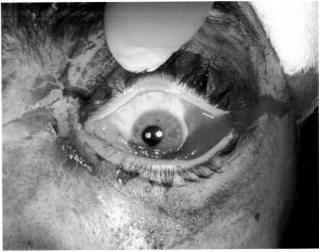

Figure 34. *Left eye proptosis, lid ecchymosis, hemorrhagic chemosis, and mid-dilated pupil indicative of retrobulbar hemorrhage. Lateral canthotomy and inferior cantholysis have been performed.*

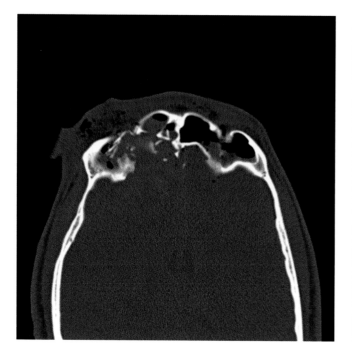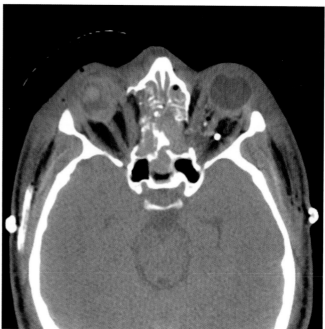

Figure 35. *Computed tomography image showing:* (Left) *Severe bilateral frontal sinus fractures and frontal lobe injury.* (Right) *Deformed right globe with intraocular hemorrhage, bilateral ethmoid fractures, and left retrobulbar hemorrhage with intraorbital foreign body. The foreign body has passed through the right orbit and both ethmoid sinuses and entered the left orbit.*

on these clinical findings, a left orbital compartment syndrome was suspected and a lateral canthotomy and inferior cantholysis were immediately performed in the emergency room. Subsequent CT scan revealed a misshapened right globe with lens disruption and vitreous hemorrhage, fractures of both ethmoid sinuses with a metallic foreign body and retrobulbar hemorrhage in the left orbit, fractures of both frontal sinuses, and a penetrating injury of the right frontal lobe (Fig. 35).

The patient was emergently taken to the operating room, where a craniotomy was performed with a partial right frontal lobectomy, cranialization of the frontal sinuses, and reconstruction of the floor of the anterior cranial fossa with titanium mesh,

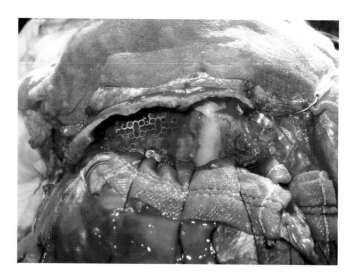

Figure 36. *Intraoperative view of frontal craniotomy showing bilateral frontal sinus cranialization and repair of floor of anterior cranial fossa.*

fibrin tissue sealant, and a pericranial graft (Fig. 36). Attention was then turned to the right eye, where a 25 mm scleral laceration was repaired with 8-0 nylon sutures after repositing the prolapsed ciliary body back into the globe (Fig. 37). The right upper lid and brow laceration were then addressed (Fig. 38). A lateral canthotomy and superior cantholysis were first performed in order to reduce the tension on the eyelid reconstruction and prevent undue pressure on the freshly repaired globe. The tarsus was then repaired with interrupted 6-0 polyglactin sutures, taking 90 percent-thickness bites of the tarsus and tying the knots on the anterior side. The lid margin was approximated at the gray line and lash line with 6-0 silk sutures. The remainder of the upper lid and brow laceration was repaired in layers with deep 5-0 polydiaxanone sutures

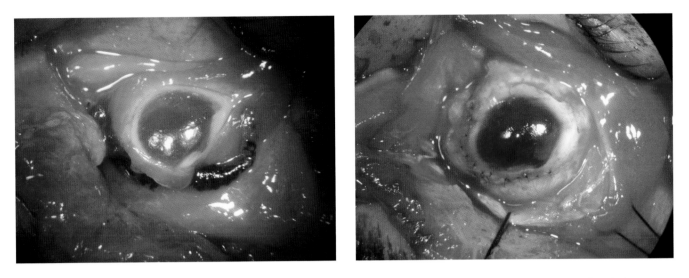

Figure 37. *Intraoperative photograph of right globe before* (Left) *and after* (Right) *scleral laceration repair. Note the prolapsed ciliary body.*

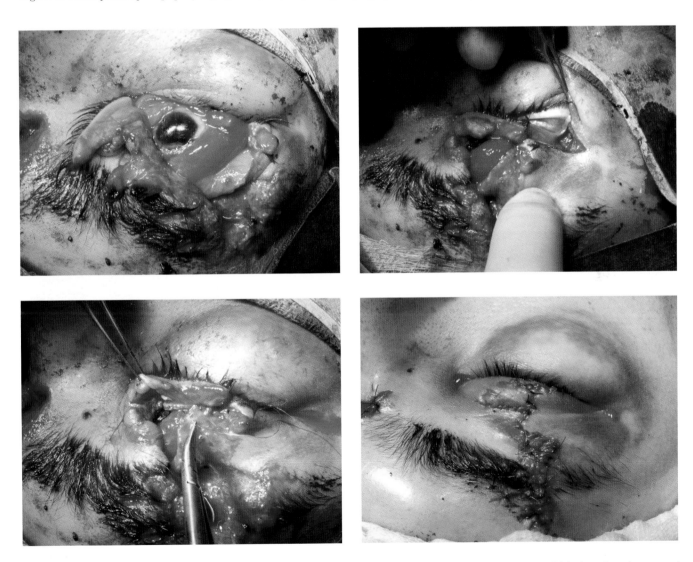

Figure 38. *Repair of complex right upper lid and brow laceration:* (Middle Left) *View of defect.* (Middle Right) *Right lateral canthotomy and superior cantholysis.* (Bottom Left) *Repair of upper tarsus.* (Bottom Right) *Completed repair of right upper lid and eyebrow.*

and interrupted 5-0 Prolene® skin sutures, taking care to properly align the brow hairs. Following surgery, the patient was promptly evacuated out-of-theater and subsequently received follow-up care at a Level V facility. His blind painful right eye was enucleated within two weeks of the injury.

This case demonstrates the complexity of the head and facial injuries that are often seen concomitantly with ocular combat injuries. The vision-threatening orbital compartment syndrome of the left eye was quickly diagnosed based on clinical findings in the absence of radiographic confirmation and appropriately treated with canthotomy and cantholysis. Surgical intervention proceeded in an orderly fashion, dealing with the intracranial injury

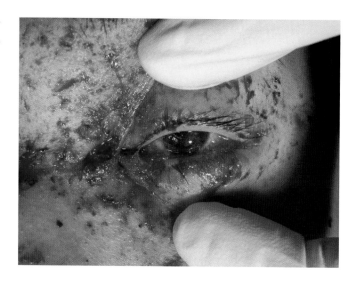

Figure 39. *Photograph showing multiple punctate facial lacerations caused by glass foreign bodies.*

first, followed by the ruptured globe repair, and finally the eyelid and brow laceration repair. Removal of the left orbital metallic foreign body was not attempted, as it posed no immediate risk to the globe and very little risk of long-term complication.

## Case 2

This 24-year-old male enlisted soldier was injured when a rocket-propelled grenade struck the windshield of his vehicle. Upon evaluation at the Level III hospital, it was apparent that he had sustained multiple glass foreign bodies to his face (Fig. 39). On CT scan, two IOFBs were present in the left eye, along with multiple

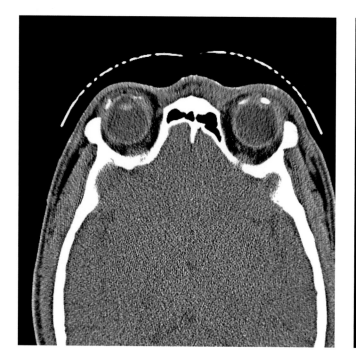
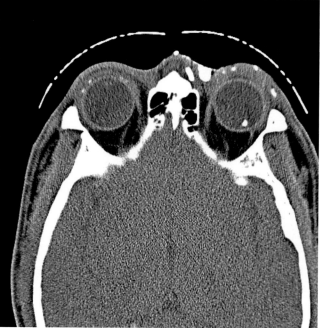

Figure 40. *Preoperative CT scan showing glass foreign bodies in the anterior segment (Left) and posterior segment (Right) of the left eye. Note multiple additional soft-tissue and subconjunctival foreign bodies.*

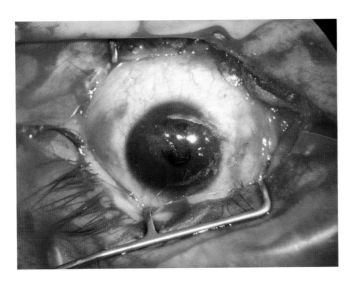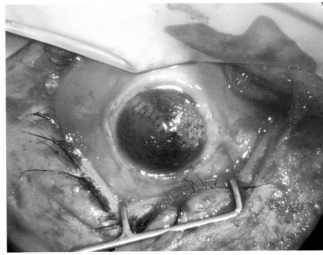

Figure 41. *Intraoperative photos before* (Left) *and after* (Right) *repair of two separate corneal lacerations, left eye. Note the cyanoacrylate glue plug over the inferonasal laceration, which obscures the underlying 10-0 nylon sutures.*

bilateral subconjunctival foreign bodies (Fig. 40). One of the foreign bodies was located in the anterior segment, and the other was in the posterior segment near the posterior pole. The patient was taken to the operating room, where the anterior chamber foreign body was easily removed through the corneal laceration it had created. The curvilinear inferotemporal laceration was repaired with multiple 10-0 nylon sutures. The second foreign body had entered the eye through the inferonasal cornea, perforated the iris and crystalline lens, and come to rest in the vitreous cavity just over the macula. The resulting stellate corneal laceration, although smaller than the first laceration, proved much more difficult to repair. A watertight closure could not be achieved with multiple 10-0 nylon sutures placed at all angles across the wound. Thus, a plug of cyanoacrylate glue was placed over the suture scaffold, with the aid of viscoelastic in the anterior chamber to prevent aqueous leakage (Figs. 41 and 42). Once a watertight seal was obtained, a bandage contact lens was placed. No attempt was made to retrieve the posterior segment foreign body. Prophylactic topical and intravenous fluoroquinolones were administered. No intravitreal antibiotics were used. The patient was evacuated to a Level V hospital, where his traumatic cataract was extracted and the retained foreign body was successfully removed by a retina specialist (Fig. 43). Visual acuity at last known follow-up was 20/25 with an aphakic rigid gas-permeable contact lens.

This case illustrates the management of corneal lacerations and IOFBs. The size of the corneal laceration does not always correlate with the difficulty of wound repair, and cyanoacrylate glue can be a valuable tool when sutures alone are inadequate in achieving a watertight closure. Foreign bodies in the anterior segment can often be safely removed, but removal of posterior segment foreign bodies should be deferred to a vitreoretinal specialist at Level IV or V facilities.

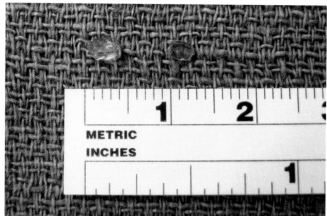

Figure 42. (Top Right) *Anterior segment and subconjunctival foreign bodies after removal.*

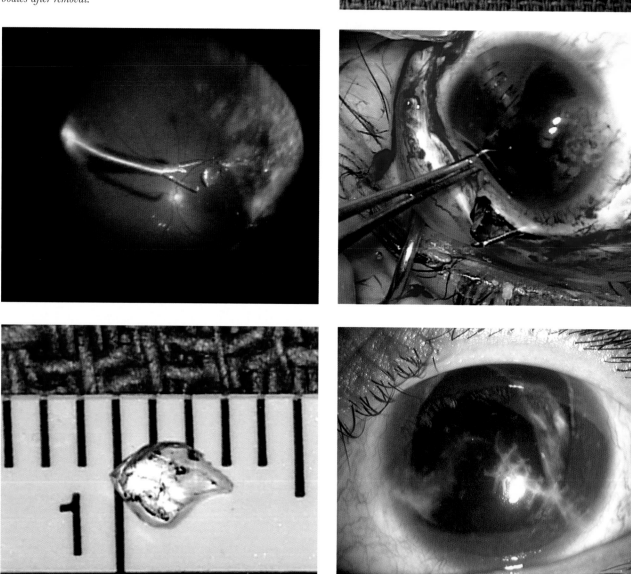

Figure 43. *Intraoperative photographs showing removal of posterior segment foreign body at Level V hospital:* (Middle Left) *IOFB being grasped with basket forceps and* (Middle Right) *removed through a scleral tunnel incision.* (Bottom Left) *IOFB after removal.* (Bottom Right) *Slit-lamp photograph at four-month postoperative visit. Images courtesy of Eric D. Weichel, M.D.*

# References

1. Wong TY, Seet MB, Ang CL. Eye injuries in twentieth century warfare: a historical perspective. Surv Ophthalmol 1997;41(6):433-459.

2. Owens BD, Kragh JF Jr, Wenke JC, et al. Combat wounds in Operation Iraqi Freedom and Operation Enduring Freedom. J Trauma 2008;64(2):295-299.

3. Mader TH, Carroll RD, Slade CS, et al. Ocular war injuries of the Iraqi insurgency, January-September 2004. Ophthalmology 2006;113(1):97-104.

4. Thach AB, Johnson AJ, Carroll RB, et al. Severe eye injuries in the war in Iraq, 2003-2005. Ophthalmology 2008;155(2):377-382.

5. Cho RI, Bakken HE, Reynolds ME, et al. Concomitant cranial and ocular combat injuries during Operation Iraqi Freedom. J Trauma 2009;67(3):516-520.

6. Hornblass A. Eye injuries in the military. Int Ophthalmol Clin 1981;21(4):121-138.

7. Handler JA, Ghezzi KT. General ophthalmologic examination. Emerg Med Clin North Am 1995;13(2):521-538.

8. Juang PS, Rosen P. Ocular examination techniques for the emergency department. J Emerg Med 1997;15(6):793-810.

9. Linden JA, Renner GS. Trauma to the globe. Emerg Med Clin North Am 1995;13(3):581-605.

10. Hutton WL, Fuller DG. Factors influencing final visual results in the severely injured eyes. Am J Ophthalmol 1994;97(6):715-722.

11. Kylstra JA, Lamkin JC, Runyan DK. Clinical predictors of scleral rupture after blunt ocular trauma. Am J Ophthalmol 1993;115(4):530-535.

12. Sheldrick JH, Vernon SA, Wilson A. Study of diagnostic accord between general practitioners and an ophthalmologist. BMJ 1992;304(6834):1096-1098.

13. Lustrin ES, Brown JH, Novelline R, et al. Radiologic assessment of trauma and foreign bodies of the eye and orbit. Neuroimaging Clin North Am 1996;6(1):219-237.

14. Otto PM, Otto RA, Virapongese C, et al. Screening test for the detection of metallic foreign bodies in the orbit before magnetic resonance imaging. Invest Radiol 1992;27(4):308-311.

15. McNicholas MM, Brophy DP, Power WJ, et al. Ocular trauma: evaluation with US. Radiology 1995;195(2):423-427.

16. Zuravleff JJ, Johnson MH. An ophthalmic surgeon's view of orbital imaging techniques. Semin Ultrasound CT MR 1997;18(6):395-402.

17. Rocha G, Brunette I, Le Francois M. Severe toxic keratopathy secondary to topical anesthetic abuse. Can J Ophthalmol 1995;30(4):198-202.

18. Kitsos G, Gartzios C, Asproudis I, et al. Central corneal thickness in subjects with glaucoma and in normal individuals (with or without pseudoexfoliation syndrome). Clin Ophthalmol 2009;3:537-542.

19. Sklar DP, Lauth JE, Johnson DR. Topical anesthesia of the eye as a diagnostic test. Ann Emerg Med 1989;18(11):1209-1211.

20. Talbot EM. A simple test to diagnose iritis. Br J Med 1987;295(6602):812-813.

21. Netland KE, Martinez J, LaCour OJ III, et al. Traumatic anterior lens dislocation: a case report. J Emerg Med 1999;17(4):637-639.

22. Spraul CW, Grossniklaus HE. Vitreous hemorrhage. Surv Ophthalmol 1997;42(1):3-39.

23. Olsen TW, Chang TS, Sternberg P Jr. Retinal detachments associated with blunt trauma. Semin Ophthalmol 1995;10(1):17-27.

24. Berlin R. Zur sogenannten commotio retinae. Klin Monatsbl Augenheilkd 1873;11:42-78.

25. Reppucci VS, Movshovich A. Current concepts in the treatment of traumatic injury to the anterior segment. Ophthalmol Clin North Am 1999;12(3):465-474.

26. Kuhn F, Maisiak R, Mann L, et al. The Ocular Trauma Score (OTS). Ophthalmol Clin North Am 2002;15(2):163-165.

27. Weichel ED, Colyer MH, Ludlow SE, et al. Combat ocular trauma visual outcomes during operations Iraqi and enduring freedom. Ophthalmology 2008; 115(12):2235-2245.

28. Barr CC. Prognostic factors in corneoscleral lacerations. Arch Ophthalmol 1983;101(6):919-924.

29. Chidiac EJ, Raiskin AO. Succinylcholine and the open eye. Ophthalmol Clin North Am 2006;19(2):279-285.

30. Mills MD, Devenyi RG, Lam WC, et al. An assessment of intraocular pressure rise in patients with gas-filled eyes during simulated air flight. Ophthalmology 2001;108(1):40-44.

31. Lincoff H, Weinberger D, Stergiu P. Air travel with intraocular gas. II. Clinical considerations. Arch Ophthalmol 1989;107(6):907-910.

32. Thompson JT. The absorption of mixtures of air and perfluoropropane after pars plana vitrectomy.

Arch Ophthalmol 1992;110(11):1594-1597.

33. Duch-Samper AM, Chaqués-Alepuz V, Menezo JL, et al. Endophthalmitis following open-globe injuries. Curr Opin Ophthalmol 1998;9(3):III:59-65.

34. Mittra RA, Mieler WF. Controversies in the management of open-globe injuries involving the posterior segment. Surv Ophthalmol 1999;44(3):215-225.

35. Colyer MH, Weber ED, Weichel ED, et al. Delayed intraocular foreign body removal without endophthalmitis during Operations Iraqi Freedom and Enduring Freedom. Ophthalmology 2007;114(8): 1439-1447.

36. Albert DM, Diaz-Rohena R. A historical review of sympathetic ophthalmia and its epidemiology. Surv Ophthalmol 1989;34(1):1-14.

37. Ward TP. Sympathetic ophthalmia. In Thach AB, ed. Ophthalmic Care of the Combat Casualty. Washington, DC: Borden Institute, Walter Reed Army Medical Center; 2003. p. 265-279.

38. DeBacker CM, Holck DEE. Enucleation in orbital trauma. In: Holck DEE, Ng JD, editors. Evaluation and treatment of orbital fractures: a multidisciplinary approach. 2nd ed. Philadelphia: Elsevier Saunders; 2006. p. 365-368.

39. Kaltreider SA, Lucarelli MJ. A simple algorithm for selection of implant size for enucleation and evisceration: a prospective study. Ophthal Plast Reconstr Surg 2002;18(5):336-341.

40. Nasr AM, Haik BG, Fleming JC, et al. Penetrating orbital injury with organic foreign bodies. Ophthalmology 1999;106(3):523-532.

41. Finklestein M, Legmann A, Rubin PA. Projectile metallic foreign bodies in the orbit: a retrospective study of epidemiologic factors, management, and outcomes. Ophthalmology 1997;104(1):96-103.

42. Khani SC, Mukai S. Posterior segment intraocular foreign bodies. Int Ophthalmol Clin 1995;35(1):151-161.

43. Punnonen E, Laatikainen L. Prognosis of perforating eye injuries with intraocular foreign bodies. Acta Ophthalmol (Copenh) 1989;67(5):483-491.

44. Packer AJ. Ocular trauma. Primary Care 1982;9(4):777-792.

45. Cohen EJ, Rapuano CL. Trauma. In: Cullom RD, Chang B, editors. The Wills eye manual: office and emergency room diagnosis and treatment of eye disease. 2nd ed. Philadelphia, PA: JB Lippincott; 1994. p. 27.

46. Fry HJ. Orbital decompression after facial fractures. Med J Aust 1967;1(6):264-266.

47. Hislop WS, Dutton GN, Douglas PS. Treatment of retrobulbar haemorrhage in accident and emergency departments. Br J Oral Maxillofac Surg 1996;34(4):289-292.

48. Hayreh SS, Kolder HE, Weingeist TA. Central retinal artery occlusion and retinal tolerance time. Ophthalmology 1980;87(1):75-78.

49. Burkat CN, Lemke BN. Retrobulbar hemorrhage: inferolateral anterior orbitotomy for emergent management. Arch Ophthalmol 2005;123(9):1260-1262.

50. Ho VH, Wilson MW, Fleming JC, et al. Retained intraorbital foreign bodies. Ophthal Plas Reconstr Surg 2004;20(3):232-236.

51. Cho RI, Kahana A, Patel B, et al. Intraoperative fluoroscopy-guided removal of orbital foreign bodies. Ophthal Plast Reconstr Surg 2009;25(3):215-218.

52. Pfister RR. Chemical injuries of the eye. Ophthalmology 1983;90(10):1246-1253.

53. Grant WM. Toxicology of the eye. 3rd ed. Springfield, MA: Charles C Thomas; 1986.

54. Herr RO, White GL Jr, Bernhisel K, et al. Clinical comparison of ocular irrigation fluids following chemical injury. Am J Emerg Med 1991;9(3):228-231.

55. Wagoner MD. Chemical injuries of the eye: current concepts of pathophysiology and therapy. Survey Ophthalmol 1997;41(4):275-313.

56. Shoff WH, Sheperd SM. Ocular trauma. In: Ferrera PC, Colucciello SA, Marx JA, et al, editors. Trauma management: an emergency medicine approach. 1st ed. St Louis, MO: Mosby; 2001. p. 197-217.

57. Villarreal PM. Traumatic optic neuropathy. A case report. Int J Oral Maxillofac Surg 2000;29(1):29-31.

58. Wang BH, Robertson BC, Girotto JA, et al. Traumatic optic neuropathy: a review of 61 patients. Plast Reconstr Surg 2001;107(7):1655-1664.

59. Levin LA, Beck RW, Joseph MP, et al. The treatment of traumatic optic neuropathy: The International Optic Nerve Trauma Study. Ophthalmology 1999;106(7):1268-1277.

# TRAUMATIC BRAIN INJURY

*Chapter 8*

**Contributing Authors**
Scott A. Marshall, MD
Randy Bell, MD
Rocco A. Armonda, MD, LTC, MC, US Army
Eric Savitsky, MD
Geoffrey S.F. Ling, MD, PhD, COL, MC, US Army

All figures and tables included in this chapter have been used with permission from Pelagique, LLC, the UCLA Center for International Medicine, and/or the authors, unless otherwise noted.

Use of imagery from the Defense Imagery Management Operations Center (DIMOC) does not imply or constitute Department of Defense (DOD) endorsement of this company, its products, or services.

**Disclaimer**
The opinions and views expressed herein belong solely to those of the authors. They are not nor should they be implied as being endorsed by the United States Uniformed Services University of the Health Sciences, Department of the Army, Department of the Navy, Department of the Air Force, Department of Defense, or any other branch of the federal government.

# Table of Contents

# Introduction

Traumatic brain injury (TBI) occurs whenever a physical force that impacts the head leads to neuropathology. This can be as simple as a minor laceration from a small fragment to decapitation. Of all the injuries to the head that are concerning, the most worrisome is TBI.

Traumatic brain injury is a leading cause of death and disability from trauma. In the United States (US), more than 50,000 patients die from TBI each year, accounting for almost one-third of all civilian trauma-related deaths.[1] Most of these injuries are a direct result of falls, motor vehicle accidents, and assaults. The cost for direct TBI medical care is estimated at more than $50 billion per year.[2,3] The majority of victims of both civilian and military TBI are young male adults.[4,5] The societal burden of TBI is staggering. Traumatic brain injury accounts for the greatest number of years lived with trauma-related disability.[5] Many victims of TBI are young and thus require extended rehabilitation and reintegration. Many will likely require medical discharge from the armed forces. The young age of many TBI victims is especially unfortunate as these patients may no longer be productive members of society at a time in their life when their potential contributions are greatest.[4]

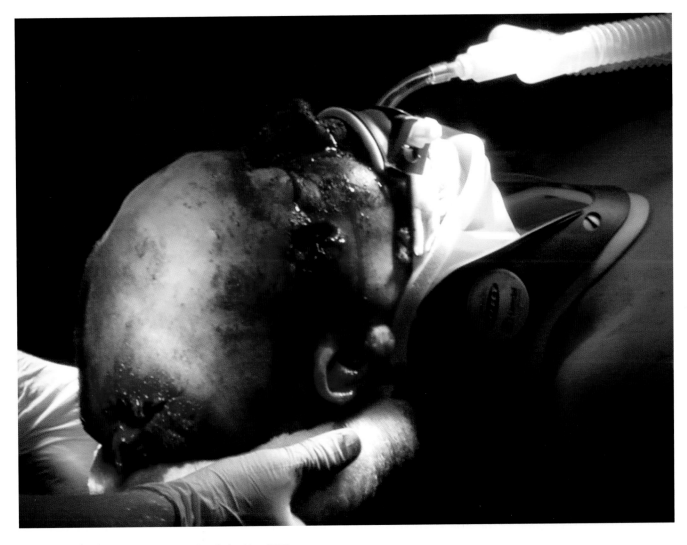

Figure 1. *A US casualty who sustained explosive blast TBI.*

Traumatic brain injury is a common battle-related injury. In the wars of the 20<sup>th</sup> century, approximately 15 to 20 percent of injuries incurred in combat involved the head.[6] Evidence suggests that this is also the case for casualties sustained in the recent wars, Operation Enduring Freedom (OEF) in Afghanistan and Operation Iraqi Freedom (OIF) (Fig. 1).[7] Some have speculated that a greater percentage of patients from these recent wars have suffered head injury than in prior conflicts.[8] This increase in prevalence is thought to be a paradoxical consequence of the remarkable improvements in medical care and protective body armor.[9] These advances have resulted in the lowest killed-to-wounded ratio in modern warfare.[10] The paradox is that with more wounded warfighters surviving, more are left with severe wounds, especially to less protected anatomical regions such as head and extremities. Thus, TBI, traumatic amputations, and other such injuries are disproportionally represented. Specifically, TBI resulting from explosive blast has become very prominent in the past several years.[11,12,13]

> Traumatic brain injury is a common battle-related injury. Treatment goals in the first 72 hours of care for the injured patient with TBI are to provide clinical stability, arrest any element of ongoing injury, preserve neurological function, and prevent medical complications secondary to multisystem trauma.

With advances in battlefield or prehospital clinical management of combat casualties, the outcomes of severe conditions such as TBI have improved. Critical elements include improved training and resources for far-forward medical providers, a highly efficient modern triage and evacuation system, and dramatically shortened length of stay in-theater prior to definitive care in the US.[14] There is evidence that the vast majority of fatal injuries incurred in combat result from injuries that would be nonsurvivable in any setting.[15] Thus, those who can be saved are being saved, even under the austere conditions of war. However, as long as there are survivors left with chronic disabilities, there is opportunity for improvements in medical care.

Treatment goals in the first 72 hours of care for the injured patient with TBI are to provide clinical stability, arrest any element of ongoing injury, preserve neurological function, and prevent medical complications secondary to severe trauma. Initially, brain injury must be suspected, and this must be followed by appropriate field management. Next, TBI patients should be triaged and evacuated to a Level III facility with advanced care capability, such as neurosurgery and neurointensive care. Subsequently, as appropriate, TBI patients are evacuated from theater to the continental US (CONUS) for advanced definitive treatment.

The purpose of this review is to outline the intricacies common to both military and civilian TBI, discuss different forms of closed and penetrating TBI, and expand upon the distinction between primary and secondary brain injuries. A review of the literature outlining various treatment algorithms, both medical and surgical, will also be provided.

## Pathophysiology of Traumatic Brain Injury

Primary brain injury is tissue destruction that occurs as a direct result of a physiologic trauma. This leads to near immediate macroscopic and cellular pathological changes. The severity and location of the primary brain injury will dictate the patient's immediate level of consciousness, mental status, and focal neurologic signs. There is no available therapy for primary brain injury at present. The focus of TBI treatment is minimizing secondary brain injury. Secondary brain injury refers to the consequences of pathological processes that begin immediately after the primary brain injury. Secondary brain injury continues for an indefinite period and can cause further dysfunction and death of neurons and glial supporting structures.

> The immediate goal of TBI treatment is minimizing secondary brain injury by optimizing cerebral blood flow. This involves mitigating elevations in ICP and addressing traumatic intracranial hemorrhage, cerebral edema, and metabolic derangements.

Quantifiably, it is widely held that most of the overall brain injury may be ascribable to secondary injury processes. Mechanisms thought to be involved in secondary brain injury include hypoxia, ischemia, free radicals, release of neurotransmitters and intracellular elements (e.g., calcium), temperature dysregulation, intracranial pressure alterations, gene activation, mitochondrial dysfunction, and inflammation.[5,16] Among these, hypoperfusion is the main cause of poor outcomes.[5,17] This is due to the susceptibility of injured neural tissue to ischemia, as it is in a hypermetabolic state following injury. This is exacerbated by dysfunction of cerebral vascular autoregulation so that there is insufficient vascular compensation for compromised cerebral perfusion. Particularly susceptible areas include the hippocampus and border zone or watershed regions such as the high parietal region. It has been hypothesized that delayed neurological dysfunction can often be attributed to the effects of delayed ischemia.[16,18] To this effect, there is evidence that a single episode of hypotension with systolic blood pressures falling below 90 mm Hg is associated with poor outcomes in severe TBI.[16,18,19] Hypoperfusion itself may result in diffuse microvascular damage and loss of blood-brain barrier integrity. This microvascular damage contributes to the prominent pattern of vasogenic edema observed after TBI.[20] Current guidelines likewise caution of the dangers of hypocapnea and hypoxia as markers for poor outcomes following TBI.[16,18,19,21]

> Hypotension (systolic blood pressure less than 90 mm Hg) leading to cerebral hypoperfusion has been linked to poor outcomes following severe TBI.

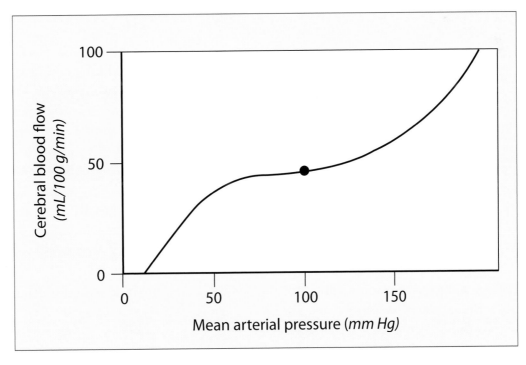

Figure 2. *Cerebral blood flow is well-autoregulated when mean arterial pressures are between 50 to 150 mm Hg.*

Research attempts at developing therapeutic strategies have focused on secondary brain injury processes while public health and technological measures have attempted to prevent primary brain injury. Currently, clinical management centers on supportive measures to mitigate secondary brain injury with particular emphasis on maintaining cerebral perfusion pressure (CPP) and tissue oxygenation, minimizing intracranial pressure (ICP) fluctuations, and treatment of cerebral edema. Various alternative experimental pharmacological therapies (e.g., free radical scavengers) and neuroprotective strategies have been investigated (e.g., therapeutic hypothermia). Unfortunately, none of these experimental therapies or strategies has been proven to effectively mitigate secondary brain injury.[22]

With regard to cerebral autoregulation, cerebral blood flow (normal values 50 to 65 milliliters [ml] per 100 grams of brain tissue per minute) is well-autoregulated when mean arterial pressures (MAPs) are between 50 to 150 mm Hg (Fig. 2). Cerebral blood flow (CBF) is a function of cerebral vascular resistance (CVR) and cerebral perfusion pressure. Since cerebral vascular resistance is proportional to the fourth power of blood vessel radius, even small changes in cerebral vessel caliber translates into significant alterations in CBF. Cerebral perfusion pressure is the pressure gradient driving CBF, and is defined as the difference between mean arterial pressure and ICP (Equation 1).

$$\text{Equation 1: CPP} = \text{MAP} - \text{ICP}$$

$$\text{Equation 2: CBF} = \text{CPP}/\text{CVR}$$

Primary brain injuries often lead to alterations in the brain's ability to autoregulate CBF even within the normal autoregulatory range.[23] This may further worsen secondary brain injury, in that loss of autoregulatory control may lead to increased CBF with changes in blood pressure and resultant increased intracranial blood volume and disruption of the blood-brain barrier with vasogenic brain edema formation. This may ultimately result in elevated ICP. Alternatively, cerebral ischemia may result if CBF is too low (i.e., less than 20 ml per 100 grams of brain tissue per minute), and the neurovasculature is unable to compensate by autoregulatory vessel dilation to maintain CBF.

It should be emphasized that hypercapnia is a potent vasodilator of cerebral microvasculature, as is hypoxemia. These states may result in cerebral hyperemia and exacerbation of preexisting elevated ICP.[24] Hyperventilation with resultant hypocapnia has a profound effect in causing cerebral microvasculature vasoconstriction.[25] This microvasculature vasoconstrictive response to hypocapnia is often well-preserved, even in the setting of devastating brain injury. Hyperventilation leading to hypocapnia will lead to a progressive decrease in ICP.[25] Loss of ICP responsiveness to hypocapnia is a poor prognostic sign. Hypocapnia will also result in decreases in CBF; every one mm Hg decrease in the partial pressure of carbon dioxide ($PCO_2$) will result in a proportionate three percent decrease in CBF.[26,27] It is important to understand the relationship between hypocapnia and CBF, as well as how hyperventilation and hypocapnia relate to ICP.

> Hyperventilation leading to hypocapnia will cause a progressive decrease in ICP. Loss of ICP responsiveness to hypocapnia is a poor prognostic sign.

Delayed cerebral swelling is the major cause of raised ICP and death. This is often the result of secondary brain injury. Persistent bleeding from damaged brain tissue, contusions, impaired autoregulation, and

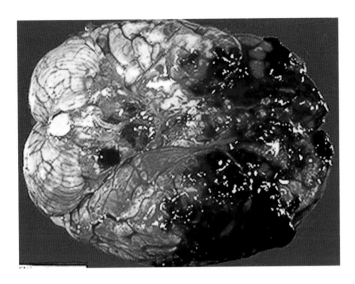

Figure 3. *Persistent bleeding from damaged brain tissue, contusions, impaired autoregulation, and breakdown of the blood-brain barrier may all contribute to brain swelling. Image courtesy of Brian J. Eastridge, MD, FACS, COL, US Army*

breakdown of the blood-brain barrier may all contribute to brain swelling (Fig. 3).[28] This swelling with resultant compression and distortion of brain parenchyma further exacerbates the injury cascade. The Monroe-Kellie doctrine is a convenient method of understanding factors leading to elevated intracranial pressures. It postulates that due to the fixed size of the intracranial compartment, an increase in volume of any of the three intracranial constituents (blood, brain, and cerebrospinal fluid) must be compensated by a decrease in one or more of the other constituents, or ICP will rise.[29,30]

Systemic complications directly related to severe head injuries are not uncommon. Neurogenic pulmonary edema is a well-described phenomenon associated with secondary brain injury.[31,32] Primary myocardial ischemia and dysrhythmias are often seen in the setting of secondary brain injury. Although the exact mechanisms are still unclear, it is theorized that these processes are the result of greatly elevated circulating catecholamine levels.[33] Brain tissue is also rich in thromboplastins, and release of these in secondary brain injury patients may result in the development of a coagulopathy.[34] The syndromes of cerebral salt wasting and the syndrome of inappropriate antidiuretic hormone secretion (SIADH) are also seen in the setting of secondary brain injury.[35,36]

## Closed Head Injury

Head injury can be broadly classified into closed versus penetrating head injury (Figs. 4 and 5). With closed head injury, the skull and overlying scalp remain intact. In closed head injury, direct impact of brain against the skull and shearing force upon neurovascular structures from rotational forces result in cell damage at the cell body and axonal level. Among civilians in the US, most closed head injury is due to motor vehicle accidents, but other causes include falls, sporting event injuries, and assault.[37] In studies analyzing US casualties in OIF, some have reported between 5 and 10 percent of all casualties sustained a closed head injury.[38] Neuronal structures strike the skull in both the direct and opposite planes of motion leading to a coup and contrecoup lesion pattern. Contusion or other injury to the brain is seen deep to the site of skull impact, as well as 180 degrees opposite the site of impact (Fig. 6). If there is a rotational component, structures will torque and twist, and thus shearing can occur. This results in diffuse axonal injury seen radiographically as punctuate hemorrhages on computed tomography (CT) or magnetic resonance imaging (MRI) at interfaces of grey and white matter. Patients with diffuse axonal injury are often in a coma after their trauma without elevations in ICP and often have unsatisfactory clinical outcomes.[5]

## Mild, Moderate, and Severe Brain Injury

The spectrum of TBI is mild, moderate, or severe. Severity is based largely on the presenting Glasgow Coma

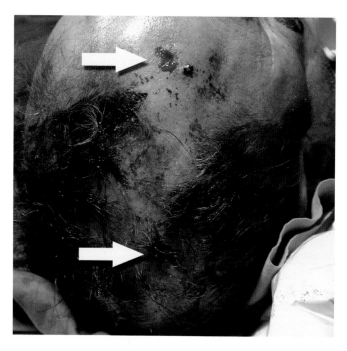

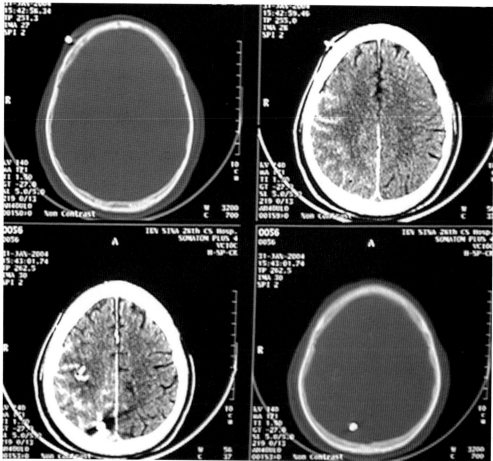

Figure 4. (Top) *The distinction between closed head injury and penetrating head injury may be difficult to make based on neurological findings. Here, one of the scalp wounds denoted by the arrows, was an entry point for a penetrating fragment that caused brain injury. Image courtesy of the Borden Institute, Office of The Surgeon General, Washington, DC.*

Figure 5. (Bottom) *Axial CT images demonstrate a right frontal extracranial fragment, traumatic subarachnoid hemorrhage, and an intracranial fragment. Image courtesy of the Borden Institute, Office of The Surgeon General, Washington, DC.*

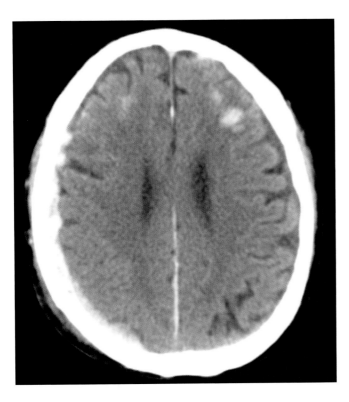

Figure 6. *Coup and contrecoup patterns of brain injury. An impact to the right parietal region has caused a left frontal intraparenchymal contusion.*

Scale (GCS) score (Table 1). These classification categories have prognostic, monitoring, and treatment implications.[39] Patients with mild TBI have an admission GCS score of greater than or equal to 13, with lower scores in this category representing more concerning injury. Mild TBI may often be referred to as concussion. These patients have experienced a brief (less than 30 min), if any, loss of consciousness or alteration in consciousness (less than 24 hrs), and presenting complaints include headache, confusion, and amnesia.[40] The spectrum of presentation and sequelae of mild TBI is broad and usually transient. When symptoms persist for three months or longer, postconcussion syndrome is diagnosed.[41] Moderate TBI is defined by an admission GCS score of 9 to 12 and is usually associated with prolonged loss of consciousness, abnormal neuroimaging, and neurological deficit.[42] Injured service members with moderate TBI will likely require rapid removal from forward areas, subsequent hospitalization, and may need neurosurgical intervention. Patients with GCS scores of 8 or less have significant neurological injury and are classified as having severe TBI. Typically, they have abnormal neuroimaging such as a CT scan demonstrating intracranial hemorrhage, often associated with a skull fracture.[42] These patients require rapid evacuation to a Level III facility and admission to the intensive care unit (ICU) for immediate airway control, breathing support with mechanical ventilation, neurosurgical evaluation, and ICP monitoring.

| BEST EYE OPENING (E) | | BEST VERBAL RESPONSE (V) | | BEST MOTOR RESPONSE (M) | |
|---|---|---|---|---|---|
| | | | | Follows commands | 6 |
| | | Oriented, alert | 5 | Localizes to pain | 5 |
| Eyes open spontaneously | 4 | Confused, appropriate | 4 | Withdrawal to pain | 4 |
| Eyes open to speech | 3 | Disoriented, inappropriate | 3 | Flexor posturing | 3 |
| Eyes open to pain | 2 | Incomprehensible speech | 2 | Extensor posturing | 2 |
| No response | 1 | No response | 1 | No response | 1 |

Table 1. *Severity of TBI is based largely on the presenting GCS score. Glasgow Coma Scale scores carry prognostic, monitoring, and treatment implications.*

## Blast Traumatic Brain Injury

Explosive blast TBI refers to TBI resulting from explosive blast exposure, and is presently classified as a subtype of TBI. The improvised explosive device (IED) is commonly implicated in explosive blast TBI in OEF and OIF.[5] Blast TBI may occur in isolation or may also be accompanied by closed head injury and/or penetrating TBI. The mechanism responsible for causing explosive blast TBI is unclear. The overpressure generated by the explosive device is the leading suspect, but other elements of the violent explosive event, such as toxins or electromagnetic pulses, might also potentially contribute.[43] Once the physical force couples to brain, the TBI itself results from a variety of local pathological effects, including impaired cerebral vascular homeostasis and formation of reactive oxygen species.[44] A recent concern is the probable large number of soldiers who have been exposed to blast and suffered a blast TBI but did not have their injury recognized or treated. This has resulted in concern over the development of psychiatric syndromes that may often be seen with blast TBI, such as post-traumatic stress disorder, anxiety, or depression. This is currently under study and the subject of much scientific and political debate.[38,45,46,47] Blast TBI is a recently recognized condition for which additional preclinical and clinical research is needed.[5]

> Psychiatric conditions such as post-traumatic stress disorder, anxiety, or depression may be seen following blast TBI.

## Second Impact Syndrome

An important caveat to the management of TBI is minimizing the risk of second impact syndrome. Though relatively uncommon, it can have devastating consequences. Second impact syndrome refers to a subsequent head injury during a recovery period from TBI that may result in significant worsening of the initial neurotrauma.[48] This has been best described among adolescents and younger TBI patients. The mechanism underlying second impact syndrome is not fully understood, and the clinical implications of second impact syndrome continues to be debated.[49,50] It is thought that impaired cerebral autoregulation, diffuse cerebral edema, and intracranial hypertension all play a role. The high mortality of second impact syndrome, up to 50 percent, is the most concerning aspect.[48] The American Academy of Neurology (AAN) guidelines for recommended periods of TBI recovery are often used to determine when soldiers with head injury may return to duty (Table 2).[40] The cited AAN guidelines are currently under review and will be updated and published in late 2011.

| SYMPTOM COMPLEX | FIRST CONCUSSION | SECOND CONCUSSION |
|---|---|---|
| Grade I: Transient confusion or cognitive impairment lasting less than 15 minutes without LOC | Remove from source of injury; frequent reevaluation; return to duty if normal cognition in 15 minutes | Return to duty in one week if no residual symptoms with physical stress or exercise |
| Grade II: Grade I symptoms but lasting greater than 15 minutes without LOC | Remove from source of injury; frequent reevaluation; no duty for one week during which medical observation continues | Return to duty in two weeks if no residual symptoms with physical stress or exercise |
| Grade III: Any degree of cognitive symptoms with LOC | Remove from source of injury; trained neurologic evaluation; consider imaging; return to duty in two weeks if asymptomatic with physical stress or exercise | Return to duty in one month if no residual symptoms with physical stress or exercise |

Table 2. *Return-to-duty guidelines following concussion. LOC, loss of conciousness. Adapted from the American Academy of Neurology Practice Parameter on Management of Concussions.*[40]

> Second impact syndrome refers to a subsequent head injury during a recovery period from TBI that may result in significant worsening of the initial neurotrauma.

## Focal versus Diffuse TBI

Closed TBI may be further classified as focal or diffuse. Focal injuries occur at the site of impact (coup injury), with neurological damage localized to those areas. This can occur wherever force is transmitted through the skull. The orbitofrontal and anterior temporal lobes are commonly affected in focal contrecoup injury. This is due to the tendency for head trauma to occur in an anterior-to-posterior direction causing the brain to move along those force vectors. As it moves, the brain traverses over the rough surface of the petrous ridge and anterior cranial fossa at the skull base leading to focal injury.

Diffuse injuries occur without the brain impacting a solid structure. This type of injury is caused by brain rotation. Because the brain is tethered by the brainstem, a severe acceleration-deceleration will cause it to rotate about this tethered axis. Axons in cerebral white matter will be disrupted, leading to axonal swelling and subsequent axonal rupture.[51] This condition is known as diffuse axonal injury. It is associated with severe neurological deficits and encephalopathy, including coma. The CT appearance of this type of injury can be delayed by up to 12 hours following initial trauma.[20] Recent evidence also suggests that the incidence of diffuse axonal injury may be higher with forces occurring in a lateral orientation, as opposed to a frontal or oblique impact common in closed head injury.[52]

## Epidural and Subdural Hematomas

In both focal and diffuse TBI, one must remain vigilant for intracranial hematomas. Such hemorrhages occur immediately or can be delayed as long as several days after the inciting trauma.[16,18] The highest risk of intracranial hematoma is within the first six to nine hours after injury.[53]

### Subdural Hematomas

Subdural hematomas are frequent occurrences in civilian neurosurgical practice (Fig. 7). Subdural hematomas account for over 15 percent of combat-related head injuries.[11] These lesions often require neurosurgical evacuation. The need for surgery is predicated on the clinical status of the patient and radiological appearance of the subdural hematoma. Subdural hematomas that require surgery are greater than 10 millimeters (mm) or cause more than five mm of midline shift with effacement of the basal cisterns. Other indications for surgery are a GCS score of 8 or less with enlarging intracranial lesions or deterioration in clinical exam.[54] This approach must take into consideration circumstances where outcomes are decidedly unfavorable such as advanced age, hematoma volume greater than 90 milliliters, presenting GCS score of 3, and time to surgery more than six hours.[55,56] There is conflicting evidence regarding optimal timing of evacuation, although most favor prompt evacuation once the indication exists.[56,57,58] Smaller subdural hematomas may be managed conservatively utilizing close neurological monitoring and early follow-up neuroimaging.[59] If there is concern that a lesion is enlarging, or that the patient's neurologic exam may decline, then immediate transfer to a facility with neurosurgical and neurointensivist care is justified. In lieu of the ability to transfer, the placement of burr holes for the evacuation of a subdural hematoma by a general surgeon has been described (Fig. 8).[60] Treacy et al. described a number of neurosurgical procedures (including burr holes) performed on patients in remote environments by general surgeons.[60] Three hundred and five procedures were performed over a 12-year

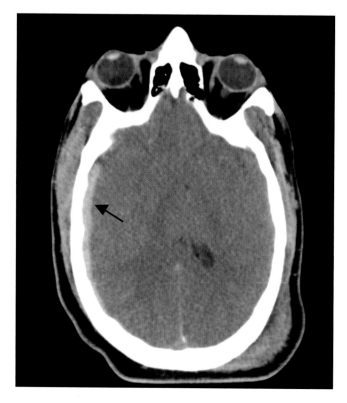

Figure 7. *Acute subdural hematoma.*

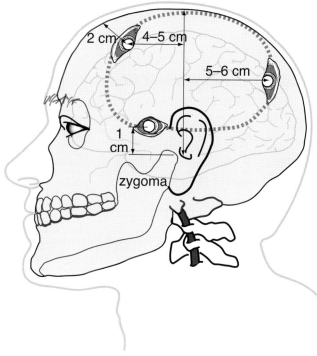

Figure 8. *Cranial landmarks and location for standard burr holes. Image courtesy of the Borden Institute, Office of The Surgeon General, Washington, DC. Illustrator: Bruce Maston.*

period (including 130 craniotomies, 88 burr holes, 33 extraventricular drains, 25 elevations of fractures, four decompressive craniectomies, three posterior fossa craniotomies, and two decompressive frontal lobectomies) for an average of over 25 procedures per year.[60] Outcomes for patients with epidural and chronic subdural hematomas were good, while poor outcomes were noted for patients with acute subdural and intracerebral hematomas.[60]

> Operative management of subdural hematomas is indicated for bleeds greater than 10 millimeters, those causing more than five millimeters of midline shift with effacement of the basal cisterns, or a GCS score of 8 or less in the context of an enlarging intracranial lesion or deteriorating clinical exam.

## Epidural Hematomas

Epidural hematomas are especially concerning, even in relatively asymptomatic patients.[61] In one case series, epidural hematomas occurred in less than 5 percent of combat-related head injury cases.[11] Classically, an epidural hematoma forms when a skull fracture occurs at the temporoparietal junction causing injury to the middle meningeal artery. Epidural hematomas have a distinctive convex lenticular appearance on CT imaging (Fig. 9). Epidural hematomas usually require neurosurgical intervention. Definitive indications for surgical evacuation include a GCS score less than 8 and a volume greater than 30 milliliters.[62] An epidural hematoma with less than 30 milliliters of volume, less than 15 mm thick, and with no more than five mm of midline shift in a patient who lacks a focal deficit can be managed nonoperatively.[62] However, as this lesion has a very high potential for progression, such patients must be followed closely with frequent neurological examination and serial CT imaging. A study of epidural hematoma patients with GCS score greater than or equal to 12 that did not meet criteria for surgery experienced an eventual surgery rate

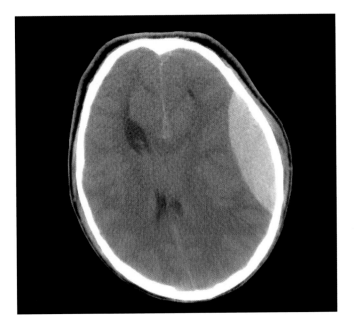

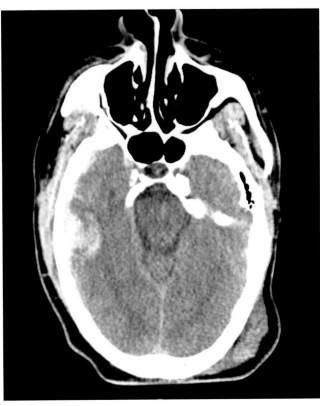

Figure 9. (Above) *Acute epidural hematoma.*

Figure 10. (Right) *Traumatic intracerebral hemorrhage.*

of less than 20 percent with no mortality.[63] The presence of a skull fracture, a six-hour delay from injury to initial CT scan, or heterogeneous density of epidural hematoma did not influence the likelihood of requiring operative management.[63]

Epidural hematomas have a very high potential for progression. If managed nonoperatively, such patients must be followed closely with frequent neurological examination and serial CT imaging.

## Traumatic Intracerebral Hemorrhage

Of the many complications of TBI, the development of traumatic intracerebral hemorrhage is one of the most clinically devastating (Fig. 10).[53,64] About 40 percent of traumatic intracerebral hemorrhages progress in size, and risk factors for enlargement include large initial size, presence of subdural hematoma, or associated subarachnoid hemorrhage.[53] One must remain aware of the occurrence of delayed traumatic intracerebral hemorrhage, which can develop up to several days after the inciting trauma. These delayed intracerebral hemorrhages are noted on CT imaging following either focal or diffuse brain injury.[16,18] More recent work has identified that CT progression to intracerebral hemorrhage associated with trauma is most likely to occur within six to nine hours after head injury.[53] Thus, imaging follow-up in conjunction with ongoing neurologic evaluation and bedside clinical monitoring is critical.[53] Indications for surgical evacuation of traumatic intracerebral hemorrhage include the presence of frontal or temporal lobe lesion greater than 50 milliliters, a GCS score of 6 to 8 with frontal or temporal lobe lesion greater than 20 milliliters, effacement of basal cisterns, or midline shift greater than five mm.[65] Traumatic intracerebral hemorrhage patients not meeting surgical criteria may be treated conservatively. This includes minimizing secondary brain injury measures, frequent neurological examinations, and repeated neuroimaging, as indicated. Eventual surgical evacuation is more likely for conservatively managed patients with worsening GCS scores, hematoma expansion greater than five milliliters or effacement of the basal cisterns.[66]

Another area of interest is the use of hemostatic agents to arrest ongoing traumatic intracerebral hemorrhage. If a traumatic intracerebral hemorrhage patient suffers from thrombocytopenia, platelet dysfunction, or coagulopathy, these factors must be corrected rapidly. However, recent trials with the use of recombinant factor VIIa (rFVIIa) for traumatic intracerebral hemorrhage have not shown mortality or outcome benefit with doses up to 200 micrograms per kilogram.[67,68]

## Herniation Syndromes

Patients with TBI and intracranial hypertension may progress to a cerebral herniation event. The skull is a fixed and rigid container almost completely filled with blood, brain, and cerebrospinal fluid (CSF). Any increase in volume from hemorrhage or edema is initially compensated by displacement of blood or CSF. When these compensatory mechanisms are exceeded, the brain will herniate out of the cranial vault, resulting in a variety of neurologic signs and symptoms (Fig. 11).

### Subfalcine, Central, and Uncal Herniation

Subfalcine herniation is a lateral shift of one frontal lobe into the contralateral side and by default occurs with any degree of midline shift of the cerebral hemispheres. The most common clinical manifestations are increasing lethargy and occasionally neurological deficits related to compromised flow to one or both anterior cerebral arteries. Unilateral anterior cerebral artery compromise classically causes weakness of the contralateral lower extremity, although involvement of the proximal arm and shoulder is reported.[69]

Uncal, or lateral transtentorial herniation, occurs when a supratentorial mass pushes the mesial temporal lobe and uncus anteriorly and downward through the tentorial opening between the ipsilateral aspect of the midbrain and the tentorium. This can result in the Kernohan's notch phenomenon, with hemiparesis ipsilateral to the side of the supratentorial lesion, and is a potentially false localizing sign.[69] Often, a unilaterally large pupil and ensuing third nerve palsy may herald this phenomenon. Radiographic findings of uncal herniation may be seen with resulting midbrain Duret hemorrhages and midbrain ischemia secondary to compromised blood flow to paramedian midbrain perforator vessels (Fig. 12).[69] Duret hemorrhages are small linear hemorrhages along the midline of the brainstem and upper pons caused by traumatic caudal displacement of the brainstem. This is usually an ominous radiographic finding.

Central herniation is downward movement of the brainstem by pressure from the supratentorial brain components. Early findings with central herniation include cranial nerve (CN) VI palsy manifesting

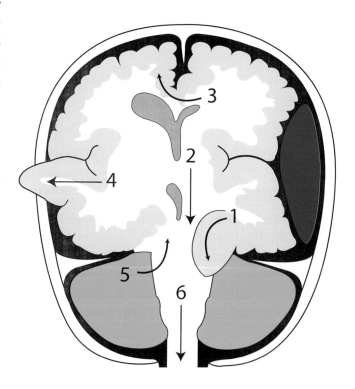

Figure 11. *Six types of brain herniation: (1) Uncal; (2) Central; (3) Subfalcine; (4) Transcranial/extracranial; (5) Upward (upward cerebellar or upward transtentorial); (6) Tonsillar (downward cerebellar).*

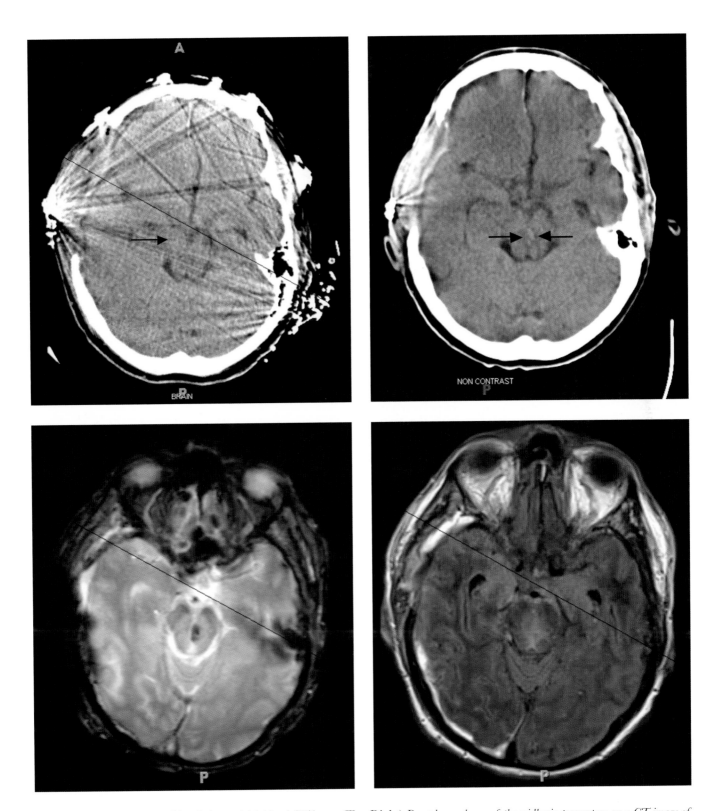

Figure 12. (Top Left) *Uncal herniation on initial head CT image.* (Top Right) *Duret hemorrhages of the midbrain tegmentum on a CT image of the same patient days later.* (Bottom Left) *Duret hemorrhages seen on MRI image.* (Bottom Right) *Duret hemorrhages and ischemic change seen on MRI image of the central midbrain.*

as lateral gaze deficits, which can be unilateral or bilateral. Like uncal herniation, if this progresses, the clinical triad of a CN III palsy (including an ipsilateral nonreactive dilated pupil), coma, and posturing can occur.[70] Occasionally, unilateral or bilateral posterior cerebral artery infarctions can occur with ongoing central or uncal herniation, due to compression of the posterior cerebral artery as it passes upwards over the tentorial notch.[71] Without aggressive management, central herniation is fatal.

## Transcranial and Paradoxical Herniation

Transcranial or extracranial herniation occurs when the brain breeches through a skull defect. Most commonly this occurs after craniectomy, as parts of the brain can shift through the surgical site (Fig. 13). This can occur in over 20 percent of postsurgical TBI patients.[72] Essentially, it represents therapeutic decompression of intracranial hypertension. Untoward complications of extracranial herniation do occur, and are related to laceration of cerebral

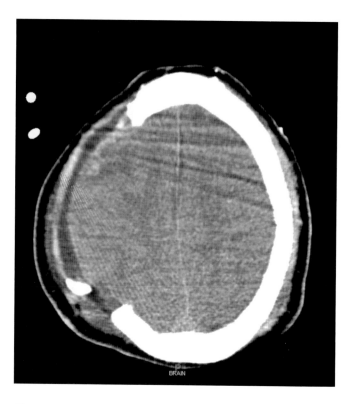

Figure 13. *Extracranial herniation through craniectomy defect.*

cortex and vascular compromise of venous drainage. Making larger rather than smaller craniectomies may minimize these complications.[72] A less recognized phenomenon is paradoxical herniation, which has been reported during lumbar cistern drainage in the setting of a craniectomy. Paradoxical herniation is when there is downward movement of brain in the setting of an overall lowered intracranial pressure.[73] Only a handful of cases of this type of herniation are reported, although this can also occur in the setting of sodium dysregulation and hypernatremia.[74] Extracranial herniation may also result from primary penetrating injury.

## Tonsillar and Upward Herniation

Tonsillar herniation occurs from downward movement of the cerebellar tonsils into the foramen magnum and compression of the lower brainstem. It can result in sudden death from compression of medullary respiratory centers and blood pressure instability.[69,71] Leading causes of this type of herniation are posterior fossa hematomas and obstruction of CSF outflow from the fourth ventricle.[71] A posterior fossa hematoma, or any significant or increasing fourth ventricular dilation, distortion, or obliteration, requires urgent neurosurgical evaluation for possible intervention to include suboccipital craniectomy and placement of an extraventricular drain.

Upward herniation is upward movement of the brain through the tentorium into the cranium. It can cause brainstem compression and can occur with excessive CSF drainage from an extraventricular drain.[75] The clinical presentation of upward herniation is not well-described, although as with all herniation syndromes, a decrease in mental status progressing to obtundation can be expected.

# Penetrating Traumatic Brain Injury

In penetrating TBI, the cranial vault is violated by a foreign body. Foreign bodies affecting soldiers in combat include shrapnel fragments and bullets of varying velocities (Fig. 14). Primary brain injury results from the projectile passing through the brain, damaging neural, vascular, and support structures along its tract. In addition to this damage, high-velocity supersonic projectiles can create a vacuum in their trail, giving rise to tissue cavitation. The rapid expansion and retraction of the vacuum cavity compresses and stretches neural and support structures, often tearing them. As the cavity may be many times larger than the projectile's tract, injury is much more severe.[76]

The majority of military penetrating TBI occurs from penetrating fragment injuries and not from fired bullets.[77] Historically, penetrating fragment-related TBI had a significantly lower overall mortality than military gunshot wound TBI.[77] In the past, the clinical management of penetrating TBI involved complete neurosurgical removal and debridement of wounds, to include retrieval of any bone and metal fragments in the brain.[77] This approach was subsequently altered following a detailed analysis of the Israeli-Lebanese conflict. This study confirmed that aggressive surgical debridement was unnecessary and may have worsened outcomes.[78]

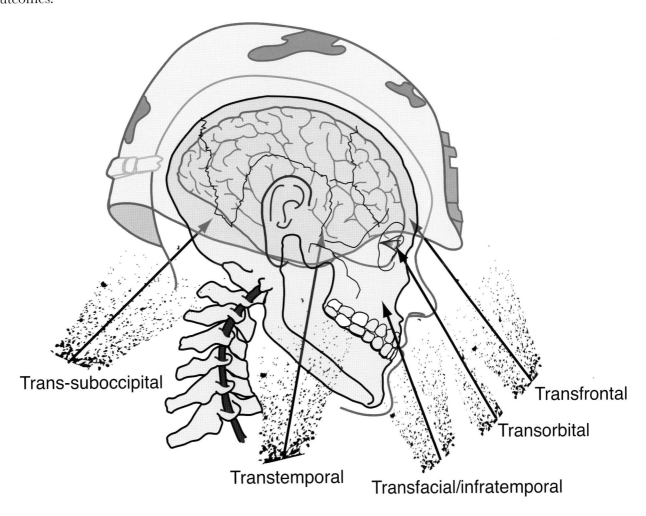

Figure 14. *Common vectors of penetrating TBI. Image courtesy of the Borden Institute, Office of The Surgeon General, Washington, DC. Illustrator: Bruce Maston.*

The majority of military penetrating TBI occurs from penetrating fragment injuries and not from fired bullets. Past clinical management of penetrating TBI involved radical wound debridement, surgical removal of fragments from the brain, and minimal decompression. Current strategies favor more conservative debridement and fragment removal coupled with more aggressive brain decompression.

Today, different management strategies are in effect, especially those based on treatment guidelines for penetrating TBI. Evidence suggests that less aggressive neurosurgical management may be warranted.[78,79] Although the level of clinical evidence does not allow for management standards to be issued, current guidelines provide clinical management options. Management options include local wound care and primary wound closure in penetrating TBI patients who have vitalized scalp without significant intracranial pathology, such as midline shift of the falx cerebri, or an intracranial hematoma requiring evacuation. If no significant mass effect is evident on CT imaging, debridement along the path of the projectile is not recommended.[79] If there is tissue devitalization and/or mass effect, then debridement is recommended prior to a primary wound closure.[79]

## Infection and Cerebrospinal Fluid Leaks

Infection following penetrating TBI is a concerning complication and can dramatically increase mortality and morbidity from head trauma.[80] The mechanism by which this occurs involves formation of a dural fistula resulting from trauma and subsequent fracture of the skull to which it is adherent. The resulting violation of the dura after penetrating TBI predisposes a patient to infection.[12,81] If temporary CSF diversion (e.g., by lumbar drain) does not lead to spontaneous closure of the CSF leak, surgical correction should be considered.[82]

While the utility of antibiotic prophylaxis following penetrating TBI is unclear, the high likelihood of wound contamination has been used to justify the prophylactic use of antibiotics.

The utility of antibiotic prophylaxis following penetrating TBI is unclear. A common practice is the use of broad-spectrum antibiotics due to the likely contamination of the wound from foreign bodies, skin, hair, and bone fragments.[80] In the authors' opinion, in lieu of standardized guidelines and better evidence-based practice on this subject, it may be worthwhile to continue broad-spectrum antibiotic coverage for these wounds and subsequently narrow antibiotics based on CSF culture data and the clinical picture of the casualty.

## Neuroimaging in Penetrating TBI

Advanced neuroimaging is often necessary in penetrating TBI patients. Acutely, CT generally provides sufficient information for appropriate surgical management. Magnetic resonance imaging should not be used in the imaging of acute TBI caused by metallic projectiles.[83] If a vascular injury is suspected, then cerebral angiography is recommended. While conventional angiography is the traditional gold standard imaging modality, computed tomography angiography is widely available and typically utilized in-theater at Level III facilities for this purpose. The sensitivity to diagnose vascular injury such as traumatic dissection of the carotid or vertebral arteries with computed tomography angiography has been reported to be similar or even superior to that of magnetic resonance imaging angiography.[84,85] In terms of other vascular pathology, the incidence of vasospasm in the setting of blast-related penetrating TBI is high, approaching

50 percent.[11] Thus, it is recommended that patients with acute penetrating TBI from explosives undergo regular noninvasive vascular assessment via transcranial Doppler, with follow-up invasive digital subtraction angiography for definitive diagnosis and endovascular intervention.[11]

---

Patients with acute penetrating TBI from explosives should undergo regular noninvasive vascular assessment via transcranial Doppler studies. Digital subtraction angiography is used for definitive diagnosis and endovascular intervention.

---

# Traumatic Brain Injury Management

An organized team approach is essential to appropriate TBI management. This begins in the field with the medic or corpsman and continues to the CSH and tertiary centers. Proper clinical management in the acute period is essential for optimal outcomes. The Guidelines for Field Management of Combat-Related Head Trauma (available at www.braintrauma.org) and Advanced Trauma Life Support (ATLS) are both useful guides.[86] After evaluation and treatment of airway, breathing, and circulatory (ABC) priorities, the far-forward careprovider must make a rapid initial neurological evaluation (disability assessment), especially determining the patient's GCS score (Table 1).[86] The GCS score is important for triage and is a quantifiable measure of impairment, which can help decide early management sequences. This initial exam helps predict outcomes of moderate and severe TBI and penetrating TBI.[39,87]

## *Initial Management (Primary Survey)*

Optimal clinical outcomes depend on proper battlefield care. It is crucial that first responders recognize the importance of airway, breathing, and circulatory management in order to optimize cerebral oxygenation and perfusion. The brain can tolerate severe hypoxia for a very limited period, and it is well-established that the duration and severity of hypoxia and hypotension in this critical early period have dramatic consequences on ultimate clinical outcome.[21,88] Thus, the goals of early resuscitation are to ensure adequate oxygen saturation (greater than 90 percent) and avoid hypotension (systolic blood pressure less than 90 mm Hg). Ensuring a secure airway and adequate ventilatory support is critical in the management of moderate and severe TBI patients. Circulation management starts with hemorrhage control in concert with damage control resuscitation.

---

Ensuring a secure airway and adequate ventilatory support is critical to the management of moderate and severe TBI patients.

---

Airway and Breathing Management

The decision to secure a reliable airway in the patient with a severe TBI is most often made by the careproviders initially evaluating and treating the patient. Rapid sequence intubation is the method of choice. It involves near simultaneous administration of a sedative agent and a neuromuscular blocking agent to induce a loss of consciousness and motor paralysis. While the benefit of rapid airway intervention in severe TBI patients is without question, the side-effect profiles of the many medications used in rapid sequence intubation warrants discussion. The issues of hemodynamic response and intracranial pressure response to endotracheal intubation become germane when dealing with severe TBI patients. The ideal agent will decrease or stabilize ICP without inducing systemic hypotension during rapid sequence intubation efforts. The more commonly used medications will be discussed with a special emphasis on any neuroprotective properties they may have.

Preoxygenation should be performed when possible. Delivering 100 percent oxygen through a nonrebreather apparatus will lead to a nitrogen washout from within the lungs. This nitrogen washout may occur over three to four minutes and may allow for several minutes of apnea before hypoxemia develops. This will minimize the chances of any transient hypoxemia during subsequent attempts at endotracheal intubation. Although there are no studies to prove preoxygenation prior to rapid sequence intubation minimizes secondary brain injury, the practice intuitively appears beneficial.[89]

Attempts at endotracheal intubation will elicit gag and cough reflexes, tachycardia, hypertension, and increased ICP. The cardiovascular responses are believed to be primarily sympathetic to the mechanical stimulation of the larynx and trachea by direct laryngoscopy and intubation. There are a variety of premedications touted as being able to blunt these responses. Lidocaine (1.5 milligrams [mg] per kilogram) administered intravenously three minutes prior to direct laryngoscopy has been advocated as an agent that may blunt reflex cardiovascular and ICP responses.[90] The ICP response to endotracheal suctioning in intubated TBI patients has been measured at approximately 22 mm Hg.[91] Studies that measured cardiovascular and ICP responses to endotracheal suctioning or endotracheal intubation using lidocaine as pretreatment to blunt these rises revealed mixed results.[90,92,93,94,95,96,97] Lidocaine has also been delivered topically and in nebulized form, in the hopes of blunting the circulatory response to intubation. The many methodologic flaws and conflicting results of these studies preclude drawing any definitive conclusions. Lidocaine did not appear to pose any short-term adverse side effects in the setting of severe TBI in any of the referenced studies. At best, lidocaine should be regarded as an agent that may have potential benefit in blunting ICP rises associated with endotracheal suctioning or intubation.

Opiates have been advocated as possibly decreasing sympathetic response to endotracheal intubation. Fentanyl has specifically been studied in the setting of severe TBI.[91,98,99,100] Results of several studies suggest it actually causes a paradoxical rise in ICP in this patient subset.[101,102] There is not enough evidence to advocate the use of fentanyl to attenuate ICP rises associated with endotracheal intubation. Some evidence suggests it actually may be harmful. Benzodiazepines are potent sedative hypnotics and have been used as adjunctive medications during RSI (rapid sequence intubation). Midazolam, with its rapid onset and short duration of action, is a popular choice. There are few studies measuring ICP and CBF responses to administration of midazolam in humans. In one of the few studies in the setting of severe TBI, Papazian et al. studied the effect of 0.15 mg per kilogram bolus midazolam intravenous infusion on ICP, MAP, and CPP. Twelve patients with severe TBI in an ICU received midazolam boluses over one minute.[103] In those patients, MAP decreased from 89 mm Hg to 75 mm Hg, CPP decreased from 71 mm Hg to 56 mm Hg, and no statistically significant change in ICP was noted. The minimum acceptable CPP in the setting of severe TBI in many treatment protocols has been set at 70 mm Hg, although current guidelines support slightly lower minimum CPP standards.[104] This study cautions against the indiscriminate use of midazolam in the setting of severe TBI, as it may cause suboptimal CPP in a subset of these patients. At present there is insufficient evidence to make any definitive conclusion regarding the neuroprotective benefit of midazolam in the setting of RSI of the severe TBI patient.

Etomidate is a short-acting, nonbarbiturate, sedative-hypnotic. A dose of 0.3 mg per kilogram administered intravenously over 30 seconds provides rapid sedation with minimal cardiovascular or respiratory depression.[105,106] It has been shown in some studies to decrease ICP, which makes it an attractive option in severe head injury patients.[107,108] It has several adverse effects; one being it may produce vomiting if not accompanied by a paralytic agent. It has also been reported to temporarily suppress adrenal function with as little as one dose.[109] There is no evidence to suggest this temporary attenuation of adrenal responsiveness is of any clinical significance. There are insufficient studies specifically measuring ICP response in head injury patients to the administration of etomidate to make definitive conclusions. However, available evidence indicates that 0.3 mg per kilogram etomidate administered intravenously over 30 seconds may be an effective adjunct in minimizing secondary brain injury in severe TBI patients.[110] Of note, given etomidate's short duration of action, additional sedatives will need to be administered to patients undergoing mechanical ventilation. Agents such as propofol and thiopental have been reported to have properties that reduce ICP rise associated with endotracheal intubation. Both agents have the propensity to induce systemic hypotension, an undesirable side effect for its relationship to CPP in the severe TBI patient.

Rapid sequence intubation involves the administration of neuromuscular blockade immediately following administration of a potent sedating agent and any pretreatment measures for ICP elevation. Succinylcholine, a rapid-acting, short duration, depolarizing neuromuscular blocking agent used at a dose of 1 to 2 mg per kilogram intravenous bolus, is the traditional first-line agent.[111] Administration of this drug has been reported to increase ICP directly, although the mechanism remains unclear.[112] Estimates of the rise in ICP as a direct result of succinylcholine administration in patients with disorders of intracranial compliance have been between 4.9 mm Hg to 12.0 mm Hg.[113,114] While the exact mechanism is speculative, it is suggested that afferent input from muscle spindle receptors to the central nervous system is responsible. Administering a defasciculating dose of a nondepolarizing neuromuscular blocking agent (pancuronium 0.01 mg per kilogram or vecuronium 0.01 mg per kilogram) intravenously three minutes prior to succinylcholine administration has been reported to blunt any subsequent rise in ICP.[113,114] An alternative to using succinylcholine is the administration of a paralytic dose of vecuronium (0.3 mg per kilogram) in an intravenous bolus fashion. This will provide intubating conditions in 100 seconds; however, this dose has the potential disadvantage of complete motor paralysis for approximately two hours and may complicate further neurologic assessment. Prolonged paralysis is thus discouraged. An alternative nondepolarizing paralytic agent with rapid-onset (one to three minutes) and intermediate duration of action (30 to 45 minutes) is rocuronium (0.6 mg per kilogram dosing). Rocuronium is not contraindicated in the setting of burns, potential hyperkalemia, and myopathies.[115,116]

> Administering a defasciculating dose of a nondepolarizing neuromuscular blocking agent intravenously three minutes prior to succinylcholine administration has been reported to blunt any subsequent rise in ICP.

Many of the pharmacological agents used to blunt intubation-related elevations in ICP must be administered several minutes prior to intubation attempts in order to achieve peak efficacy. Combat casualty careproviders must use their judgment in these scenarios. Will several minutes of potential hypercarbia or hypoxemia result by waiting for these premedication drugs with theoretical benefit to take effect? Would the resultant rise in ICP from increased CBF offset any benefit these medications provide? While minimizing transient elevations in ICP with premedication or appropriate muscle blockading agents during RSI is theoretically appealing, no definitive proof linking this to improved neurologic outcomes exists.

## Head Position

The traditional practice of elevating the head of TBI patients in order to minimize ICP has been challenged. Advocates of a supine position argued it would allow for higher cerebral perfusion pressures and optimized CBF. Rosner et al. measured the effect of head elevation from zero to 50 degrees on ICP and CPP. They concluded that zero degree head elevation maximized CPP.[117] Durward et al. studied the effect of head elevation at 0, 15, 30, 60 degrees on ICP and CPP. They concluded that 15 to 30 degrees of elevation reduced ICP while maintaining CPP. Further elevations of the head to 60 degrees caused an increase in ICP and a significant decrease in CPP.[118] Feldman et al. measured ICP, CPP, CBF, and mean carotid pressures on head injury patients at zero and 30 degrees head elevation. They found mean ICP values of 14.1 mm Hg at 30 degrees elevation increased to a mean ICP value of 19.7 mm Hg at zero degrees elevation. Mean carotid pressures decreased from 89.5 mm Hg to 84.3 mm Hg when patients went from zero degrees to 30 degrees elevation, and no differences in CPP or CBF were noted.[119] From this data, it appears that elevating the head of severe TBI patients to greater than 30 degrees may be detrimental to CBF. Elevation of the head up to 30 degrees may be of some benefit in selected patients with TBI with respect to decreasing ICP, although it may be at the expense of diminished CPP and CBF. Once ICP monitoring is instituted, a more accurate assessment of the optimal degree of head elevation in the patient with severe TBI patient may be made. Of note, any consideration of head position changes need to take into account the stability of the cervical spine or potential for injury.

> Elevation of the head up to 30 degrees may be of some benefit in selected patients with TBI with respect to decreasing ICP, although it may be at the expense of diminished CPP and CBF.

Compromised venous drainage can exacerbate intracranial hypertension. It is prudent to always assume an occult cervical spine injury in any TBI patient with altered mental status or blunt injury above the clavicle until ruled out by radiographic imaging.[86] The cervical spine should be immobilized with a rigid neck collar during the initial survey. The neck collar serves a dual purpose. It protects the cervical spine and keeps the head midline. Spinal injuries concomitant with TBI are not uncommon, as a recent retrospective review of head injury casualties from OEF/OIF included a 16 percent incidence of spinal column trauma of various types.[12] In a recent retrospective review of the epidemiology of spinal trauma in polytrauma patients, 8 percent had associated spinal injuries, and the percentages of cervical, thoracic, lumbar, and sacral injuries were 35, 19, 37, and 27 percent, respectively.[120] It is important to immobilize the spine of a polytrauma patient when spinal instability is suspected, and remain vigilant for exam findings, which may be explained by occult spinal cord injury.

> Assume an occult cervical spine injury is present in any TBI patient with altered mental status or blunt injury above the clavicle, until it is ruled out by radiographic imaging and clinical assessment.

## Secondary Survey

The secondary survey of a trauma patient follows the primary survey and includes a more detailed yet rapid neurologic examination. Examining the patient and detailing the extent of neurologic impairment is essential. Ideally, this can be accomplished in advance of sedation and/or paralysis for endotracheal intubation and other procedures. The diagnosis of TBI is made on history and physical examination. Neuroimaging provides supportive information. It is important to remember that altered mental status or obtundation may be due to other causes, including impaired ventilation, oxygenation, perfusion, glycemic derangement, or medication/toxin exposure in addition to occult head injury. These conditions must be considered during the initial trauma evaluation.[86]

## *TBI Management Guidelines and Options*

The overriding concept of management of the moderate and severe TBI patient is the prevention of secondary injury. In the initial hours after the inciting trauma, this involves mitigating elevations in ICP, traumatic intracranial hemorrhage, cerebral edema, and metabolic derangements. Treatment guidelines for the management of severe TBI published by the Brain Trauma Foundation have been instrumental in improving care through guiding therapy with evidenced-based recommendations.[121] Guidelines for the prehospital and field management of brain injury are also published, and all three sets of guidelines can be obtained from the Brain Trauma Foundation free of charge (www.braintrauma.org).

### Airway Management and Ventilation

Ensuring adequate oxygenation and appropriate ventilation of the head-injured patient is vital. Oxygenation and ventilation goals should be to maintain adequate oxygenation with partial pressure of oxygen in arterial blood ($PaO_2$) greater than 60 mm Hg, and avoid either hypocarbia or hypercarbia by maintaining a $PCO_2$ in the normal range, except for brief periods of hyperventilation discussed below.[21,122]

> Oxygenation and ventilation goals should be to maintain adequate oxygenation with $PaO_2$ greater than 60 mm Hg, and avoid either hypocarbia or hypercarbia by maintaining a $PCO_2$ in the normal range.

In the field, oxygen saturation should be greater than or equal to 90 percent. Hypoxic episodes with saturations lower than this are associated with worse outcomes.[123,124] Absolute indications for inserting an artificial airway are a GCS score of 8 or less or suspicion that the patient's ability to ventilate or protect his or her airway is compromised. Oral endotracheal intubation is preferred in Level III facility settings. Nasotracheal intubation is not recommended in the setting of significant head trauma. The possibility exists for increasing ICP due to stimulation of the nares as well as displacing occult skull fractures through nasopharyngeal manipulation.[125,126] Another advantage to intubation is to ensure the maintenance of eucapnea ($PCO_2$ of 35 to 40 mm Hg), as hypercapnea will induce increased ICP.[127]

### Role of Hyperventilation

Acute hyperventilation has traditionally been a first-line intervention in rapidly decreasing ICP. As the ability to monitor CBF, cerebral metabolism, and cerebral ischemia has improved, new information regarding potential pitfalls of hyperventilation has emerged. Recent studies have noted that while hyperventilation acutely decreases ICP, it also decreases CBF, and in many cases may induce cerebral ischemia.[25,27,128,129] Severe TBI patients have been found to have either increased or reduced CBF during the early phases of their injuries. Both states may be associated with elevated ICP. While hyperventilating the TBI patient with increased CBF may be desirable, hyperventilation may induce cerebral ischemia in patients with reduced CBF. In certain patients with increased CBF, hyperventilation has lead to decreased CBF in uninjured areas of the brain, while creating a relative increase in CBF to areas of injured brain. This localized increase in CBF to injured areas of brain is thought to occur due to the diminished responsiveness of the injured brain's microvasculature to hypocapnia.

Optimal titration of hyperventilation therapy requires close monitoring of objective indicators of cerebral ischemia.[130,131] Objective indicators of cerebral ischemia or CBF include measurement of jugular venous saturations, thermal diffusion flowmetry, transcranial Doppler ultrasounds, and xenon-enhanced CT scans. These methods of measuring cerebral ischemia or CBF are not widely available to CCC providers. This has led to the recommendation that hyperventilation only be used in settings of documented elevated ICP and as a temporary and last-line treatment to decrease elevated ICP refractory to other means, such as sedation, paralysis, CSF drainage, lowering of brain metabolism, and osmotic therapy.

> Hyperventilation should only be used as a temporary and last-line measure to decrease elevated ICP refractory to other means, such as sedation, paralysis, CSF drainage, lowering of brain metabolism, and osmotic therapy. Physicians should use a $PCO_2$ level of 30 to 32 mm Hg as their target when they decide to institute hyperventilation therapy in the setting of severe head injury.

Prolonged hyperventilation has been clearly associated with exacerbation of cerebral ischemia.[132] Very brief durations of hyperventilation may be acceptable only as a temporizing measure until other means of managing increased ICP are readied. If hyperventilation is continued for longer than 12 hours, metabolic compensation negates the ameliorative effects of respiratory alkalosis caused by a hypocapnic state, and continued hyperventilation may be harmful.[127] The recommended goal for baseline $PCO_2$ levels is normocapnia in the 35 to 40 mm Hg range, but during an impending herniation event, hyperventilation will acutely lower $PCO_2$ and ICP within seconds. Based on available data, physicians should use a $PCO_2$ level of 30 to 32 mm Hg as their target when they decide to institute hyperventilation therapy in the setting of severe head injury. The current recommended $PCO_2$ is to strictly avoid levels below 25 mm Hg.[125,127]

## Hemodynamic Management

The objective of hemodynamic therapy in TBI is to ensure adequate brain perfusion. The specific treatment goals are systolic blood pressure greater than or equal to 90 mm Hg, CPP greater than or equal to 60 mm Hg, and euvolemia. As discussed above, CPP is MAP minus ICP (Equation 1). Although CPP is neither a direct measure of CBF nor regional cerebral flow, it is indicative of the overall adequacy of brain perfusion, especially in the context of elevated ICP.

Blood pressure management may be challenging in combat-injured patients. Often, the patient is in hemorrhagic shock due to accompanying injuries such as traumatic extremity amputation. As such, hypotension is common and independently associated with TBI, poor outcome, and mortality.[16,133] Systolic blood pressures less than 90 mm Hg has an especially deleterious effect. When compared to hypoxemia, low systolic blood pressure is associated with a worse outcome.[17] With head injury, the ability of the neurovasculature to autoregulate is impaired, and thus regional cerebral blood flow becomes directly dependent on systemic blood pressure.[125] Experimental models show that the injured brain is highly susceptible to even subtle ischemic states.[134] It is therefore imperative to avoid even short episodes of hypotension after TBI. Overall fluid balance of head injured patients is also important. Retrospective data suggests that TBI patients who were volume depleted by about 600 milliliters developed worse outcomes.[135]

> Hypotension is common in combat casualties. Hypotension following severe TBI has been associated with poor outcomes and increased mortality.

Hemostasis of the obvious soft-tissue head wound is usually obtained with direct pressure dressing or a field dressing such as HemCon® or QuikClot®. Crystalloid fluids are used for fluid resuscitation in the field phase of the treatment of the brain-injured patient. Later, blood products may be transfused as needed. Analysis of data from OEF and OIF indicates that hemorrhagic shock is best treated with red blood cells and plasma using a 1:1 ratio based on volume.[15] Colloid and hypotonic fluids are relatively contraindicated in TBI. Colloid fluids containing albumin have been shown to increase mortality.[136] Hypotonic fluids, such as half-normal saline and lactated Ringer's, have the potential to exacerbate cerebral edema.[125]

> Colloid and hypotonic fluids are relatively contraindicated in TBI. Colloid fluids containing albumin have been shown to increase mortality, while hypotonic fluids, such as half-normal saline and lactated Ringer's, have the potential to exacerbate cerebral edema.

Cerebral perfusion pressure goals are best met with intravenous fluids. If CPP cannot be maintained with intravenous fluids alone, vasoactive pharmacologic agents may be considered. Norepinephrine and phenylephrine are often used, as they are thought to have minimal effect on cerebral vasomotor tone. If vasopressors are used, then continuous hemodynamic monitoring is needed.[76] Aggressive use of vasopressor agents has been associated with increased incidence of acute respiratory distress syndrome; however, this complication potentially could have been the result of exceeding CPP levels of 70 mm Hg.[137]

## Goals for ICP Management

The goal for ICP management in brain-injured patients is to maintain a normal ICP which is generally less than 20 cm $H_2O$ or 15 mm Hg. Data suggest that elevations over 25 mm Hg are associated with poor outcomes, and thus interventions should be aimed at reducing ICP to less than this amount.[138] Current guidelines recommend instituting measures to control ICP when pressures of 20 mm Hg are reached and aggressive means employed to prevent ICP elevations over 25 mm Hg.[139] One must keep in mind the achievable CPP based on MAP and ICP during therapy, as many interventions to decrease ICP may also have systemic effects on peripheral hemodynamics. The maintenance of a CPP of at least 60 mm Hg is strongly recommended.[104] This is often accomplished with the use of vasopressor agents, although complications, including higher incidence of adult respiratory distress syndrome, may result from overshooting the goal CPP to greater than 70 mm Hg with vasopressors and intravenous fluids, as previously discussed.[137]

## Intracranial Pressure and External Ventricular Drains

The management of ICP is paramount in neurocritical and neurosurgical care. If ICP progresses unchecked, it will culminate in cerebral herniation. Simple therapeutic measures should be instituted in every moderate to severe TBI patient so as to minimize increasing ICP. Such simple interventions include keeping the head midline, avoiding any circumferential neck dressings for wound hemostasis or securing the endotracheal tube, and avoiding placement of internal jugular central venous lines into the dominant internal jugular vein. All of these will optimize venous outflow from the head.[42] The Trendelenburg position should not be used as it will do the opposite.[140]

All TBI patients with suspected elevated ICP should have an ICP monitor placed. Options include an intraventricular catheter, intraparenchymal fiberoptic or solid-state monitor, subdural bolt, and epidural fiber optic catheter. The most invasive is the intraventricular catheter. It provides the most accurate measurement of ICP as it is placed into the third ventricle that is almost at the center of the cranial vault.[141] It is also the most consistently reliable as it can be zeroed. The other methods are less invasive as they either require only minimal or no penetration of brain parenchyma. As closed systems, they have a lower incidence of infection but, unfortunately, also are subject to measurement drift as they cannot be zeroed. Another benefit of the intraventricular catheter is that it provides a treatment option for ICP management. The intraventricular catheter is also known as an external ventricular drain, as it can be used for CSF removal.[141] If hydrocephalus is seen on CT, an external ventricular drain is the best option (Fig. 15).

> There is evidence that with proper training, placement of an external ventricular drain or other ICP monitors can be done safely by non-neurosurgeons.

Indications for placing an ICP monitor include a patient with a GCS score less than or equal to 8 (after resuscitation) and an acute abnormality on CT, such as traumatic intracerebral hemorrhage, compression of the basal cisterns, or evidence of contusion.[142] If a patient has two of the following: systolic blood pressure less than 90 mm Hg, motor posturing on exam, and/or is greater than or equal to 40 years of age, then an ICP monitor should likewise be placed or strongly considered.[142] Typically a neurosurgeon places these devices. However, there is evidence that with proper training, placement of an external intraventricular drain or other ICP monitors can be done safely by neurointensivists and other non-neurosurgeons (Fig. 16).[143,144] It should be stated that this is not yet a mainstream position, and that access to the cranial vault should ideally only occur with neurosurgical oversight.

## Hypertonic Saline and Other Medical ICP Management Options

Initial medical intervention for elevated ICP includes avoidance of exacerbating factors such as fever, seizures, venous outflow obstruction, hyperglycemia, or hypercarbia. The next line of therapy involves osmotic therapy. Several agents have been used for this purpose in the past, but currently mannitol and hypertonic saline (HTS) are the mainstays of osmotic or hyperosmolar therapy.

### *Role of Mannitol*

Mannitol is an osmotically active agent that has long been used in the management of elevated ICP.[145] The mechanism of its action involves multifactorial pathways to lower ICP.[146] It has volume expansion and rheologic properties making red blood cell mediated oxygen delivery to brain cells more effective. This in turn may stimulate reflex cerebral microvasculature vasoconstriction.[147,148] Irrespective of the mechanism of action of mannitol, its effectiveness in reducing ICP is well documented.[147] It will consistently decrease ICP by approximately 20 to 35 percent within 10 to 20 minutes of intravenous administration. The ICP reduction effect of mannitol typically lasts at least two hours.[149,150,151] A common fear of inducing acute hypotension in the multiple trauma patient by infusing mannitol precludes its use by many physicians. However, in multiple studies, mannitol infusion resulted in acute increases in central venous pressure and mean arterial pressures.[146,148,150] The osmotic diuresis leading to hypotension was rarely noted. When hypotension did occur, it occurred several hours later and was mild and easily treated with volume replacement. Mannitol appears to be a safe and effective drug in acutely reducing ICP in severe TBI patients.

> Mannitol can decrease ICP by approximately 20 to 35 percent within 10 to 20 minutes of intravenous administration, and its effects last for two hours.

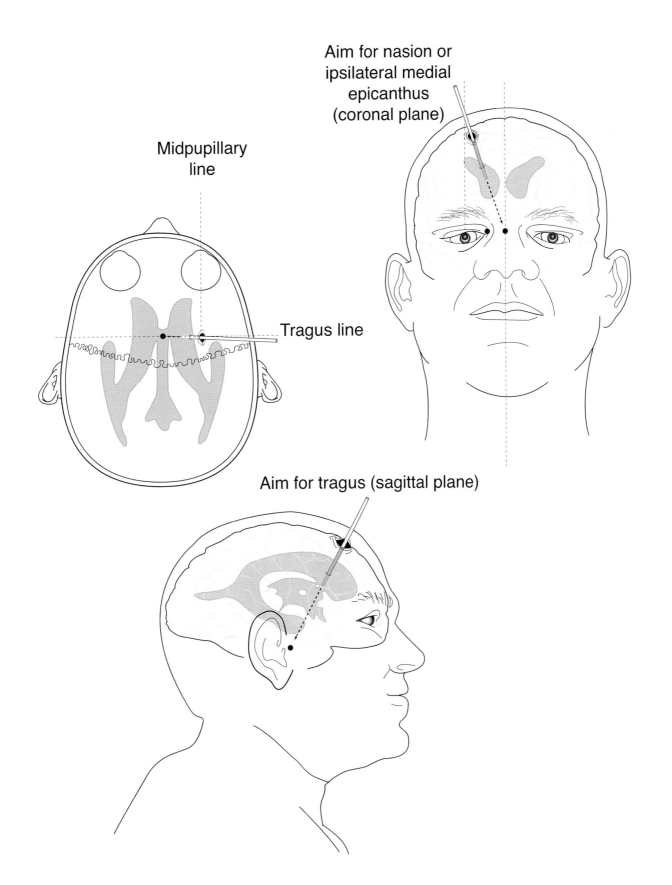

Midpupillary
line

Tragus line

Aim for nasion or
ipsilateral medial
epicanthus
(coronal plane)

Aim for tragus (sagittal plane)

Figure 15. *Landmarks for placement of intraventricular catheter. Adapted image courtesy of the Borden Institute, Office of The Surgeon General, Washington, DC. Illustrator: Bruce Maston.*

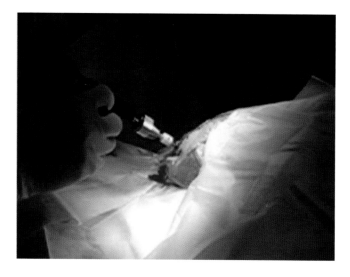

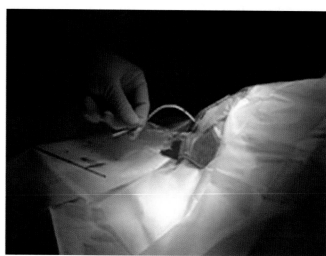

Figure 16. *An intraventricular catheter provides the most accurate measurement of ICP and is a valuable treatment option for ICP management.* (Top Left) *A hole is drilled through the skull.* (Top Right) *The intraventricular catheter is advanced into the third ventricle at the center of the cranial vault.* (Bottom Right) *If needed, CSF can be removed if necessary.*

Mannitol should be given intravenously via a peripheral or central intravenous line at a dose of 0.25 to 1.0 grams per kilogram. Small doses of mannitol (0.25 grams per kilogram) have been shown to effectively reduce ICP in patients with TBI.[152] Earlier data shows that mannitol use in TBI correlates with decreased ICP and improvements in CBF and CPP.[149] Past recommendations for mannitol to be given as bolus infusions rather than continuous are no longer supported. Still, in common clinical practice, a single bolus dose is most widely used.[153] So long as serum osmolality is followed closely, additional doses of mannitol can be given. A serum osmolality of 320 milliosmole (mOsm) per liter is generally accepted as a treatment endpoint, although some investigators advocate that slightly higher levels can be tolerated with caution.[154]

### Hypertonic Saline (HTS)

Another option for hyperosmolar therapy is HTS. Studies using 7.5% and 23.4% HTS provide evidence of clinical benefit.[155,156] Recent data support the use of bolus doses of 30 to 60 ml of 23.4% HTS to emergently treat a herniation event.[156] An additional benefit of using 23.4% HTS is that its ameliorative effect on ICP lasts longer than mannitol.[157] When used, 23.4% HTS must be administered via a central venous line over ten to fifteen minutes to prevent hypotension and phlebitis. A commonly used initial treatment goal is to achieve serum sodium levels 145 to 155 milliequivalents (mEq) per liter, which is equivalent to a serum osmolality of 300 to 320 mOsm per liter in most patients.[140] A continuous intravenous infusion of 2% or 3% HTS can be used to maintain high serum osmolality. When doing so, it is suggested that the fluid be made as a 50%:50% mix of sodium chloride and sodium acetate so as to prevent hyperchloremic metabolic acidosis. At 2% concentration, HTS can be given through a peripheral intravenous catheter, but at 3% or higher, it must be given via a central line due to its potential to cause phlebitis. The infusion rate is set based on a particular patient's intravascular needs. Typically, a maintenance rate of 75 ml per hour is used. However, these solutions can be administered in 250 ml boluses to treat episodes of intracranial hypertension or systemic hypotension.

Studies using 7.5% and 23.4% HTS provide evidence of clinical benefit in reducing ICP in cases of refractory intracranial hypertension.

If continuous infusions of hypertonic solutions are used, serum sodium should be monitored frequently, at least every six hours. Rapid drops in serum sodium are to be avoided so as not to precipitate cerebral edema.[140] Dehydration must also be avoided.[135] Generally, HTS therapy is maintained for the first four to seven days after injury. After the peak edema period elapses, HTS infusion can be switched to normal saline or terminated while observing for the slow return to normonatremia.

## Other Pharmacologic Agents to Reduce ICP

If ICP remains poorly controlled after the efforts described above, then induced pharmacologic coma can be considered. The postulated effect of pharmacologic coma on ICP is through reduction of cerebral metabolism with concomitant reductions in CBF and reduced tissue oxygen demand. The most commonly used agent for pharmacological coma is pentobarbital. This drug can be administered intravenously at a loading dose of 5 mg per kilogram, followed by an infusion of 1 to 3 mg per kilogram per hour. There is a high-dose regimen that begins with an intravenous loading dose of 10 mg per kilogram over 30 minutes followed by 5 mg per kilogram per hour infusion for three hours, followed by 1 mg per kilogram per hour titrated to therapeutic goals, which are either burst suppression on continuous electroencephalography (EEG) monitoring or a reduction in ICP.[76] If burst suppression is not obtained with this dose, then a smaller loading dose and increased rate can be given until a satisfactory EEG tracing is seen or ICP is controlled. Other barbiturates may be used including the much shorter acting thiopental, whose half-life of five hours is suited for short-term therapy of elevations in ICP.[140] Thiopental doses of 200 to 500 mg can be given via bolus intravenous push while monitoring for hypotension.

Another option for pharmacological coma is propofol, which is given at an intravenous loading dose of 2 mg per kilogram, followed by a titrated infusion of up to 100 micrograms (mcg) per kilogram per minute. The use of propofol for this clinical indication is controversial. Long-term and high-dose propofol infusions have been associated with the development of hypotension and a newly described metabolic disorder termed propofol infusion syndrome.[158] This consists of renal failure, rhabdomyolysis, hyperkalemia, myocardial failure, metabolic acidosis, lipemia, hepatomegaly, and death. The mechanism for this is not fully understood, but significant caution must be used in any infusion over 5 mg per kilogram per hour or treatment lasting longer than 48 hours.[159] In a study of propofol used for ICP reduction, there was a failure to show a six-month outcome benefit.[160] If propofol is used for induction of a pharmacological coma (and resultant ICP reduction), continuous EEG monitoring will be required to monitor the electrical activity of the brain.

## Induced Hypothermia

Induced hypothermia for TBI remains controversial but promising. Recent animal data shows promise for induced hypothermia with improved neurophysiologic metrics in an asphyxial brain injury model.[161] There is also data in brain trauma that induced mild hypothermia (33 to 35 degrees) may improve outcomes as far out as two years following head injury.[162] Current use of prophylactic hypothermia for treatment of ICP in severe TBI is a second-tier therapy but may be helpful in refractory intracranial hypertension. If utilized, modalities of induction of hypothermia include skin-applied gel cooling systems and intravenous methods, as well as traditional air-circulating cooling blankets, iced gastric lavage, and surface ice packing.[140] The goal of maintaining normothermia and avoiding hyperthermia in TBI patients, however, remains strongly recommended.[5]

## Decompressive Craniectomy

Decompressive craniectomy is an emerging clinical approach to the early intervention and management of TBI.[163] The reported experience to date is conflicting. In a study of 57 young patients (age less

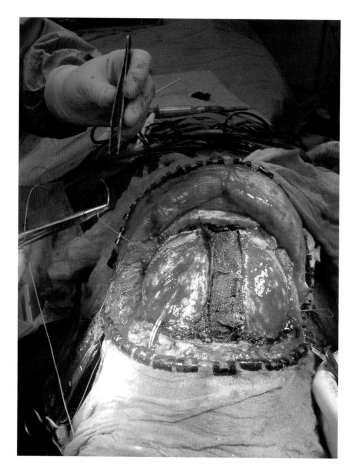

Figure 17. *Early decompressive craniectomy in a patient with blast TBI.*

than 50) with severe TBI, early decompressive craniectomy was associated with a good outcome, defined as social rehabilitation, in 58 percent of patients. The authors reported a relatively low mortality of less than 20 percent.[164] A retrospective French study reported a similar outcome in only 25 percent of severe TBI patients.[165] Older data from the Trauma Coma Data Bank has suggested that even though radiographic improvement occurred, there is no significant improvement in patient outcome after craniectomy.[166] One of the difficulties in interpreting the available data is the lack of agreement as to how the procedure is to be performed (e.g., release the dura or not, timing of surgery, cutoff age, and TBI severity on presentation) (Fig. 17).[167]

> The authors' OEF and OIF neurosurgical experience supports the practice of early decompressive hemicraniectomy for treatment of severe blast TBI. From a practical military standpoint, this may obviate the need to use more conventional methods to control ICP, such as pharmacologic coma.

Currently, two trials enrolling an estimated combined number of over 800 patients are underway. The Randomized Evaluation of Surgery with Craniectomy for Uncontrollable Elevation of Intra-Cranial Pressure (RESCUEicp) and the Decompressive Craniectomy (DECRA) trials may better elucidate the role of decompressive craniectomy in severe TBI. The RESCUEicp trial is the larger of the two and is a multicenter trial in Europe comparing decompressive craniectomy to medical management in TBI.[168] The DECRA trial has a smaller planned enrollment and is being conducted in Australia, New Zealand, Canada, and

Saudi Arabia. The authors' OEF and OIF neurosurgical experience supports early hemicraniectomy for treating severe blast TBI.

### Current Use of Decompressive Craniectomy with Intractable Intracranial Hypertension

From a practical military standpoint, craniectomy provides an additional measure of safety for ICP control. Early decompressive craniectomy may obviate the need to use more conventional methods to control ICP such as pharmacological coma, which is difficult to execute in a deployed and hostile setting due to the limited number of neurological critical care specialists and lack of EEG support in a war zone. In a recent paper comparing GCS scores of patients at the time of head trauma and at discharge, TBI patients who underwent a craniectomy had lower initial GCS scores than those who underwent craniotomy, but at discharge their GCS scores were not significantly different.[11] This study implies that although these patients were worse initially, they improved after decompressive craniectomy to the point where they appeared indistinguishable from those who initially presented with a better neurologic exam. In the combat setting, decompressive craniectomy may be a practical, though aggressive, approach to ICP management. Future studies on larger cohorts of patients and with more rigorous study design may either support or refute this practice (Fig. 18).

## Anticonvulsant Use in TBI

Traumatic brain-injured patients are at risk for both early (less than seven days) and late (more than seven days) post-traumatic seizures. This risk is worsened by traumatic intracranial hemorrhage.[169] A seizure in the acute phase can exacerbate the injury. Phenytoin, a well-established antiepileptic drug, has been shown

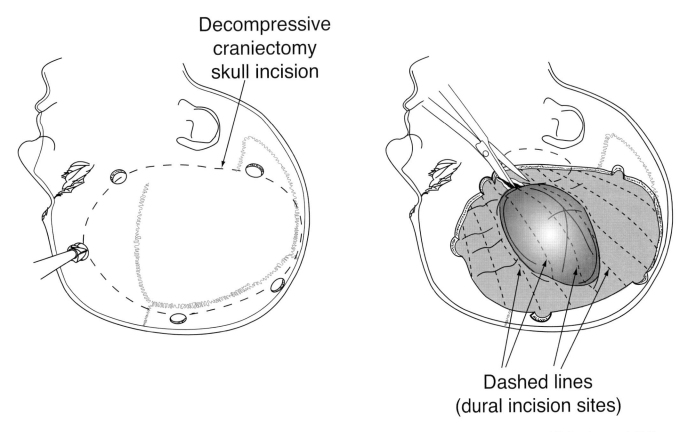

Figure 18. *Decompressive craniectomy bone flap and exposed hematoma. Bone may be cut using a power craniotome, or a Hudson brace and Gigli saw. Adapted image courtesy of the Borden Institute, Office of The Surgeon General, Washington, DC. Illustrator: Bruce Maston.*

to be beneficial in reducing the risk of seizures during the first week after TBI.[170] Carbamazepine, phenobarbital, and valproate are also effective antiepileptic drugs.[171] Unfortunately, no antiepileptic drug has been shown to prevent the development of late post-traumatic seizures. Studies have shown that when followed for 15 years after significant TBI, approximately 50 percent of patients will develop late seizures.[172] As 50 percent will not, the recommended approach is to stop antiepileptic drug therapy after the first seven days, and only reinstitute treatment should late seizures manifest.[173] The potential for cognitive side effects of phenytoin make prolonged prophylactic use of this medication less attractive.[174] If a patient is unable to take medications orally, alternatives to phenytoin and fosphenytoin are valproate and levetiracetam, as all are available in intravenous form. Levetiracetam has not undergone rigorous human clinical TBI trials but has been shown to be effective in preclinical TBI models.[175]

There is little evidence to support or refute the use of antiepileptic drugs for prevention of post-penetrating TBI seizures. The risk of seizure following penetrating TBI is much higher than nonpenetrating TBI, and thus antiepileptic drugs are prescribed by most providers.[176] Management options include the use of antiepileptic drugs during the first seven days after penetrating TBI and then to discontinue their use.[177] Should the patient suffer a late seizure, the antiepileptic drug therapy can be restarted. Therapeutic options are phenytoin, fosphenytoin, carbamazepine, valproate, or phenobarbital.[173]

> The risk of seizures following penetrating TBI is much higher than nonpenetrating TBI. Hence, antiepileptic drugs, such as phenytoin, are frequently administered for at least the first seven days following injury.

## Critical Care and Air Evacuation

After initial emergency care, patients with moderate and severe TBI require close neurological and physiological monitoring. This is best done in the ICU of a Level III care facility, where monitors and advanced clinical practice nurses are present. Evidence demonstrates improved outcomes when specialized neurological intensive care teams, employing evidence-based clinical care, guide management.[178] The presence of other traumatic injuries may require additional care from trauma, orthopedic, craniofacial and other specialists. In this critical injury period, the best measure of efficacy of treatment or worsening of condition is the neurologic examination. Thus, regular clinical neurological examination by skilled practitioners is needed. In the acute period, it may be as often as every hour and then less frequently if the patient remains stable. Intracranial pressure and CPP measurements should be made continuously if an ICP monitor is indicated. However, even in the presence of ICP monitoring, the importance of the clinical examination and neurological assessment cannot be overstated. The highest risk period for deterioration is in the first few days after TBI. The majority of conversion to traumatic intracerebral hemorrhage occurs usually within the first nine hours, and generally the peak period of cerebral edema is from 48 to 96 hours after TBI.[53] Thereafter, these processes wane, and there is clinical improvement with better ICP control.[76]

> Evidence demonstrates improved outcomes in patients with moderate and severe TBI when specialized neurological intensive care teams apply evidence-based clinical care. This is best done in the ICU of Level III care facilities.

Current military policy supports the principle of rapid out-of-theater evacuation to fixed medical facilities, although the decision to transfer the severely injured soldier with TBI via air evacuation may still be difficult. As discussed above, both the peak period of cerebral edema, as well as the likely conversion of TBI to traumatic intracerebral hemorrhage will occur in the hours and days after the initial trauma. For this reason, it is wise to have the injured service member out-of-theater and en route to a medical center that is part of the casualty evacuation system. Although the risk of transferring a patient who may become unstable during air evacuation is disconcerting, a recent review of the Air Force Critical Care Air Transport Team's (CCATT) safety record and census of trauma and nontrauma-related air evacuations is reassuring.[179] During the period of study, air evacuations via CCATT teams from OIF to Landstuhl, Germany, no inflight or 24-hour post-flight fatalities were reported among flights occurring over a one-year period for the flight time of approximately five hours. In this study, 17 percent of combat casualties had neurologic injury, and 9 percent of these patients had an ICP monitor in place with resultant increases in ICP during flight occurring in 3 percent of patients. Although the authors of this study credit the in-theater medical teams with proper preparation of trauma-related casualties for air evacuation, there is data to support the current doctrine of rapid removal of casualties from theater.[179] This policy has been credited with improved rates of fatalities of soldiers wounded in combat during the conflicts in Iraq and Afghanistan.[180]

## Other Management Considerations

Other important considerations include preventing secondary complications of critical illness including venous thromboembolism, gastric stress ulcers, and decubitus ulcers. Injured and immobilized patients are at high risk for developing deep venous thrombosis with subsequent venous thromboembolism. The optimal approach in severe TBI with intracranial hemorrhage is uncertain. Sequential compression devices on the lower extremities are minimally invasive and are not associated with worsening intracranial hemorrhage. Thus, they should be placed as soon as possible. The optimal timing of introduction of unfractionated or low molecular weight heparin for venous thromboembolism prophylaxis in head trauma is less clear.

However, if there are no contraindications to heparin use (e.g., ongoing coagulopathy, worsening thrombocytopenia, or ongoing hemorrhage) then treatment should be started as soon as possible, ideally within the first 36 hours of injury.[181] A practical guide is to obtain CT imaging of the brain after a period of 24 to 36 hours, and if no increase in hemorrhage or new hemorrhage has occurred, then subcutaneous heparin can be started. In the setting of any degree of increasing traumatic intracerebral hemorrhage, the risks and benefits of heparin must be weighed on an individual basis. The routine placement of inferior vena cava filters is controversial, and placement is currently supported only by a low-level recommendation in patients with a GCS score of less than 8 and contraindications to anticoagulation.[181,182]

Gastric stress ulcers may be prevented using either H2-receptor antagonists or proton-pump inhibitors.[183] Either one of these medications should be routinely used for gastric stress ulceration prophylaxis in severe TBI patients, although the tendency for H2-receptor antagonists to cause thrombocytopenia may limit their usefulness.[184] Prevention of skin breakdown is a concern in all severely injured trauma patients, and care must be taken to reduce the likelihood of decubitus ulcers through frequent repositioning, vigilant nursing care, and good skin hygiene practices.

# Summary

Medical management of the combat TBI patient is challenging. The field and hospital care of TBI is largely confined to supportive efforts to minimize secondary brain injury for optimal neurologic recovery. This is accomplished through maintaining cerebral perfusion, controlling ICP, and preventing morbidity associated with critical illness. Routine or prolonged hyperventilation, as discussed previously, is harmful and should be avoided.[27] As new pharmacologic and medical approaches are introduced, there will be increasing opportunity to better manage these patients and enhance their long-term neurologic outcomes.

# References

1. Sosin DM, Sniezek JE, Thurman DJ. Incidence of mild and moderate brain injury in the United States, 1991. Brain Inj 1996;10(1):47-54.

2. Sosin DM, Sniezek JE, Waxweiler RJ. Trends in death associated with traumatic brain injury, 1979 through 1992. Success and failure. JAMA 1995;14;273(22):1778-1780.

3. Thurman DJ. Epidemiology and economics of head trauma. In: Miler L, Jayes R, editors. Head trauma: basic, preclinical, and clinical directions. New York: Wiley and Sons; 2001. p. 1193-1202.

4. Rimel RW, Giordani B, Barth JT, et al. Disability caused by minor head injury. Neurosurgery 1981;9(3):221-228.

5. Maas Al, Stocchetti N, Bullock R. Moderate and severe traumatic brain injury in adults. Lancet Neurol 2008;7(8):728-741.

6. Bellamy RF. The medical effects of conventional weapons. World J Surg 1992;16(5):888-892.

7. Rustemeyer J, Kranz V, Bremerick A. Injuries in combat from 1982-2005 with particular reference to those to the head and neck: a review. Br J Oral Maxillofac Surg 2007;45(7):556-560.

8. Okie S. Traumatic brain injury in the war zone. N Engl J Med 2005;352(20):2043-2047.

9. Warden D L, French L. Traumatic brain injury in the war zone. N Engl J Med 2005;353(6):633-634.

10. Patel TH, Wenner KA, Price SA, et al. A U.S. Army forward surgical team's experience in Operation Iraqi Freedom. J Trauma 2004;57(2):201-207.

11. Armonda RA, Bell RS, Vo AH, et al. Wartime traumatic cerebral vasospasm: recent review of combat casualties. Neurosurgery 2006;59(6):1215-1225.

12. Bell RS, Vo AH, Neal CJ, et al. Military traumatic brain and spinal column injury: a 5-year study of the impact blast and other military grade weaponry on the central nervous system. J Trauma 2009;66(4 Suppl):S104-111.

13. Zoroya G. Key Iraq wound: brain trauma. USA Today 2005;March 3.

14. Sariego J. CCATT: a military model for civilian disaster management. Disaster Manag Response 2006;4(4):114-117.

15. Holcomb JB, McMullin NR, Pearse L, et al. Causes of death in U.S. Special Operations Forces in the global war on terrorism: 2001-2004. Ann Surg 2007;245(6):986-991.

16. Chesnut RM, Marshall LF, Klauber MR, et al. The role of secondary brain injury in determining outcome from severe head injury. J Trauma 1993;34(2):216-222.

17. Barton CW, Hemphill JC, Morabito D, et al. A novel method of evaluating the impact of secondary brain insults on functional outcomes in traumatic brain-injured patients. Acad Emerg Med 2005;12(1):1-6.

18. Chesnut RM, Marshall LF. Management of severe head injury. In: Ropper A, editor. Neurological and neurosurgical intensive care. 3rd ed. New York: Raven Press; 1993. p. 203-246.

19. Jiang JY, Gao GY, Li WP, et al. Early indicators of prognosis in 846 cases of severe traumatic brain injury. J Neurotrauma 2002;19(7):869-874.

20. Salazar AM, Johnson RT, editors. Current therapies in neurologic disease. 3rd ed. Philadelphia, PA: B.C. Decker, Inc.; 1990. p. 202-208.

21. Brain Trauma Foundation; American Association of Neurological Surgeons; Congress of Neurological Surgeons; Joint Section on Neurotrauma and Critical Care, AANS/CNS, Bratton SL, Chestnut RM, Ghajar J, et al. Guidelines for the management of severe traumatic brain injury. I. Blood pressure and oxygenation. J Neurotrauma 2007;24 Suppl 1:S7-13.

22. Brain Trauma Foundation; American Association of Neurological Surgeons; Congress of Neurological Surgeons; Joint Section on Neurotrauma and Critical Care, AANS/CNS, Bratton SL, Chestnut RM, Ghajar J, et al. III. Prophylactic hypothermia. J Neurotrauma 2007;24 Suppl 1:S21-25.

23. Bouma GJ, Muizelaar JP, Bandoh K, et al. Blood pressure and intracranial pressure-volume dynamics in severe head injury: relationship with cerebral blood flow. J Neurosurg 1992;77(1):15-19.

24. Bouma GJ, Muizelaar JP, Choi SC, et al. Cerebral circulation and metabolism after severe traumatic brain injury: the elusive role of ischemia. J Neurosurg 1991;75(5):685-693.

25. Fortune JB, Feustel PJ, Graca L, et al. Effect of hyperventilation, mannitol, and ventriculostomy drainage on cerebral blood flow after head injury. J Trauma 1995;39(6):1091-1097.

26. Obrist WD, Langfitt TW, Jaggi JL, et al. Cerebral blood flow and metabolism in comatose patients with acute head injury. Relationship to intracranial hypertension. J Neurosurg 1984;61(2):241-253.

27. Muizelaar JP, Marmarou A, Ward JD, et al. Adverse effects of prolonged hyperventilation in patients with severe head injury: a randomized clinical trial. J Neurosurg 1991;75(5):731-739.

28. Sawauchi S, Abe T. The effect of haematoma, brain injury, and secondary insult on brain swelling in traumatic acute subdural haemorrhage. Acta Neurochir (Wien) 2008;150(6):531-536.

29. Monroe A. Observations on the structure and functions of the nervous systems. Edinburgh: Creech and Johnson;1783.

30. Kellie G. An account of the appearances observed in the dissection of two of three individuals presumed to have perished in the storm of the 3d, and whose bodies were discovered in the vicinity of Leith on the morning of the 4th, November 1821; with some reflections of the pathology of the brain. Edinburgh Trans Med Chir Sci 1824;1:84-169.

31. Simmons RL, Martin AM Jr, Heisterkamp CA III, et al. Respiratory insufficiency in combat casualties. II. Pulmonary edema following head injury. Ann Surg 1969;170(1):39-44.

32. Rogers FB, Shackford SR, Trevisani GT, et al. Neurogenic pulmonary edema in fatal and nonfatal head injuries. J Trauma 1995;39(5):860-866.

33. Shivalkar B, Van Loon J, Wieland W, et al. Variable effects of explosive or gradual increase in intracranial pressure on myocardial structure and function. Circulation 1993;87(1):230-239.

34. Stein SC, Chen XH, Sinson GP, et al. Intravascular coagulation: a major secondary insult in nonfatal traumatic brain injury. J Neurosurg 2002;97(6):1373-1377.

35. Dóczi T, Tarjanyi J, Huszka E, et al. Syndrome of inappropriate secretion of antidiuretic hormone (SIADH) after head injury. Neurosurgery 1982;10(6 Pt 1):685-688.

36. Harrigan MR. Cerebral salt wasting syndrome: a review. Neurosurgery 1996;38(1):152-160.

37. Jagger J. Prevention of brain trauma by legislation, regulation, and improved technology: a focus on motor vehicles. J Neurotrauma 1992;9 Suppl 1:S313-316.

38. Hoge CW, McGurk D, Thomas JL, et al. Mild traumatic brain injury in U.S. Soldiers returning from Iraq. N Engl J Med 2008;358(5):453-463.

39. Perel P, Arango M, Clayton T, et al. Predicting outcome after traumatic brain injury: practical prognostic models based on large cohort of international patients. BMJ 2008;336(7641):425–429.

40. American Academy of Neurology. Practice parameter: the management of concussion in sports (summary statement). Report of the Quality Standards Subcommittee. Neurology 1997;48(3):581-585.

41. American Psychiatric Association. Diagnostic and statistical manual of mental disorders, 4th ed. Text revision. Washington, DC: American Psychiatric Association; 2000.

42. Geocadin RG. Traumatic brain injury. In: Bhardwaj A, Mirski MA, Ulatowski JA, editors. Handbook of neurocritical care. 1st ed. Totowa, NJ: Humana Press; 2004. p. 73-89.

43. Ling GSF. Personal communications, 2009.

44. DeWitt DS, Prough DS. Blast-induced brain injury and posttraumatic hypotension and hypoxemia. J Neurotrauma 2009;26(6):877-887.

45. Schneiderman AI, Braver ER, Kang HK. Understanding sequelae of injury mechanisms and mild traumatic brain injury incurred during the conflicts in Iraq and Afghanistan: persistent postconcussive symptoms and posttraumatic stress disorder. Am J Epidemiol 2008;167(12):1446-1452.

46. Martin EM, Lu WC, Helmick K, et al. Traumatic brain injuries sustained in the Afghanistan and Iraq wars. Am J Nurs 2008;108(4):40-47.

47. Bryant RA. Disentangling mild traumatic brain injury and stress reactions. N Engl J Med 2008;358(5):525-527.

48. Snoek JW, Minderhoud JM, Wilmink JT. Delayed deterioration following mild head injury in children. Brain 1984;107(Pt 1):15-36.

49. Ropper AH, Gorson KC. Clinical practice. Concussion. N Engl J Med 2007;356(2):166-172.

50. McCrory PR, Berkovic SF. Second impact syndrome. Neurology 1998;50(3):677-683.

51. Meythaler JM, Peduzzi JD, Eleftheriou E, et al. Current concepts: diffuse axonal injury-associated traumatic brain injury. Arch Phys Med Rehabil 2001;82(10):1461-1471.

52. Zwahlen RA, Labler L, Trentz O, et al. Lateral impact in closed head injury: a substantially increased risk for diffuse axonal injury—a preliminary study. J Craniomaxillofac Surg 2007;35(3):142-146.

53. Narayan RK, Maas AI, Servadei F, et al. Progression of traumatic intracerebral hemorrhage: a prospective observational study. J Neurotrauma 2008;25(6):629-639.

54. Bullock MR, Chesnut R, Ghajar J, et al. Surgical Management of Traumatic Brain Injury Author Group. Surgical management of acute subdural hematomas. Neurosurgery 2006;58(3 Suppl):S16-24.

55. Koc RK, Akdemir H, Oktem IS, et al. Acute subdural hematoma: outcome and outcome prediction. Neurosurg Rev 1997;20(4):239-244.

56. Sakas DE, Bullock MR, Teasdale GM. One-year outcome following craniotomy for traumatic hematoma in patients with fixed dilated pupils. J Neurosurg 1995;82(6):961-965.

57. Valadka AB, Robertson CS. Surgery of cerebral trauma and associated critical care. Neurosurgery 2007;61(1 Suppl):203-220.

58. Seelig JM, Becker DP, Miller JD, et al. Traumatic acute subdural hematoma: major mortality reduction in comatose patients treated within four hours. N Engl J Med 1981;304(25):1511-1518.

59. Croce MA, Dent DL, Menke PG, et al. Acute subdural hematoma: nonsurgical management of selected patients. J Trauma 1994;36(6):820-82; discussion 826-827.

60. Treacy PJ, Reilly P, Brophy B. Emergency neurosurgery by general surgeons at a remote major hospital.

ANZ J Surg 2005;75(10):852-857.

61. Paterniti S, Fiore P, Macri E, et al. Extradural haematoma. Report of 37 consecutive cases with survival. Acta Neurochir (Wien) 1994;131(3-4):207-210.

62. Bullock MR, Chesnut R, Ghajar J, et al. Surgical Management of Traumatic Brain Injury Author Group. Surgical management of acute epidural hematomas. Neurosurgery 2006;58(3 Suppl):S7-15; discussion Si-iv.

63. Chen TY, Wong CW, Chang CN, et al. The expectant treatment of "asymptomatic" supratentorial epidural hematomas. Neurosurgery 1993;32(2):176-179.

64. Clifton GL, Grossman RG, Makela ME, et al. Neurological course and correlated computerized tomography findings after severe closed head injury. J Neurosurg 1980;52(5):611-624.

65. Bullock MR, Chesnut R, Ghajar J, et al. Surgical Management of Traumatic Brain Injury Author Group. Surgical management of traumatic parenchymal lesions. Neurosurgery 2006;58(3 Suppl):S25-46.

66. Chang EF, Meeker M, Holland MC. Acute traumatic intraparenchymal hemorrhage: risk factors for progression in the early post-injury period. Neurosurgery 2006;58(4):647-656.

67. Narayan RK, Maas Al, Marshall LF, et al. Recombinant factor VIIA in traumatic intracerebral hemmorrhage: results of a dose-escalation clinical trial. Neurosurgery 2008;62(4):776-786.

68. Mayer SA, Brun NC, Begtrup K, et al. Efficacy and safety of recombinant activated factor VII for acute intracerebral hemorrhage. N Engl J Med 2008;358(20):2127-2137.

69. Brazis PW, Masdeu JC, Biller J. Localization in clinical neurology. 5th ed. Lippincott Williams & Wilkins; 2007. p. 521-555.

70. Chesnut RM, Gautille T, Blunt BA, et al. The localizing value of asymmetry in pupillary size in severe head injury: relation to lesion type and location. Neurosurgery 1994;34(5):840-845.

71. Blumenfeld H. Neuroanatomy through clinical cases. Sinauer Associates, Inc; 2002. p. 137-151.

72. Yang XF, Wen L, Shen F, et al. Surgical complications secondary to decompressive craniectomy in patients with a head injury: a series of 108 consecutive cases. Acta Neurochir (Wien) 2008;150(12):1241-1247; discussion 1248.

73. Vilela MD. Delayed paradoxical herniation after a decompressive craniectomy: case report. Surg Neurol 2008;69(3):293-296.

74. Marshall SA, Ling GSF. Personal communications, 2009.

75. Prabhakar H, Umesh G, Chouhan RS, et al. Reverse brain herniation during posterior fossa surgery.

J Neurosurg Anesthesiol 2003;15(3):267-269.

76. Ling GS, Marshall SA. Management of traumatic brain injury in the intensive care unit. Neurol Clin 2008;26(2):409-426.

77. Hammon WM. Analysis of 2187 consecutive penetrating wounds of the brain from Vietnam. J Neurosurg 1971;34(2 Pt 1):127-131.

78. Brandvold B, Levi L, Feinsod M, et al. Penetrating craniocerebral injuries in the Israeli involvement in the Lebanese conflict, 1982-1985. Analysis of a less aggressive surgical approach. J Neurosurg 1990;72(1):15-21.

79. Pruitt BA Jr. (Eds). Guidelines for the Management of Penetrating Brain Injury. Surgical management of penetrating brain injury. J Trauma 2001;51(2 Suppl):S16-25.

80. Pruitt BA Jr. (Eds). Guidelines for the Management of Penetrating Brain Injury. Antibiotic prophylaxis for penetrating brain injury. J Trauma 2001;51(2 Suppl):S34-40.

81. Aarabi B, Taghipour M, Alibaii E, et al. Central nervous system infections after military missile head wounds. Neurosurgery 1998;42(3):500-507.

82. Pruitt BA Jr. (Eds). Guidelines for the Management of Penetrating Brain Injury. Management of cerebrospinal fluid leaks. J Trauma 2001;51(2 Suppl):S29-33.

83. Pruitt BA Jr. (Eds). Guidelines for the Management of Penetrating Brain Injury. Neuroimaging in the management of penetrating brain injury. J Trauma 2001;51(2 Suppl):S7-11.

84. Provezale JM, Sarikaya B. Comparison of test performance characteristics of MRI, MR angiography, and CT angiography in the diagnosis of carotid and vertebral artery dissection: a review of the medical literature. AJR AM J Roentgenol 2009;193(4):1167-1174.

85. Vertinsky AT, Schwartz NE, Fischbein NJ, et al. Comparison of multidetector CT angiography and MR imaging of cervical artery dissection. AJNR Am J Neuroradiol 2008;29(9):1753-1760.

86. American College of Surgeons Committee on Trauma. Advanced trauma life support program for doctors. 8th ed. Chicago, IL: American College of Surgeons; 2008.

87. Pruitt BA Jr. (Eds). Guidelines for the Management of Penetrating Brain Injury. Prognostic indicators. J Trauma 2001;51(2 Suppl):S50.

88. Pigula FA, Wald SL, Shackford SR, et al. The effect of hypotension and hypoxia on children with severe head injuries. J Pediatr Surg 1993;28(3):310-315; discussion 315-316.

89. Fujimori M, Virtue RW. The value of oxygenation prior to induced apnea. Anesthesiology 1960;21:46-49.

90. Lev R, Rosen P. Prophylactic lidocaine use preintubation: a review. J Emerg Med 1994;12(4):499-506.

91. White PF, Schlobohm RM, Pitts LH, et al. A randomized study of drugs for preventing increases in intracranial pressure during endotracheal suctioning. Anesthesiology 1982;57(3):242-244.

92. Chraemmer-Jørgensen B, Høilund-Carlsen PF, Marving J, et al. Lack of effect of intravenous lidocaine on hemodynamic responses to rapid sequence intubation of general anesthesia: a double-blind controlled trial. Anesth Analg 1986;65(10):1037-1041.

93. Donegan MF, Bedford RF. Intravenously administered lidocaine prevents intracranial hypertension during endotracheal suctioning. Anesthesiology 1980;52(6):516-518.

94. Yano M, Nishiyama H, Yokota H, et al. Effect of lidocaine in ICP response to endotracheal suctioning. Anesthesiology 1986;64(5):651-653.

95. Wilson IG, Meiklejohn BH, Smith G. Intravenous lidocaine and sympathoadrenal responses to laryngoscopy and intubation. The effect of varying time of injection. Anaesthesia 1991;46(3):177-180.

96. Tam S, Chung F, Campbell M. Intravenous lidocaine: optimal time of injection before tracheal intubation. Anesth Analg 1987;66(10):1036-1038.

97. Bedford RF, Persing JA, Poberskin L, et al. Lidocaine or thiopental for rapid control of intracranial hypertension? Anesth Analg 1980;59(6):435-437.

98. Trindle MR, Dodson BA, Rampil IJ. Effects of fentanyl versus sufentanil in equianesthetic doses on middle cerebral artery blood flow velocity. Anesthesiology 1993;78(3):454-460.

99. Jones R, Gage A. Use of fentanyl in head injured patients. Ann Emerg Med 1994;23(2):385-386.

100. Helfman SM, Gold MI, DeLisser EA, et al. Which drugs prevent tachycardia and hypertension associated with tracheal intubation: lidocaine, fentanyl, or esmolol? Anesth Analg 1991;72(4):482-486.

101. Sperry RJ, Bailey PL, Reichman MV, et al. Fentanyl and sufentanil increase intracranial pressure in head trauma patients. Anesthesiology 1992;77(3):416-420.

102. Tobias JD. Increased intracranial pressure after fentanyl administration in a child with closed head trauma. Pediatr Emerg Care 1994;10(2):89-90.

103. Papazian L, Albanese J, Thirion X, et al. Effect of bolus doses of midazolam on intracranial pressure and cerebral perfusion pressure in patients with severe head injury. Br J Anaesth 1993;71(2):267-271.

104. Brain Trauma Foundation; American Association of Neurological Surgeons; Congress of Neurological Surgeons; Joint Section on Neurotrauma and Critical Care, AANS/CNS, Bratton SL, Chestnut RM, Ghajar J, et al. Guidelines for the management of severe traumatic brain injury. IX. Cerebral perfusion

thresholds. J Neurotrauma 2007;24 Suppl 1:S59-64.

105. Johnson DM, King RW, Bohnett M. The safety and efficacy of etomidate as an adjunct to endotracheal intubation in the ED. Acad Emerg Med 1994;1:318.

106. Burton JH. Etomidate. Acad Emerg Med 1995;2(1):72-74.

107. Dearden NM, McDowall DG. Comparison of etomidate and althesin in the reduction of increased ICP after head injury. Br J Anesth 1985;57(4):361-368.

108. Renou AM, Vernheit J, Macrez P, et al. Cerebral blood flow and metabolism during etomidate anesthesia in man. Br J Anesth 1978;50(10):1047-1051.

109. Lundy JB, Slane ML, Frizzi JD. Acute adrenal insufficiency after a single dose of etomidate. J Intensive Care Med 2007;22(2):111-117.

110. Batjer HH. Cerebral protective effects of etomidate: experimental and clinical aspects. Cerebrovasc Brain Metab Rev 1993;5(1):17-32.

111. Thompson JD, Fish S, Ruiz E. Succinylcholine for endotracheal intubation. Ann Emerg Med 1982;11(10):526-529.

112. Haldin M, Wahlin A. Effect of succinylcholine on intraspinal fluid pressure. Acta Anesthesia Scand 1959;3:155-161.

113. Minton MD, Grosslight K, Stirt JA, et al. Increases in intracranial pressure from succinylcholine. Prevention by nondepolarizing blockade. Anesthesiology 1986;65(2):165-169.

114. Stirt JA, Grosslight KR, Bedford RF, et al. "Defasciculation" with metocurine prevents succinylcholine-induced increases in intracranial pressure. Anesthesiology 1987;67(1):50-53.

115. Xue FS, Liao X, Liu JH, et al. A comparative study of the dose-response and time course of action of rocuronium and vecuronium in anesthetized adult patients. J Clin Anesth 1998;10(5):410-415.

116. Hunter JM. Rocuronium: the newest aminosteroid neuromuscular blocking drug. Br J Anaesth 1996;76(4):481-483.

117. Rosner MJ, Coley IB. Cerebral perfusion pressure, intracranial pressure, and head elevation. J Neurosurg 1986;65(5):636-641.

118. Durward QJ, Amacher AL, Del Maestro RF, et al. Cerebral and cardiovascular responses to changes in head elevation in patients with intracranial hypertension. J Neurosurg 1983;59(6):938-944.

119. Feldman Z, Kanter MJ, Robertson CS, et al. Effect of head elevation on intracranial pressure, cerebral perfusion pressure, and cerebral blood flow in head-injured patients. J Neurosurg 1992;76(2):207-211.

120. Vives MJ, Kishan S, Asghar J, et al. Spinal injuries in pedestrians struck by motor vehicles. J Spinal Disord Tech 2008;21(4):281-287.

121. Brain Trauma Foundation; American Association of Neurological Surgeons; Congress of Neurological Surgeons; Joint Section on Neurotrauma and Critical Care, AANS/CNS, Carney NA, Ghajar J. Guidelines for the management of severe traumatic brain injury. Introduction. J Neurotrauma 2007;24 Suppl 1:S1-2.

122. Warner KJ, Cuschieri J, Copass MK, et al. Emergency department ventilation effects outcome in severe traumatic brain injury. J Trauma 2008;64(2):341-347.

123. Miller JD, Sweet RC, Narayan R, et al. Early insults to the injured brain. JAMA 1978;240(5):439-442.

124. Redan JA, Livingston DH, Tortella BJ, et al. The value of intubating and paralyzing patients with suspected head injury in the emergency department. J Trauma 1991;31(3):371-375.

125. Stiver SI, Manley GT. Prehospital management of traumatic brain injury. Neurosurg Focus 2008;25(4):E5.

126. Marlow TJ, Goltra DD Jr, Schabel SI. Intracranial placement of a nasotracheal tube after facial fracture: a rare complication. J Emerg Med 1997;15(2):187–191.

127. Brain Trauma Foundation; American Association of Neurological Surgeons; Congress of Neurological Surgeons; Joint Section on Neurotrauma and Critical Care, AANS/CNS, Bratton SL, Chestnut RM, Ghajar J, et al. Guidelines for the management of severe traumatic brain injury. XIV. Hyperventilation. J Neurotrauma 2007;24 Suppl 1:S87-90.

128. Sheinberg M, Kanter MJ, Robertson CS, et al. Continuous monitoring of jugular venous saturation in head injured patients. J Neurosurg 1992;76(2):212-217.

129. Darby JM, Yonas H, Marion DW, et al. Local "inverse steal" induced by hyperventilation in head injury. Neurosurgery 1988;23(1):84-88.

130. Chan KH, Dearden NM, Miller JD, et al. Multimodality monitoring as a guide to treatment of intracranial hypertension after severe brain injury. Neurosurgery 1993;32(4):547-552; discussion 552-553.

131. Cruz J. On-line monitoring of global cerebral hypoxia in acute brain injury. J Neurosurg 1993;79(2):228-233.

132. Marion DW, Firlik A, McLaughlin MR. Hyperventilation therapy for severe traumatic brain injury. New Horiz 1995;3(3):439-447.

133. Schreiber MA, Aoki N, Scott BG, et al. Determinants of mortality in patients with severe blunt head

injury. Arch Surg 2002;137(3):285-290.

134. Jenkins LW, Moszynski K, Lyeth BG, et al. Increased vulnerability of the mildly traumatized rat brain to cerebral ischemia: the use of controlled secondary ischemia as a research tool to identify common or different mechanisms contributing to mechanical and ischemic brain injury. Brain Res 1989;477(1-2):211-224.

135. Clifton GL, Miller ER, Choi SC, et al. Fluid thresholds and outcome from severe brain injury. Crit Care Med 2002;30(4):739-745.

136. SAFE Study Investigators; Australian and New Zealand Intensive Care Society Clinical Trials Group; Australian Red Cross Blood Service; George Institute for International Health, Myburgh J, Cooper DJ, Finfer S, et al. Saline or albumin for fluid resuscitation in patients with traumatic brain injury. N Engl J Med 2007;357(9):874-884.

137. Contant CF, Valadka AB, Gopinath SP, et al. Adult respiratory distress syndrome: a complication of induced hypertension after severe head injury. J Neurosurg 2001;95(4):560-568.

138. Ratanalert S, Phuenpathom N, Saeheng S, et al. ICP threshold in CPP management of severe head injury patients. Surg Neurol 2004;61(5):429-434; discussion 434-435.

139. Brain Trauma Foundation; American Association of Neurological Surgeons; Congress of Neurological Surgeons; Joint Section on Neurotrauma and Critical Care, AANS/CNS, Bratton SL, Chestnut RM, Ghajar J, et al. Guidelines for the management of severe traumatic brain injury. VIII. Intracranial pressure thresholds. J Neurotrauma 2007;24 Suppl 1:S55-58.

140. Raslan A, Bhardwaj A. Medical management of cerebral edema. Neurosurg Focus 2007;22(5):E12.

141. Brain Trauma Foundation; American Association of Neurological Surgeons; Congress of Neurological Surgeons; Joint Section on Neurotrauma and Critical Care, AANS/CNS, Bratton SL, Chestnut RM, Ghajar J, et al. Guidelines for the management of severe traumatic brain injury. VII. Intracranial pressure monitoring technology. J Neurotrauma 2007;24 Suppl 1:S45-54.

142. Brain Trauma Foundation; American Association of Neurological Surgeons; Congress of Neurological Surgeons; Joint Section on Neurotrauma and Critical Care, AANS/CNS, Bratton SL, Chestnut RM, Ghajar J, et al. Guidelines for the management of severe traumatic brain injury. VI. Indications for intracranial pressure monitoring. J Neurotrauma 2007;24 Suppl 1:S37-44.

143. Ehtisham A, Taylor S, Bayless L, et al. Placement of external ventricular drains and intracranial pressure monitors by neurointensivists. Neurocrit Care 2008;10(2):241-247.

144. Harris CH, Smith RS, Helmer SD, et al. Placement of intracranial pressure monitors by non-neurosurgeons. Am Surg 2002;68(9):787-790.

145. Wise BL, Chater N. The value of hypertonic mannitol solution in decreasing brain mass and lowering

cerebro-spinal-fluid pressure. J Neurosurg 1962;19:1038-1043.

146. Brown FD, Johns L, Jafar JJ, et al. Detailed monitoring of the effects of mannitol following experimental head injury. J Neurosurg 1979;50(4):423-432.

147. Muizelaar JP, Wei EP, Kontos HA, et al. Mannitol causes compensatory cerebral vasoconstriction and vasodilation in response to blood viscosity changes. J Neurosurg 1983;59(5):822-828.

148. Rosner MJ, Coley I. Cerebral perfusion pressure: a hemodynamic mechanism of mannitol and the postmannitol hemogram. Neurosurgery 1987;21(2):147-156.

149. Mendelow AD, Teasdale GM, Russel T, et al. Effect of mannitol on cerebral blood flow and cerebral perfusion pressure in human head injury. J Neurosurg 1985;63(1):43-48.

150. Muizelaar JP, Lutz HA III, Becker DP. Effect of mannitol on ICP and CBF and correlation with pressure autoregulation in severely head-injured patients. J Neurosurg 1984;61(4):700-706.

151. Cruz J, Miner ME, Allen SJ, et al. Continuous monitoring of cerebral oxygenation in acute brain injury: injection of mannitol during hyperventilation. J Neurosurg 1990;73(5):725-730.

152. Marshall LF, Smith RW, Rauscher LA, et al. Mannitol dose requirements in brain-injured patients. J Neurosurg 1978;48(2):169-172.

153. Brain Trauma Foundation; American Association of Neurological Surgeons; Congress of Neurological Surgeons; Joint Section on Neurotrauma and Critical Care, AANS/CNS, Bratton SL, Chestnut RM, Ghajar J, et al. Guidelines for the management of severe traumatic brain injury. II. Hyperosmolar therapy. J Neurotrauma 2007;24 Suppl 1:S14-20.

154. Diringer MN, Zazulia AR. Osmotic therapy: fact and fiction. Neurocrit Care 2004;1(2):219-233.

155. Oddo M, Levine JM, Frangos S, et al. Effect of mannitol and hypertonic saline on cerebral oxygenation in patients with severe traumatic brain injury and refractory intracranial hypertension. J Neurol Neurosurg Psychiatry 2009;80(8):916-920.

156. Koenig MA, Bryan M, Lewin JL III, et al. Reversal of transtentorial herniation with hypertonic saline. Neurology 2008;70(13):1023-1029.

157. Ware ML, Nemani VM, Meeker M, et al. Effects of 23.4% sodium chloride solution in reducing intracranial pressure in patients with traumatic brain injury: a preliminary study. Neurosurgery 2005;57(4):727-736.

158. Smith H, Sinson G, Varelas P. Vasopressors and propofol infusion syndrome in severe head trauma. Neurocrit Care 2009;10(2):166-172.

159. Brain Trauma Foundation; American Association of Neurological Surgeons; Congress of Neurological

Surgeons; Joint Section on Neurotrauma and Critical Care, AANS/CNS, Bratton SL, Chestnut RM, Ghajar J, et al. Guidelines for the management of severe traumatic brain injury. XI. Anesthetics, analgesics, and sedatives. J Neurotrauma 2007;24 Suppl 1:S71-76.

160. Kelly DF, Goodale DB, Williams J, et al. Propofol in the treatment of moderate and severe head injury: a randomized, prospective double-blinded pilot trial. J Neurosurg 1999;90(6):1042-1052.

161. Jia X, Koenig MA, Shin HC, et al. Improving neurological outcomes post-cardiac arrest in a rat model: immediate hypothermia and quantitative EEG monitoring. Resuscitation 2008;76(3):431-442.

162. Qiu WS, Liu WG, Shen H, et al. Therapeutic effect of mild hypothermia on severe traumatic head injury. Chin J Traumatol 2005;8(1):27-32.

163. Rosenfeld JV, Cooper DJ, Kossmann T, et al. Decompressive craniectomy. J Neurosurg 2007;106(1):195-196.

164. Guerra WK, Gaab MR, Dietz H, et al. Surgical decompression for traumatic brain swelling: indications and results. J Neurosurg 1999;90(2):187-196.

165. Albanèse J, Leone M, Alliez JR, et al. Decompressive craniectomy for severe traumatic brain injury: evaluation of the effects at one year. Crit Care Med 2003;31(10):2535-2538.

166. Münch E, Horn P, Schürer L, et al. Management of severe traumatic brain injury by decompressive craniectomy. Neurosurgery 2000;47(2):315-322.

167. Pompucci A, De Bonis P, Pettorini B, et al. Decompressive craniectomy for traumatic brain injury: patient age and outcome. J Neurotrauma 2007;24(7):1182-1188.

168. Hutchinson P, Timofeev I, Grainger S, et al. The RESCUEicp decompressive craniectomy trial. Crit Care 2009;13(Suppl 1):P85.

169. Annegers JF, Coan SP. The risks of epilepsy after traumatic brain injury. Seizure 2000;9(7):453-457.

170. Temkin NR, Haglund MM, Winn HR. Causes, prevention, and treatment of post-traumatic epilepsy. New Horiz 1995;3(3):518-522.

171. Temkin NR. Antiepileptogenesis and seizure prevention trials with antiepileptic drugs: meta-analysis of controlled trials. Epilepsia 2001;42(4):515-524.

172. Agrawal A, Timothy J, Pandit L, et al. Post-traumatic epilepsy: an overview. Clin Neurol Neurosurg 2006;108(5):433–439.

173. Brain Trauma Foundation; American Association of Neurological Surgeons; Congress of Neurological Surgeons; Joint Section on Neurotrauma and Critical Care, AANS/CNS, Bratton SL, Chestnut RM, Ghajar J, et al. Guidelines for the management of severe traumatic brain injury. XIII. Antiseizure prophylaxis. J

Neurotrauma 2007;24 Suppl 1:S83-86.

174. Naidech AM, Kreiter KT, Janjua N, et al. Phenytoin exposure is associated with functional and cognitive disability after subarachnoid hemorrhage. Stroke 2005;36(3):583-587.

175. Wang H, Gao J, Lassiter TF, et al. Levetiracetam is neuroprotective in murine models of closed head injury and subarachnoid hemorrhage. Neurocrit Care 2006;5(1):71-78.

176. Temkin NR. Preventing and treating posttraumatic seizures: the human experience. Epilepsia 2009;50 Suppl 2:10-13.

177. Pruitt BA Jr. (Eds). Guidelines for the Management of Penetrating Brain Injury. Antiseizure prophylaxis for penetrating brain injury. J Trauma 2001;51(2 Suppl);S41-43.

178. Patel HC, Menon DK, Tebbs S, et al. Specialist neurocritical care and outcome from head injury. Intensive Care Med 2002;28(5):547-553.

179. Mason PE, Eadie JS, Holder AD. Prospective observational study of United States (US) Air Force Critical Care Air Transport Team Operations in Iraq. J Emerg Med 2008;28(5):547-553.

180. Grissom TE, Farmer JC. The provision of sophisticated critical care beyond the hospital: lessons from physiology and military experiences that apply to civil disaster medical response. Crit Care Med 2005;33(1 Suppl):S13-21.

181. Rogers FB, Cipolle MD, Velmahos G, et al. Practice management guidelines for the prevention of venous thromboembolism in trauma patients: the EAST practice management guidelines work group. J Trauma 2002;53(1):142-164.

182. Marion DW. Head and spinal cord injury. Neurol Clin 1998;16(2):485-502.

183. Daley RJ, Rebuck JA, Welage LS, et al. Prevention of stress ulceration: current trends in critical care. Crit Care Med 2004;32(10):2008-2013.

184. Ropper AH, Gress DR, Diringer MN, et al. Head injury. In: Ropper AH, Gress DR, Diringer MN, et al., editors. Neurological and neurosurgical intensive care. 4th ed. Philadelphia, PA: Lippincott Williams & Wilkins; 2004. p. 189-207.

# EXTREMITY INJURY
*Chapter 9*

**Contributing Authors**
John F. Kragh, Jr., MD, COL, MC, US Army
Jess M. Kirby, MD, MAJ, MC, US Army
James R. Ficke, MD, COL, MC, US Army

All figures and tables included in this chapter have been used with permission from Pelagique, LLC, the UCLA Center for International Medicine, and/or the authors, unless otherwise noted.

Use of imagery from the Defense Imagery Management Operations Center (DIMOC) does not imply or constitute Department of Defense (DOD) endorsement of this company, its products, or services.

**Disclaimer**
The opinions and views expressed herein belong solely to those of the authors. They are not nor should they be implied as being endorsed by the United States Uniformed Services University of the Health Sciences, Department of the Army, Department of the Navy, Department of the Air Force, Department of Defense, or any other branch of the federal government.

# Table of Contents

# Introduction

Combat casualty care (CCC) poses unique challenges. "Special experience is required to handle war injuries" and a good trauma surgeon is not necessarily a good war surgeon.[1] The goal of this chapter is to translate lessons learned during Operation Enduring Freedom (OEF) and Operation Iraqi Freedom (OIF) into a useful guide for managing combat casualties with extremity injuries.

- A majority (54 percent to 82 percent) of casualties at far-forward hospitals have extremity injuries.[2,3]
- The severity of limb injury encountered during CCC is far greater than that encountered in civilian care (Fig. 1).
- General surgeons often need to perform orthopaedic procedures such as complex wound debridement, external fixation of fractures, and fasciotomy for compartment syndrome.
- Extremity injury care underscores one of the most obvious differences between military and civilian scope of practice for nonorthopaedic CCC providers.

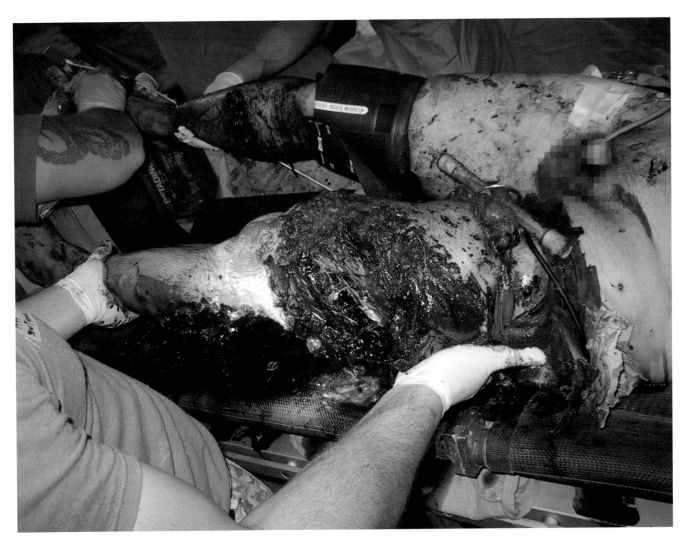

Figure 1. *The severity of limb injury encountered during CCC is far greater than that encountered in civilian care. Image courtesy of Harold Bohman, MD, CAPT, MC, US Navy.*

# Burden of Extremity Injury

Extremity injuries in battle casualties are common, disabling, and costly.[2,4,5] Much of war surgery is orthopaedic related. Extremity injuries were noted in 54 percent of casualties from OEF and OIF.[2] Furthermore, the casualties with extremity injuries consume the most care at the first hospital as evidenced by operating room time used, proportion of surgeries performed, and number of occupied beds.[3] Data collected from 2003 to 2006 in OIF indicate that extremity injuries have increased in severity (Fig. 2).[6] Despite the increase in injury severity, more casualties with more severe limb injuries are surviving and undergoing rehabilitation in large part due to improved CCC.

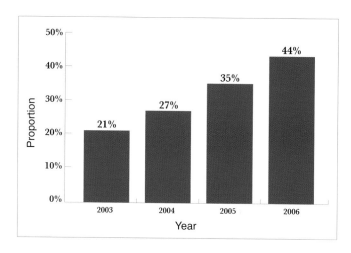

Figure 2. *Annual proportion of US casualties with severe limb injuries during OEF and OIF.*

> Extremity injuries were noted in 54 percent of casualties from OEF and OIF.

Extremities are particularly vulnerable to combat-specific injury mechanisms like parachuting and fast-roping injuries, which are similar to falls from height.[7,8,9,10] The proportion of casualties with major limb trauma has doubled during the course of the OIF (from 21 percent to 44 percent).[11] In OEF and OIF, battlefield casualties with limb injuries consume about 65 percent of inpatient care, cause the greatest number of disabled soldiers, and result in the greatest projected disability costs.[5]

Extremity injury is of great importance as casualties can be saved with proper care and, conversely, endangered with inappropriate care (Fig. 3). The scope of practice for most careproviders expands when one goes to war. In the words of Sir Robert Jones who was knighted for his CCC in World War I, "the War has taught the orthopaedic surgeon that he has to be more of a general surgeon; it has taught the general surgeon that he should be more of an orthopaedist."[12] Extremity injury care is a prime example of this expanded scope of practice, as nonorthopaedists are often responsible for providing limb-saving interventions and care. Orthopaedic workload at times necessitates nonorthopaedic trained surgeons to perform extremity procedures such as: (1) complex wound debridement; (2) external fixation of fractures; and (3) fasciotomy for compartment syndrome (Fig. 4). These procedures are technically challenging, and if performed late or not at all, they are associated with increased mortality and morbidity rates.[13,14] Other critical interventions include applying extremity tourniquets and managing traumatic amputations.

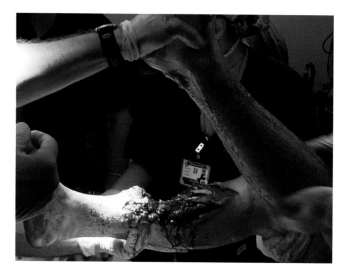

Figure 3. *Nonorthopaedists are often responsible for providing limb-saving interventions and care.*

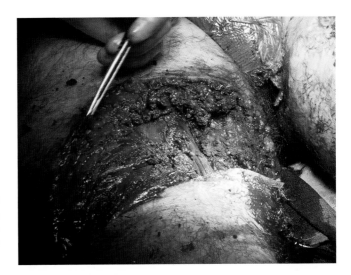

Figure 4. *General surgeons often need to perform orthopaedic procedures such as:* (Top Right) *complex wound debridement,* (Bottom Left) *external fixation of fractures, and* (Bottom Right) *fasciotomy for compartment syndrome. Fasciotomy image courtesy of Defense Imagery Management Operations Center (DIMOC).*

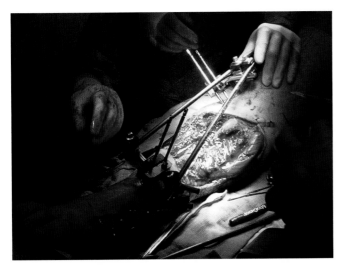

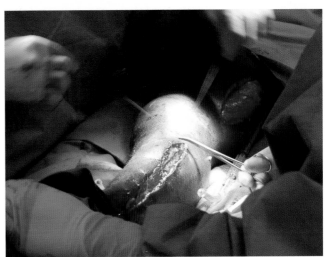

General surgeons often need to perform orthopaedic procedures such as complex wound debridement, external fixation of fractures, and fasciotomy for compartment syndrome.

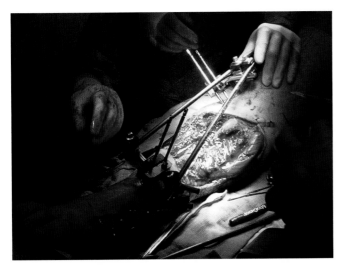

Figure 5. *White board demonstrating numerous combat casualties with multiple injuries. Image courtesy of the Borden Institute, Office of The Surgeon General, Washington, DC.*

Combat casualties with multiple injuries can rapidly overwhelm orthopaedic service capacity (Fig. 5). Orthopaedists should anticipate this challenge and be prepared to help manage trauma system resources according to a preexisting protocol. Delegating cases, training colleagues, extending care through ancillary careproviders, and delegating nonorthopaedic tasks (e.g., casualty triage) to others will maximize available orthopaedic resources. In the setting of multiple casualties, the scope of practice for orthopaedists widens to include burn care, escharotomies, assisting in damage control surgery and resuscitation, and soft-tissue repairs, flaps, and reconstructions.

# Extremity Injury-Associated Mortality

A common preventable cause of battlefield death is limb hemorrhage.

- Casualty fatality rates have remained at an all-time low, while injury severity has increased because of lifesaving care such as emergency tourniquet use and improved patient resuscitation.
- A persistent, difficult to manage cause of death is limb hemorrhage too proximal for tourniquet or direct pressure control.
- United States (US) military hospital casualty death rates (casualties who died of wounds received in action, after arrival at a hospital) are 5 percent despite high injury severity.
- The orthopaedist is considered the subject matter expert on musculoskeletal injures, tourniquet use, and proximal limb hemorrhage.

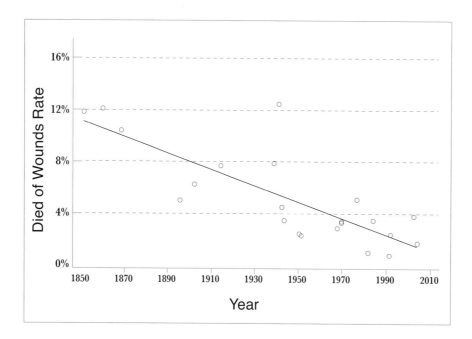

Figure 6. *Rates over time of casualties who died of wounds.*

Battlefield survival is at an all-time high for US casualties during OEF and OIF. Casualty fatality rates have remained at an all-time low while the injury severity has increased because of lifesaving care such as improved body armor, emergency tourniquet use, and improved patient resuscitation.[15,16,17,18] Orthopaedic trauma was the main cause of death in about 7 percent of casualties who were killed in action before arrival at a hospital in recent wars (e.g., Somalia, Vietnam), and the most common mechanism of death in this cohort was exsanguination.[19,20,21,22] Those casualties who died of wounds received in action after arrival at a hospital died of a myriad of traumatic sequelae. These included exsanguination, shock, and sepsis.[20] The rate of those who died of wounds, usually above 10 percent prior to 1900, has decreased with treatment advancements. As of 2009, the rate of those who died of wounds is about 5 percent (Fig. 6).[23,24,25,26]

Varying definitions of combat casualties who died of wounds make historical comparisons between individual wars difficult. Casualty statistics come predominantly from the war victors of modern nations, so there is a reporting bias. Although died of wounds is a phrase with a commonly accepted innate meaning, its operational definition is very specific and less appreciated. Died of wounds received in hostile action is a specific casualty category; it excludes victims of a terrorist activity and includes those who die of wounds or other injuries received in action after having reached a medical treatment facility. The died of wounds rate generally goes up when prehospital care is optimized, as the casualties arriving alive at the first hospital generally are more severely injured than if prehospital care is suboptimal. If prehospital care is suboptimal, the killed in action rate generally goes up, and the died of wounds rate goes down.[27]

Battlefield tourniquet use has been shown to be a lifesaving intervention when tourniquets are applied for limb exsanguination (Fig. 7).[15,28] The proportion of casualties dying from isolated limb exsanguination has dropped from 7 percent to 2 percent during the course of OEF and OIF. This decrease in mortality is likely due to improved resuscitation, better battlefield bandages, and more frequent use of tourniquets in the prehospital setting.[6,15,17]

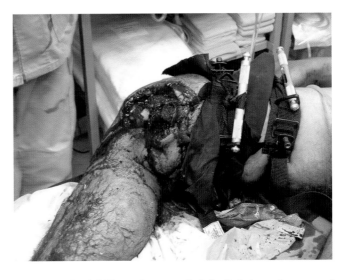

Figure 7. *Battlefield tourniquets applied for limb hemorrhage control are a lifesaving intervention. If one tourniquet is ineffective, side-by-side (in sequence longitudinally) dual tourniquet use may be effective. Image courtesy of the Borden Institute, Office of The Surgeon General, Washington, DC.*

The incidence of combat casualties suffering extremity wounds that arrive alive at CCC facilities has not changed much over time. Improved survival to hospital discharge is likely the result of resuscitation improvements, more rapid evacuation, body armor, and early forward surgery.[29,30] The proportion of survivors with extremity wounds increases when body armor is used compared to when it is not used. The greater lethality of head and torso war wounds results in casualties killed in action, disproportionate to casualties with isolated limb injury. The proportion of casualties arriving alive at the hospital with extremity injuries is 54 percent in OEF and OIF.[2] This is similar to the average projected body surface area for the extremities (61 percent) vulnerable to penetrating trauma in adult males proposed by Burns and Zuckerman.[4,30] Prolonged evacuation times due to tactical situations or other reasons generally increase the rates of those killed in action and generally decrease the rates of those who died of wounds in a delayed fashion. Shorter evacuation times usually reverse the aforementioned trends.[25,29] Recent medical advancements and body armor may have saved preferentially more torso-wounded casualties.[29]

> The proportion of casualties dying from isolated limb exsanguination has dropped from 7 percent to 2 percent during the course of OEF and OIF. This decrease in mortality is likely due to improved resuscitation, better battlefield bandages, and more frequent use of tourniquets in the prehospital setting.

Case fatality rates for limb trauma patients admitted to hospitals have changed dramatically in the last century.[31] For example, case fatality rates for femur fractures have dropped from 80 percent in early World War I to less than 1 percent recently because of such advancements as the use of the Thomas splint before arrival at a hospital, intramedullary nailing, and early mobilization rather than bed rest and traction.[25,32] Gas gangrene, tetanus infections, and wound sepsis, common in World War I, are uncommon in OEF and OIF because of improved surgical debridement, wound irrigation, tetanus immunization, and antibiotic advancements.[6,25]

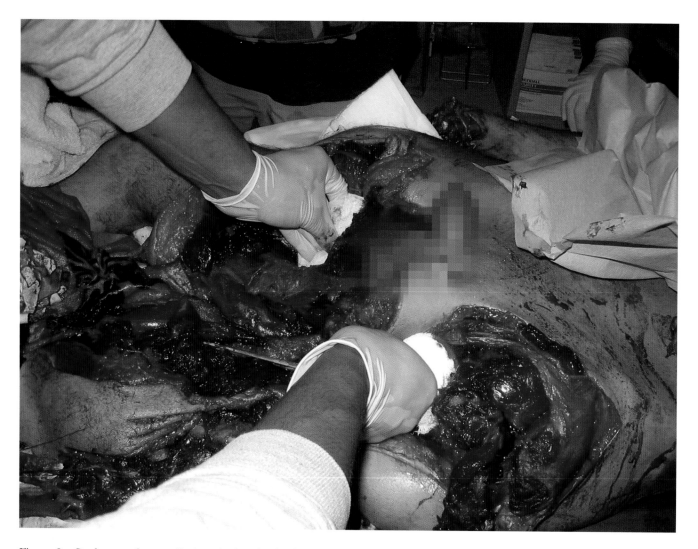

Figure 8. *Combat casualty mortality is predominantly related to vascular trauma and hemorrhage. Note pressure being applied to bilateral transected femoral arteries in this casualty. Image courtesy of the Borden Institute, Office of The Surgeon General, Washington, DC.*

Combat casualty mortality is predominantly related to vascular trauma and hemorrhage for those killed in action and those who died of wounds.[6,25] Observational data indicate that the type of tissue injured (e.g., artery, vein, or muscle), location (proximal versus distal) of the wound, and the mass of tissue wounded are associated with trauma outcomes such as death and survival.[25,33] For example, pelvic vessel disruption has had intermediate lethality between femoral and thoracoabdominal vessel disruption.[25] Proximal traumatic amputations are more lethal than distal amputations, and traumatic amputations of the lower limbs are more lethal than those of the upper limbs.[25] Multiple traumatic amputations are more lethal than single amputations.[20] These findings all converge on the idea that for combat casualties, the larger vessels bleed more, and greater tissue loss is associated with greater blood loss and higher mortality (Fig. 8).

> Observational data indicate that the type of tissue injured (e.g., artery, vein, or muscle), location of the wound (proximal versus distal), and the mass of tissue wounded are associated with trauma outcomes such as death and survival.

Hemorrhage control (in general) and tourniquet use (in particular) have been associated with improved combat casualty survival.[15,34,35] Emboli and intravascular clots, including deep venous thrombosis, pulmonary embolism, air embolus, and missile emboli, are uncommon but potentially preventable causes of extremity injury-associated death.[20] Multiple organ failure and sepsis are additional causes of death that are potentially preventable.[6,20,25]

Since the majority of the combat casualties suffer extremity trauma, orthopaedists are a cornerstone of CCC. Orthopaedists should prepare to train, educate, and extend the scope of practice of other CCC providers and ancillary staff regarding orthopaedic trauma. The orthopaedist is considered the subject matter expert on musculoskeletal injures, tourniquet use, and proximal limb hemorrhage control.

## Emergency Tourniquet Application

Tourniquet use is probably the single most obvious difference in practice between combat and civilian casualty care.[35]

- The objective of emergency tourniquet use is to extinguish the distal pulse, thereby controlling bleeding distal to the site of tourniquet application.
- Tourniquets provide maximal benefit the earlier they are applied following difficult to control extremity hemorrhage.
- Improvised (windlass) tourniquets should be applied only when scientifically designed tourniquets are absent. A windlass is a lever that can be wound to tighten a tourniquet.
- Tourniquets work better when applied distally (forearms and calves) than when applied more proximally (upper arms or thighs).
- Remove clothing and other underlying materials prior to tourniquet application (when possible) to ensure a tight and secure tourniquet fit.
- Remove the clothing surrounding a tourniquet to enable identification of all surrounding wounds and injuries.
- Do not apply tourniquets directly over joints as compression of vascular structures and bleeding control is limited by overlying bone.
- If one tourniquet is ineffective, side-by-side (in sequence longitudinally) dual tourniquet use may be effective.

The current indication for emergency tourniquet use in combat is any compressible limb wound that the first responder assesses as possibly lethal.[36] Tourniquet use for this indication has demonstrated favorable results following optimization of tourniquet design, training, doctrine, casualty evacuation, and tourniquet research.[15,28] The goals of emergency tourniquet use are to control bleeding and to extinguish the distal pulse. Timing and speed of application are vital because tourniquet placement before shock onset saves about 20-fold more casualties than placement after shock onset (96 percent survival with use before onset of shock versus 4 percent survival after onset of shock). Early prehospital tourniquet application saves about 11 percent more lives than delayed in-hospital use.[15] Tourniquet use in combat is recommended before casualty extraction or transport.[36]

> Tourniquets provide maximal benefit the earlier they are applied for difficult to control extremity hemorrhage. Tourniquet placement before the onset of shock is associated with 96 percent survival versus 4 percent survival after the onset of shock.

How tourniquets are applied has direct patient survival implications. Loose, misplaced, unattended, and broken devices have been associated with loss of hemorrhage control and death.[15,35] Materials under a tourniquet should be removed at the first opportunity to ensure optimal tourniquet constriction.[36] Periodic reassessment of tourniquets and casualties is vital. For example, a thigh tourniquet can loosen during patient transport or manipulation and thus permit rebleeding, especially when there is clothing or gear between the tourniquet and the skin.[36] A previously tight thigh tourniquet can loosen after exsanguination from non-extremity bleeding (e.g., chest, abdomen, or pelvis injuries). A significant loss of total body blood volume (e.g., 3.75 liters) will diminish the thigh circumference (volume) under and proximal to the tourniquet and will cause tourniquet loosening. Hence serial evaluations and tourniquet retightening are vital, when indicated.[36] However, reassessment should not include loosening and reapplication until surgeons are prepared to directly address the source of hemorrhage.

> The objective of emergency tourniquet use is to extinguish the distal pulse, thereby controlling bleeding, distal to the site of tourniquet application.

Clothing about a tourniquet should be removed at the first opportunity (when the tactical situation permits) to allow detection of all wounds. Undetected wounds are associated with uncontrolled hemorrhage and death.[36] Surveys are cursory when the applier and the casualty are under gunfire. Hastily performed casualty examinations often miss injuries; hence, casualties should be routinely reexamined at each level of care. Scientifically designed, laboratory tested, and clinically validated tourniquets should be used whenever possible.[36,37] The Combat Application Tourniquet (C-A-T®) is the most effective prehospital tourniquet (of tourniquets that have undergone clinical trials), and the Emergency & Military Tourniquet (EMT) is the most effective emergency department tourniquet.[36] Tourniquet effectiveness was defined by stopping visible bleeding and elimination of a palpable pulse (Fig. 9). Improvised windlass tourniquets should only be used when well-designed and clinically validated tourniquets are unavailable. A windlass is a lever that can be wound to tighten a tourniquet.

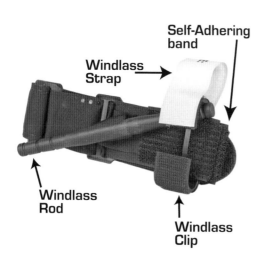
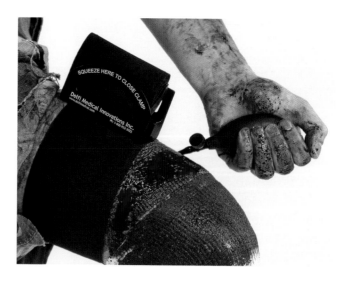

Figure 9. *The indication for emergency tourniquet use in combat is any compressible limb wound that the first responder assesses as potentially lethal. (Left) The Combat Application Tourniquet® is effective in a prehospital setting. (Right) The Emergency & Military Tourniquet is effective in an emergency department setting. Images courtesy of North American Rescue, LLC and Delfi Medical Innovations, Inc.*

> Improvised (windlass) tourniquets should be applied only when scientifically designed tourniquets are unavailable.

Tourniquet use over the distal segment of Hunter's canal near the knee should be avoided because prominent bones and tendons risk ineffectiveness. Tourniquets work well, provided they are applied proximal to wounds. They work better on the forearm or calf area and need not be reserved for the thigh or upper arm as is sometimes recommended for control of distal limb hemorrhage.[36] A common misconception is that a tourniquet has a lower effectiveness on two-boned segments (forearm and lower leg) than on one-boned segments (upper arm and thigh). A tourniquet actually has higher, rather than lower, effectiveness on two-boned limb segments.[36] The main determinant of effectiveness in well-designed tourniquets is the ratio of device width-to-limb circumference.[36,38] If one tourniquet is ineffective, then side-by-side (in sequence longitudinally) use can extinguish the distal pulse and stop bleeding, as such use widens the compressed area.

> If one tourniquet is ineffective, side-by-side (in sequence longitudinally) dual tourniquet use may be effective.

Misconceptions regarding tourniquets are rampant and take time and effort to correct.[36,38,39,40] Tourniquet education, training, and doctrine are vital and should be refined based on clinical evidence. Orthopaedists are looked to for tourniquet advice because they commonly use tourniquets during their day-to-day surgical practice. Orthopaedists are often asked to educate CCC providers on how and when tourniquets should be applied and how to detect and manage tourniquet-related problems. Orthopaedists may even be asked to build and steward tourniquet programs (i.e., find, order, store, test, clean, and fix devices, educate users, and document adverse events).[15,36]

Combat Application Tourniquet (C-A-T®): Application Steps (see Appendix 1)

(1) Route band around injured limb

(2) Pass band through the outside slit

(3) Pull band tight

(4) Twist windlass rod until bleeding has stopped and distal pulse is extinguished

(5) Lock the rod with the clip

(6) Secure the rod with the strap

(7) Record time tourniquet was applied

# Limb Compartment Syndrome

- Compartment syndrome continues to cause significant morbidity in OEF and OIF.
- Over-resuscitation with crystalloids can cause compartment syndrome.
- Compartment syndrome is a clinical diagnosis.
- Pressure manometry-based diagnosis of compartment syndrome in combat settings is unreliable.
- Lethal mistakes include delayed or limited fasciotomy skin incisions.
- Fasciotomy is not indicated in patients with prolonged compartment syndromes (warm ischemia duration exceeding 12 hours).

## Introduction

Compartment syndrome is a significant cause of combat-related morbidity in OEF and OIF and is highly varied in its presentation.[11] For US military casualties with limb injury in OEF and OIF, the incidence of compartment syndromes at or before arrival at Landstuhl Regional Medical Center, Germany, is 15 percent (Kragh, in press).[11] Combat casualty careproviders must often manage multiple cases of compartment syndrome prior to mastering the subtleties of diagnosis, treatment, and developing the ability to identify injured limbs at risk for developing the condition.[13]

> Compartment syndrome continues to cause significant morbidity in OEF and OIF, with an incidence of 15 percent at or before arrival at Landstuhl Regional Medical Center, Germany.

## Definition, Mechanisms, and Risk

Compartment syndrome is defined as an increased interstitial pressure within an enclosed osteofascial space (compartment) that reduces capillary blood perfusion below a level necessary for tissue viability.[41] As with all ischemia-reperfusion syndromes, duration of ischemia affects severity. Two basic mechanisms that cause compartment syndrome are an increase in the volume of tissue within an enclosed space and a decrease in the size of the enclosed space.

The compartment syndrome is common with injuries such as fractures that have severe swelling or bleeding.[41] Interestingly, open fractures have a higher rate of compartment syndrome than closed fractures despite the fascial rents seen with open fractures (Fig. 10). This is likely due to the higher injury force seen with open fractures resulting in greater tissue trauma, swelling, and bleeding.[41] The occurrence of compartment syndrome in a fractured limb has recently been associated with slower subsequent fracture healing rates.[42] The interstitial pressure of limbs also plays an important role in the mobilization of interstitial fluids into the intravascular space in response to distant hemorrhage and the tamponade of local intracompartmental hemorrhage.

The list of causes or risk factors for compartment syndrome is long and diverse (Appendix 2).[41] In combat casualties, more than one contributing factor is often present. Current data indicate that the most obvious determinant of fasciotomy frequency in OEF and OIF is the injury severity of the limb wound, based on the Abbreviated Injury Scale (AIS) of the most severe extremity wound.[11] Limb interstitial tissue pressures increase with resuscitation.[41] Hence, care must be taken to avoid excessive administration of crystalloid fluids that can worsen compartment syndrome. The overall injury severity score (ISS), frequency of tourniquet use, shock, and hypoperfusion also confer compartment syndrome risk.[11]

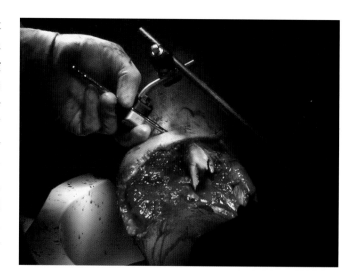

Figure 10. *Open fractures have a higher rate of compartment syndrome than closed fractures despite the fascial rents seen with open fractures.*

> Over-resuscitation with crystalloids can cause compartment syndrome.

## Clinical Findings

The classic findings seen with acute limb ischemia (i.e., pain, pallor, paresthesias, pulselessness, and poikilothermia) are not clinically reliable for the diagnosis of compartment syndrome and often manifest only in the late stages of compartment syndrome.[41] The finding of distal limb pulselessness is due to compression of arteries within the compartment. Civilian literature reports that pulselessness is a late clinical finding in compartment syndrome.[41] The authors' experiences in OIF revealed similar findings. Pulselessness is rarely seen, and it is usually a late finding when it is documented. In an alert and cooperative patient, compartment syndrome is manifest by pain out of proportion to the physical injury observed. The pain is typically worse with passive stretch of the muscles within the ischemic compartment. This pain on passive stretch is a sensitive indicator of compartment syndrome as it occurs early in its course; however, it is not specific.[43,44] While a palpably tense compartment is a specific clinical finding, it is not highly sensitive.[45] Sensory symptoms such as paresthesias are often an early indicator of nerve ischemia.[46]

> Compartment syndrome is a clinical diagnosis. Clinicians must weigh the mechanism of injury and suggestive clinical findings, including pain with passive stretch, palpable tenseness of the affected compartment, and neurovascular examination to arrive at the diagnosis.

The time of onset of compartment syndrome is often hours following injury, but it can occasionally present within minutes of injury.[47] The authors have seen florid compartment syndrome cases in OIF that presented within 15 to 45 minutes of injury with pulselessness that was rapidly reversed following fasciotomy.[47] Clinical findings in casualties with compartment syndromes can be classified as early and late. Early findings such as a palpably tense compartment, pain out of proportion to the injury, and pain with passive stretch of involved muscles are due to the elevated hydrostatic pressure within the fascial compartment.[41] Late findings of paresthesias and paralysis are due to the duration of tissue ischemia, particularly of nerves and muscle, respectively. Permanent nerve palsy is uncommon with compartment syndrome. The etiology of extremity weakness may be difficult to differentiate clinically from myopathy of ischemia-reperfusion, which is common and associated with the duration of ischemia.[41] The pressure gradient applied to the nerve (such as with a tourniquet) deforms the nerve at the point of maximal gradient (e.g., at the tourniquet edge) and is the cause of the nerve palsy. Nerve palsy clinically resolves slower than nerve ischemia but usually completely resolves.[36] Nerve ischemia is zonal, not focal, and is rarely severe in the emergency setting. It is associated with prolonged ischemia time.[36] Muscle is the tissue most sensitive to the duration of ischemia, the nerve is less so.

The rate of limb swelling is greatest early after injury, as tissue compartments are more pliable. Limbs typically reach maximum swelling 36 to 48 hours following injury.[48] Resolution of limb swelling occurs over a similar duration.[49] Comorbidities such as hemorrhagic shock and treatments (e.g., tourniquets and resuscitation) may alter swelling timelines, such that maximal swelling occurs up to five days following injury. This can result in discordant total body fluid intake and output measurements.[49] This means that compartment syndrome can be absent early at a forward treatment facility, yet occur from one to four days later during evacuation to rearward hospitals.[13] Furthermore, even if a fasciotomy is performed at a forward hospital, continued swelling can cause recurrent compartment syndrome if the release was not complete. This occurrence is associated with increased amputation and mortality rates.[13] The degree of swelling is also associated with the degree of injury and the degree of over-resuscitation, particularly with fluids more dilute than plasma.[13,49]

Recurrent compartment syndrome can be seen with incomplete release of compartments and is associated with increased amputation and mortality rates.

Prevention and identification of compartment syndrome are difficult. Historically, under-resuscitation was associated with acute renal failure. Subsequently, over-resuscitation with excessive fluids was linked to excessive limb edema and compartment syndromes, even in uninjured limbs.[50,51] Over-resuscitation leading to limb compartment syndrome is analogous to over-resuscitation leading to abdominal compartment syndrome.[50,52] Modern resuscitation has evolved towards physiologically-based targets (e.g., controlled hypotension with adequate perfusion), rather than simply replacing the estimated volume of blood loss with crystalloid fluids. Over-resuscitation has become less common recently.[16,53]

## Diagnosis

The diagnosis of compartment syndrome in war is based on clinical findings. Clinicians must weigh the mechanism of injury (e.g., blast) and suggestive clinical findings, including pain with passive stretch, palpable tenseness of the affected compartment, and neurovascular examination to arrive at the diagnosis. Common laboratory tests suggestive (but not diagnostic) of late or missed compartment syndrome, include elevated serum levels of creatinine kinase and urine myoglobinuria.[41] Due to limited sensitivity and specificity of clinical and laboratory findings, the diagnosis of compartment syndrome in the civilian sector is highly dependent on measuring tissue compartment pressures.[54] It is common civilian practice to measure compartment pressure before and after fasciotomy to confirm both the diagnosis and the efficacy of fascial release.[54] The accuracy of manometric-based diagnosis of compartment syndrome is unreliable in combat settings, and its use is not recommended.[47] Limb tissues such as muscle compartments are not incompressible matter (such as water) and do not transmit pressures fully or immediately like incompressible fluids. Time and distance attenuate high pressures within limb tissues. Failure to measure tissue pressure in proximity (e.g., within five centimeters) to the zone of peak pressure may result in a serious underestimation of the maximum compartment pressure.[55]

Manometric-based diagnosis of compartment syndrome in combat settings is unreliable and not recommended.

Even the methods and pressure threshold used for diagnosis are controversial. Pressures are indirect indicators of ischemia, and the amplitude of the pressure does not account for the ischemic duration, individual tolerance of ischemia, variations of anatomic compartments, and location of measurement versus pathology, such as fracture site.[54] No consensus exists on whether the pressure threshold within the compartment should be 30 or 45 mm Hg (4 to 6 kilopascals) or whether the difference between the intracompartmental pressure from the blood pressure such as the diastolic blood pressure (delta pressure) should be 30 or 40 mm Hg (4 to 5.33 kilopascals).[54] There is

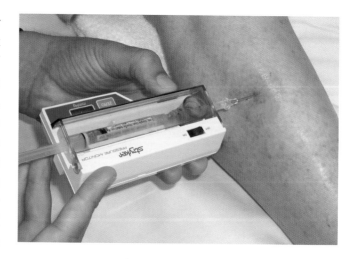

Figure 11. *Manometric-based diagnosis of compartment syndrome in combat settings is unreliable.*

even a lack of consensus regarding the type of catheters (slit, wick, and ultrafiltration) that should be used to measure compartmental pressures (Fig. 11).[43]

Observation and serial clinical examination of patients with limb trauma and equivocal compartment syndrome clinical findings are common in civilian settings. In such cases, recent interventions (e.g., aggressive fluid resuscitation) combined with mechanism of injury and evolving physical findings, such as a palpably tense compartment, can facilitate early diagnosis. In the mentally impaired (e.g., sedated, intubated, or unconscious) casualty, diagnosis of compartment syndrome is difficult because the clinical examination is less sensitive. Similarly, in combat settings, serial examinations may be impossible or unreliable because patients are often evacuated long distances under austere conditions. In such scenarios, prophylactic fasciotomies are recommended prior to transport based on clinical findings, extent of soft-tissue injury, anticipated resuscitation, and potential ischemia time.[56] Circular casts, which are common in civilian settings, are usually avoided in war, since evacuation over distances and time without close monitoring permit the onset of compartment syndrome without detection or treatment.[13,57]

> Delayed attempts at therapeutic fasciotomies are suboptimal and are associated with increased morbidity and mortality. Certain clinical findings – wounds with extensive soft-tissue injury, anticipated lengthy resuscitation, and potential extended ischemia time – should prompt prophylactic fasciotomies prior to evacuation of patients.

Failure to detect compartment syndrome early risks rhabdomyolysis, renal failure, Volkmann's ischemic contracture (ischemic muscle necrosis), and permanent limb dysfunction.[41] Delayed attempts at therapeutic fasciotomies are suboptimal and are associated with increased morbidity and mortality.[13]

## Treatment

The definitive treatment for acute compartment syndrome is therapeutic fasciotomy. When compartment syndrome is risked or is impending during the lag time from injury to syndrome onset, the fasciotomy is termed prophylactic.[47]

Evidence indicates a delayed fasciotomy is not indicated for casualties with a prolonged compartment syndrome (i.e., warm ischemia duration greater than 12 hours).[14,58] Fasciotomy in this subset of patients will increase infection rates and will decrease survival.[47] An algorithm for clinical decision making on compartment syndrome management in a combat setting is provided in Figure 1 within Appendix 2.

> Fasciotomy is not indicated for casualties with a prolonged compartment syndrome (i.e., warm ischemia duration greater than 12 hours).

Temporizing measures such as removing circumferential dressings or casts, removing sutures from tightly bound closures, and placing the affected limb at the level of the heart to balance inflow and venous return do no harm but are inadequate to treat an established compartment syndrome. In a casualty, marked elevation or dependence of the injured limb relative to the heart can increase risk of compartment syndrome, especially if the casualty is at risk for or is in hemorrhagic shock.[41] Extremity elevation is contraindicated because it decreases arterial blood flow and the arteriovenous pressure gradient and thus worsens the ischemia.[59]

Marked elevation or depression of the injured limb relative to the heart can increase the risk of compartment syndrome.

The sequelae of neglected or delayed treatment of compartment syndrome are ischemic contractures, nerve injury (due to nerve ischemia), potential amputation, systemic effects of myonecrosis, and death.[13,54] The morbidity risk and sequelae of compartment syndrome and fasciotomy are outlined in detail in Table 1.

| MORBIDITY RISK AND SEQUELAE OF COMPARTMENT SYNDROME AND FASCIOTOMY | |
|---|---|
| Potential Morbidity: Compartment Syndrome and Early Fasciotomy | Skin scar, scaly skin, ulceration, tethered tendons |
| | Postoperative arterial or graft thrombosis, thromboembolic disease wound infection, nonhealing fasciotomy wounds |
| | Limb swelling or chronic edema, shape change of limb, muscle hernia |
| | Pain, paresis or paralysis, paresthesia |
| | Coverage challenge: primary closure, delayed primary closure, skin graft, flap |
| | Possible repair of arterial injury worsening ischemia-reperfusion injury |
| Potential Sequelae List: Compartment Syndrome with Late or Incomplete Fasciotomy | Mortality, sepsis, multiple organ failure, acute kidney failure |
| | Myonecrosis, myoglobinemia, myoglobinuria, or rhabdomyolysis |
| | Paresis or paralysis |
| | Stiffness or contracture |
| | Limb amputation, tissue loss (e.g., muscle debridement) |

Table 1. *Morbidity risk and sequelae of compartment syndrome and fasciotomy.*

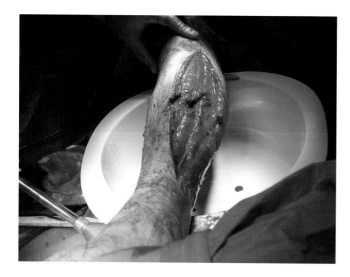

Figure 12. *The fasciotomy skin incision should be long, approximating the proximal to distal length of the compartment to be released. Image courtesy of the Borden Institute, Office of The Surgeon General, Washington, DC.*

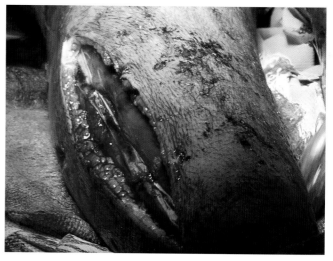

Figure 13. *Limited fasciotomy skin incisions, as seen above, should be avoided.*

## FASCIOTOMY SURGICAL STEPS (LEG AS AN EXAMPLE)

1. Initiate surgical positioning (supine); palpate bony landmarks and septum between anterior and lateral compartments.

2. Plan and mark incisions for dermotomies; do not use one-incision technique; use two-incision technique.

3. Make a medial skin incision: longitudinal posterior to tibia margin; avoid saphenous vein and nerve; from proximal tibia near the pes anserinus to the proximal ankle flexor retinaculum; do not use short skin incisions.

4. Make a lateral skin incision: near the septum between the anterior and the lateral compartments; avoid the superficial peroneal nerve from the proximal tibia margin near iliotibial band insertion on Gerdy's tubercle to the proximal ankle extensor retinaculum; do not use short skin incisions.

5. Expose the lateral leg fascia for a visual and palpable check of bony landmarks and septum between the anterior and the lateral compartments.

6. Divide the lateral fascia transversely at the septum to confirm entry into both the anterior and the lateral compartments. Extend this fasciotomy anterior and posterior enough for confirmation; use instrument or finger to confirm entry into both compartments.

7. Divide the lateral leg fascia longitudinally from the transverse fasciotomy; do this both proximally and distally for both the anterior and the lateral compartments.

8. Anterior compartment fasciotomy goes from the proximal tibia margin near the iliotibial band insertion on Gerdy's tubercle to the proximal ankle extensor retinaculum. Partially release one-quarter inch of the retinaculum; do not use short fascia incisions.

9. Superficial medial fasciotomy releases the posterior superficial compartment and goes from the proximal tibia margin near the pes to the proximal ankle flexor retinaculum. Partially release one-quarter inch of the retinaculum; do not use short fascia incisions.

10. Deep medial fasciotomy releases the deep posterior compartment and goes along the posterior medial tibia margin. Release the medial soleus margin from the tibia; check especially deep and proximal.

11. Check muscle bulge after fasciotomy; palpably confirm the adequacy of all releases.

Table 2. *Fasciotomy surgical steps using the leg as an example.*

## Fasciotomy Techniques

Extremity fasciotomy can be performed as an emergent bedside procedure but is preferably undertaken in the operative suite where anesthesia, sterile conditions, adequate lighting, and appropriate equipment are readily available (Table 2). Skin incisions (dermotomies) provide nearly no compartment release in and of themselves. The fasciotomy skin incision should be long because fasciotomy will need to span the length of the compartment itself.[54] The skin incision approximates the proximal to distal length of the compartment to be released (Figs. 12 and 13). Long skin incisions permit proper palpation and inspection of the compartment pressure and fascial release. Fasciotomies in civilian settings are often shorter because injury severities and compartment syndromes are less severe than in military settings and because reassessments are easier. A detailed outline of compartment names and corresponding main muscle groups and diagnostic and procedural codes used for CCC documentation are provided in Table 4 within Appendix 2. An operative note template for dictation, surgical planning, and data collection is provided in Table 5 within Appendix 2.

---

Limited fasciotomy skin incisions should be avoided. Skin incisions should be long, as a fasciotomy will need to span the length of the compartment itself.

---

### Lower Leg Fasciotomy

For the lower extremities, the common compartments that need release are in the lower leg (calf) and thigh. The four compartments of the lower leg consist of the anterior, lateral, superficial posterior, and deep posterior compartments. These compartments are typically released with longitudinal medial and lateral incisions (two skin incisions) (Fig. 14). One skin incision versus two skin incisions risks incomplete

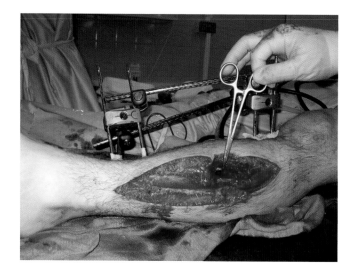
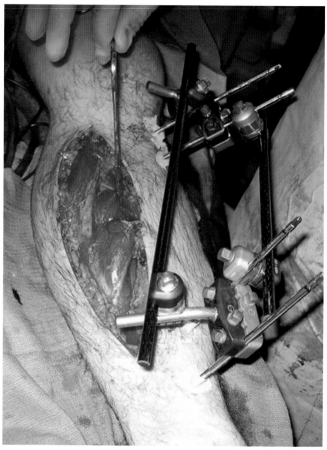

Figure 14. *The four compartments of the lower leg are typically released with longitudinal lateral and medial skin incisions as demonstrated in the adjacent images. Images courtesy of the Borden Institute, Office of The Surgeon General, Washington, DC.*

fascial release since it is associated with both an inadequate inspection and inadequate palpation of muscles and fascia; this includes an inadequate check of the completeness of the release. The lower leg compartments are the ones most commonly released late, and should be released earlier in such cases prior to swelling reaching its maximum at the index surgery.[13] The anterior leg compartment fasciotomy in war can include a partial (five millimeter) release of the proximal portion of extensor tendon retinaculum near the ankle. This should ensure that the distal extent of the fasciotomy is sufficiently complete.

> A double-skin incision technique should be used to release the four compartments of the lower leg in combat casualties.

### Thigh Fasciotomy
The thigh has three large compartments (anterior, posterior, and adductor), which are released with longitudinal medial and lateral incisions. The lateral thigh incision, used to access both the anterior and the posterior thigh compartments, can be extended to release the hip abductor muscles, tensor fascia lata, and gluteal muscles (Fig. 15).[41]

### Upper Arm Fasciotomy
The upper arm contains three compartments: one anterior, one posterior, and one for the deltoid muscle. These compartments are typically approached with medial and lateral skin incisions, and the lateral incision may also be extended to include release of the deltoid compartment.[41]

### Forearm Fasciotomy
In the forearm, the three compartments are dorsal, volar, and mobile wad muscles. The forearm fascial release is typically through one volar skin incision and one dorsal skin incision. The volar skin incision provides access to the mobile wad, superficial, and deep volar musculature and may be extended distally for the carpal tunnel release. The dorsal skin incision is used to release the contents of the dorsal forearm compartment. Individual forearm muscle epimysium, the layer of connective tissue that ensheaths an entire muscle, may be as robust as the superficial fascia of the forearm resulting in elevated pressures within individual muscle belly sheaths. Thus, each muscle belly, especially volar, should be inspected for possible release (epimysiotomy) in addition to release of the forearm fascia (Fig. 16).[41]

### Hand Compartment Fasciotomy
Hand compartments can be released through five skin incisions: two dorsally-based incisions over the index and ring finger metacarpals; one radial incision over the thenar muscles; one ulnar incision over the hypothenar muscles; and the final skin incision for the carpal tunnel release (Fig. 17).[41] Carpal tunnel release is commonly performed too late. The carpal tunnel should be released at the index surgery before swelling has reached its maximum.[13]

## Conclusions
Short skin incisions and incomplete fasciotomies risk mortality and morbidity.[13] Long skin incisions should be made to ensure adequate exposure of the deepest portion of the wound.[60] A single skin incision of the lower leg for a four-compartment fasciotomy may work well in civilian care, but it has not worked well in war. A double-skin incision technique should be used in combat casualties. Orthopaedists serve patients well if they make themselves widely available for consultation regarding combat casualties at risk for compartment syndrome.

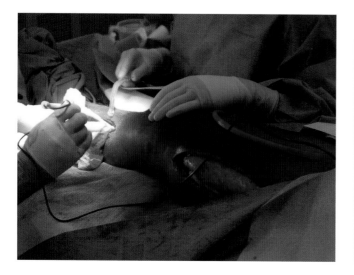

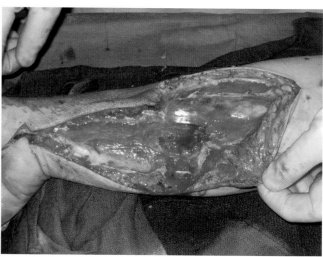

Figure 15. *The lateral thigh incision can be used to access the anterior and posterior thigh compartments and can be extended to release the hip abductor muscles, tensor fascia lata, and gluteal muscles. Image courtesy of Defense Imagery Management Operations Center (DIMOC).*

Figure 16. *Volar forearm debridement and fasciotomy. Each muscle belly should be inspected for possible release (epimysiotomy) in addition to release of the forearm fascia. Image courtesy of the Borden Institute, Office of The Surgeon General, Washington, DC.*

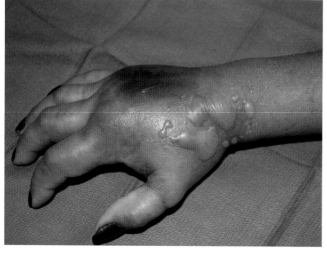

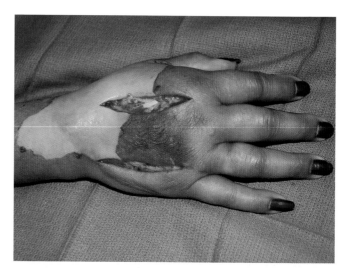

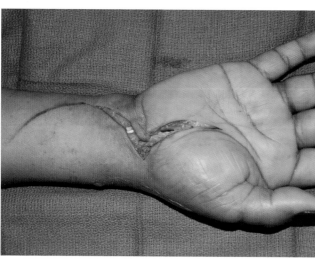

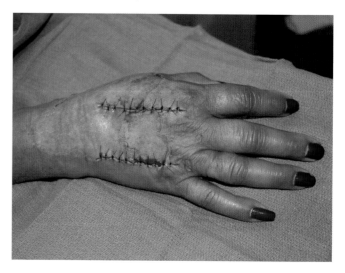

Figure 17. (Middle Left) *Hand compartment syndrome.* (Middle Right) *Dorsal skin incisions.* (Bottom Left) *Carpal tunnel release.* (Bottom Right) *Skin closure at 96 hours. Images courtesy of Rady Rahban, MD.*

# Traumatic Limb Amputations

- Blast injury is a common cause of traumatic limb amputation.
- Traumatic limb amputations may be multiple and can result in lethal hemorrhage.
- Careproviders should provide immediate lifesaving interventions and avoid becoming distracted by visually disturbing limb amputations.
- The distal segments of amputated limbs should be checked for viable autologous vein graft sources before disposal.
- Traumatic fasciotomies are not a substitute for the purposeful and complete surgical release of compartment fascia.
- The preservation of vital tissues achieved through atypical delayed surgical amputations may result in better functional outcomes than limb shortening in order to get a conventional wound closure.

## *Introduction*

The term amputation can refer to an injury, an emergent procedure, a delayed procedure in planned staged care, a delayed procedure for treatment or prevention of a complication, an elective procedure perhaps for limb dysfunction, or an outcome. Thus, the context of usage for the term amputation should be made explicitly clear in medical communications and records by the provider and coder (Appendix 3). Care notes are often written with indelible markers on adhesive tape applied to the casualty in order to get important information to rearward hospitals when records are otherwise at risk of being lost (Fig. 18).

Historically, most major limb amputations in combat settings were injuries as the result of extensive limb trauma, a surgery for consequence of severe infection, or a surgery for irreparable major arterial injury.[61,62,63] The percentage of limbs lost because of major vascular trauma and severe infection had decreased in modern warfare. However, the greater use of explosive weapons in OEF and OIF has resulted in a steady number of limbs lost because of massive blast injuries.[64] Traumatic limb amputation accounts for 7.4 percent of major limb injuries in OEF and OIF; it was 8.3 percent in the Vietnam War.[61,64]

> Blast injury is a common cause of traumatic limb amputation; traumatic limb amputation accounts for 7.4 percent of major limb injuries in OEF and OIF.

Limb salvage can occur when war surgeons use damage control vascular surgery principles and a team approach to injury triage and patient resuscitation.[65,66,67] It is important to note that surgical amputation (when indicated) should not be considered a failure of care, but rather, a key step of maximizing limb function. After debridement of all nonviable tissues, a reconstructive mindset and approach by careproviders are critical. A second operation to check the wound for possible debridement should be routinely planned 24 to 48 hours after the initial debridement, depending on the amount of initial tissue destruction and wound contamination. A fracture proximal to a traumatic amputation should be stabilized and is not an indication for more proximal amputation since successful fixation can help retain a longer and possibly more functional residual limb. The principle is to retain the maximum number of options for definitive care.[63]

## *Initial Assessment*

The closer the limb is to the explosion, the higher the likelihood of amputation. Casualties closer to

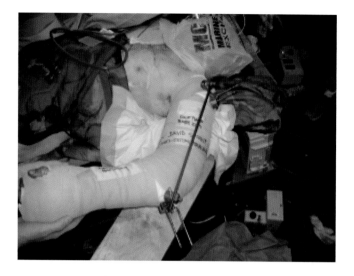 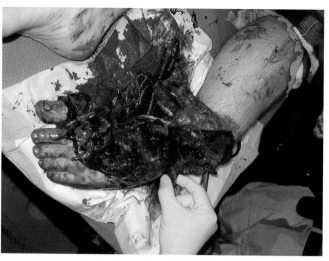

Figure 18. *Improvised patient information communication strategy. Patient information is written directly onto the dressing of a patient emerging from surgery. Image courtesy of Harold Bohman, MD, CAPT, MC, US Navy.*

Figure 19. *Although traumatic limb amputations are devastating injuries, patient morbidity and mortality can be minimized with appropriate management. Image courtesy of the Borden Institute, Office of The Surgeon General, Washington, DC.*

explosions may have multiple amputations. The amputation site generally correlates with lesion severity as in the Abbreviated Injury Scale (AIS); more proximal lesions are more severe and lethal. Traumatic limb amputations are visually very disturbing, even to seasoned careproviders and can distract CCC providers from delivering optimal patient care (Fig. 19). Traumatic limb amputations are devastating injuries; however, if appropriately managed, patient morbidity and mortality can be minimized.[15,63]

The initial therapeutic approach to the patient with a traumatic amputation should follow the same protocol as with all combat casualties. The emphasis should be placed on identifying and treating immediately life-threatening conditions first. Once immediate life-threats are mitigated, further evaluation of a traumatic limb amputation is warranted. The zone of injury may be wide and not limited to the direct penetrating portion of the explosion, as the blunt effects may be proximal to the open wound. The degree of wound contamination can be severe.

> Traumatic limb amputations may be multiple and can result in lethal hemorrhage. Careproviders should provide immediate lifesaving interventions and avoid becoming distracted by visually disturbing limb amputations.

Severe limb injuries, like subtotal traumatic amputations and mangled limbs, have been evaluated using a scale and assigned a score in order to help assess treatment options, such as the likelihood of successful limb salvage. Such efforts have been limited in their ability to predict outcomes or dictate care.[68] Similarly, the prognostic value of the insensate foot in association with limb salvage or surgical amputation has been evaluated. Researchers concluded that the insensate foot at presentation is neither prognostic of long-term plantar sensory status nor functional outcome, and should not be a component of a limb-salvage decision algorithm.[69] Two small case series have described how the technique of shortening and angulation of extremities with significant soft-tissue and bone loss can facilitate soft-tissue coverage.[70,71] Delayed gradual distraction of the shortened extremities is performed with a hinged circular external fixator. Further studies of this promising technique are required.

## Initial Resuscitation

Massive extremity hemorrhage is often an immediate life-threat in patients with traumatic proximal limb amputations.[36] An appropriately applied tourniquet on the residual proximal limb can be a first-line lifesaving intervention in such patients.[15] Proximal surgical control of the vascular structures can control distal sources of hemorrhage. Following the control of active limb hemorrhage, the patient can be evaluated for other life-threatening conditions followed by resuscitation of the casualty and the residual limb. Tactical situations such as extraction of casualties entrapped within vehicles (under enemy fire) may present unusual circumstances for prehospital surgical amputation. The amputated limb should accompany the casualty and should be assessed as a possible source of autologous vein graft harvesting.[66] Ideally, only the treating surgeon should discard the distal limb in order to ensure its therapeutic value to patient care has been fully assessed.

An amputated limb should be assessed as a possible source of autologous vein graft harvesting and discarded only after its therapeutic value to patient care has been fully considered.

### Primary (Completion) Amputation

In traumatic limb amputations, the nonviable distal portion is often attached to the proximal portion by a small skin bridge or a few intact tendons that span a segment of lost tissue. Transecting such bridging tissue is called a primary or completion amputation (Fig. 20). Primary amputation is indicated if the limb cannot be reconstructed or salvaged. This procedure is occasionally done in the emergency department, but it is typically performed during the first visit to the operating room. Other indications for primary (completion) amputation include: (1) ischemic limbs with irreparable vascular injury; (2) hemorrhage control refractory to other means; and (3) enabling lifesaving resuscitation in a patient whose injury physiologic burden (e.g., ongoing shock, hypothermia, acidosis, coagulopathy, or infection) will not permit limb salvage.[63] The latter exemplifies when limb-salvage techniques are beyond the physiologic capacity of the patient.[65]

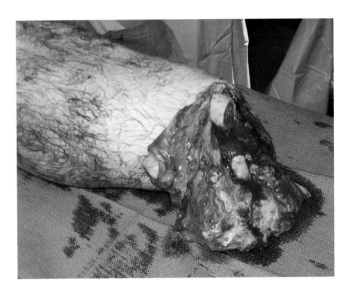

Figure 20. *Primary amputation is indicated if a limb cannot be reconstructed or salvaged. Image courtesy of the Borden Institute, Office of The Surgeon General, Washington, DC.*

Primary amputation is indicated if a limb cannot be reconstructed or salvaged. Primary amputation indications include ischemic limbs with irreparable vascular injury, hemorrhage control refractory to other means, or when limb salvage is beyond the physiologic capacity of the patient.

### Wound Debridement

Successful debridement depends on the surgeon's capacity to assess tissue for viability and the ability of the surgeon to remove contaminants.[72] Wounds associated with traumatic limb amputation are often grossly contaminated and contain nonviable tissue in need of surgical debridement and copious irrigation (Fig. 21). During surgical debridement, all viable and uncontaminated tissues, however random in nature, should be retained with the hope of preserving maximal limb length and function.[73] Retention of maximum nerve length, especially in the upper extremity, has value since targeted reinnervation is possible later.[74] Therefore, in the initial surgery, resection of nerves should not be routinely performed.

> During surgical debridement for completion amputation, all viable and uncontaminated tissues should be retained with the hope of preserving maximal limb length and function.

Certain types of wound contaminants may require special care. Oil-laden wounds may require soap or an additive that may safely aid in the removal of what is not water-soluble. Unfortunately, there is little data to determine best practices. White phosphorus is a chemical that is in some munitions used for illumination. White phosphorus is actually a yellow, waxy chemical that ignites spontaneously when exposed to air.[75] It is used as a filling for various projectiles, as a smoke-producing agent, and has an incendiary effect. White phosphorous smoking wounds can be covered in saline, but this only temporarily staves off recombustion. There is a thermal component to the injury when there is combustion as it is an exothermic process. Most of the cutaneous injury resulting from white phosphorus burns is due to the

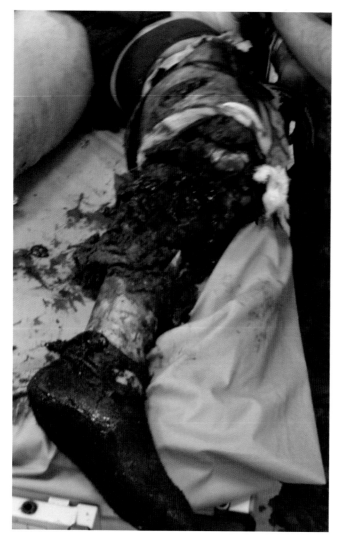

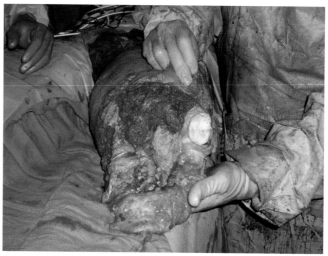

Figure 21. (Left) *Wounds associated with traumatic limb amputation are often grossly contaminated and contain nonviable tissue in need of surgical debridement and copious irrigation.* (Above) *During surgical debridement, all viable tissues should be retained with the hope of preserving maximal limb length and function. Images courtesy of Glenn J. Kerr, MD, MAJ, MC, US Army.*

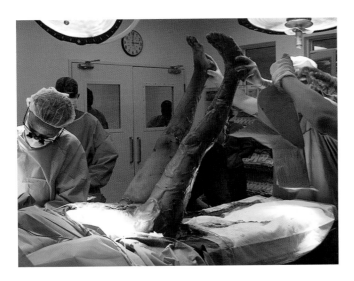

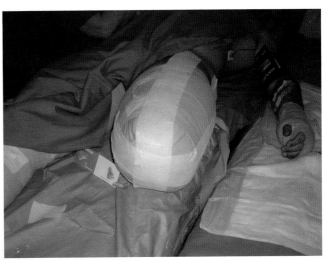

Figure 22. *Surgical limb preparation should be quite proximal because the zone of injury or planes of traumatic dissection may be more proximal than suspected on physical examination.*

Figure 23. *Combat extremity wounds should not be closed primarily. This residual proximal limb wound was dressed with bulky dry dressings. Image courtesy of Glenn J. Kerr, MD, MAJ, MC, US Army*

ignition of clothing and is treated as a conventional burn. Copper sulfate was once recommended for aid in locating the white phosphorus during debridement, but this is no longer recommended as copper sulfate use is associated with fatal hemolysis.[75] If copper sulfate solutions are used, they should be washed away immediately and not used as a wet dressing. White phosphorus-injured patients should be dressed with saline-soaked dressings to prevent reignition of the phosphorus by contact with the air.[76] Members of the US Army Burn Center have patented a gel for use in treatment of white phosphorus wounds, but there is little data regarding its use in a combat setting.

## Fasciotomy

Fasciotomy is often necessary in limbs with traumatic amputations. It would be a mistake to think that surgical fasciotomies are not necessary following traumatic amputations. While traumatic limb amputations create fascial disruptions, these traumatic fasciotomies (disruptions) do not adequately reduce intracompartmental pressures and do not equate to a surgical fasciotomy. Traumatic fasciotomies are not a substitute for the purposeful and complete surgical release of compartment pressures.[41] The injury proximal to

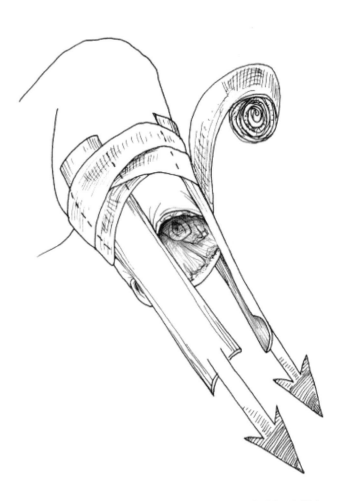

Figure 24. *Skin traction remains an option to preserve limb length if there is a planned four (or more) day interval between surgeries. Image courtesy of the Borden Institute, Office of The Surgeon General, Washington, DC. Illustrator: Jessica Shull.*

the amputation may also warrant fascial release. The fascial compartments of the residual proximal limb should be examined and fasciotomies performed if necessary for treatment or prevention of compartment syndrome.

> Traumatic fasciotomies are not a substitute for the purposeful and complete surgical release of compartments.

## Surgical Amputation and Wound Care

Surgical limb preparation should be very proximal (sometimes more proximal than the groin or axilla) because the zone of injury or planes of traumatic dissection are more proximal than suspected on physical examination (Fig. 22). Proximal control of arteries may require access to the pelvis, abdomen, or chest. Use of a tourniquet during the surgery is common to help with hemorrhage control. Ligation of distal major artery and vein injuries is indicated to avoid rebleeding after resuscitation, transport, limb mobilization, or dressing changes. Traumatic nerve stumps have gentle traction applied and are sharply transected proximal to the zone of injury and proximal enough so that the nerve retracts under soft-tissue. Large nerves, such as the sciatic nerve, may require ligation if the vessels within them bleed. Failure to ligate such nerves may risk rebleeding.

Combat extremity wounds are not closed primarily. The skin can often be loosely approximated with a few sutures to keep some skin tension and coverage while allowing drainage from the open wounds during transport (Fig. 23). Skin traction remains an option to preserve limb length if there is a planned four or more day interval between surgeries. Skin traction technique and postoperative management are described well in the Emergency War Surgery Manual (Figs. 24 and 25).[63] The residual proximal limb should be dressed with bulky dry dressings. While data are limited to anecdotal reports by war surgeons, negative-pressure wound therapy appears best avoided at the initial surgery for wounds at risk for rebleeding. Negative-pressure wound dressings can be considered after the casualty and wounds are stable without bleeding for 48 hours (following initial resuscitation) (Fig. 26).

## Delayed Amputation

Indications for delayed limb amputation may include complications like refractory wound sepsis, failed

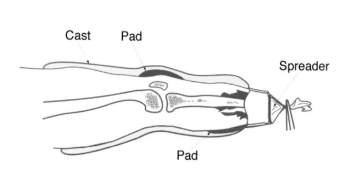

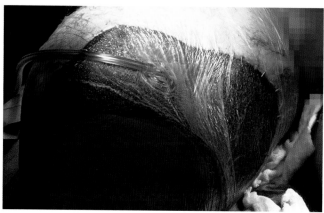

Figure 25. *A bivalved transportation cast (prior to patient transport) allows for continuous traction. Image courtesy of the Borden Institute, Office of The Surgeon General, Washington, DC. Illustrator: Jessica Shull.*

Figure 26. *Negative-pressure wound dressings can be considered after the casualty is stable and wounds are without bleeding for 48 hours following initial resuscitation.*

flap coverage or limb salvage (due to vascular or musculoskeletal causes), and selective amputation to optimize limb function (e.g., relieve pain or prosthetic fitting).[77] Selective amputation is performed when the distal salvaged limb function is less than that with a prosthetic. This decision is typically deferred to the definitive treatment facility after discussion with the casualty. Standard, conventional amputation levels were developed mostly from patients with diabetic vasculopathies. These standard civilian-based practices do not apply to most combat casualties. Positive outcomes have been documented for amputees undergoing delayed surgical amputations of atypical configurations (level and flaps).[77] Atypical surgical amputations do not employ standard or traditional levels of bony cuts, standard (textbook) skin incisions, or typical musculofascial flaps to cover the cut bone and conform to conventional prosthetic fittings.[77]

Initial efforts to maximally salvage viable tissue following atypical limb amputations enable broader future treatment options for the distal limb. Thus, preservation of viable tissues appears to result in better outcomes than limb shortening in order to get a typical wound closure.[77] Open guillotine amputations have fallen out of favor and are only performed based on the specific margins of tissue loss or necrosis.[77] The US Army recommends performing atypical amputations so that rearward care can optimize outcomes.[78] Tissue viability is used to determine the extent of debridement. The initial surgery is performed without regard for the likely subsequent amputation level.

> The preservation of vital tissues achieved through atypical delayed surgical amputations may result in better functional outcomes than limb shortening performed in order to get a conventional wound closure.

Atypical stump flaps (sometimes called flaps of opportunity) can be used in later surgeries to close the wound when it is ready for closure (Fig. 27). Such flaps are not fashioned during the initial surgery. For example, short (as little as one- to two-centimeter stumps) and even incomplete transtibial stumps can help avoid problems with through-the-knee amputations like the retraction of tendons or skin that may force more proximal amputation later for definitive wound closure.

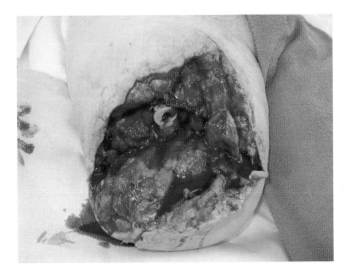 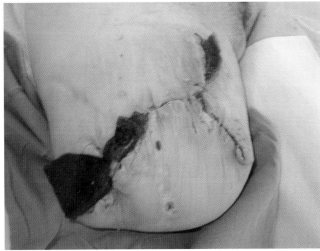

Figure 27. *Atypical stump flaps (sometimes called flaps of opportunity) can be used in later surgeries to close the wound when it is ready for closure. Images courtesy of Robert R. Granville, MD, COL, MC, US Army.*

## *Rehabilitation*

Rehabilitation services at specialized amputee centers have been documented to result in improved outcomes.[79] Besides the surgical reconstruction of residual limbs (flaps, bone grafting, amputation revision), casualties undergo a comprehensive evaluation and treatment plan for a broad spectrum of issues like traumatic brain injury, tympanic membrane rupture, and psychological and social screening. Currently in the US military, a physiatrist is often the leader of the rehabilitation team. Each casualty is routinely assigned a case manager for coordination of the myriad of medical and administrative issues they will face. Casualties are sent to the most appropriate facility based on injury severity. Rehabilitative care may be provided at a small base and hospital (simple injuries) or may occur at a tertiary medical center (complex injuries). One tertiary care center is San Antonio Military Medical Center (formerly Brooke Army Medical Center), which is a Level I trauma center with a burn center and a rehabilitative and amputee center called the Center for the Intrepid.[80,81,82] In summary, refinements in traumatic amputation care, amputation surgery, and aftercare have led to improved patient outcomes.[83,84]

# Combat Casualty Wound Care

- The management of combat wounds differs from civilian wound care.
- Combat wounds differ in degree and number from wounds occurring in the civilian sector.
- Combat wounds evolve more rapidly than civilian wounds and require more frequent reevaluation following injury.
- Initial postoperative dressings on blast injuries should routinely be dry, bulky dressings.

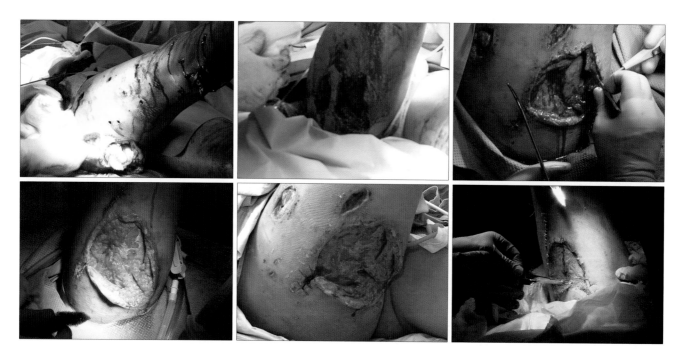

Figure 28. *Combat wounds evolve more rapidly than civilian wounds and require more frequent reevaluation following injury. Over time, bleeding and swelling ensue and resolve, while tissues can become devitalized and revitalized. This sequence of images shows the initial wound on day one* (Top Left) *and evolution* (Left to Right) *of the wound in response to multiple debridements over a two-week timeframe* (Bottom Right).

## Introduction

War wounds are often the result of higher-energy mechanisms than those in civilian sector. As such, combat wound size, severity, and lethality are often greater.[56] Combat-associated wounds evolve in the hours to days following the initial injury. What one careprovider sees at the point-of-injury often differs substantially from what is seen at the forward hospital (hours later) and then the rearward hospitals (days later) (Fig. 28). Over time, bleeding and swelling ensue and resolve while tissues can become devitalized and revitalized. Wound edema typically peaks at one to two days following the initial injury.[48,56] However, the consequences of initial treatments (e.g., tourniquet ischemia reperfusion and resuscitation fluid edema) may delay the timing of maximal edema to five days.[56] Both the magnitude of tissue edema and the variability of the time lag from initial injury to maximal edema can be startling to careproviders who have minimal CCC experience.[13]

> Combat wounds evolve more rapidly than civilian wounds and require more frequent reevaluation following injury.

## Extremity Resuscitation and Wound Management

Following injury (battle conditions permitting), initial wound treatment involves covering of wounds with sterile dry dressing bandages and splinting of bony injuries to prevent further injury.[85] Combat casualty care providers should address obvious life-threatening priorities first. The life-over-limb principle always applies. Uncontrolled limb wound hemorrhage is often identified as an immediate priority. Hemorrhage control options include: (1) manual direct pressure over the wound or proximal pressure points; (2) limb elevation; (3) hemostatic dressings; and (4) extremity tourniquet application. Tourniquets, a hemorrhage control adjunct to damage control resuscitation, provide maximal benefit the earlier they are applied following difficult to control extremity wound hemorrhage.[15]

Once the patient has been evacuated from the point-of-injury to the next echelon of care, the combat casualty should be reassessed. Immediate life-threats need to be addressed, including the control of any persisting wound hemorrhage. Subsequent to addressing immediate life-threats, limb wound management should consist of neurovascular examination of the limb, wound inspection, and wound irrigation with the goal of removing gross contamination.[85] If limb salvage is an option, limb perfusion must be optimized

### CARE OF A COMBAT LIMB WOUND

- Control hemorrhage; tourniquets are temporary adjuncts
- Prevent or treat shock, hypothermia, and coagulopathy
- Immobilize limb fractures and joint dislocations to minimize further injury
- Limit wound contamination to reduce infection risk
- Debride wounds by removing devitalized tissue, while maximally retaining viable tissue
- Keep wounds clean by repeated irrigation and debridement
- Cover wounds to reduce infection risk
- Prevent deep venous thrombosis and emboli
- Provide reconstructive care to maximize casualty and limb function
- Provide limb care within comprehensive rehabilitation

Table 3. *Key steps in the care of a combat limb wound.*

and further injury must be prevented. Immediate priorities include: (1) diagnosis and treatment of vascular injury and compartment syndrome; (2) shunting, vein grafting, or primary repair of arterial injuries; (3) immobilization of unstable bony injuries; and (4) prevention of wound infection. A summary of key steps in the care of combat limb wounds is provided in Table 3.

## Special Wounds

### Vascular Injury

The optimal management of extremity vascular injuries sustained in war requires collaboration between orthopaedists, general surgeons, and vascular surgeons. The process may involve temporizing vascular shunts, definitive repairs, or vascular reconstructions (Fig. 29).[86] The challenge of emergently addressing extremity vascular injury repair can tax a trauma system's personnel, supplies, and operative resources.[87] Ideally the regional trauma system serves to direct available resources towards providing optimal care. Optimal management of these complex injuries requires up-front planning, coordination of care, and frequent process improvements.

> Vascular injuries may be treated with temporizing vascular shunts or limited vascular procedures at Level II facilities, whereas definitive repairs or vascular reconstructions can be provided at Level III facilities.

Currently in the US military, Forward Surgical Teams can perfuse limbs with shunts or perform limited vascular procedures. Most Combat Support Hospitals (Level III facilities) provide extensive limb revascularization capacity. The scope of practice for orthopaedic surgeons and general surgeons in war broadens and demands that they perform more vascular procedures than they would otherwise perform in more controlled environments. Damage control principles should be applied to the care of acute wartime vascular injuries with emphasis on the effective correction of physiologic shock.[65,66] To this end, surgical time must be limited to essential resuscitative procedures, with the goal of returning to the operating room after physiologic parameters are restored and stabilized. A detailed discussion of vascular injury repair is provided in the Damage Control Surgery chapter.

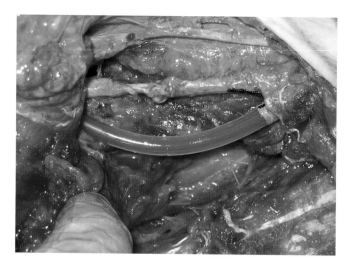

Figure 29. *Temporizing vascular shunt placed in the brachial artery at a Level II facility. Image courtesy of the Borden Institute, Office of The Surgeon General, Washington, DC.*

### Muscle, Tendon, and Ligament

Skeletal muscle repair is an uncommon surgical task in early CCC, but it is sometimes needed after the first debridement and surgery. Complete disruption or transection of a muscle belly or tendon can lead to morbidity without surgical repair. Hence, if no agonist muscle exists (or is too small), surgical repair may be indicated for improved future muscle strength, patient satisfaction, or cosmetic results.[88] Also, the need to cover underlying tissues such as nerve, tendon, or bone may also prompt surgical repair of muscle transections. Recent advancements in skeletal muscle repair have emphasized epimysium-based suturing.[89,90,91,92,93] Crushed limbs or those entrapped and ischemic for prolonged times pose management difficulties. A delayed fasciotomy (greater than 12 hours following injury) may increase sepsis and mortality rates compared to conservative care.[14]

Ligament repair can be done early, but not necessarily at the first surgery, for complete disruption of major ligaments leading to joint instability. Large ligaments with joint instability may be repaired end-to-end, oversewn, reinforced, or reinserted anatomically into their bony origins with nonabsorbable suture when the wound is clean. In the setting of gross wound contamination, a knee-bridging external fixator and serial surgical debridements prior to primary ligament repair or reconstruction are indicated. Serial assessment of joint stability and stiffness over time can help guide follow-on care.

Blood vessels, tendons, nerves, bone, and open joint spaces should be covered throughout care, at least temporarily by loose apposition of the surrounding tissue or skin so that the delicate tissues do not dry out. This drying (with resultant stiffness) risk is greatest in exposed segments of immobilized open joints.[94] However, good results with motion of open joints can be attained if the joint is mechanically stable.[94] All other soft-tissue wounds should be left open so that drainage may occur.

> Blood vessels, tendons, nerves, bone, and open joint spaces should be covered by loose apposition of the surrounding tissue or skin, so that the delicate tissues do not desiccate. All other soft-tissue wounds should be left open so that drainage may occur.

## Open Joint Injury

A penetrating wound near a joint such as the knee may cause a traumatic arthrotomy, a communication between the wound and joint space where foreign matter or bacterial contamination may remain in the joint and lead to septic arthritis (Fig. 30). Retained foreign matter or contamination in diarthrodial (freely moveable) joints is an indication for early surgical debridement and irrigation of the joint space and wound.

If a traumatic arthrotomy is suspected, a saline load test can be performed to help ascertain if the wound communicates with the joint space. A saline load test is the needle administration of sterile normal saline into the joint space through an uncontaminated route through the skin and soft-tissues. Enough saline is injected into the joint space to cause visible leakage if traumatic arthrotomy is present. The leakage may be seen in the wound if there is enough saline and limited blood and other obscurants. The saline load test is positive if the leakage is detected and negative if not detected. The saline load test has limitations in clinical practice. In a study, false positive clinical results occurred in 39 percent and false negative results in

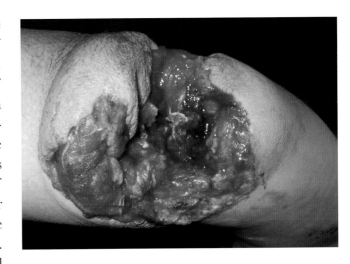

Figure 30. *Traumatic arthrotomy with extensive soft-tissue and bone injuries of the elbow due to a gunshot wound. Image courtesy of the Borden Institute, Office of The Surgeon General, Washington, DC.*

43 percent of casualties; there were no complications from the use of the test.[95] In several studies using the saline load test to evaluate small lacerations around the knee, saline loads of less than 145 to 194 milliliters were of questionable sensitivity. The authors concluded small volume saline load tests should not be used to rule out open knee injuries.[96,97] The injection of methylene blue has traditionally been used as an alternative agent for detecting open joint injuries. The performance characteristics of intraarticular injection of methylene blue for detecting open joint injuries remain poorly defined. Of note, the use of high-dose intravenous methylene blue as a diagnostic agent (for alternative procedures) has been linked to a variety of neuropsychiatric adverse side effects.[98,99,100,101] These rare cases were possibly associated with concomitant patient use of medications affecting serotonin metabolism.

> If doubt exists as to whether a wound communicates with a major joint space, the principle of exploration of the traumatic wound, followed by debridement and irrigation, should be practiced.

## Nerve Repair

Penetrating war trauma with associated peripheral nerve injury is uncommon.[4] When such injuries occur, they can be severe, require complicated care, and result in persistent disability.[102,103] Historically, advances in nerve repair, grafting, tendon transfers, and rehabilitation have been developed in part through CCC.[103]

The 1988 edition of the Emergency War Surgery Manual provides a detailed discussion of the management of peripheral nerve injury.[104] It details arteriovenous fistulas, clots and contusions, missile fragments, and causalgia associated with nerve injury. The 2004 edition of the Emergency War Surgery Manual discourages primary repair of peripheral nerve injuries in war wounds and advocates for prevention of desiccation by soft-tissue coverage of the nerve.[105] Specifically, debridement of nerve is not indicated except for grossly destroyed areas of the nerve and trimming frayed edges.[105] Recent advancements in the field of targeted reinnervation in the setting of upper extremity amputations have led to the goal of limiting initial nerve debridement to just the nonviable portions and preserving nerve length so that reinnervation, if chosen, is assisted with longer nerve stumps.[74] Surgeon experience is needed for the surgical repair of peripheral nerves. Loupe magnification is recommended for surgeons, and fascicular and epineurial repair appears prudent in most simple cases. The tagging of nerve with a fine, monofilament, nonabsorbable suture (e.g., 6-0 nylon) is not mandatory but can assist in identifying nerves during later surgeries.

> Primary repair of nerve injuries should not be performed in combat settings. Initial objectives include judicious debriding of nonviable neural tissue and avoiding desiccation by ensuring adequate soft-tissue coverage of wounds. Definitive nerve repair can be accomplished at rearward facilities following patient evacuation.

# War Wound Closure

- Extremity combat wounds should not be closed primarily.
- Cover bone, tendons, nerves, vessels, or joints with loosely apposed skin to prevent desiccation of underlying tissue and minimize risk of wound contamination.
- Wound closure decreases nosocomial infections, but closure too early risks wound infections associated with devitalized tissue.
- Zig-zag use of suture or vessel loops can provide wide wounds with some tension in order to aid in closure.

## Introduction

No extremity wound sustained during combat should be closed primarily at the first debridement because the risk of infection from residual contamination is very high.[105] The one exception is closing soft-tissues over open joint injuries following thorough joint washout and wound debridement in an operating room. Definitive closure of combat wounds can be done in several ways: (1) delayed primary closure; (2) negative-pressure wound dressings; (3) skin grafting; (4) local or free tissue transfer; and (5) healing by secondary intention. One or a combination of the above methods may be selected based on the nature and location of the wound, material available, and skill of the careprovider and treating facility resources.[106] From non-US casualties treated in a Combat Support Hosptial in Iraq, gram-negative bacteria were the most commonly isolated pathogens.[107] Cultures of respiratory fluid yielded positive results earlier than cultures of wound or blood samples and potentially serve as an earlier marker of future infections. Continued aggressive infection control for all casualties is needed.[107]

> With the exception of open joint injuries, no extremity wound sustained during combat should be closed primarily.

## Timing of Wound Closure

While primary closure of wounds within the strict controls of mature civilian trauma centers has shown good results, primary closure of war wounds is deemed inappropriate by experts in CCC.[108,109,110] Preparation of a wound for closure requires clinical judgment and is based upon: (1) the appearance of the tissue (i.e., clean, granulating, healthy tissue versus foul smelling and purulent tissue); (2) the absence of active infection; and (3) the ability to achieve a tension-free closure.

Classically, war wounds are not closed primarily since the wounds are often severe and contaminated. Occasionally the US Army has had to mandate delayed closure guidelines, such as in World War II.[111] Part of the problem is that the surgeon cannot see all types of contamination such as bacteria or fine particulate matter.[72] Another problem is that the wound core may include obviously nonviable tissue but there is a surrounding zone of tissue that may be devitalized but not dead, such that there is limited perfusion, a so-called zone of stasis that may evolve and swell over time.[72] The surrounding zone of stasis may be susceptible to over-resuscitation or may be responsive to negative-pressure therapies that may reduce swelling locally.[72]

> Timing of wound closure is dependent upon the appearance of the tissue, absence of infection, and ability to achieve a tension-free closure.

## Wound Closure Techniques

Delayed primary closure of war wounds can be effectively performed after planned, staged wound debridements.[56] The stapling of a zig-zag pattern of suture or vessel loops across wide wounds with some tension can aid in closure by keeping the skin from passively retracting further (Fig. 31). Mild drainage and granulation can occur before closure. Such suture patterns can be periodically retightened by pulling on the suture and adding a staple in incremental closure, perhaps avoiding an operative visit.

Early in OEF and OIF, CCC providers became familiar with negative-pressure wound dressing devices,

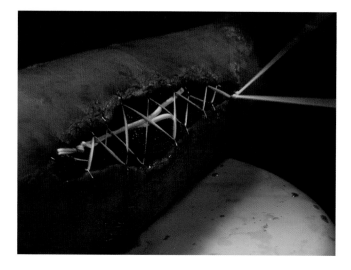

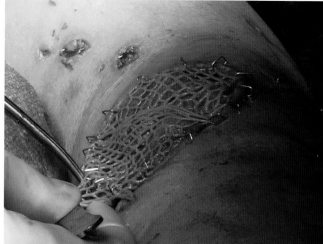

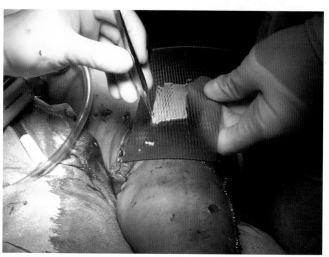

Figure 31. (Top Left) *The stapling of a zig-zag pattern of suture or vessel loops across wide wounds can aid in closure by keeping the skin from passively retracting further. Such patterns may be periodically retightened through increased tension.*

Figure 32. (Top Right) *In areas of skin loss with adequate muscle or granulation tissue coverage, a skin graft may be the treatment selected to cover the wound.*

Figure 33. (Bottom Right) *Meshing of the skin allows for greater graft coverage, improved conformity of the graft, and drainage of serous fluid.*

as did civilian careproviders in the US. As familiarity and positive clinical outcomes became common, more frequent use ensued for a wider spectrum of wounds.[56] In areas of skin loss with adequate muscle or granulation tissue coverage, a skin graft may be the treatment selected to cover the wound. Most commonly, a meshed split-thickness (0.015 inch) graft is used over the exposed soft-tissues.[56] Meshing the graft allows for more area coverage per donor site harvested, but more highly meshed grafts will contract more as they heal and are less cosmetically acceptable (Fig. 32).[56] Full-thickness skin grafting is considered for areas such as the palms of the hand where contracture of the graft is undesirable (Fig. 33). The skin graft may also be used in combination with delayed primary closure of a wound to first make the area needing a skin graft smaller. After serial debridements, the wound edges are approximated primarily, and then a skin graft is used to cover areas that cannot be closed because of tissue loss.

Local rotational tissue transfer (local flaps) can be a reliable way to achieve wound closure in areas lacking muscle or granulation tissue coverage (Fig. 34).[56] Common reliable rotational flaps in the lower extremity include the medial and lateral gastrocnemius flaps, soleus flap, and the reverse sural artery flap (Fig. 35).[56] In the upper extremity, the radial forearm flap is reliable.[56] Free tissue transfer or flaps are options as well, but it must be remembered that the zone of injury in war wounds is often larger than the open wound itself.[56] This makes flap anastomosis within the zone of injury complicated.[106,110,112]

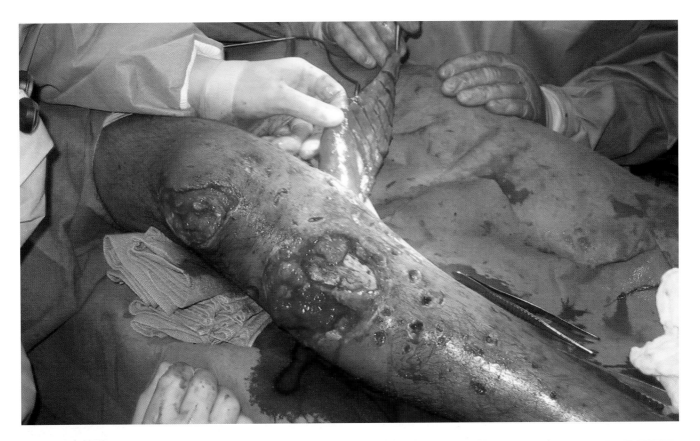

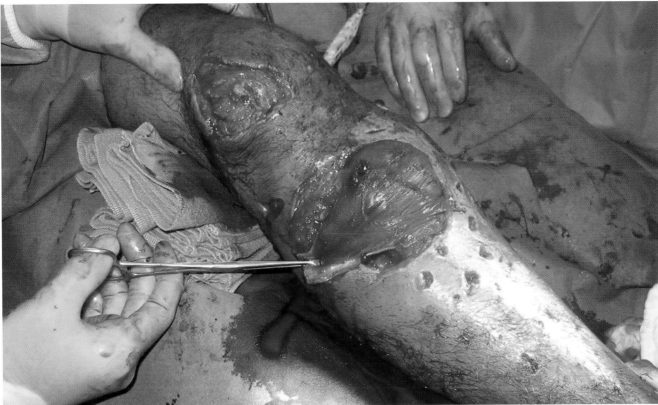

Figure 34. *Gastrocnemius muscle flap:* (Top) *A large anterior leg wound with exposed tibia due to fragmentation injury.* (Bottom) *The gastrocnemius was exposed, divided, and passed through a subcutaneous tunnel to cover the defect. Images courtesy of the Borden Institute, Office of The Surgeon General, Washington, DC, and Michael Shaun Machen, MD, COL, MC, US Army.*

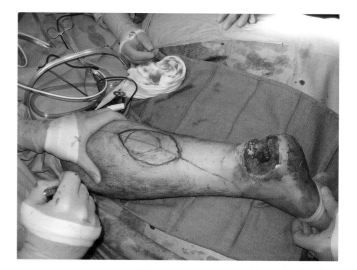

Figure 35. *Sural nerve flap:* (Right) *Fragmentation injury to the heel of the foot with exposed bone.* (Bottom Left) *A segment of skin, subcutaneous fat, and fascia are fashioned at the midcalf.* (Bottom Right) *A flap is rotated and sutured into place. Images coaaurtesy of the Borden Institute, Office of The Surgeon General, Washington, DC, and Michael Shaun Machen, MD, COL, MC, US Army.*

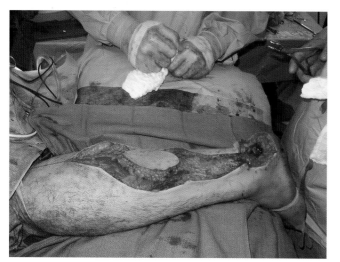

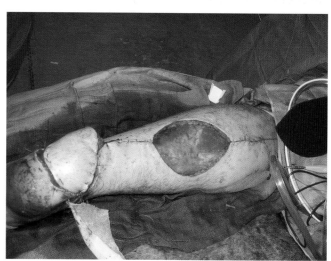

> Definitive closure of combat wounds can be achieved through delayed primary closure, negative-pressure wound dressings, skin grafting, local or free tissue transfer, or healing by secondary intention.

## Wound Coverage

The timing of wound coverage is complex. As previously noted, war wounds and their management differ significantly from wounds seen in the civilian sector. Early coverage of war wounds is often associated with inadequate wound debridement and increased infection rates, while delayed coverage is also associated with increased nosocomial infection rates.[110] More studies need to be done to define optimal wound coverage practices and minimize complications such as nonunion, flap failure, and infection.[110]

> Early coverage of war wounds is often associated with inadequate wound debridement and increased infection rates, while delayed coverage is associated with increased nosocomial infection rates.

# Preventing War Wound Infections

## *Wound Debridement and Irrigation*

- All war wounds should be considered dirty and contaminated.
- Thorough wound debridement and irrigation are the main defenses against combat wound infection.
- Recent evidence shows that high-pressure pulsatile lavage traumatizes wounds and complicates healing.
- Copious low-pressure irrigation balances the need for contaminant removal with maintaining structural integrity of viable tissues.

## Introduction

Although the sepsis rate in trauma is roughly 0.75 percent, the mortality of such cases is about 4 percent.[113] As such, the prevention of infection is an important imperative in trauma systems.[85] After casualty evacuation from the point-of-injury to a safe area, the CCC provider can evaluate the wound and manually remove or irrigate away gross contamination. Initial wound irrigation is sometimes performed in the prehospital setting before reapplication of a wound dressing.[114] The nonoperative debridement and irrigation of wounds as a bedside procedure can be done in the emergency department. The process typically consists of superficial wound inspection with lavage or irrigation of blood, debris, and loose bone fragments. Irrigation is often done at the first inspection of the wound to limit emergency department dressing changes. The promptness of the initial wound irrigation may have a slight effect on decreasing infection risk, but studies supporting this conclusion are limited.[115] All but the smallest and most superficial of war wounds should undergo such irrigation. Wound infections tend to increase hospital length of stay, cost of care, and complication rates.[107,113,114]

## Wound Flora

The bacteria within a war wound are often thought to contaminate the wound at the time of injury or soon thereafter.[113,114] The natural history of such wound flora is not clearly known, but there are seasonal and geographic variations.[113,114] The flora change over time and this likely occurs as a result of host, injury, treatment, and yet undefined reasons.[113,114] Early wound flora is a mix of gram-positive and gram-negative bacteria including anaerobes.[116] By day five, *Pseudomonas aeruginosa* is commonly noted.[116] Later-stage flora includes gram-negative bacteria such as *Pseudomonas aeruginosa*, *Klebsiella pneumonia*, and *Proteus* spp.[116]

Early in OEF, the extremity infection rate was reported as 3.8 percent (two of 52 casualties) but another report noted 77 percent (27 of 35) of deep cultures of tibia fractures were positive, and five went on to amputation with four associated with ongoing infections.[116,117,118] According to a review by Yun (from 2003 and 2006) there were 2,854 OEF or OIF admissions to Brooke Army Medical Center; 664 (23 percent) patients were admitted to the orthopaedic service with approximately 13 percent developing osteomyelitis. A total of 25 percent of these patients developed recurrent osteomyelitis.[116,119] Gram-negative bacterial pathogens were primarily responsible for the initial infections. Of those who had subsequent recurrent infections, initial gram-negative pathogens were typically eradicated and the subsequent infections were the result of gram-positive infections, primarily staphylococcus species. Murray et al. pointed out that the latter-stage infections were the result of nosocomial infections and were not present at the time of initial injury.[116]

## Wound Irrigation

Wound irrigation and debridement are the most common of all surgical procedures in war hospitals, particularly for limb wounds. The sheer number of these cases taxes the system, surgeons, and perioperative services.[3] The volume of such cases leads to familiarity but also breeds complacency. The skill, diligence, and experience needed to do these procedures optimally are paramount to reducing infections.

### Timing of Irrigation

Early irrigation in contaminated wound model experiments has resulted in superior bacterial removal than when delayed irrigation is used.[115] Clinical evidence supports early irrigation within six to eight hours of injury.[116] The optimal time to repeat irrigation is unclear. Given that bacteria counts rebound in wound models within 48 hours, performing serial wound irrigation every two days is a reasonable choice.[113,114,115,116,120,121]

> Clinical evidence supports early irrigation of wounds within eight hours of injury.

### Volume of Irrigation

Copious initial wound irrigation should be performed to minimize bacterial contamination, which will decrease subsequent wound infection rates.[77] The actual amount of fluid required is debatable, but ideally enough is used so that any gross material is removed and the wound grossly appears clean.[85] Current US military (Joint Trauma Theater System) wound irrigation guidelines recommend nine liters or more of sterile saline be used for large traumatic wounds, six liters or more for moderate-size wounds, and three liters as a minimum for small traumatic wounds.[77,122] These are ideal amounts, and the amount and type of irrigant may be constrained by actual supplies and resources. Recent evidence indicates that the irrigant volume decreases bacterial load in an approximation of a natural logarithmic decay. A point of diminishing returns occurs near nine liters for average-size wounds.[77,121]

### Irrigants and Additives

Traditionally, the preferred wound irrigant has been sterile saline or sterile water.[77] Recent studies have demonstrated that potable (drinking) water may also be used.[85,123] Appendix 4 provides the Joint Trauma Theater System (JTTS) Clinical Practice Guidelines (CPG) for Irrigation in War Wounds recommended by the United States Army Central Command. Additives (e.g., antibiotics, surfactants, soaps, or antiseptics) to irrigants have been used with the intent of decreasing local bacterial contamination.[122] Many of these additives are potentially cytotoxic to the cells of the wound.[109] There is no evidence to suggest additives to standard wound irrigants are more beneficial than irrigants without additives. Wound irrigant additive use for war wounds is not recommended.[77,121,122] The optimal irrigant temperature is unclear, but casualty hypothermia should be avoided, so warm irrigants should be chosen as indicated.

> There is no evidence to suggest additional benefit to supplementing standard wound irrigation solutions with chemical additives.

### Irrigation Devices

High-pressure lavage devices should be avoided because they can cause further tissue injury and push contamination deeper between tissue planes.[77,122] Copious low-pressure irrigation balances the need for contaminant removal while protecting wounded tissues (Appendix 4).[115,120,122,123] Low-pressure pulsatile

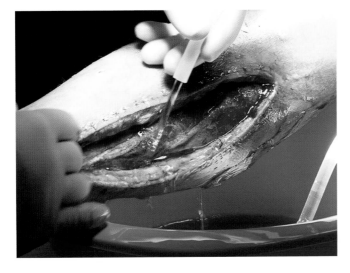

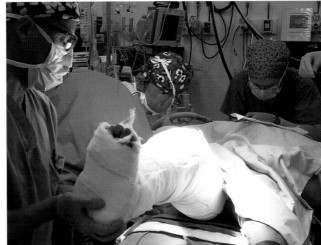

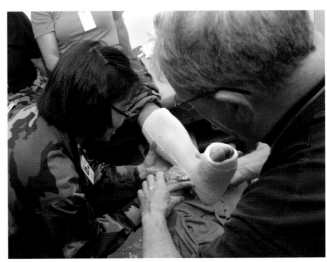

Figure 36. (Top Left) *Copious low-pressure wound irrigation should be performed to minimize bacterial contamination. High-pressure lavage should be avoided.*

Figure 37. (Top Right) *Initial postoperative dressings of blast injuries should be bulky dry dressings, which will allow absorption of the copious amounts of wound drainage.*

Figure 38. (Bottom Right) *Plaster casts must be bivalved and the cast padding cut down to the skin to prevent excessive pressure on the enclosed limb. Image courtesy of Defense Imagery Management Operations Center (DIMOC).*

lavage, gravity-fed irrigation, and manual bulb-syringe irrigation are currently all techniques successfully used in CCC (Fig. 36).[77,12,]

High-pressure lavage devices should be avoided because they can further tissue injury and drive contaminants deeper between tissue planes.

## Wet-to-Dry Dressing Debridement

Initial postoperative dressings on blast injuries should be dry, bulky dressings, which will be able to absorb the copious amounts of wound drainage seen early in this injury pattern (Fig. 37).[56,77] As the wound begins to drain less, a wet-to-dry debridement dressing change schedule can be started, if superficial debridement is desired. The use of wet-to-dry dressings is a debridement technique in which dry dressings are removed two or three times daily and replaced with damp, sterile ones. As the damp dressing dries, local tissue adheres. When this dressing is removed, it also removes the superficial wound serous drainage and provides a small amount of superficial debridement.[56,77]

Initial postoperative dressings on blast injuries should be bulky dry dressings.

Reevaluation of wounds should occur frequently since wounds evolve with time. Dressing wounds tightly with gauze may prohibit drainage and risk infection.[60] Initial postoperative limb dressings should be made with the injury severity in mind. Severe injuries can swell so much that dry, bulky dressings are needed to permit swelling while absorbing copious serous wound drainage.

When plaster casts are applied for the immobilization of fractures, two lateral longitudinal half-inch segments should be removed from the cast's entire length (bivalving) and the circular dressings cut down to the skin (Fig. 38). This procedure prevents undue pressure on the enclosed limb when swelling occurs.[41] The military air evacuation system in OEF and OIF prohibits casts that are not split (bivalved) in this manner because of the risk of limb swelling during aeromedical transport.[57]

> Circumferential plaster casts should be bivalved to prevent excessive pressure on the enclosed limb.

## Surgical Wound Debridement

Following evacuation of the casualty to a facility with surgical capability, early and assertive surgical debridement of grossly contaminated and nonviable tissues is the first step in infection control.[113,114,116] Inadequate wound debridement has been cited as the most common cause of war wound infection.[116] War wound surgery involves careful exploration of all wounds (i.e., closed wounds, entry and exit wounds, missile tracks between entry and exit, and secondary missile tracks caused by fragmentation of the munitions after entering the body).[60]

> Inadequate wound debridement has been cited as the most common cause of war wound infection. Fasciotomy is often integral to debridement.

A systematic approach to wound evaluation will help the surgeon avoid missing areas of a large wound. This involves: (1) starting by exploring the most superficial wound first; (2) debriding the skin and subcutaneous tissue; (3) then debriding muscle and fascia; (4) fasciotomy and hematoma removal; and (5) finishing deep wound debridement of periosteum and bone. Fasciotomy is often integral to debridement. Debridement's core meaning includes unbridling the wound, which includes removal of expanding hematomas and relieving compartment pressure. Diligent wound exploration is required to avoid iatrogenic injury to the traversing vessels and nerves within the wound. In the authors' experience a geographic approach to wound evaluation, dividing it into quadrants and addressing all pathology in each quadrant before moving to the next one, has been successful.

The broad spectrum of foreign matter found within war wounds is remarkable. Over time, CCC providers will document everything from blast injury victim bone fragments to palm dates and even insects within war wounds (Table 4). Of note, the anatomic location of a foreign body does not indicate what path it took to get there. For example, a casualty in OIF with a traumatic amputation above the left knee was found to have a large foreign body in his right chest on radiography (Fig. 39). The foreign body was initially thought to be something on the cassette he was lying upon, until a repeat chest radiograph reconfirmed its presence. An 18 x 2 x ¼ inch explosion-related fragment had entered his right lung via his abdomen from his knee wound. The missile track was confirmed surgically. It traversed the bladder, rectum, kidney, intestines, liver, diaphragm, and lung. Missile tracks following blast injuries are notoriously difficult to precisely and reliably identify.

| FOREIGN MATTER IDENTIFIED DURING DEBRIDEMENT |
| --- |
| • Dirt, soil, mud, sand, rocks, road debris, dust, and compost |
| • Bullets, shrapnel, ordnance fragments, uniform bits, clothing, and equipment |
| • Other casualty items blasted into the wound, bones, clothing, boots, kit, and gear |
| • Animal matter such as insects, worms, carcass fragments, excrement, and leather |
| • Plant matter such as wood, grass, leaves, roots, and nuts |
| • Manmade items: glass, car or building parts, concrete, pipes, nails, batteries, nuts, bolts, screws, and metal can parts |
| • Water, sewage, water plants, and frog fragments |
| • Chemical matter, phosphorous, acids, liquids, and smoked or charred items |

Table 4. *Foreign matter identified in explosion-related wounds.*

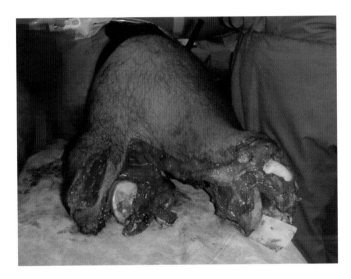

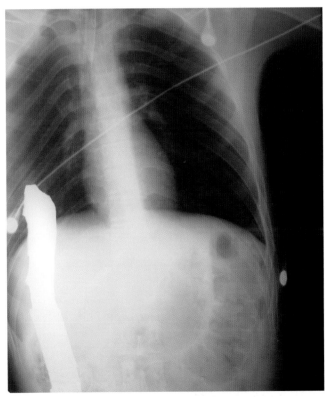

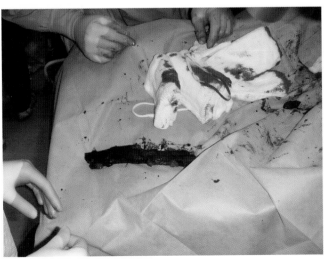

Figure 39. *Missile tracks following blast injuries are difficult to identify:* (Top Left) *Combat casualty with a traumatic amputation above the left knee.* (Top Right) *Foreign body noted on chest radiograph.* (Bottom Left) *Explosion-related fragment that had entered the chest cavity via the casualty's abdomen from the knee wound. Images courtesy of John B. Holcomb, MD, COL(Ret.), MC, US Army.*

Missile tracks following blast injuries are difficult to reliably identify. Large missile fragments in soft-tissue wounds are often removed, whereas small fragments are only removed if they are readily accessible.

Sharp surgical debridement of devitalized and grossly contaminated tissues is the primary surgical means of infection prevention.[114,124] However, the innate meaning of devitalized (that which is less than fully vital) is operationally problematic, as devitalized tissues range from bruised or edematous to blackened eschar. Muscle rigor, a feature of rigor mortis, is rarely seen in the living casualty.[36,125] Analyzing how effectively surgeons classify viable versus nonviable tissue during debridement efforts is rarely researched. Ensuring CCC providers new to war are adequately trained in this process is critical.[60,126]

Generous surgical extension of the wound in order to see the damaged tissues adequately (around the wound recesses) is important. This process enables complete inspection and removal of devitalized tissues and foreign material that may have traveled along or through fascial planes.[60] Such extension of traumatic wounds often includes longitudinal skin incisions and compartmental fasciotomy. Fascia is generously released.[54] Judicious excision of skin margins, often just a millimeter or two, will remove devitalized or grossly contaminated edges while maintaining as much cover as practical (Fig. 40). Grossly contaminated skin edges are often identified following irrigation and removal of dried blood. The skin edges' white fibrous strands are often covered with dark particulate debris such as sand. Contaminants tightly adhere to these fibers, which can be a millimeter or longer. These contaminated and difficult to clean fibrous strands are useless and risk infection.

There is little beyond expert opinion on which to base tissue fragment management recommendations.[127] Large missile fragments (shrapnel) in soft-tissue wounds are typically removed, whereas small fragments are removed only if they are easily accessible.[60] If iatrogenic trauma would result from the removal of smaller fragments, they are allowed to remain in place.[60] Shrapnel is a term used classically for fragments from preformed antipersonnel munitions, but is now commonly used by lay people to indicate metal fragments from explosive shells.

When wound tracks from entry-to-exit are long relative to their width, debris such as bone fragments and blood clots can be debrided without fully opening the wound. This can be accomplished by passing

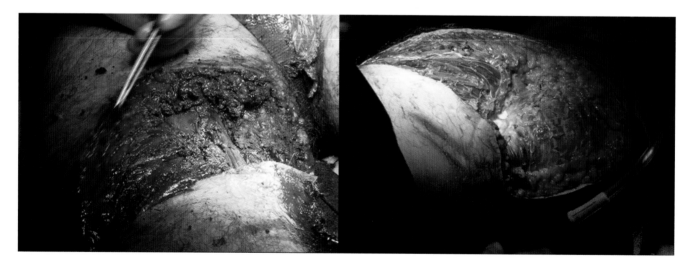

Figure 40. *Early and assertive surgical debridement of nonviable tissue is a critical step in infection control.*

a small but long surgical sponge across the track, often by a clamp, such that the wound floss can help pull the debris out the dependent opening. Similarly, the dependent opening can be used for drainage, and if the opening is not large enough for adequate drainage, then it can be enlarged. If the track is blind in that it has no exit, and the entry is not dependent, then a counterincision can be made in a dependent area. The dependent drainage by gravity is usually for the casualty in the supine position, and can simplify care while decreasing complications.

Wound drains are routinely placed by surgeons in war wounds with the intent of decreasing infection rates. While data are limited, existing studies suggest that open surgical drains are associated with more complications (e.g., infections) as compared to no drains or closed drains.[128] A Cochrane review of closed drains following orthopaedic surgery in a civilian patient population concluded there is insufficient evidence to support the routine use of closed suction drainage following orthopaedic surgery.[129] Further studies are required to better define the role of surgical drains for war wounds.

### Assessing Muscle Viability
The most challenging and problematic tissue to debride in wounded limbs is skeletal muscle. Muscle, in particular, can be judged as living or dead roughly based on the four C's of muscle viability. These include (1) color (red versus pale or brown); (2) consistency (not waxy or stewed); (3) contractility (on being pinched with the tips of a forceps); and (4) capacity to bleed (capillary bleeding when cut).[126] Tissue discoloration or staining from surface hemorrhage on wound surfaces or small hemorrhages within tissue such as skeletal muscle should be differentiated from large hematomas, contamination, and tissue ischemia. Color is not as reliable as the other C's. Dead muscles can bleed from larger blood vessels within the skeletal muscle itself, so this capacity to bleed should be differentiated from the capacity to bleed from capillaries.[14] The former is a false positive indicator of viable tissue, while the latter is a true indicator of tissue viability. Muscle injury, particularly when large and associated with ischemia, can be associated with coagulopathy. Hence, careproviders must be aware that slow, venous oozing from cut muscle may also be a false positive indicator of tissue viability. Medications such as aspirin, nonsteroidal antiinflammatory drugs, and anticoagulants may accentuate such bleeding in casualties.[130]

> Muscle viability can be assessed based on the four C's: color, consistency, contractility, and capacity to bleed.

### Massive Wounds (Upper Thigh and Buttock)
Massive wounds of the upper thigh and buttock are problematic in two aspects; control of hemorrhage and determination of the amount of muscle to be excised (Fig. 41).[36] The wound may be too proximal for a tourniquet. Oozing may persist and may be associated with coagulopathy in need of correction.[35,131] Placement of an emergency tourniquet as proximal as possible, while still partially covering the wound, can be temporarily effective in hemorrhage control. However, this approach risks failing to extinguish the arterial pulse and may lead to complications (e.g., expanding hematomas and compartment syndrome).[36] Surgical preparation with the tourniquets in place, within the operative field, can maintain hemorrhage control and allow more time for surgical team preparation.[15,36,65,66,67] In large wounds of the buttock and upper thigh, repeat wound inspection on the second or third postoperative day are indicated. These repeat inspections during staged debridements and irrigations can ensure any remaining devitalized tissue is recognized sooner for further debridement.[56]

In large, complex wounds it is difficult to determine the amount of muscle to excise. Residual devitalized tissue in wounds risk infection. With high-energy mechanisms, damage along fascial planes and between muscle bundles occurs, which may further devitalize deep muscle as some muscle perfusion comes from adjacent planes. Surgeons digitally probing for debris or hematomas should be aware that the technique of using their fingers to circumferentially dissect around small muscles can damage vasculature structures. Muscles like the sartorius in the thigh can be inadvertently stripped of their segmental blood supply through circumferential digital dissection, resulting in muscle necrosis and infection. The intramuscular vascular patterns of muscles are poorly known.[132] After sharp debridement, copious low-pressure wound irrigation can be used to remove loose debris, missile fragments, and decrease wound surface bacterial contamination (Appendix 4).[115,121,122,123]

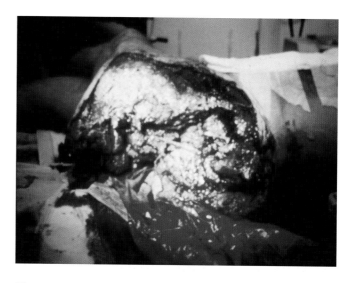

Figure 41. *Hemorrhage from massive wounds of the upper thigh and buttock may be difficult to control, and determining the amount of muscle to debride is often difficult. Images courtesy of John B. Holcomb, MD, COL (Ret.), MC, US Army.*

## Negative-Pressure Wound Dressings

- Negative-pressure wound dressings are commonly used in OEF and OIF.
- Appropriately applied and managed negative-pressure wound dressings result in improved wound healing rates.
- Placement of a negative-pressure dressing should occur only after thorough debridement of devitalized and contaminated tissues.
- A wound vacuum device is available and approved for aeromedical transport use in OEF and OIF.

Negative-pressure wound dressings have been used successfully in the treatment of war injuries.[133,134] The negative-pressure dressing provides a closed environment for the wound and resorbs the large amounts of serous fluids that drain from blast injuries.[135] This closed system may reduce hospital-acquired infections because these wounds are less prone to repeated inspection and manipulation.

| Negative-pressure wound dressings are commonly used in OEF and OIF. |
| --- |

Inappropriate use of negative-pressure wound dressings has been associated with infectious complications. Placement of a negative-pressure dressing should occur only after thorough debridement of devitalized and contaminated tissues.[56,133] Use of the negative-pressure dressing overlying dead tissues can create a closed space. This closed space creates an ideal environment for abscess formation, which would lead to local and potential systemic infectious complications.[56] This closed wound environment provides the ideal media for bacterial growth if the vacuum device fails, or is left in place too long between debridements.[136] Loss of vacuum suction or tube blockage can have similar outcomes as device failure.[134] If suction is lost, the tube or dressing can be cut to allow drainage or the negative-pressure dressing can be replaced by dry bulky dressings. As previously mentioned, based on anecdotal reports by war surgeons, negative-pressure wound therapy appears best avoided at the initial surgery for wounds at risk for rebleeding. Negative-pressure wound dressings can be considered after the casualty and wounds are stable without bleeding for 48 hours (following initial resuscitation).

> Placement of a negative-pressure dressing should occur only after thorough debridement of devitalized and contaminated tissues. Negative-pressure dressings should be avoided in wounds at risk for rebleeding.

Negative-pressure wound therapy can facilitate the delayed closure of large traumatic wounds. It does so by decreasing the size of the wound over time. The device applies tension to the skin and removes third-space fluids. The device can be an adjunct in split-thickness skin grafting. During OEF and OIF, a wound vacuum device (The V.A.C. Freedom® Therapy System, Kinetic Concepts, Inc. or KCI, San Antonio, TX) was approved for aeromedical transport in OEF and OIF. The wound vacuum assisted closure or V.A.C., is a proprietary label for KCI's negative-pressure wound therapy system, a common one used currently in the US military. Devices have to be approved by the military for safe aircraft use prior to implementation during aeromedical transportation in casualty care.

## Antibiotic Impregnated Pellets and Cement Bead Therapy

An adjunctive measure that can be used with or without the negative-pressure dressings is antibiotic-impregnated beads (Fig. 42). Such beads are usually made of polymethylmethacrylate, a type of bone cement, with a heat stable antibiotic additive such as tobramycin. The polymerization of the polymethylmethacrylate powder with the liquid catalyst is exothermic in forming the cement, so the antibiotic powder needs to be heat stabile, or it will be inactivated in bead formation. Antibiotic bead pouch use reduces bacterial growth in an anaerobic environment.[116] Antibiotic beads may offer some benefit in the prevention of infection at the local site, but no data exists on their efficacy in war wounds or long-term effect on wound infection.[116]

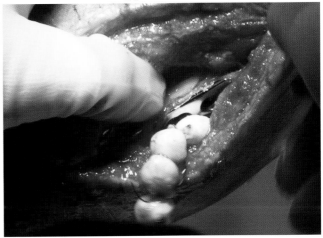

Figure 42. *Antibiotic beads may offer some benefit in the prevention of local infection, but definitive data are lacking on their efficacy in war wounds.*

Preparation of antibiotic bead pouches consumes valuable time and operative resources; ideally these should be prepared ahead of time.[116] Effective local antibiotic delivery can be obtained with both commercially available calcium sulfate pellets and with handmade polymethylmethacrylate beads.[137] Tobramycin-impregnated calcium sulfate pellets have been shown to effectively prevent infection in a contaminated wound model.[138]

## Antibiotics and Tetanus Immunization

- Systemic antibiotic administration should occur within three hours of sustaining combat wounds.
- Antibiotic guidelines for routine combat wounds should be followed.

- Ensuring up-to-date tetanus immunization status following combat wounds is important to eliminating tetanus infections.
- The main risk for developing wound infection in casualties is the severity of the injury.

## Prophylaxis

Prevention of infection in war wounds is an important goal.[139] Injury severity and wound management practices are important determinants of subsequent infection.[128] The benefits and risks of current antibiotic wound prophylaxis practices to prevent infections in combat casualties have yet to be fully defined.[85,140] Early wound cleansing and surgical debridement, antibiotics, bony stabilization, and maintenance of infection control measures are essential to diminish or prevent infections.[85] Antibiotic prophylaxis or therapy is an adjunct to adequate surgical debridement of war wounds.[116] Prophylactic antibiotics have been associated with high rates of drug-resistant organisms.[116]

Initial care of combat wounds occurs at the point-of-injury, where a sterile bandage may be applied and oral antibiotic administered as prophylaxis.[139] Prophylactic antibiotics in tactical CCC settings have been recommended for all open wounds. If the evacuation time of the casualty is expected to be more than three hours, the use of oral antibiotics is recommended within three hours of injury.[85] Recommendations for initial antibiotic prophylaxis in OEF and OIF for open extremity wounds with oral antibiotics are moxifloxacin (400 milligrams orally, one single dose in the field) or as an alternative levofloxacin (500 milligrams orally, one single dose in the field), but empiric evidence is scant regarding effectiveness or outcomes.[85]

> Prophylactic antibiotics in tactical CCC settings have been recommended for all open wounds and should be administered within three hours of sustaining combat wounds.

Antibiotic recommendations for OEF and OIF casualties with open fractures arriving at a treatment facility that possesses intravenous antibiotic supplies are one gram of cefazolin (also known as cephazolin) intravenously every eight hours for 72 hours. An alternative to cefazolin is clindamycin (900 milligrams intravenously every eight hours for 72 hours). The clindamycin dosing used in war wounds differs from 450 milligrams every six hours civilian sector dosing. Clinical evidence supporting this practice is limited. Subsequent use of antibiotics (beyond 72 hours) should be reserved for treatment of documented infections, as opposed to prophylaxis, in order to limit the selection of multidrug-resistant organisms. In patients who present more than 72 hours after injury, or are injured with antipersonnel land mines (implying soil contamination), metronidazole should be added as well to the treatment for 48 hours intravenously and then orally until delayed primary wound closure is complete.[85] Evidence is scant regarding effectiveness or outcomes of aforementioned recommendations.

Wounds should only be cultured routinely when an infection is suspected. Antibiotic selection is ideally based on results of wound cultures and bacterial antibiotic sensitivities. Recent hospital and regional bacterial flora should influence antibiotic selection. Temporal and geographic variations occur with the organisms isolated from combat wounds.[113,114] Longstanding systematic tetanus immunization programs for US military personnel have largely prevented tetanus infections.[113] New cases of tetanus in military personnel are rarely seen today.[113,114] If a combat casualty (e.g., host national) has not received a primary immunization series against tetanus infection, primary tetanus immunization and passive prophylaxis (tetanus immune globulin) should be administered.[85]

All penetrating combat wounds should be considered tetanus-prone, and patients should be provided a tetanus toxoid booster immunization if more than five years have passed since their most recent tetanus immunization.

## Fracture Management

- Fractures stabilization decreases pain, eases wound care, and improves soft-tissue and vascular repair outcomes.
- Initial fracture stabilization is performed in a damage control manner in war and is not definitive.
- Most hand and foot fractures can be adequately stabilized for transport with simple splints applied over dressings.
- External fixators can loosen with patient transport; so the clamps should be periodically retightened (e.g., 24 to 48 hours) after application.

### *Introduction*

Extremity trauma with bony fractures is a common war injury.[60] About 26 percent of casualties with

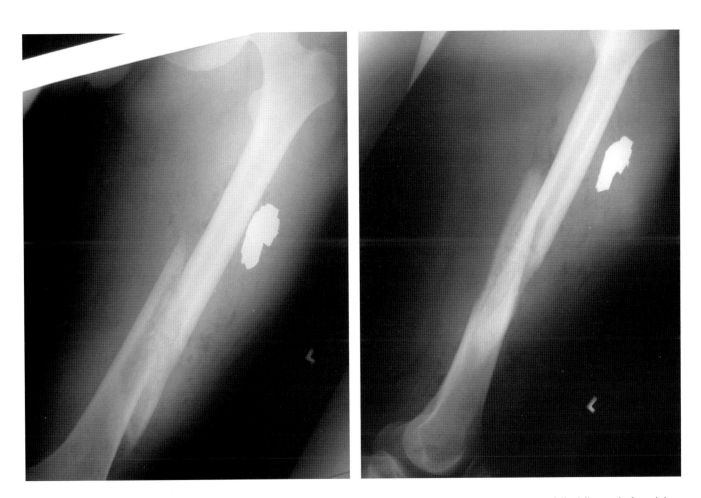

Figure 43. *Radiographic evaluation of the traumatized limb should (at a minimum) include biplanar radiographs to fully delineate the bony injury. Here, (Left) PA and (Right) lateral radiographs demonstrate a midfemoral fracture and the metallic fragment that caused the injury. Images courtesy of the Borden Institute, Office of The Surgeon General, Washington, DC.*

extremity wounds in OIF have a fracture. The majority of these injuries (82 percent) are open fractures where the soft-tissue envelope around the fracture has been physically disrupted, and the bone has been exposed to the external environment.[2,4] Inexperienced providers can underestimate wounds by thinking that a skin wound does not communicate with a nearby fracture when it actually does, so a high index of suspicion should persist pending orthopaedic evaluation.

Eighty-two percent of extremity fractures in OIF are open fractures.

Radiographic evaluation of the traumatized limb should (at a minimum) include biplanar radiographs to fully delineate the bony injury (Fig. 43). Stabilization of these fractures has several benefits, including patient comfort, protection of the surrounding soft-tissues, protection of vascular repairs, and improved wound care.[116] The goals of fracture management in the combat setting are to prevent infection, preserve options for limb reconstruction or limb salvage, and prevent further tissue injury and hemorrhage during patient treatment and transport.[57] Simple, early management of fractures can avoid long-term complications such as osteomyelitis and nonunion.

Goals of fracture management in the combat setting are to prevent infection, preserve options for limb reconstruction or limb salvage, and prevent further tissue injury and hemorrhage during patient treatment and transport.

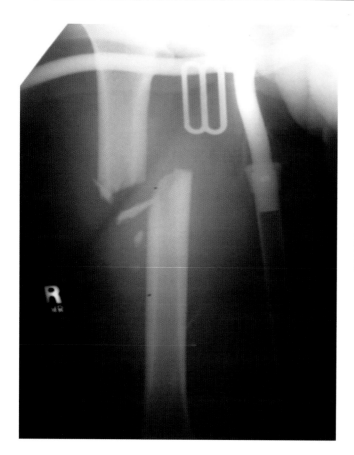

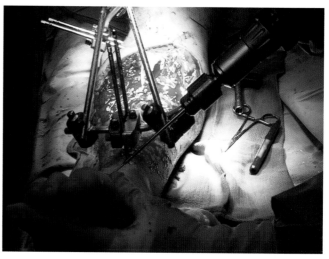

Figure 44. (Left) *Limb deformity due to displaced fractures can compromise the vascular supply to the distal limb. If compromised perfusion is detected, immediate longitudinal traction should be applied.*

Figure 45. (Above) *When possible, fixation devices should be placed in a location that avoids traversing the traumatic wound or hematoma itself.*

## Initial Fracture Wound Management

Initial limb deformity due to displaced fractures can compromise the vascular supply to the distal limb (Fig. 44). The CCC provider should respond to the limb with compromised perfusion and displaced fracture with longitudinal limb traction, which will grossly realign the limb at its proper length, thereby reducing the fracture shortening and typically improving distal perfusion. The fracture reduction can be maintained with manual traction if necessary; or if supplies and time allow, temporary plaster splints can be applied to hold the limb out-to-length.

In this type of unstable skeletal injury, the distal pulses should be checked frequently and more definitive fracture fixation should be sought. If fracture reduction is successfully performed and the vascular supply to the distal extremity remains compromised, an arterial injury should be assumed until proven otherwise. Careproviders are advised to immediately transfer such cases to an echelon of care capable of providing vascular repair (typically a Level III facility). Periarticular fracture reduction is also important for limb perfusion, length, soft-tissue balance, joint surface reduction, and follow-on care.

> If vascular supply distal to a skeletal injury remains compromised following successful fracture reduction, arterial injury should be assumed present and the casualty transferred to a Level III facility for further evaluation.

## Initial Fracture Stabilization

Initial fracture stabilization should be viewed as part of limb resuscitation and not definitive fixation.[141] Care should be taken to first do no further harm by ensuring the placement of fixation devices is away from nerves and vessels. When possible, to minimize risk of infection, fixation devices should be placed in a location that avoids traversing the traumatic wound or hematoma itself (Fig. 45). Half-pin frame external fixators, K-wires (Kirschner wires), splints, and skeletal traction can all be used for fracture stabilization.[142] Skeletal traction is fast but limited to patients not needing further evacuation because traction must be removed for transport. External splints allow for noninvasive fracture stabilization and provide a cradle for the injured soft-tissue envelope (Fig. 46). The disadvantage of splinting is the potential for loss of fracture reduction with motion in the splint and the inability to easily inspect the wounds underlying the splint unless it is removed.

> Initial fracture stabilization should be viewed as part of damage control limb resuscitation and not as definitive fixation.

External fixators and K-wires provide skeletal fixation and are indicated for long-bone and periarticular fractures in which stability cannot be achieved by splinting.[77] Commonly, the fixator will be applied concurrently with a vascular procedure to provide a stable limb and protect the site of vascular repair or shunting (Fig. 47). Segmental metacarpal and metatarsal fractures with bony loss can be spanned longitudinally with K-wires to reduce soft-tissue contractures during transport. Such wires can be straight or have 90-degree bends to block the fractures' ends out at their reduced positions for optimal soft-tissue lengths (Fig. 48). There is no single, ideal form of resuscitation fixation, but the options used should first do no further harm and, second, provide a stable extremity for transport out of the theater of operations.[77]

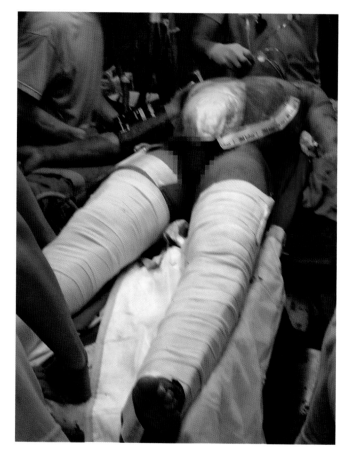

Figure 46. (Right) *External splints allow for noninvasive fracture stabilization. In this combat casualty, additional surgery was deferred until the patient was stable. Image courtesy of the Borden Institute, Office of The Surgeon General, Washington, DC.*

Figure 47. (Bottom Left) *This open femur fracture was rapidly stabilized with external fixation while a shunt of the superficial femoral artery was placed. The external fixator provided added protection to the site of vascular shunting.*

Figure 48. (Bottom Right) *Segmental metacarpal and metatarsal fractures with bony loss can be spanned longitudinally with K-wires to reduce soft-tissue contractures. The K-wire is bent four times (90-degree corners) so when the ends are inserted in the bone marrow, the corners hold the soft-tissues out the length of the bone depth.*

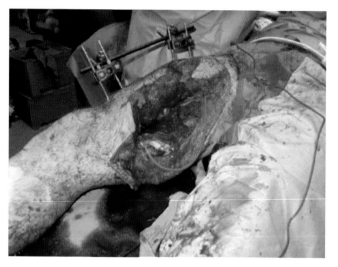

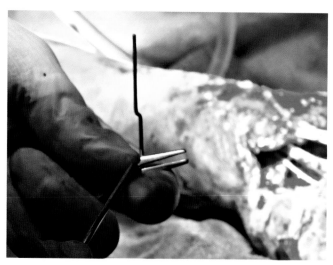

External fixators and K-wires provide skeletal fixation. They are indicated for long-bone and periarticular fractures in which stability cannot be achieved by splinting.

## *Open Fracture Management*

The approach to an open fracture should proceed with similar tenets as for other contaminated wounds. Initial open fracture wound irrigation can be performed as part of the wound inspection in the emergency department. This initial inspection and irrigation should not be considered definitive treatment. Copious intraoperative wound irrigation and sharp surgical debridement are indicated with adjunctive, broad-spectrum, intravenous antibiotic prophylaxis (Fig. 49).[77,116] Nonviable tissues, including bone fragments stripped of their soft-tissues, should be removed (Fig. 50). An exception to this removal may include retention of large articular bony fragments regardless of soft-tissue attachments as long as they are not grossly contaminated and appear suitable for articular reconstruction.[77]

Internal fixation of fractures should be delayed until the patient has been resuscitated and the soft-tissue injury has been treated.[77] With rapid aeromedical evacuation of combat casualties to Level IV and V facilities, there are no compelling indications for internal fracture fixation of US and coalition forces in-theater during OEF and OIF. Internal fixation of host nation patients after a clean wound bed has been obtained has been performed in OEF and OIF.[77] Certain fracture types (e.g., displaced femoral neck and talus fractures) have, in the past, been considered a dilemma for CCC providers, as delay in fracture reduction was believed to increase risk of avascular necrosis. Recent studies have shown no difference in results, and therefore the increased risk, and often increased reduction difficulty, favor early evacuation and fixation out-of-theater.

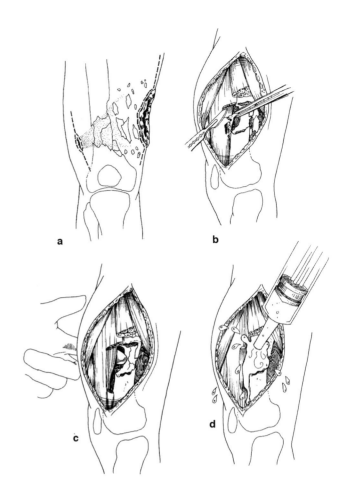

Figure 49. *The approach to an open fracture should proceed with similar tenets as for other contaminated wounds. Copious intraoperative wound irrigation and sharp surgical debridement are indicated with adjunctive broad-spectrum intravenous antibiotic prophylaxis. Image courtesy of the Borden Institute, Office of The Surgeon General, Washington, DC. Illustrator: Jessica Shull.*

> With rapid aeromedical evacuation of combat casualties to Level IV and V facilities, there are no compelling indications for internal fracture fixation of US and coalition forces in-theater during OEF and OIF.

Most of the initially placed frames will eventually be removed or modified to allow for definitive fracture fixation.[143,144] Bony stabilization of the extremities is indicated to hold alignment of the long bones to prevent laceration of soft-tissue structures by the fracture surfaces, prevent injury to vascular shunts or grafts, and provide comfort to patients during transport. External splinting may be appropriate for more distal fractures. Such fractures are closed, low-energy, and stable fractures. External splinting can also serve as an adjunct to external fixation (e.g., a posterior leg splint to keep the foot out of equinus with a half-pin frame on a tibia fracture). If a circumferential cast is used, it and the cast padding must be bivalved prior to aeromedical evacuation.

## External Fixation of Extremity Fractures

External fixation is invasive and is generally reserved for long-bone and periarticular fractures not amenable to splinting. External fixation preserves access to the wound and soft-tissues for serial evaluation

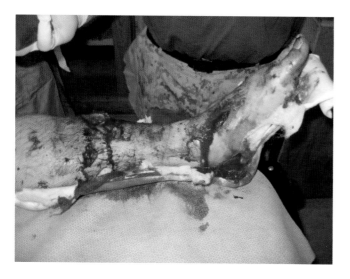

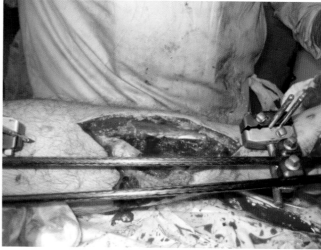

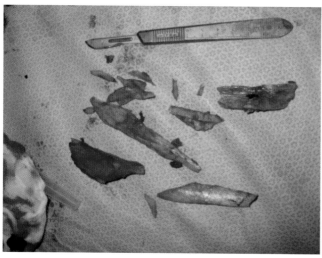

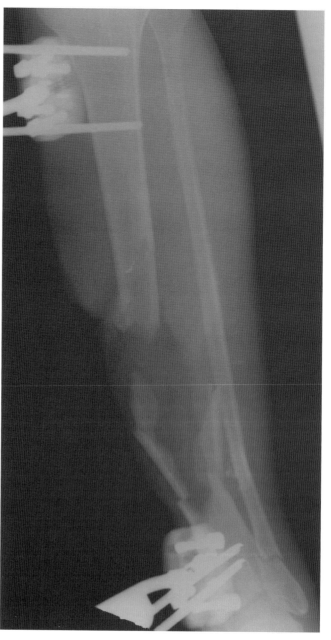

Figure 50. *Open fracture management:* (Top Left) *Casualty with open tibial and fibular fractures at presentation.* (Top Right) *Appearance of wound following irrigation, sharp surgical debridement, removal of nonviable tissue, and external fixation.* (Bottom Left) *Bone fragments stripped of their soft-tissues.* (Bottom Right) *Radiographic appearance of the injured limb following external fixation.*

and debridement while providing rigid skeletal fixation, and it may save time during damage control interventions.[109] Disadvantages of external fixation are the potential for iatrogenic vessel or nerve injury, pin site infections, lack of soft-tissue support, and possibly fewer surgical options if pin complications occur.[77,145] General surgeons should be familiar with the standard constructs of external fixation for use in initial care of battle casualties and have a thorough understanding of limb anatomy to ensure safe pin placement.[57] External fixation constructs may be applied without fluoroscopy and without the need for power tools.

> General surgeons should be familiar with the standard constructs of external fixation for use in initial care of battle casualties and have a thorough understanding of limb anatomy to ensure safe pin placement.

For effective external fixation, a minimal number of pins should be used to provide skeletal stability during resuscitation. This stabilization is commonly performed with two half-pins on both proximal and distal sides of the fracture (Fig. 51). Other factors that can make the external fixator frames more rigid are bony cortical contact of the reduced fracture edges, larger diameter half-pins, pin pairs spread farther apart (each pair on either side of the fracture), number of bars used in the frame, use of bars in multiple planes in the frame, and lessening the distance from the bone to the closest bar.[142]

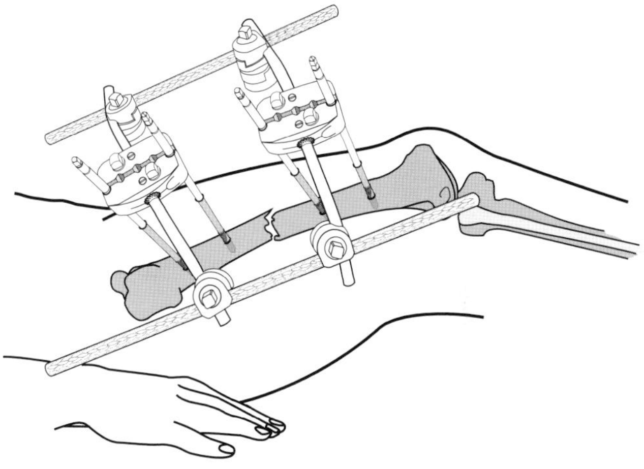

Figure 51. *Stabilization with external fixation is commonly performed with two half-pins on both proximal and distal sides of the fracture. Image courtesy of the Borden Institute, Office of The Surgeon General, Washington, DC. Illustrator: Bruce Maston.*

Basic principles of external fixation dictate that the half-pins used should be bicortical (as opposed to unicortical) with avoidance of all neurovascular structures, joints, open wounds, fractures, and fracture hematoma.[142,145] As with any fracture work, care must be paid to the surrounding neurovascular structures before, during, and after provisional fracture reduction.

> Principles of external fixation dictate that half-pins should be bicortical (as opposed to unicortical) and should avoid all neurovascular structures, joints, open wounds, fractures, and fracture hematomas.

External fixation of a distal femur fragment at distal Hunter's canal involves placing the half-pin tip in close proximity to neurovascular structures. Care must be exercised to avoid inadvertent injury to the superficial femoral artery as it courses through Hunter's canal.[145] Distal pulses should be reevaluated if limb manipulation is performed and after external fixation pins are placed. Clinical examination of peripheral nerves is important because external fixation pins can injure nerves.[145] An excellent atlas for review of safe tissue intervals for placement of external fixation half-pins is the Atlas for the Insertion of Transosseous Wires and Half-Pins: Ilizarov Method.[142]

## Upper Extremity Fracture Fixation

Upper extremity fractures are typically stabilized with splints or external fixators. Most fractures of the hand and upper extremity can be managed with external splints applied to the injured limbs (Fig. 52).

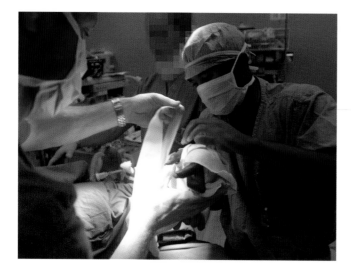 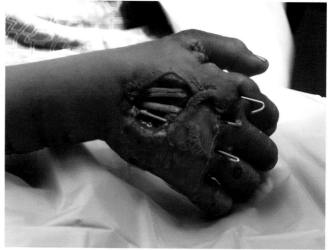

Figure 52. *Most fractures of the hand and upper extremity can be managed with external splints applied to the injured limbs. Image courtesy of Defense Imagery Management Operations Center (DIMOC).*

Figure 53. *In this pediatric hand injury with segmental loss of multiple metacarpal shafts, K-wires were used to preserve bony length.*

These splints should be well-padded. If the splints span across the wrist, they should place the wrist and hand in the neutral or safe position (wrist is placed in 20 degrees of extension, metacarpophalangeal joints are positioned at 70 degrees of flexion, and interphalangeal joints are straight), whenever possible. External fixation of upper extremity fractures can be of value in cases with marked soft-tissue injury, vascular shunt or repair, and segmental bone loss. Additionally, metacarpal fractures with bony loss may benefit from internal K-wire fixation to maintain bony length and prevent soft-tissue contracture during evacuation out of theater and initial limb resuscitation and wound debridements.[77] With external fixation of smaller diameter bones, the inserted pin diameter size should be kept to less than one-third of the diameter of the bone to limit the risk of fracture upon half-pin removal. When severe bony loss shortens the injured limb (e.g., segmental loss of multiple metacarpal shafts), K-wires (0.065 inch) can be placed in the proximal and distal bone fragments after four 90-degree bends are made at the desired bone length in order to keep limb length ideal during planned staged care (Fig. 53). If the hand maintains its good perfusion, it can be relatively resistant but not immune to infections and infected hardware. Fixation of hand fractures is often delayed until the wounds are clean and otherwise generally follows most civilian care principles. The priority in hand injuries in war are restoring perfusion and providing soft-tissue care followed by fracture care.

External fixation of humerus fractures should be reserved for those fractures with risk of vascular or neurologic injury due to fracture displacement. Often a coaptation splint or cuff and collar sling can suffice in simple fracture patterns, but if vascular structures have been shunted or repaired, more rigid skeletal fixation is indicated. Bony loss around the elbow joint may also be an indication for spanning external fixation, as this injury treated with a splint may displace and put traversing arteries and nerves at risk. Forearm fractures can also be managed with splinting or external fixation depending on the degree of soft-tissue injury, vascular status, and risk of displacement in a splint.

## Lower Extremity Fracture Fixation

Similar to the upper extremity injuries, lower extremity fractures are amenable to splinting or external fixation depending on the soft-tissue injury, risk of fracture displacement, and risk to vascular structures or repairs if the fractures displace. Foot injuries can be treated in a similar fashion as hand fractures;

K-wires can be fashioned to maintain metatarsal length if segmental loss is present. A plantar or posterior splint can be used for simple fracture patterns of the ankle and feet. If a splint is used across the ankle joint, the ankle should be placed in neutral dorsiflexion. Tibia fractures should be closely evaluated for presence of or potential to develop compartment syndromes. Simple closed fractures can be treated in a splint but may need additional time in-theater to allow for serial compartment checks during the first 24 to 48 hours of fracture swelling. Commonly, open tibia fractures are initially treated with external fixation. This allows for wound care, protection of neurovascular structures, and patient comfort during evacuation. Injuries of the proximal tibia and distal femur may warrant a knee-spanning external fixation to prevent knee dislocation or fracture displacement.

## Femur Fracture Fixation

Femur fractures can present with a markedly shortened, floppy limb with severe hemorrhage (both internal and external to the limb).[146] Restoration of the bony length reduces pain, blood loss, and risk of neurovascular injury from the sharp bony fracture surfaces.[146] Initially external traction splints can achieve some stability and bony alignment for safe patient transport (Fig. 54). For example, a Thomas splint, which is similar to the modern Hare traction splint, is the only other first-aid device besides the tourniquet evidenced to save lives of the limb injured (Fig. 55).[146] However, these traction splints rely on pressure on the ischial tuberosity proximally for their mechanical effect to hold the limb out to length. If such splints are misused or unattended, risk of sciatic nerve compression and possible risk of tourniquet-like effect by tight straps can occur. Such problems underscore the importance of periodic reassessment and adjustment of splints.

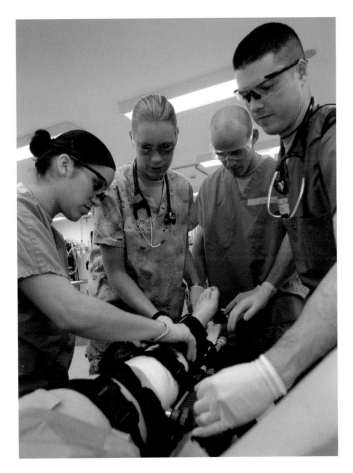

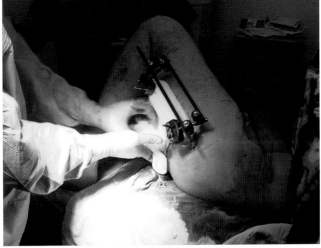

Figure 54. (Left) *An external traction splint can help stabilize and align displaced femur fractures. Image courtesy of Defense Imagery Management Operations Center (DIMOC).*

Figure 55. (Above) *Restoration of the bone length reduces pain, blood loss, and risk of neurovascular injury from sharp fracture fragments.*

Proximal tibial or distal femoral traction pins can be used to bring the femoral fracture out to length as well, but they cannot be used routinely during interhospital patient transport (Fig. 56). Hip spica casting of femur fractures should be avoided because wound access and visibility are poor, and the heavy logistical burden outweighs the benefit of the cast.[147] A common form of femoral fracture immobilization is half-pin external fixation in a unilateral frame configuration (Fig. 57). Safe areas for half-pin placements are from anterior in the thigh to lateral in the thigh (i.e., half-pin placement across the anterolateral quadrant is safe).[142,148] Care must be taken to avoid placing pins into the knee joint, as this risks septic arthritis and iatrogenic cartilage injury. Care in not overdrilling the pins through the far cortices and into the distal Hunter's canal is needed to avoid arterial injury.[145] Hip or knee-spanning frames may be used as well for very proximal and distal fractures, respectively.

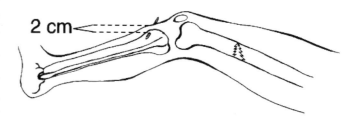

Figure 56. *Proximal tibial or distal femoral traction pins can be used to bring a femoral fracture out to length. Image courtesy of the Borden Institute, Office of The Surgeon General, Washington, DC.*

## Pelvic Fracture Fixation

The evaluation of patients sustaining pelvic trauma is a critical component of trauma care. Severe pelvic injuries result from high-energy trauma and are associated with a variety of injuries. A multidisciplinary

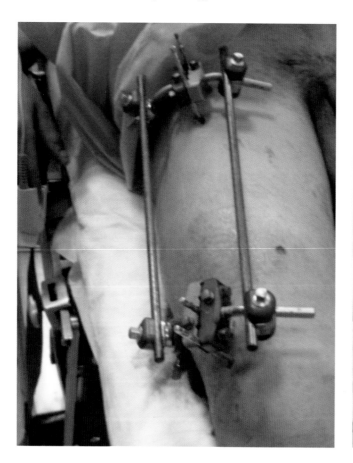
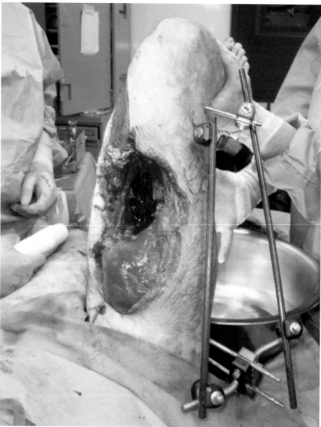

Figure 57. *For femoral fracture immobilization, half-pins may be safely placed across the anterolateral quadrant of the thigh. Images courtesy of David Carmack, MD, and Michael Shaun Machen, MD, COL, MC, US Army.*

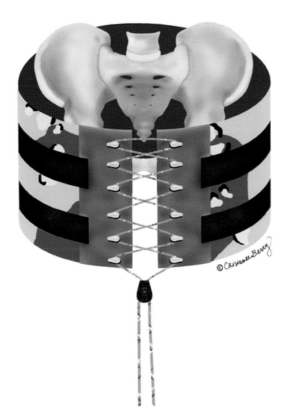

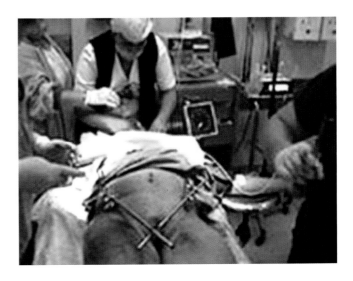

Figure 58. (Left) *Pelvic stability may be improved with application of a pelvic binder or bed sheet around the patient's hips. Image courtesy of Pelvic Binder, Inc.*

Figure 59. (Below) *Selective use of external fixation of the pelvis should be considered in patients with mechanical pelvic instability and persistent hemorrhage. Image courtesy of Trauma.org.*

approach to the early care of the casualty with pelvic trauma is important. Further discussion of acute surgical issues associated with pelvic trauma is provided in the Damage Control Surgery chapter.

> Early pelvic stabilization can control hemorrhage and reduce mortality.

Pelvic fractures in combat settings can present with severe and difficult to control hemorrhage.[149] The goals of resuscitation are to first stop the bleeding in the pelvis and then identify all open wounds. A patient with a pelvic fracture needs a thorough external and internal physical examination (including rectum and vagina) to identify any open fractures. The sources of bleeding from a pelvic fracture are venous, arterial, and bony fracture surfaces themselves. Errors in early assessment or management can increase mortality.[150] Fecal contamination and associated injuries can complicate care.

> Patients with a pelvic fracture need a thorough external and internal physical examination (including rectum and vagina) to identify open pelvic fractures.

If the pelvic fracture pattern is unstable, initial stability may be improved with a pelvic binder or sheet around the patient's hips (greater trochanters) to reduce motion in an unstable pelvis (Fig. 58).[77] Pelvic binders should be avoided in lateral compression fractures because they add to the compression laterally by their pressure on the greater trochanters; in this way, pelvic binders can worsen fracture displacement.[151]

Eastridge et al. noted the importance of pelvic fracture pattern in guiding management in a civilian patient population suffering from pelvic ring disruption and hemorrhagic shock.[149] These authors noted that

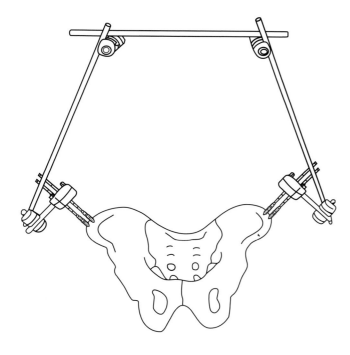

Figure 60. *External fixator placement in the iliac crests allows for the most direct control of the pelvis. Image courtesy of the Borden Institute, Office of The Surgeon General, Washington, DC.*

casualties with signs of ongoing shock with stable pelvic fracture patterns and hemoperitoneum require celiotomy as the initial intervention, as the site of major hemorrhage is predominantly intraperitoneal. In patients with unstable fracture patterns, even in the presence of hemoperitoneum, consideration should be given to angiography before celiotomy.[149] Extraperitoneal pelvic packing has been used as an adjunctive measure to angiographic embolization to achieve direct hemostasis and control venous bleeding following massive traumatic pelvic hemorrhage.[151,152] Further studies are required to define the utility of this approach. Interventional radiology capacity (therapeutic angiography) is limited in OEF and OIF, thus making pelvic packing a primary consideration in patients with massive pelvic hemorrhage.

If pelvic mechanical instability and hemodynamic instability persist, selective use of external fixation of the pelvis should be considered.[151] Rigid bony stability may allow for hemostasis, as the hematoma and vessels may be protected from further injury during initial management.[151] Of note, external fixators can displace pelvic fractures with posterior element (sacroiliac joint) instability and result in anterior pelvic compression and posterior pelvic element distraction, which can exacerbate pelvic hemorrhage (Fig. 59).[151] This phenomenon is possible with overcompression of the anterior ring resulting in diastasis of the posterior injury.

An anterior pelvic fixator can be placed without power tools and without fluoroscopic assistance. The half-pins can be tightened into a T-handled chuck for bony insertion as the half-pin's threads can cut into bone. The half-pins that are specifically designed with blunt tips for pelvic bone insertion in the Stryker's Hoffman® II External Fixation System are commonly used in the US military. The blunt tipped half-pins tend to stay within the bone between the two tables of the pelvic bone instead of sharply cutting through the inner or outer tables, and thereby with more bony purchase have better skeletal fixation. Through a skin incision and finger dissection yielding direct digital palpation of the inner and outer cortices of the pelvis with the surgeon's thumb and forefinger, half-pins are typically inserted through the bone cortex two to four centimeters posterior to the anterior superior iliac spines aligned with and between the inner and outer tables of the pelvis. This distance posterior to the anterior superior iliac spine has the greatest amount of bone available for optimal pin placement and will avoid the lateral femoral cutaneous nerve (Fig. 60).

### Open Pelvic Trauma

Open pelvic fractures are uncommon in war.[153] When they do occur, they can present with severe hemorrhage that is difficult to control. Open pelvic fractures often result from penetrating trauma that causes less skeletal instability but higher rates of arterial hemorrhage relative to closed pelvic fractures (Figs. 61 and 62). Damage control surgery such as emergent laparotomy, proximal control of vessels, and pelvic packing may be indicated, although there is little evidence to guide management. The resuscitation

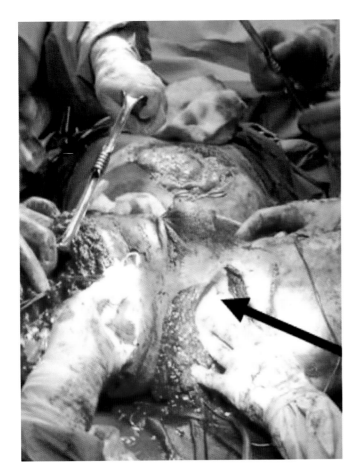

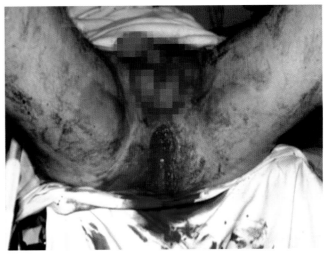

Figure 61. (Left) *Open pelvic fractures can present with severe hemorrhage that is difficult to control. This casualty required 200 units of blood in 24 hours. Image courtesy of Leopoldo C. Cancio, MD, FACS, COL, MC, US Army.*

Figure 62. (Below) *Open pelvic fractures require immediate hemorrhage control, aggressive and thorough debridement, pelvic stabilization, and a diverting colostomy in the presence of wounds at risk for fecal soliage. Image courtesy of Raymond F. Topp, MD, LTC, MC, US Army.*

requirements in such cases can be extreme and mortality rates high.[153] If the open fracture has radiographic findings suggestive of pelvic fracture instability commonly associated with blunt trauma, then the principles of care from blunt pelvic trauma still probably apply as discussed previously.[149] However, additional principles of open pelvic trauma may also apply and include consideration for massive transfusion and pelvic packing.[152,154]

> Open pelvic fractures are uncommon in war. When present, they require immediate hemorrhage control, aggressive and thorough debridement, pelvic stabilization, and a diverting colostomy in the presence of wounds at risk for fecal soilage.

## Associated Injuries

### *Genitourinary Complications*
The genitourinary injuries found in association with pelvic injuries are discussed in the Damage Control Surgery chapter.

### *Hip Dislocations*
Hip dislocations are often associated with pelvic (e.g., acetabular fractures) trauma.[155] Hip dislocations are classified as posterior (80 to 90 percent), anterior (10 to 15 percent) and central (2 to 4 percent). All hip dislocations must be regarded as true orthopaedic emergencies (Fig. 63). Following a hip dislocation, traction on the blood vessels supplying the femoral head can result in ischemia. Prompt reduction of hip dislocations is necessary to minimize the incidence of avascular necrosis of the femoral head.[156]

Classic teaching is that all hip dislocations should be reduced within six hours.[157,158] The sooner the hip is reduced the better. The longer a hip is dislocated, the greater the risk of avascular necrosis. The timing and method of reduction depend on the patient's condition, the type of dislocation, and associated fractures. Adequate relaxation ensures the greatest chance for success. Patients will need to undergo deep sedation.

> All hip dislocations must be regarded as true orthopaedic emergencies. Prompt reduction of hip dislocations is necessary to minimize the incidence of avascular necrosis of the femoral head.

Most anterior hip dislocations reduce easily with traction in line with the deformity. Posterior hip dislocations may be reduced by the Allis or Stimson maneuvers. In the Allis maneuver, an assistant stabilizes the anterior superior iliac spines while the patient is supine. First the knee is flexed, then the hip is flexed, and traction is applied below the knee pulling it upward. The leg is internally and externally rotated until reduction is achieved. The Stimson maneuver requires the patient to lie prone with the affected extremity completely off the table or stretched. The hip and knee are flexed to 90 degrees, and downward pressure is placed on the flexed knee. The leg is gently externally and internally rotated until reduction is accomplished.

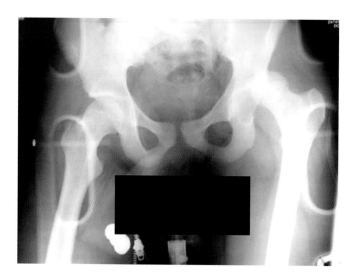

Figure 63. *Example of a left hip dislocation. All hip dislocations should be treated as true orthopaedic emergencies and reduced as soon as possible.*

Following hip reduction, an abduction pillow is placed between the patient's thighs and holds them widely apart to maintain the reduction. A post-reduction hip radiograph should be obtained to confirm adequate reduction and document any fracture fragments. Occasionally, a hip dislocation may be irreducible due to the incarceration of a tendon, joint capsule, or fracture fragment. These cases will need closed reduction under general anesthesia or open (i.e., operative) reduction.

### Acetabular Fractures

Fractures of the acetabulum represent 20 percent of all pelvic fractures.[159] There are four types of acetabular fractures: posterior rim, transverse, iliopubic (i.e., anterior column) and ilioischial (i.e., posterior column). Posterior rim fractures represent the most common form of acetabular fracture. They are almost always associated with posterior hip dislocations. Transverse acetabular fractures may be associated with central hip dislocations. Iliopubic column acetabular fractures may be associated with central or anterior hip dislocations. Ilioischial column fractures have an associated sciatic nerve injury in 25 to 30 percent of cases.[160] The general treatment of acetabular fractures includes analgesia, CT imaging with thin sections to further characterize the injury, hospitalization, and orthopaedic consultation. The goal of treating acetabular fractures is to reestablish the normal femoral head and acetabular relationship. Associated hip dislocations require prompt reduction to avoid long-term complications.

# Summary

The frequency and severity of extremity injuries in OEF and OIF are substantial. Extremity injury care underscores one of the most obvious differences between military and civilian scope of practice for nonorthopaedic CCC providers. Combat casualty careproviders need to have a solid understanding of the general principles of combat extremity wound and injury management. General surgeons will often need to perform orthopaedic procedures such as complex wound debridement, external fixation of fractures, and fasciotomy for compartment syndrome. For experienced orthopaedists, the means and goals of CCC differ slightly in context. For example, host nation casualty management is aimed more towards providing definitive care, to the extent local logistical constraints allow. Definitive care of US military casualties is typically deferred to Level V facilities. Balancing ideal versus practical casualty care in a combat theatre will challenge even the most seasoned careprovider.

# References

1. Hamdan TA. Missile injuries of the limbs: an Iraqi perspective. J Am Acad Orthop Surg 2006;14(10 Spec No.):S32-36.

2. Owens BD, Kragh JF Jr, Wenke JC, et al. Combat wounds in Operation Iraqi Freedom and Operation Enduring Freedom. J Trauma 2008;64(2):295-299.

3. Cho JM, Jatoi I, Alarcon AS, et al. Operation Iraqi Freedom: surgical experience of the 212th Mobile Army Surgical Hospital. Mil Med 2005;170(4):268-272.

4. Owens BD, Kragh JF Jr, Macaitis J, et al. Characterization of extremity wounds in Operation Iraqi Freedom and Operation Enduring Freedom. J Orthop Trauma 2007;21(4):254-257.

5. Masini BD, Waterman SM, Wenke JC, et al. Resource utilization and disability outcome assessment of combat casualties from Operation Iraqi Freedom and Operation Enduring Freedom. J Orthop Trauma 2009;23(4):261-266.

6. Kelly JF, Ritenour AE, McLaughlin DF, et al. Injury severity and causes of death from Operation Iraqi Freedom and Operation Enduring Freedom: 2003-2004 versus 2006. J Trauma 2008;64(2 Suppl):S21-26; discussion S26-27.

7. Kragh JF Jr, Jones BH, Amaroso PJ, et al. Parachuting injuries among Army Rangers: a prospective survey of an elite airborne battalion. Mil Med 1996;161(7):416-419.

8. Kragh JF Jr, Taylor DC. Parachuting injuries: a medical analysis of an airborne operation. Mil Med 1996;161(2):67-69.

9. Kragh JF Jr, Taylor DC. Fast-roping injuries among Army Rangers: a retrospective survey of an elite airborne battalion. Mil Med 1995;160(6):277-279.

10. Erpelding JM, Taylor DC, Kragh JF Jr. Extremity trauma in wartime: lessons learned from recent conflicts. Techniques in Orthopaedics 1995;10(3):171-175.

11. Kragh JF Jr, Wade CE, Baer DG, et al. Orthopaedic trauma in the current war: severity, fasciotomy, and tourniquets. J Orthop Trauma In press 2010.

12. Watson F. The Life of Sir Robert Jones. London: Hodder & Stoughton;1934.

13. Ritenour AE, Dorlac WC, Fang R, et al. Complications after fasciotomy revision and delayed compartment release in combat patients. J Trauma 2008;64(2 Suppl):S153-161; discussion S161-162.

14. Reis ND, Better OS. Mechanical muscle-crush injury and acute muscle-crush compartment syndrome: with special reference to earthquake casualties. J Bone Joint Surg Br 2005;87(4):450-453.

15. Kragh JF Jr, Walters TJ, Baer DG, et al. Survival with emergency tourniquet use to stop bleeding in major limb trauma. Ann Surg 2009;249(1):1-7.

16. Ennis JL, Chung KK, Renz EM, et al. Joint Theater Trauma System implementation of burn resuscitation guidelines improves outcomes in severely burned military casualties. J Trauma 2008;64(2 Suppl):S146-S151; discussion S151-S152.

17. Holcomb JB, Wade CE, Michalek JE, et al. Increased plasma and platelet to red blood cell ratios improves outcome in 466 massively transfused civilian trauma patients. Ann Surg 2008;248(3):447-458.

18. Eastridge BJ, Jenkins D, Flaherty S, et al. Trauma system development in a theater of war: experiences from Operation Iraqi Freedom and Operation Enduring Freedom. J Trauma 2006;61(6):1366-1372; discussion 1372-1373.

19. Bellamy RF. The causes of death in conventional land warfare: implications for combat casualty care research. Mil Med 1984;149(2):55-62.

20. Bellamy, RF. Combat trauma overview. In: Textbook of military medicine. Part IV. Surgical combat casualty care: Anesthesia and perioperative care of the combat casualty. Washington, DC: Office of the Surgeon General, Borden Institute; 1995. p. 1-42.

21. Maughon JS. An inquiry into the nature of wounds resulting in killed in action in Vietnam. Mil Med 1970;135(1):8-13.

22. Mabry RL, Holcomb JB, Baker AM, et al. United States Army Rangers in Somalia: an analysis of combat casualties on an urban battlefield. J Trauma 2000;49(3):515-528; discussion 528-529.

23. Keggi KJ, Southwick WO. Early care of severe extremity wounds: a review of the Vietnam experience and its civilian applications. Instr Course Lect 1970;19:183-203.

24. Feltis JM J. Surgical experience in a combat zone. Am J Surg 1970;119(3):275-278.

25. Beebe GW, DeBakey ME, editors. Battle casualties. Springfield, IL: Charles C Thomas; 1952.

26. Beebe GW, DeBakey ME. Battle casualties: incidence, mortality, and logistic considerations. Ann Intern Med 1953;38(6):1345-1346.

27. Holcomb JB, Stansbury LG, Champion HR, et al. Understanding combat casualty care statistics. J Trauma 2006;60(2):397-401.

28. Kragh JF Jr, Baer DG, Walters TJ. Extended (16-hour) tourniquet application after combat wounds: a case report and review of the current literature. J Orthop Trauma 2007;21(4):274-278.

29. Bellamy RF. A note on American combat mortality in Iraq. Mil Med 2007;172(10):I, 1023.

30. Burns BD, Zuckerman S. The wounding power of small bomb and shell fragments. British Ministry of Supply, Advisory Council on Scientific Research and Technical Developments; 1942.

31. Holcomb JB, McMullin NR, Pearse L, et al. Causes of death in U.S. Special Operations Forces in the global war on terrorism: 2001-2004. Ann Surg 2007;245(6):986-991.

32. Brav EA. Military contributions to the development of orthopaedic surgery by the Armed Forces, U.S.A. Since World War I. Clin Orthop Relat Res 1966;44:115-126.

33. Grant RT, Reeve EB. Observations on the general effects of injury in man: with special reference to wound shock. Medical Research Council Special Report Series No. 277. London: HM Stationery Office; 1951. p. 3-67.

34. Artz CP, Howard JM, Sako Y, et al. Clinical experiences in the early management of the most severely injured battle casualties. Ann Surg 1955;141(3):285-296.

35. Beekley AC, Sebesta JA, Blackbourne LH, et al. Prehospital tourniquet use in Operation Iraqi Freedom: effect on hemorrhage control. J Trauma 2008;64(2 Suppl):S28-37.

36. Kragh JF Jr, Walters TJ, Baer DG, et al. Practical use of emergency tourniquets to stop bleeding in major limb trauma. J Trauma 2008;64(2 Suppl):S38-49; discussion S49-50.

37. Klenerman L. The tourniquet manual. London: Springer-Verlag; 2003.

38. Brodie S, Hodgetts TJ, Ollerton J, et al. Tourniquet use in combat trauma: UK military experience. J R Army Med Corps 2007;153(4):310-313.

39. Parker P, Clasper J. The military tourniquet. J R Army Med Corps 2007;153(1):10-12.

40. Hodgetts TJ, Mahoney PF. The military tourniquet: a response. J R Army Med Corps 2007;153(1):12-15.

41. Mubarak SJ, Hargens AR. Compartment syndromes and Volkmann's contracture. Philadelphia, PA: Saunders; 1981. p. 50-57.

42. Balian B, Ennis O, Moorcroft CI, et al. Factors affecting healing in closed tibia fractures. American Academy of Orthopaedic Surgeons meeting; Las Vegas, NV; 2009.

43. Elliott KG, Johnstone AJ. Diagnosing acute compartment syndrome. J Bone Joint Surg Br 2003;85(5):625-632.

44. Rorabeck CH, Macnab I. The pathophysiology of the anterior tibial compartmental syndrome. Clin Orthop 1975;113:52-57.

45. Ulmer T. The clinical diagnosis of compartment syndrome of the lower leg: are clinical findings

predictive of the disorder. J Orthop Trauma 2002;16(8):572-577.

46. McQueen MM, Christie J, Court-Brown CM. Acute compartment syndrome in tibial diaphyseal fractures. J Bone Joint Surg Br 1996;78(1):95-98.

47. Kragh JF. Joint Theater Trauma System (JTTS) Clinical Practice Guideline. Compartment syndrome (CS) and the role of fasciotomy in extremity war wounds. 2009 Apr 30 [cited 2010 May 5]. Available from: URL: http://www.usaisr.amedd.army.mil/cpgs.html.

48. Tull F, Borrelli J Jr. Soft-tissue injury associated with closed fractures: evaluation and management. J Am Acad Orthop Surg 2003;11(6):431-438.

49. Cope O, Moore FD. The redistribution of body water and the fluid therapy of the burned patient. Ann Surg 1947;126(6):1010-1045.

50. Tremblay LN, Feliciano DV, Rozycki GS. Secondary extremity compartment syndrome. J Trauma 2002;53(5):833-837.

51. Kosir R, Moore FA, Selby JH et al. Acute lower extremity compartment syndrome (ALECS) screening protocol in critically ill trauma patients. J Trauma 2007;63(2):268-275.

52. Madigan MC, Kemp CD, Johnson JC, et al. Secondary abdominal compartment syndrome after severe extremity injury: are early, aggressive fluid resuscitation strategies to blame? J Trauma 2008;64(2):280-285.

53. Revell M, Greaves I, Porter K. Endpoints for fluid resuscitation in hemorrhagic shock. J Trauma 2003;54(5 Suppl):S63-67.

54. Tornetta P III. Templeman D. Compartment syndrome associated with tibial fracture. Instr Course Lect 1997;46:303-308.

55. Heckman MM, Whitesides TE Jr, Grewe SR, et al. Compartment pressure in association with closed tibial fractures. The relationship between tissue pressure, compartment, and the distance from the site of the fracture. J Bone Joint Surg Am 1994;76(9):1285-1292.

56. Nessen SC, Lounsbury DE, Hetz SP, editors. Soft-tissue Trauma and Burns. In: War Surgery in Afghanistan and Iraq: A Series of Cases, 2003-2007. Washington, DC: Department of the Army, Office of the Surgeon General, Borden Institute; 2008. p. 205-248.

57. US Department of Defense (US DoD) Extremity fractures. In: Emergency War Surgery, Third United States Revision. Washington, DC: Department of the Army, Office of the Surgeon General, Borden Institute; 2004. p. 23.1-23.21.

58. Sheridan GW, Matsen FA III. Fasciotomy in the treatment of the acute compartment syndrome. J Bone Joint Surg Am 1976;58(1):112-115.

59. Matsen FA III, Wyss CR, Krugmire RB Jr, et al. The effects of limb elevation and dependency on local arteriovenous gradients in normal human limbs with particular reference to limbs with increased tissue pressure. Clin Orthop Relat Res 1980;150:187-195.

60. Bronwell AW, Artz CP, Sako Y. Recent advances in medicine and surgery based on professional medical experiences in Japan and Korea 1950-1953. Debridement in Medical Science Publication No. 4. US Army Medical Service Graduate School. Washington, DC: Walter Reed Army Medical Center; 19-30 Apr, 1954.

61. Stansbury LG, Branstetter JG, Lalliss SJ. Amputation in military trauma surgery. J Trauma 2007;63(4):940-944.

62. US Department of Defense (US DoD). General Considerations of Forward Surgery. In: Emergency War Surgery, Second United States Revision. Washington, DC: Department of the Army, Office of the Surgeon General, Borden Institute; 1988.

63. US Department of Defense (US DoD). Amputations. In: Emergency War Surgery, Third United States Revision. Washington, DC: Department of the Army, Office of the Surgeon General, Borden Institute; 2004. p. 25.1-25.8.

64. Stansbury LG, Lalliss SJ, Branstetter JG, et al. Amputations in U.S. military personnel in the current conflicts in Afghanistan and Iraq. J Orthop Trauma 2008;22(1):43-46.

65. Fox CJ, Gillespie DL, Cox ED, et al. The effectiveness of a damage control resuscitation strategy for vascular injury in a combat support hospital: results of a case control study. J Trauma 2008;64(2 Suppl):S99-106; discussion S106-107.

66. Fox CJ, Gillespie DL, Cox ED, et al. Damage control resuscitation for vascular surgery in a combat support hospital. J Trauma 2008;65(1):1-9.

67. Fox CJ, Mehta SG, Cox ED, et al. Effect of recombinant factor VIIa as an adjunctive therapy in damage control for wartime vascular injuries: a case control study. J Trauma 2009;66(4 Suppl):S112-119.

68. Bosse MJ, MacKenzie EJ, Kellam JF, et al. A prospective evaluation of the clinical utility of the lower-extremity injury-severity scores. J Bone Joint Surg Am 2001;83-A(1):3-14.

69. Bosse MJ, McCarthy MJ, Jones AL, et al. The Lower Extremity Assessment Project (LEAP) Study Group. The insensate foot following severe lower extremity trauma: an indication for amputation? J Bone Joint Surg Am 2005;87(12):2601-2608.

70. Hsu JR, Beltran MJ; Skeletal Trauma Research Consortium. Shortening and angulation for soft-tissue reconstruction of extremity wounds in a combat support hospital. Mil Med 2009;174(8):838-842.

71. Gulsen M, Ozkan C. Angular shortening and delayed gradual distraction for the treatment of asymmetrical bone and soft-tissue defects of tibia: a case series. J Trauma 2009;66(5):E61-66.

72. Webb LX, Dedmond B, Schlatterer D, et al. The contaminated high-energy open fracture: a protocol to prevent and treat inflammatory mediator storm-induced soft-tissue compartment syndrome (IMSICS). J Am Acad Orthop Surg 2006;14(10 Spec No.):S82-86.

73. Langworthy MJ, Smith JM, Gould M. Treatment of the mangled lower extremity after a terrorist blast injury. Clin Orthop 2004;422:88-96.

74. O'Shaughnessy KD, Dumanian GA, Lipschutz RD, et al. Targeted reinnervation to improve prosthesis control in transhumeral amputees. A report of three cases. J Bone Joint Surg Am 2008;90(2):393-400.

75. Barillo DJ, Cancio LC, Goodwin CW. Treatment of white phosphorus and other chemical burn injuries at one burn center over a 51-year period. Burns 2004;30(5):448-52.

76. US Department of Defense (US DoD). Burn injuries. In: Emergency War Surgery, Third United States Revision. Washington, DC: Department of the Army, Office of the Surgeon General, Borden Institute; 2004. p. 28.1-28.15.

77. Nessen SC, Lounsbury DE, Hetz SP, editors. Orthopedic Trauma. In: War Surgery in Afghanistan and Iraq: A Series of Cases, 2003-2007. Washington, DC: Department of the Army, Office of the Surgeon General, Borden Institute; 2008. p. 249-316.

78. Hayda RA, Ficke JR. Wartime amputation instructional video [Digital video disc]. Washington, DC: Department of the Army; Feb 2002.

79. Dougherty PJ. Wartime amputee care. In: Smith DG, Michael JW, Bowker JH, editors. Atlas of amputations and limb deficiencies: surgical, prosthetic, and rehabilitation. 3rd ed. Rosemont, IL: American Academy of Orthopaedic Surgeons; 2004. p. 77-97.

80. Smith DG, Granville RR. Moderators' summary: amputee care. J Am Acad Orthop Surg 2006;14(10 Spec No.):S179-182.

81. Gajewski D, Granville R. The United States Armed Forces Amputee Patient Care Program. J Am Acad Orthop Surg 2006;14(10 Spec No.):S183-187.

82. Potter BK. Scoville CR. Amputation is not isolated: an overview of the US Army Amputee Patient Care Program and associated amputee injuries. J Am Acad Orthop Surg 2006;14(10 Spec No.):S188-90.

83. Rehabilitation of the injured combatant, Vol 1. Textbook of military medicine. Washington, DC: Department of the Army, Office of The Surgeon General, Borden Institute; 1998.

84. Rehabilitation of the injured combatant, Vol 2. Textbook of military medicine. Washington, DC: Department of the Army, Office of The Surgeon General, Borden Institute; 1999.

85. Hospenthal DR, Murray CK, Andersen RC, et al. Guidelines for the prevention of infection after combat-related injuries. J Trauma 2008;64(3 Suppl):S211-S220.

86. Vertrees A, Fox CJ, Quan RW, et al. The use of prosthetic grafts in complex military vascular trauma: a limb salvage strategy for patients with severely limited autologous conduit. J Trauma 2009;66(4):980-983.

87. Fox CJ, Starnes BW. Vascular surgery on the modern battlefield. Surg Clin North Am 2007;87(5):1193-1211.

88. Kragh JF Jr, Basamania CJ. Surgical repair of acute traumatic closed transection of the biceps brachii. J Bone Joint Surg Am 2002;84-A(6):992-998.

89. Kragh JF Jr, Svoboda SJ, Wenke JC, et al. Suturing of lacerations of skeletal muscle. J Bone Joint Surg Br 2005;87(9):1303-1305.

90. Kragh JF Jr, Svoboda SJ, Wenke JC, et al. The role of epimysium in suturing skeletal muscle lacerations. J Am Coll Surg 2005;200(1):38-44.

91. Chance JR, Kragh JF Jr, Agrawal CM, et al. Pullout forces of sutures in muscle lacerations. Orthopaedics 2005;28(10):1187-1190.

92. Kragh JF Jr, Svoboda SJ, Wenke JC, et al. Epimysium and perimysium in suturing in skeletal muscle lacerations. J Trauma 2005;59(1):209-212.

93. Kragh JF Jr, Svoboda SJ, Wenke JC, et al. Passive biomechanical properties of sutured mammalian muscle lacerations. J Invest Surg 2005;18(1):19-23.

94. Burkhalter WE, editor. Orthopaedic surgery in Vietnam. Medical Department, United States Army. Washington, DC: Office of the Surgeon General and Center of Military History; 1994.

95. Voit GA, Irvine G, Beals RK. Saline load test for penetration of periarticular lacerations. J Bone Joint Surg Br 1996;78(5):732-733.

96. Nord RM, Quach T, Walsh M, et al. Detection of traumatic arthrotomy of the knee using the saline solution load test. J Bone Joint Surg Am 2009;91(1):66-70.

97. Keese GR, Boody AR, Wongworawat MD, et al. The accuracy of the saline load test in the diagnosis of traumatic knee arthrotomies. J Orthop Trauma 2007;21(7):442-443.

98. Vutskits L, Briner A, Klauser P, et al. Adverse effects of methylene blue on the central nervous system. Anesthesiology 2008;108(4):684-692.

99. Mathew S, Linhartova L, Raghuraman G. Hyperpyrexia and prolonged postoperative disorientation following methylene blue infusion during parathyroidectomy. Anaesthesia 2006;61(6):580-583.

100. Sweet G, Standiford SB. Methylene-blue-associated encephalopathy. J Am Coll Surg 2007;204(3):454-458.

101. Ng BK, Cameron AJ, Liang R, et al. Serotonin syndrome following methylene blue infusion during parathyroidectomy: a case report and literature review. Can J Anaesth 2008;55(1):36-41.

102. Omer GE Jr, Spinner M, Van Beeks AL, editors. Management of peripheral nerve problems. 2nd ed. Philadelphia: W.B. Saunders; 1998.

103. Sunderland S. Nerves and nerve injuries. New York: Churchill Livingston; 1978.

104. US Department of Defense (US DoD). Wounds and Injuries of Peripheral Nerves. In: Emergency War Surgery, Second United States Revision. Washington, DC: Department of the Army, Office of the Surgeon General, Borden Institute; 1988.

105. US Department of Defense (US DoD). Soft-tissue injuries. In: Emergency War Surgery, Third United States Revision. Washington, DC: Department of the Army, Office of the Surgeon General, Borden Institute; 2004. p. 22.1-22.15.

106. Kumar AR. Standard wound coverage techniques for extremity war injury. J Am Acad Orthop Surg 2006;14(10 Spec No.):S62-65.

107. Moran KA, Murray CK, Anderson EL. Bacteriology of blood, wound, and sputum cultures from non-US casualties treated in a combat support hospital in Iraq. Infect Control Hosp Epidemiol 2008;29(10):981-984.

108. Rajasekaran S, Dheenadhayalan J, Babu JN, et al. Immediate primary skin closure in type-III A and B open fractures: results after a minimum of five years. J Bone Joint Surg Br 2009;91(2):217-224.

109. Manring MM, Hawk A, Calhoun JH, et al. Treatment of war wounds: a historical review. Clin Orthop Rel Res 2009;467(8):2168-2191.

110. Sherman R, Rahban S, Pollak AN. Timing of wound coverage in extremity war injuries. J Am Acad Orthop Surg 2006;14(10 Spec No.):S57–61.

111. Noe A. Extremity injury in war: a brief history. J Am Acad Orthop Surg 14(10 Spec No.):S1-6.

112. Levin LS. New developments in flap techniques. J Am Acad Orthop Surg 2006;14(10 Spec No.):S90-93.

113. Murray CK. Infectious disease complications of combat-related injuries. Crit Care Med 2008;36(7 Suppl):S358-364.

114. Murray CK, Roop SA, Hospenthal DR, et al. Bacteriology of war wounds at the time of injury. Mil Med 2006;171(9):826-829.

115. Owens BD, Wenke JC. Early wound irrigation improves the ability to remove bacteria. J Bone Joint Surg Am 2007;89(8):1723-1726.

116. Murray CK, Hsu JR, Solomkin JS, et al. Prevention and management of infections associated with combat-related extremity injuries. J Trauma 2008;64(3 Suppl):S239-251.

117. Lin DL, Kirk KL, Murphy KP, et al. Evaluation of orthopaedic injuries in Operation Enduring Freedom. J Orthop Trauma 2004;18(8 Suppl):S48-53.

118. Johnson EN, Burns TC, Hayda RA, et al. Infectious complications of open type III tibial fractures among combat casualties. Clin Infect Dis 2007;45(4):409-415.

119. Yun HC, Branstetter JG, Murray CK. Osteomyelitis in military personnel wounded in Iraq and Afghanistan. J Trauma 2008;64(2 Suppl):S163-168; discussion S168.

120. Owens BD, Wenke JC, Svoboda SJ, et al. Extremity trauma research in the United States Army. J Am Acad Orthop Surg 2006;14(10 Spec No.):S37-40.

121. Owens BD, White DW, Wenke JC. Comparison of irrigation solutions and devices in a contaminated musculoskeletal wound survival model. J Bone Joint Surg Am 2009;91(1):92-98.

122. Joint Theater Trauma System Clinical Practice Guidelines. Initial management of war wounds: wound debridement and irrigation. 2010 Mar 1 [cited 2010 May 5]. Available from: URL: http://www.usaisr.amedd.army.mil/cpgs.html.

123. Svoboda SJ, Owens BD, Gooden HA, et al. Irrigation with potable water versus normal saline in a contaminated musculoskeletal wound model. J Trauma 2008;64(5):1357-1359.

124. Bowyer G. Débridement of extremity war wounds. J Am Acad Orthop Surg 2006;14(10 Spec No.):S52-56.

125. Rose CA, Hess OW, Welch CS. Vascular injuries of the extremities in battle casualties. Ann Surg 1946;123(2):161-179.

126. Artz CP, Sako Y, Scully RE. An evaluation of the surgeon's criteria for determining the viability of muscle during debridement. AMA Arch Surg 1956;73(6):1031-1035.

127. Peyser A, Khoury A, Liebergall M. Shrapnel management. J Am Acad Orthop Surg 2006;14(10 Spec No.):S66-70.

128. Simchen E, Raz R, Stein H, et al. Risk factors for infection in fracture war wounds (1973 and 1982 wars, Israel). Mil Med 1991;156(10):520-527.

129. Parker MJ, Livingstone V, Clifton R, et al. Closed suction surgical wound drainage after orthopaedic surgery. Cochrane Database Syst Rev 2007;3:CD001825.

130. Kauvar DS, Wade CE. The epidemiology and modern management of traumatic hemorrhage: US and international perspectives. Crit Care 2005;9 (Suppl 5):S1-9.

131. Nelson DE. Coagulation problems associated with multiple transfusions secondary to soft-tissue injury. USARV Medical Bulletin 1968;3(5):40-49.

132. Bowden RE, Gutmann E. The fate of voluntary muscle after vascular injury in man. J Bone Joint Surg Am 1949;31B(3):356-68.

133. Leininger BE, Rasmussen TE, Smith DL, et al. Experience with wound VAC and delayed primary closure of contaminated soft tissue injuries in Iraq. J Trauma 2006;61(5):1207-1211.

134. Lalliss SJ, Branstetter JG, Murray CK, et al. Infection rates in U.S. military personnel using vacuum-assisted closure. Plast Reconstr Surg 2007;120(2):574-575;author reply 575-576.

135. Webb LX. New techniques in wound management: vacuum-assisted wound closure. J Am Acad Orthop Surg 2002;10(5):303-311.

136. Berkowitz MJ, Rediske MW, Chance MJ, et al. Technique tip: creation of a vacuum-assisted closure system for wound management in an austere environment. Foot Ankle Int 2007;28(3):388-391.

137. Wenke JC, Owens BD, Svoboda SJ, et al. Effectiveness of commercially-available antibiotic-impregnated implants. J Bone Joint Surg Br 2006;88(8):1102-1104.

138. Thomas DB, Brooks DE, Bice TG, et al. Tobramycin-impregnated calcium sulfate prevents infection in contaminated wounds. Clin Orthop Relat Res 2005;441:366-371.

139. Butler F, O'Connor K. Antibiotics in tactical combat casualty care 2002. Mil Med 2003;168(11):911-914.

140. Holtom PD. Antibiotic prophylaxis: current recommendations. J Am Acad Orthop Surg 2006;14(10 Spec No.):S98-100.

141. Mazurek MT, Burgess AR. Moderators' summary: stabilization of long bones. J Am Acad Orthop Surg 2006;14(10 Spec No.):S113-117.

142. Catagni, MA. Atlas for the insertion of transosseous wires and half-pins: Ilizarov method. 2nd ed. Memphis, TN: Smith & Nephew Orthopaedics; 2003.

143. Dougherty PJ, Silverton C, Yeni Y, et al. Conversion from temporary external fixation to definitive fixation: shaft fractures. J Am Acad Orthop Surg 2006;14(10 Spec No.):S124–127.

144. Della Rocca GJ, Crist BD. External fixation versus conversion to intramedullary nailing for definitive management of closed fractures of the femoral and tibial shaft. J Am Acad Orthop Surg 2006;14(10 Spec No.):S131-135.

145. Topp RF, Hayda R, Benedetti G, et al. The incidence of neurovascular injury during external fixator placement without radiographic assistance for lower extremity diaphyseal fractures: a cadaveric

study. J Trauma 2003;55(5):955-958.

146. Kirkup J. Foundation lecture. Fracture care of friend and foe during World War I. ANZ J Surg 2003;73(6):453-459.

147. McHenry T, Simmons S, Alitz C, et al. Forward surgical stabilization of penetrating lower extremity fractures: circular casting versus external fixation. Mil Med 2001;166(9):791-795.

148. Mehta S, Sankar WN, Born CT. External fixation of the pelvis and extremities. Philadelphia, PA: Lippincott Williams & Wilkins; 2005.

149. Eastridge BJ, Starr A, Minei JP, et al. The importance of fracture pattern in guiding therapeutic decision-making in patients with hemorrhagic shock and pelvic ring disruptions. J Trauma 2002;53(3):446-450; discussion 450-451.

150. Giannoudis PV, Pape HC. Damage control orthopaedics in unstable pelvic ring injuries. Injury 2004;35(7):671-677.

151. Hak DJ, Smith WR, Suzuki T. Management of hemorrhage in life-threatening pelvic fracture. J Am Acad Orthop Surg 2009;17(7):447-457.

152. Tötterman A, Madsen JE, Skaga NO, et al. Extraperitoneal pelvic packing: a salvage procedure to control massive traumatic pelvic hemorrhage. J Trauma 2007;62(4):843-852.

153. US Department of Defense (US DoD). Pelvic Injuries. In: Emergency War Surgery, Third United States Revision. Washington, DC: Department of the Army, Office of the Surgeon General, Borden Institute; 2004. p. 21.1-21.4.

154. Joint Theater Trauma System (JTTS) Clinical Practice Guideline. Pelvic fracture care. 2008 Nov 12 [cited 2010 May 5]. Available from: URL: http://www.usaisr.amedd.army.mil/cpgs.html.

155. Alonso JE, Volgas DA, Giordano V, et al. A review of the treatment of hip dislocations associated with acetabular fractures. Clin Orthop Relat Res 2000;Aug(377):32-43.

156. Yang EC, Cornwall R. Initial treatment of traumatic hip dislocations in the adult. Clin Orthop Relat Res 2000;Aug(377):24-31.

157. Rodríguez-Merchán EC. Osteonecrosis of the femoral head after traumatic hip dislocation in the adult. Clin Orthop Relat Res 2000;Aug(377):68-77.

158. Cash DJ, Nolan JF. Avascular necrosis of the femoral head 8 years after posterior hip dislocation. Injury 2007;38(7):865-867.

159. Gibbs MA, Bosse MJ. Pelvic ring fractures. In: Ferrera PC, Colucciello SA, Marx JA, et al, editors. Trauma management: an emergency medicine approach. St Louis, MO: Mosby; 1998. p. 330-333.

160. Hillyard RF, Fox J. Sciatic nerve injuries associated with traumatic posterior hip dislocations. Am J Emerg Med 2003;21(7):545-548.

# Appendices

1.  Combat Application Tourniquet (C-A-T®) Application Steps

2.  Joint Theater Trauma System Clinical Practice Guideline — Compartment Syndrome (CS) and the Role of Fasciotomy in Extremity War Wounds

3.  Glossary and Classification of Amputations

4.  Joint Theater Trauma System Clinical Practice Guideline — Irrigation of War Wounds

# Combat Application Tourniquet®

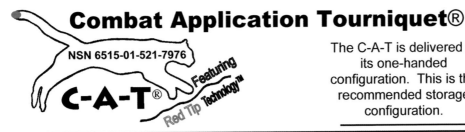

NSN 6515-01-521-7976

C-A-T® *Featuring Red Tip Technology*™

The C-A-T is delivered in its one-handed configuration. This is the recommended storage configuration.

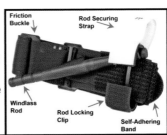

Friction Buckle | Rod Securing Strap | Windlass Rod | Rod Locking Clip | Self-Adhering Band

## Instructions for Use: Two-handed Application

**1** Route the band around the limb and pass the red tip through the

inside slit of the buckle. Pull the band tight.

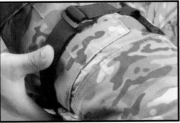

**2** Pass the red tip through the outside slit of the buckle.

The friction buckle will lock the band in place.

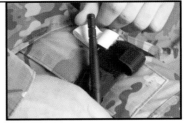

**3** Pull the band <u>very tight</u> and securely fasten the band back on itself.

When the band is pulled tight, no more then 3 fingers will fit between the band and the limb.

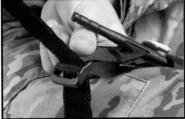

**4** Twist the rod until bright red bleeding has stopped

and the distal pulse is eliminated.

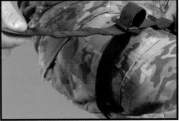

**5** Place the rod inside the clip locking it in place. Check for bleeding.

and distal pulse. If bleeding is not controlled, apply a second tourniquet proximal to the first and reassess.

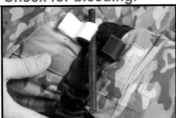

**6** Secure the rod inside the clip with the strap.

Prepare the patient for transport and reassess. Record the time of application.

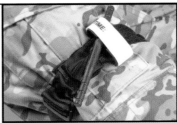

## Using the Friction Buckle

For two-handed application or when *the band becomes dirty*, use the friction buckle to lock the band in place.

**1** Pass the red tip through the

inside slit of the buckle. Pull the band tight.

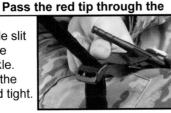

**2** Pass the red tip through the

outside slit of the buckle.

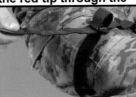

**3** Pull the band tight

and securely fasten the band back on itself.

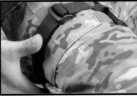

The Combat Application Tourniquet® is Patent Pending

RAW-18050

1

Licensed and manufactured by:
Composite Resources Inc.
803.366.9700 www.composite-resources.com

# Instructions for Use: One-handed Application

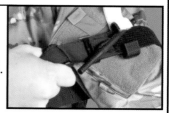

The C-A-T is delivered in its one-handed configuration. This is the recommended storage configuration.

Friction Buckle
Rod Securing Strap
Windlass Rod
Rod Locking Clip
Self-Adhering Band

**1** Insert the wounded limb through the loop formed by the band.

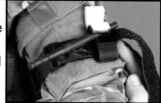

**2** Pull the band tight and securely fasten the band back on itself.

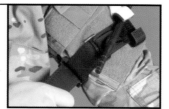

**3** Adhere the band around the limb. Do not adhere the band past the rod clip.

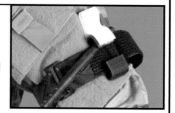

**4** Twist the rod until bright red bleeding has stopped and the distal pulse is eliminated.

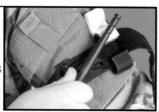

**5** Place the rod inside the clip locking it in place. Check for bleeding and distal pulse

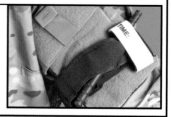

**6** Adhere the band over the rod, inside the clip, and fully around the limb.

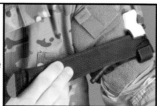

**7** Secure the rod and band with the strap. Prepare for transport and reassess.

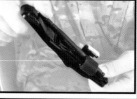

## Storing in the One-Handed Configuration

**1** Pass the red tip through the inside slit in the buckle.

Pull 6" of band through, fold it back and adhere the band to itself.

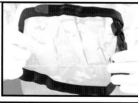

**2** Flatten the loop formed by the band

Place the buckle in the middle of the flattened band.

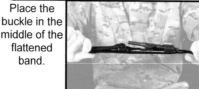

**3** Fold the C-A-T in half placing the buckle at one end

The C-A-T is now ready to be placed in your medical kit.

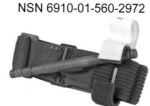

EMS Orange
PN 30-0023

Trainer Blue
NSN 6910-01-560-2972

Exclusive distribution in the U.S. by:
**North American Rescue Inc.   1-888-689-6277**
www.NARescue.com   info@NARescue.com
**NSN 6515-01-521-7976**

2

## Joint Theater Trauma System Clinical Practice Guideline

# COMPARTMENT SYNDROME (CS) AND THE ROLE OF FASCIOTOMY IN EXTREMITY WAR WOUNDS

| Original Release/Approval | 30 Apr 09 | Note: This CPG requires an annual review. | |
|---|---|---|---|
| Reviewed: | Apr 09 | Approved: | 30 Apr 09 | |
| Supersedes: | This is a new CPG | | |
| ☐ Minor Changes *(or)* | ☐ *Changes are substantial and require a thorough reading of this CPG* *(or)* |
| ☐ Significant Changes: | |

1. **Goal**. Provide an overview of CS and present a standardized approach to guide providers in the evaluation and treatment of patients with extremity war wounds, including the role of prophylactic and therapeutic fasciotomy.

2. **Background**. Compartment syndrome (CS) is a common, controversial, and disabling problem in the current war. Recent research indicates proper detection of compartment syndrome is lifesaving; and lethal if late.[1] The operational definition of compartment syndrome is a clinical syndrome wherein high pressure within a myofascial space reduces perfusion and decreases tissue viability. Therapeutic fasciotomy is indicated for established compartment syndrome, and prophylactic fasciotomy is indicated for risk of compartment syndrome.[2-4] Fasciotomy during lag phase between injury and syndrome onset is prophylactic. Early detection is challenging, so prophylactic fasciotomy is routine when compartment syndrome is likely; but the circumstances for prophylactic fasciotomy are unclear. Injury, treatment, and casualty variables affect risk (Tables 1 and 2).[1-7] Variable importance and their time lags differ widely, but the main factors are limb injury severity (particularly vessel injuries), and overall casualty injury severity (particularly shock) with a lesser factor being over-resuscitation (particularly >5 liters of crystalloid). Some factors are interrelated, e.g. in rats functional loss resulting from tourniquet use is worsened by additional hemorrhage in fast-twitch but not slow twitch muscles. Surveys indicate surgeons with more education and experience are willing to perform fasciotomy more often, and the fasciotomy rate has increased five-fold in the current war. Initially, the rate was too low, but the optimal rate is unknown. Other variables may affect limb ischemia-reperfusion with swelling. In and of itself, injury swelling maximizes in 1 to 2 days, additional swelling from post-injury ischemia-reperfusion (e.g., revascularization, shock, tourniquet use) appears to delay maximal limb swelling further; perhaps to 2 to 3 days post injury. Problems with compartment syndrome include morbidity and mortality (Table 3). High altitude (including normal AE aircraft cabin pressure), in and of itself, is not a contributor to compartment syndrome. Once the decision has been made to perform a prophylactic or therapeutic fasciotomy, a complete fasciotomy must be performed. There is evidence to support complete compartment release by full-length skin and fascial incisions is superior to limited fasciotomy.

3. **Evaluation and Treatment.**

   a. The signs and symptoms of CS are the classic 5 P's which include: pain on passive stretch of muscle often out of proportion to that of the injury as expected by the provider; palpably tense muscle compartments; paralysis; paresthesias or sensory deficit; pulsessness.[2] Pain is sensitive and early given a cooperative casualty, but it is not

Guideline Only/Not a Substitute for Clinical Judgment

April 2009

Page 1 of 10

Compartment Syndrome (CS) and the
Role of Fasciotomy in Extremity War Wounds

EXTREMITY INJURY | 471

specific. Palpably tense muscle is specific but not sensitive, and usually there is some swelling; rigor is differentiated by stiffness. Paralysis and paresthesias are generally late and least helpful acutely. Pulselessness is seen virtually never in civilian compartment syndrome, but occurs rarely in war, sometimes within minutes of an arterial injury or an expanding hematoma.

b. The most common compartment syndrome is in the anterior leg.[1-2] About 45% of all compartment syndromes are caused by tibia fracture, and Volkmann's contracture occurs in 1% to 10% of cases of CS. Open fractures, even with traumatic fasciotomy, have higher CS rates than closed fractures because they are more severe, with more swelling and more often injured arteries. The most commonly missed compartment syndromes are the anterior and deep posterior compartments of the leg. The most commonly incompletely released compartments are also in the leg.[1]

c. Passive stretch pain (e.g., ankle dorsiflexion), palpation of muscles for tenseness, and pulse quality. Pressure monitoring by manometer does not diagnose reliably CS in theater, so the diagnosis remains a clinical, not a laboratory, diagnosis. Since there is currently no sensitive or specific technique for establishing the diagnosis of compartment syndrome, a fasciotomy should be considered in a patient with significant mechanism of injury and clinical findings suspicious for compartment syndrome.

d. When monitoring patients for the development of CS, serial clinical examinations are repeated hourly when risk is high and less frequent when low. Provider experience and training improve detection. Documentation is important for later providers and performance improvement. The methods of manometric monitoring of compartments and the clinically significant thresholds to identify compartment syndrome are, at present, not known. A new manometer drains fluid.

e. In one study, burns sustained in combat have been associated with an increased fasciotomy rate.[1] **In the absence of crush injury, fracture, multiple trauma, over-resuscitation, electrical injury or similar indications, prophylactic fasciotomies on burned extremities may increase morbidity and mortality and are not indicated.** (For additional information on escharotomy and fasciotomy in the management of patients with extremity burns, see "Burn Care" JTTS CENTCOM CPG, 21 Nov 08).

f. When established limb compartment syndromes prolonged, complications (mortality, infection) are frequent according to the best evidence available[6]. These casualties may meet indications for resuscitation, urine alkalinization, mannitol use, and intensive support. Such conservative care has led to better outcomes than fasciotomy in casualties with closed injuries with mechanically crushed muscle (see Figure 1 and Reis & Better, 2005). So for compartment syndromes that last more than 12 hours (warm ischemia) and the muscle appears to be dead, there may be better outcomes with conservative care than fasciotomy.

4. **Author:** COL John Kragh is the primary author of this CPG.

Guideline Only/Not a Substitute for Clinical Judgment

April 2009

Page 2 of 10

Compartment Syndrome (CS) and the
Role of Fasciotomy in Extremity War Wounds

472 | EXTREMITY INJURY

## 5. References.

[1] Ritenour AE, Dorlac WC, Fang R, et al. Complications after fasciotomy revision and delayed compartment release in combat patients. *J Trauma*. 2008;64(2 Suppl):S153-61; discussion S161-2. Landstuhl cohort. Inadequate fasciotomy risks mortality. Surgeons should have this.

[2] Mubarak SJ, Hargens AR. Compartment Syndromes and Volkmann's Contracture. Saunders, Philadelphia, 1981. First book on compartment syndrome, a dated classic.

[3] US Army, Medical Research and Materiel Command. Compartment Syndrome: Diagnosis and Surgical Management DVD, 2008. 90 minutes, how to do surgery.

[4] Office of The US Army Surgeon General, Health Policy and Services (HP&S) Directorate, All Army Action Order, Complications after fasciotomy revision and delayed compartment release in combat patients. 15 May 2007. Ritenour message.

[5] Klenerman L. The Tourniquet Manual. London: Springer; 2003. The only book on tourniquets which increase the risk of compartment syndrome somewhat especially if used incorrectly such as a venous tourniquet.

[6] Reis ND. Better OS. Mechanical muscle-crush injury and acute muscle-crush compartment syndrome : with special reference to earthquake casualties. J Bone Joint Surg Br. 87(4) :450-3, 2005. Late fasciotomy risks infection and mortality.

[7] Walters TJ, Kragh JF, Kauvar DS, Baer DG. The combined influence of hemorrhage and tourniquet application on the recovery of muscle function in rats. J Orthop Trauma. 22(1) :47-51, 2008. Risk factors are interrelated.

# Approved by CENTCOM JTTS Director, JTS Director and Deputy Director and CENTCOM SG

Guideline Only/Not a Substitute for Clinical Judgment

April 2009

Page 3 of 10

Compartment Syndrome (CS) and the
Role of Fasciotomy in Extremity War Wounds

EXTREMITY INJURY | 473

## APPENDIX A
## TABLES & FIGURES

| Table 1. Risks for Acute Traumatic Compartment Syndrome* | |
|---|---|
| Decreased Compartment Volume | Tight cast or dressing, closure of prior fasciotomy, excess traction |
| | External limb compression or crush particularly in obtunded or incapacitated casualty |
| | Frostbite, burns or electric injury (may include escharotomy) |
| Increased Compartment Contents | Edema accumulation: embolism, intravascular thrombosis, replantation, venous tourniquet, injections, extravasation, infiltration, ergotamine ingestion ischemia-reperfusion, swelling, artery injury or spasm, revascularization procedures, prolonged arterial tourniquet use, shock hypoperfusion, angiography and catheterization, limbs positioned well above heart, mal-positioned joints (ankle dorsiflexion,) or stretched muscles |
| | Prolonged immobilization and limb compression particularly with obtunded or drugged casualty, some surgical positioning |
| | Hemorrhage, hemophilia, coagulopathy, anticoagulation, vessel injury |
| | Fractures particularly tibia fractures in adults, supracondylar humerus fractures in children displaced, comminuted, or open fractures increase hemorrhage, swelling, and CS risk |
| | Popliteal cyst, long leg brace |
| *Modified from reference 2 | |

Guideline Only/Not a Substitute for Clinical Judgment
April 2009
Page 4 of 10

Compartment Syndrome (CS) and the
Role of Fasciotomy in Extremity War Wounds

474 | EXTREMITY INJURY

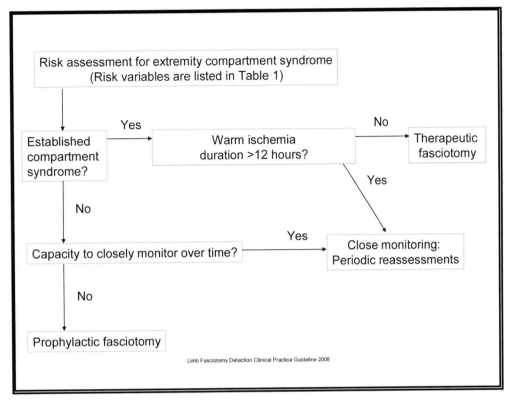

**Figure 1.**
**Algorithm for Clinical Decision Making**
**on Compartment Syndrome in a Deployed Setting**

| Table 2.<br>Healthcare Record Data in the Setting of<br>Compartment Syndrome During War |
| --- |
| Was the fasciotomy prophylactic (compartment syndrome absent) or therapeutic (compartment syndrome present)? |
| When was the fasciotomy indicated and when was the injury?<br>When was the procedure (to determine treatment lag)? |
| Was the casualty able to be followed closely? If so, what was the clinical course? Was the casualty alert, intubated, or head injured?<br>Was there a nerve injury or nerve block/regional anesthetic? |
| What was the injury or risk factors, e.g., ischemia-reperfusion, that indicated the procedure? |

Guideline Only/Not a Substitute for Clinical Judgment

April 2009

Page 5 of 10

Compartment Syndrome (CS) and the
Role of Fasciotomy in Extremity War Wounds

EXTREMITY INJURY | 475

| Table 2. (continued) Healthcare Record Data in the Setting of Compartment Syndrome During War |
| --- |
| What are the sources of ischemia-reperfusion in the injury and care of this case? |
| Associated injuries altering risk of compartment syndrome: shock, occult hypoperfusion, hypoxia, nerve dysfunction, impaired, obtunded, or uncooperative casualty, arterial injury or ischemia, fractures with soft tissue injury, over-resuscitation syndrome, coagulopathies (including hemophilia, etc.), hematoma formation, crush injury, capillary leak syndrome, and prolonged compression. |
| What were the surgical findings and muscle compartment response to the procedure? |
| What was the technique (dermotomy, fasciotomy, surgical approach, length of fasciotomy)? |
| Was there retinaculotomy or epimysiotomy? List names of all compartments released. |
| What delimited the fasciotomy extent, e.g., anterior leg fascia goes from the proximal tibial crest near Gerdy's tubercle to the anterior ankle extensor retinaculum (crural ligament)? |
| List associated procedures: debridement, irrigation, fracture fixation, etc. |
| Planned care: staged? Closure, repeat debridement, delayed primary, skin graft, or flap. |

| Table 3. Morbidity Risk and Sequelae of Compartment Syndrome and Fasciotomy | |
| --- | --- |
| Potential Morbidity: Compartment Syndrome and Early Fasciotomy | skin scar, scaly skin, ulceration, tethered tendons |
| | postoperative arterial or graft thrombosis, thromboembolic disease |
| | wound infection, nonhealing fasciotomy wounds |
| | limb swelling or chronic edema, shape change of limb, muscle hernia |
| | pain, paresis or paralysis, paresthesia |
| | coverage challenge: primary closure, delayed primary closure, skin graft, flap |

April 2009

| Table 3. (continued)<br>Morbidity Risk and Sequelae<br>of Compartment Syndrome and Fasciotomy | |
| --- | --- |
| | possible repair of arterial injury worsening ischemia-reperfusion injury |
| Potential Sequelae List: Compartment Syndrome with Late or Incomplete Fasciotomy | mortality, sepsis, multi-organ failure, acute kidney failure |
| | myonecrosis, myoglobinemia, myoglobinuria, or rhabdomyolysis |
| | paresis or paralysis |
| | stiffness or contracture |
| | limb amputation, tissue loss, e.g., muscle debridement |

| Table 4.<br>Data Sheet: Compartment Names, Main Muscles, and Diagnosis and Procedure Codes | | | | |
| --- | --- | --- | --- | --- |
| Compartment | Main muscle(s) | Left or Right | Wound Notes, Compartment Syndrome (CS), Diagnoses, Indications, & Findings | Procedure(s) and Tissue Response to Procedure |
| | | | 958.91: traumatic CS of upper extremity<br>958.92: traumatic CS of lower extremity<br>958.99: traumatic CS of other sites<br>958.90: CS, unspecified<br>Prophylactic (CS absent) or therapeutic (CS present)<br>Artery, vein, clot, & hematoma findings in compartment on exploration | 83.12: fasciotomy of hand<br>83.14: fasciotomy, division of fascia<br>83.09: incision of fascia<br>86.09: escharotomy dermotomy, epimysiotomy<br>Response: muscles bulged through fasciotomy, no bulge, pulse returned after absence |
| Deltoid | deltoid | | | |
| Arm, Anterior | biceps, brachialis | | | |

Guideline Only/Not a Substitute for Clinical Judgment

April 2009

Page 7 of 10

Compartment Syndrome (CS) and the
Role of Fasciotomy in Extremity War Wounds

EXTREMITY INJURY | 477

| | | | | | |
|---|---|---|---|---|---|
| | **Table 4. (continued)** | | | | |
| | **Data Sheet: Compartment Names, Main Muscles, and Diagnosis and Procedure Codes** | | | | |
| **Compartment** | **Main muscle(s)** | **Left or Right** | **Wound Notes, Compartment Syndrome (CS), Diagnoses, Indications, & Findings** | **Procedure(s) and Tissue Response to Procedure** |
| Arm, Posterior | triceps | | | |
| Forearm, volar | flexors | | | |
| Forearm, dorsal | extensors | | | |
| Forearm, mobile wad | brachioradialis | | | |
| Hand, interossei | interossei | | | |
| Hand, central palmar | flexors | | | |
| Hand, hypothenar | digiti minimi | | | |
| Hand, thenar | thumb muscles | | | |
| Gluteus maximus | gluteus maximus | | | |
| Gluteus medius | other glutei | | | |
| Tensor fascia lata | tensor | | | |
| Thigh, anterior | quadriceps | | | |
| Thigh, posterior | hamstrings | | | |
| Thigh, adductor | adductors | | | |
| Leg, anterior | tibialis anterior | | | |
| Leg, lateral | peronei | | | |
| Leg, deep posterior | tibialis posterior | | | |
| Leg, superficial | gastrocnemius | | | |

Guideline Only/Not a Substitute for Clinical Judgment

April 2009

Compartment Syndrome (CS) and the
Role of Fasciotomy in Extremity War Wounds

| | | | **Table 4. (continued)** Data Sheet: Compartment Names, Main Muscles, and Diagnosis and Procedure Codes | | |
| --- | --- | --- | --- | --- |
| **Compartment** | **Main muscle(s)** | **Left or Right** | **Wound Notes, Compartment Syndrome (CS), Diagnoses, Indications, & Findings** | **Procedure(s) and Tissue Response to Procedure** |
| posterior | | | | |
| Foot, interossei | interossei | | | |
| Foot, central | flexors | | | |
| Foot, lateral | digiti minimi | | | |
| Foot, medial | great toe muscles | | | |
| Iliacus | iliacus, psoas | | | |

| **Table 5.** Operative Note Template for Dictation, Surgical Planning, or Data Collection | |
| --- | --- |
| 1. Patient | 2. Surgeon |
| 3. Date of Surgery | 4. Anesthesia |
| 5. EBL: | 6. Tubes |
| 7. Specimens | 8. Complications |
| 9. Implants, Devices | |
| 10. Indication for operation:<br>　　established compartment syndrome (therapeutic)<br>　　risk of compartment syndrome developing (prophylactic) | |
| 11. Preoperative wound appearance:<br>　　size (volume of damaged tissue: large surgeon hand ~500ml)<br>　　depth, location, contamination material or matter | |
| 12. Preoperative imaging findings:<br>　　soft tissue injury seen & fracture | |

Guideline Only/Not a Substitute for Clinical Judgment

April 2009

Compartment Syndrome (CS) and the
Role of Fasciotomy in Extremity War Wounds

| Table 5. (continued) |
|---|
| **Operative Note Template for Dictation, Surgical Planning, or Data Collection** |
| 13. <u>Examination under anesthesia, fluoroscopy, and surgical exploration findings:</u><br><br>    distal pulse status<br><br>    wound size, depth, location, contamination, materials or matter; burn eschar location and depth<br><br>    vessel status, pulse, limb perfusion, capillary refill, congestion, edema, color of skin, warmth<br><br>    clot presence, intravascular or extra vascular site, size (volume), location<br><br>    hematoma presence<br><br>    compartment hardness: soft, hard<br><br>        epimysiotomy (if done by muscle name or compartment if known)<br><br>        retinaculotomy (if done by name, e.g., partial proximal ankle extensor<br><br>        retinaculotomy extended from anterior leg compartment fasciotomy<br><br>        result of fasciotomy and procedure (distal perfusion and pulse; gap in fasciotomy edges on release in cm; bulging out of muscles in compartment)<br><br>        compartments soft or hard<br><br>        muscle color, consistency, contractility, capacity to bleed |
| 14. <u>Patient condition, status, disposition and plan:</u> |
| 15. <u>Key note for air evacuation: "Patient has been monitored for X hours after injury/surgery and has not had progression of signs or symptoms of compartment syndrome."</u> |

Guideline Only/Not a Substitute for Clinical Judgment

April 2009

Page 10 of 10

Compartment Syndrome (CS) and the
Role of Fasciotomy in Extremity War Wounds

480 | EXTREMITY INJURY

# Glossary and Classification of Amputations

## *Mechanism*
- Traumatic amputations are injuries, not procedures.

## *Timing of amputation procedure*
- Originally, the use of primary, secondary, and intermediate amputation dealt with the timing of suppuration, but recently the usage of primary has generally meant early and secondary meant late.
- Primary amputation is a procedure done at the first surgery; it means the same as a debridement amputation or completion amputation (terms which are less specific). Synchronous amputations: multiple amputations when occurring simulateneously as when two or more operative teams work together on different limbs.

## *Degree of amputation (limb transection)*
- Partial (or subtotal) traumatic amputation is preferable to near complete amputation since complete traumatic amputation is confusable with completion amputation which is a procedure. Total traumatic amputation is preferable to complete traumatic amputation.
- Open traumatic amputation is the norm, but closed traumatic amputations occur rarely while involving disruption of most of the limb yet have intact skin.
- Site of major amputation
- On physical examination before the results of the radiographs are available, providers can simply use the word 'about' (as in 'amputation about the knee') instead of speculating what exactly the amputation site may be.
- Trans-pelvic
- Through the hip
- Transfemoral is preferable to above knee which is less specific
- Through the knee
- Transtibial is preferable to below knee which is less specific.
- Through the ankle
- Fore quarter (interscapulothoracic)
- Hind quarter (interilioabdominal or internnominoabdominal)
- Major amputation: amputation of upper extremity proximal to the wrist and lower extremity proximal to the ankle ('proximal' is more precise than 'above').
- Minor amputation: amputation of the smaller parts such as fingers, toes, hands or feet.

## *Number of limbs*
- Single amputation: amputation of one limb only
- Double amputation: amputation of two limbs
- Triple amputation: amputation of three limbs
- Quadruple amputation: amputation of four limbs

## *Surgical Technique*
- The 'guillotine amputation' technique was a rapid procedure that was done with a circular sweep of the knife and cut of the saw through bone transverse to the long axis of the limb with the cross-section being left open when the primary closure was not indicated. The guillotine amputation label

was later superseded by the open circular amputation which actually permitted the different tissue cuts to be at different levels. The current preferred term is open, length-preserving amputation in order to emphasize the principle of preserving the maximum distal tissue as practical instead of following an arbitrary or transverse direction that wastes normal tissue.

*Appendix 4*

| **IRRIGATION OF WAR WOUNDS:** |||
| **Wound Debridement, Washout and Irrigation** |||
| Original Release/Approval | 2 Oct 2006 | Note: This CPG requires an annual review. |
| Reviewed: Apr 2009 | Approved: 6 May 2009 | |
| Supersedes: | Irrigation of War Wounds, 19 Nov 2008 | |
| ☒ Minor Changes *(or)* | ☐ Changes are substantial and require a thorough reading of this CPG *(or)* ||
| ☐ Significant Changes | ||

**1. Goal:** To review indications for and the procedures associated with battle related wound debridement, washout, and irrigation.

**2. Background.** Wound debridement, washout and irrigation are the surgical procedures most performed in the combat theater. Given the power of today's munitions, prompt removal of devitalized tissue, debris, blood and bacteria is imperative not only to prevent local wound complications, but also may decrease the incidence of systemic effects associated with such wounds. **While the degree of initial debridement is left to the operating surgeon, care must be given to ensuring all devitalized tissue is removed while at the same time attempting to preserve as much soft tissue as possible for reconstructive surgery at higher echelons of care. This is best accomplished via serial debridement and washouts.** Though high pressure pulsatile lavage devices (HPPL) are used extensively in civilian institutions, they should not be used in the combat theater as they may contribute to increased tissue damage and result in a rebound increase in bacterial load, as opposed to that seen with the simple bulb syringe method of washout and irrigation.[1]

**3. Evaluation and Treatment.**

a. Devices: **Simple bulb irrigation or gravity irrigation is the preferred method for wound washout and irrigation.** In addition, the bulb and syringe method is more widely available and is significantly less expensive. Large bore gravity-run tubing is the suggested choice for a quick method of irrigation, since it accepts two bags at once, yet still gentle in nature. Example of the large bore tubing is Baxter's Y-Type TUR Irrigation Set, used for urologic cystoscopy, 2C4005, Deerfield, IL: NSN 3218654401; UI 20/case.

b. Fluids: Current research demonstrates that normal saline, sterile water and potable tap water have similar usefulness, efficacy and safety. Sterile isotonic solutions are readily available and remain the fluid of choice for washout and irrigation. If unavailable, sterile water or potable tap water can be used.[2]

c. Volume: Bacterial loads drop logarithmically with increasing volumes of 1, 3, 6, and 9 liters of irrigation. Sufficient volumes should be utilized to remove all visible debris. The current recommendations are as follows: 1-3 liters for small volume wounds, 4-8 liters for moderate wounds, and 9 or more liters for large wounds or wounds with evidence of heavy contamination.

Guideline Only/Not a Substitute for Clinical Judgment
May 2009
Page 1 of 2   Irrigation of War Wounds: Wound Debridement, Washout and Irrigation

EXTREMITY INJURY | 483

d. <u>Timing of debridement and irrigation</u>: Early wound irrigation facilitates the ability to decrease bacterial load.[3] Wounds should undergo debridement and irrigation as soon as feasible after life threatening injury. **Depending on the nature of the wound and the degree of contamination, all battle-related wounds should be washed out at least once every 48 hours.** Obviously, those wounds with more significant contamination will require more frequent washouts, and strong consideration should be given to performing a washout in the period just prior to aeromedical evacuation.

e. <u>Closure</u>: **Though no hard and fast rules exist for the closure of battle injuries, experience over the last seven years indicates that if the wound was caused by some form of munitions or battle-related trauma, it should initially be left open and allowed to heal by secondary intention or undergo delayed primary closure after several evaluations.**

4. **Responsibilities**: It is the trauma team leader's responsibility to ensure compliance with CPG adherence.

5. **References**:

[1] Svoboda SJ, Bice TG, Gooden HA,et al. Comparison of bulb syringe ad pulsed lavage irrigation with use of bioluminescent musculoskeletal wound model. J Bone Joint Surg Am 2006; 88(10): 2167-74

[2] Owens, BD, White DW, Wenke JC. Comparison of irrigation solutions and devices in a contaminated musculoskeletal wound survival model. J Bone Joint Surg Am 2009; 91 (1): 92-8.

[3] Owens, BD, Wenke JC. Early wound irrigation improves the ability to remove bacteria. J Bone Joint Surg AM 2007; 89 (8); 1723-6

[4] *Emergency War Surgery Handbook*, 3rd US Revision, 2004.

# Approved by CENTCOM JTTS Director, JTS Director and Deputy Director and CENTCOM SG

Guideline Only/Not a Substitute for Clinical Judgment
May 2009
Page 2 of 2      Irrigation of War Wounds: Wound Debridement, Washout and Irrigation

484 | EXTREMITY INJURY

# SPINAL TRAUMA
## *Chapter 10*

**Contributing Authors**
Raymond F. Topp, MD, LTC, MC, US Army
Eric Savitsky, MD
William P. Cranston, PA, CPT, SP, US Army

All figures and tables included in this chapter have been used with permission from Pelagique, LLC, the UCLA Center for International Medicine, and/or the authors, unless otherwise noted.

Use of imagery from the Defense Imagery Management Operations Center (DIMOC) does not imply or constitute Department of Defense (DOD) endorsement of this company, its products, or services.

**Disclaimer**

The opinions and views expressed herein belong solely to those of the authors. They are not nor should they be implied as being endorsed by the United States Uniformed Services University of the Health Sciences, Department of the Army, Department of the Navy, Department of the Air Force, Department of Defense, or any other branch of the federal government.

# Table of Contents

# Introduction

Combat casualty care (CCC) providers play a vital role in the diagnosis and initial management of acute spinal injury patients. Combat casualty care frequently presents patient care challenges that are beyond the scope of Advanced Trauma Life Support (ATLS) training.[1] Failure to recognize and appropriately manage unstable spinal injuries may result in the development or the progression of neurologic injury.[2] The optimal management of spinal injuries is dictated by a CCC provider's skill set, support staff, and access to equipment necessary to achieve desired outcomes.

Two broad categories of spinal trauma on the battlefield are penetrating and blunt injuries. Penetrating spinal injuries in combat are most often the result of gunshot wounds or fragmentation injuries from blast mechanisms.[3,4,5] Blunt trauma can result from falls, tertiary injury from blasts, combat vehicle collisions, and numerous other mechanisms. The early identification and management of open spinal injuries are critical. A direct path from the skin through the dura defines an open spinal injury. All spinal injuries associated with penetrating trauma should be deemed open spinal injuries, until proven otherwise (Fig. 1). Conversely, blunt

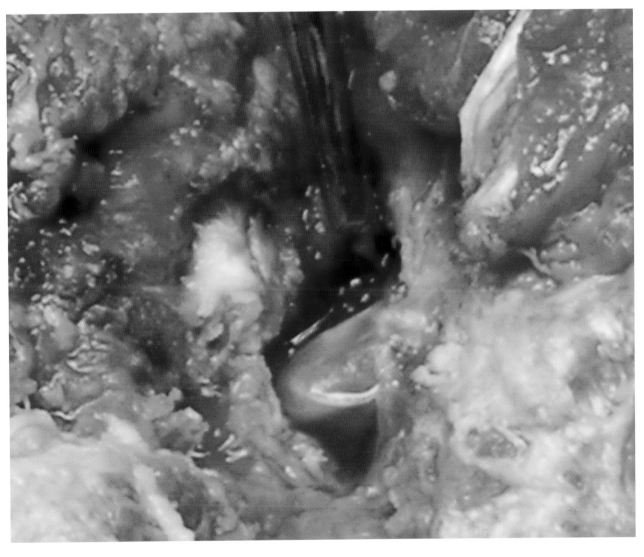

Figure 1.  *Pediatric host nation patient with penetrating trauma to his back.  Here, exposed spinal cord with cerebrospinal fluid leak is noted at the lumbar (L3) level. The spine was stable with only posterior spinal column involvement. Image courtesy of the Borden Institute, Office of The Surgeon General, Washington, DC.*

trauma leading to spinal injury, needs to be classified on a case-by-case basis based on physical findings (e.g., open wound in proximity to spinal injury). Regardless of the etiology, spinal trauma represents a critical wounding pattern that increases the morbidity and mortality of soldiers injured on the battlefield.[6]

All soldiers injured on the battlefield, including soldiers with spinal cord injuries, are treated within the Health Service Support (HSS) system. This system comprises established levels of CCC. Each level of care, starting at the point of injury to medical centers within the continental United States (CONUS), varies in respective capacity to manage spinal trauma. Each level of care (Level I thru Level V) is designed to deliver a progressively greater degree of care and resources. Careproviders working in Level I thru Level III facilities will face the challenge of providing initial care for a significant number of penetrating spinal trauma casualties. This will be a markedly different experience for CCC providers trained in civilian centers, where blunt trauma mechanisms of spinal injury predominate.[7,8,9] This chapter will discuss the varying levels of CCC, relevant anatomical considerations and spinal cord injury patterns, and the optimal management of the spinal injury patient within a CCC environment.

# Epidemiology

As of June 2010, 37,669 combatants were listed as wounded in action from Operation Enduring Freedom (OEF) and Operation Iraqi Freedom (OIF). Total soldier deaths from these two conflicts over the same time period was 5,425. In an attempt to report and study the injuries from this conflict, Holcomb et al. have created the Joint Theater Trauma Registry (JTTR) database. From this database, the rate of spine injury from OEF and OIF is 1.4 percent.[10] Therefore, CCC providers will need to be proficient in the management of combatants with spine injuries.

# Levels of Combat Casualty Care

Civilian medical care for spinal injuries relies on the ability of emergency medical services (EMS) personnel to stabilize spinal injuries and directly transport the patient, using spinal immobilization, to a trauma center for definitive care. Typically, the civilian transport process takes less than an hour. In extenuating circumstances, if the patient is located in a remote location at the time of injury, transport time may be extended to several hours. In contrast, CCC provided from the point of injury to CONUS medical centers proceeds through varying stages of care. Typically, it takes 72 to 96 hours for a combat casualty to reach a Level V facility (Fig. 2).[11,12,13] Combat casualty care is not only complicated by long distance air evacuation (AIREVAC) through multiple facilities and careproviders, but also by unpredictable weather conditions and the inherent hostility of the battlefield.

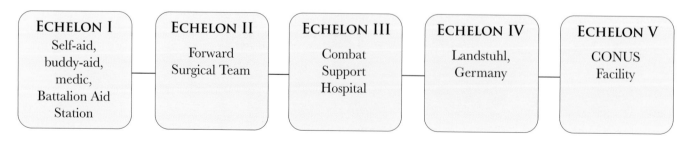

Figure 2. *Evacuation chain for combat casualties.*

## Level I

Level I CCC refers to the initial care an injured soldier receives in the battlefield. This level of care is often provided by a combat medic trained at an emergency medical technician–basic (EMT-B) level. There are times when a careprovider with a higher level of training (e.g., special forces medic, physician assistant, or physician) is present at the point of injury. However, CCC providers at this level are limited by available resources and their environment. Level I care is often provided while the initial conflict or battle is in progress (Fig. 3). Casualty evacuation (CASEVAC) times may be delayed because of the ensuing battle or the hostility of the terrain.

> Because of the possibility of exposing themselves to hostile fire, CCC providers may not be able to safely provide proper spinal immobilization for those injured on the battlefield (e.g., care-under-fire scenario). It is recommended that spinal immobilization be performed once the injured soldier has been moved to a safer location, such as a casualty collection point.

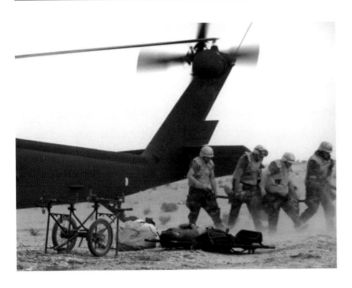

Figure 3. *On the battlefield (e.g., care-under-fire scenario), preservation of the lives of the casualty and medic is of paramount importance. Spinal immobilization of the injured soldier is performed once they have been moved to a safer location. Image courtesy of the Borden Institute, Office of The Surgeon General, Washington, DC.*

Although battlefield heroics often prevail, careproviders risk injury or death by exposing themselves to direct fire from the enemy in order to provide CCC. Current ATLS guidelines recommend all patients with an injury above the clavicle or a head injury resulting in a loss of consciousness be immobilized in a semi-rigid cervical collar and a backboard.[1] This is not always appropriate on the battlefield because proper placement of a cervical collar and spinal immobilization could involve multiple personnel exposing themselves to hostile fire, thereby increasing the likelihood of more injured soldiers. In a retrospective study of penetrating trauma to the neck in the Vietnam War, Arishita et al. discovered that roughly 1.4 percent of the casualties treated with cervical spine precautions actually had a spinal injury that would have benefited from cervical spine immobilization.[14] The authors concluded that mandatory cervical spine immobilization of all penetrating neck trauma sustained in an environment hostile to careproviders had an unfavorable risk-to-benefit ratio. For this reason, it is recommended that spinal immobilization be performed once the injured soldier has been moved to a safer location, such as a casualty collection point.

> Studies performed in civilian and combat settings suggest that most patients with normal neurological exams following penetrating trauma to the neck will not have a mechanically destabilized spinal column.[15,16]

## Level II

Level II care expands upon Level I care by providing a designated CCC facility that is more removed from direct conflict. This facility is staffed with greater numbers of careproviders with access to laboratory and medical imaging technology. Radiographic studies are usually limited to plain radiography and hand-carried ultrasonography. Computed tomography (CT) and magnetic resonance imaging (MRI) are typically not available at these facilities. The main mission of Level II facilities is to recognize and treat injuries that compromise a casualty's airway, breathing, and the circulatory system. Treatment initiated at this level typically follows the established protocols found in ATLS.[1] Combat casualties with suspected unstable spinal injuries undergo spinal immobilization at Level II facilities. Spinal injury patients who are experiencing neurogenic shock are treated with supportive care. Operative interventions aimed at stabilizing spinal injuries are not typically performed at these facilities.

## Level III

Level III care facilities are represented by a field hospital environment such as a Combat Support Hospital (CSH), described as a Mobile Army Surgical Hospital (MASH) in previous conflicts. Level III facilities provide highly trained and specialized careproviders, extensive medical imaging capacity (e.g., CT scans), laboratory support, and blood bank services. In addition, they provide dedicated operating rooms with specialized surgical capabilities, and it is not uncommon to have vascular surgeons, neurosurgeons, orthopaedic surgeons, and trauma surgeons available.

This is the first CCC environment where more definitive stabilization of life-threatening injuries can be achieved. With regard to spinal injury, this level of care allows for better delineation of spinal column injury via CT imaging. Computed tomography has the ability to detect even the most subtle bone pathology. In addition, as the patient is further evaluated, tertiary examination of the casualty often confirms or refutes the presence of spinal injury. Once a spine injury is recognized, a Level III CSH provides the human and logistical resources needed to maintain strict spinal immobilization and ensure optimal patient transportation. If the patient cannot be treated definitively at this level with subsequent return-to-duty, the primary mission of the CSH is to stabilize all injuries such that the casualty can tolerate intertheater air evacuation to a higher level of care.

## Level IV

Level IV facilities (e.g., Landstuhl Medical Center in Germany) are major medical centers that have the capacity to diagnose and treat complex injuries. They are often located out-of-theater and provide maintenance of stabilization and ongoing resuscitation. These treatment facilities provide a broad spectrum of specialty and subspecialty medical care, advanced diagnostic capability (e.g., MRI, angiography suites, nuclear medicine), surgical interventions, and stabilization prior to the patient reaching Level V care.

## Level V

Level V facilities (e.g., Brooke Army Medical Center-BAMC) provide stabilization, definitive care, and reconstructive surgical capabilities. Level V is the highest level of medical treatment available to combat casualties. Definitive surgical repair and reconstruction of all injuries is provided at this level of care. With regard to spine injuries, definitive stabilization optimally occurs at Level V, unless it is medically necessary to perform at preceding levels of care (e.g., a case of progressive neurologic deterioration with documented cord compression).

Unless it is medically necessary to perform an operation at preceding levels of care (e.g., progressive neurologic deterioration with documented cord compression), a definitive stabilization procedure optimally occurs at Level V facilities.

Battlefield spinal injuries will challenge CCC providers. Given the limited capabilities to recognize and definitively treat spinal trauma in Level I and II settings, the main goal of management is to maintain spinal immobilization and initiate spinal cord resuscitation pending better delineation of spinal injury. Level III facilities will enable optimal radiographic imaging of spinal injuries, while definitive surgical stabilization typically occurs at Level IV and V facilities.

## Emergency Management

Forty-seven percent of patients with spinal trauma and 64 percent of patients with spinal cord injuries have concomitant injuries in civilian studies.[17,18] Head, chest, and long-bone injuries are the most frequently associated injuries. Similarly, a majority of spinal injuries sustained in combat environments will be associated with concurrent injuries.[3,4,5,6]

In the setting of multiple trauma, in which most spinal injuries occur, assessment and management of airway, breathing, and circulatory system compromise take priority. The assessment and management of airway, breathing, and circulation issues and the simultaneous identification of neurologic disability with exposure of the casualty constitute the primary survey. Immediately

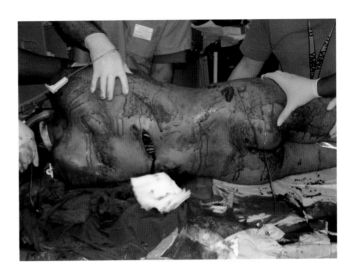

Figure 4. *Open spinal injury. Image courtesy of Joint Combat Trauma Management Course, 2007.*

following initial stabilization, a careful neurologic examination is warranted. Spinal cord injuries have important physiologic consequences. A cervical or high thoracic spinal cord injury often results in a loss of phrenic and/or intercostal nerve function with resultant compromise of diaphragmatic and chest wall excursion. This is of special concern in patients with concurrent head, chest wall, or lung injury. All patients with high-level spinal cord injuries require close observation to ensure that ventilation and oxygenation remain adequate.

All patients with high-level spinal cord injuries require close observation to ensure that ventilation and oxygenation remain adequate.

Once primary survey issues are addressed, a secondary survey is performed. The secondary survey consists of performing a focused physical examination. Palpation of the entire spinal column and a more detailed neurological exam are performed during the secondary survey. Spinal injuries are typically documented during this phase of casualty management. Special attention must be paid to identifying physical findings suggestive of open spinal injuries (e.g., open wound in proximity to spinal injury) and detecting neurologic deficits suggestive of spinal injury (Fig. 4). The neurologic exam does not have to be extensive but should document the basic sensory and motor function of the combat casualty.

A direct path from the skin through the dura defines an open spinal injury. All spinal injuries associated with penetrating trauma should be deemed open injuries, until proven otherwise.

| 0 | Total paralysis |
|---|---|
| 1 | Palpable or visible contraction |
| 2 | Active movement, full range of motion, gravity eliminated |
| 3 | Active movement, full range of motion, against gravity |
| 4 | Active movement, full range of motion, against gravity and provides some resistance |
| 5 | Active movement, full range of motion, against gravity and provides normal resistance |
| 5* | Muscle able to exert, in examiner's judgment, sufficient resistance to be considered normal if identifiable factors were not present |
| NT | Not testable. Patient unable to reliably exert effort or muscle unavailable for testing due to factors such as immobilization, pain on effort, or contracture |

Table 1. *American Spinal Injury Association Muscle Grading Score.*

In a responsive patient, light touch examination attempts to localize the lowest dermatome with normal sensation equilaterally. The sensation of pain may be of limited utility, as most casualties will have been made more comfortable with the use of narcotics or may have altered mental status due to concurrent injuries. However, motor function can be readily assessed in a cooperative patient. An intact motor level is recorded as that level that maintained enough muscular function to resist gravity (3 out of 5 motor strength) (Table 1).[19] Special attention must be paid to documenting rectal tone, sacral sensation, and bowel and bladder function to avoid missing injuries to the terminal spinal cord (conus medullaris) and cauda equina.

Neurologic assessment in unresponsive patients is much more limited. The exam consists of observing spontaneous movements, the patient's motor responses to painful stimuli, the presence or absence of deep tendon reflexes, and rectal sphincter tone.

A complete secondary survey includes careful examination of the entire length of the patient's spine. This is performed by gently logrolling the patient to his or her side while supporting the patient's spine with a cervical collar and in-line immobilization (Fig. 5). The patient's back should be inspected for open wounds, deformity, and ecchymosis. The spine should be palpated for a step-off or interspinous widening. The locations of lacerations and abrasions on the skull may help determine the mechanism of cervical injuries. Occipital lacerations suggest flexion injuries,

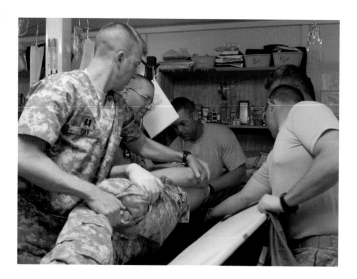

Figure 5. *During the secondary survey, patients should be logrolled, and the entire length of their backs should be inspected for tenderness, open wounds, deformities, or ecchymoses. Image courtesy of Defense Imagery Management Operations Center (DIMOC).*

whereas frontal or superior injuries suggest extension or axial compression, respectively. The presence of a single spinal injury does not preclude careful evaluation of the rest of the spine. Eight to 28 percent of patients with a spinal column injury have additional noncontiguous spinal injuries, and it has been noted that up to 30 percent of these injuries are not initially recognized.[20,21,22,23,24] The upper and lower extremities are examined for motor function by nerve root level. Tables 2 and 3 outline how upper and lower extremity spinal nerve roots relate to muscle function, sensation, and reflex activity. The motor examination also includes a digital rectal examination for voluntary or reflex bulbocavernosus anal sphincter contraction.

Eight to 28 percent of patients with a spinal column injury have additional noncontiguous spinal injuries, and up to 30 percent of these injuries are not initially recognized.

| Root | Reflex | Muscles | Sensation |
| --- | --- | --- | --- |
| C5 | Biceps | Deltoid, biceps | Lateral arm |
| C6 | Brachioradialis | Wrist extension, biceps | Lateral forearm, thumb, index finger |
| C7 | Triceps | Wrist flexion, finger extension, triceps | Middle finger |
| C8 | | Finger flexion | Medial forearm |
| T1 | | Finger abduction | Medial arm |

Table 2. *Upper extremity spinal nerve roots with respective muscle function, sensation, and reflex activity.*

| Root | Reflex | Muscles | Sensation |
| --- | --- | --- | --- |
| L1, L2 | | Hip flexion | Inguinal crease (L1), anterior thigh (L2) |
| L2, L3 | | Knee extension | Anterior thigh (L2), anterior thigh just above knee (L3) |
| L4 | Patellar tendon | Ankle dorsiflexion | Medial leg, medial foot |
| L5 | None | Extensor hallucis longus extension | Lateral leg, foot dorsum |
| S1 | Achilles tendon | Ankle flexion | Lateral foot, sole |

Table 3. *Lower extremity spinal nerve roots with respective muscle function, sensation, and reflex activity.*

Areas of sensory deficit should be accurately recorded, dated, and timed on the medical record progress note or spinal injury flow sheet and demarcated with ink at the affected level on the patient's skin.

The sensory examination includes testing of dermatomal pattern skin sensation. The light touch sensation of a cotton-tipped applicator (Q-tip®) rubbed lightly over the skin is a quick and reliable examination maneuver. Sensation should also be tested in the perianal region. The areas of sensory deficit should be accurately recorded, dated, and timed on the medical record progress note or a spinal injury flow sheet. It is also recommended that the sensory level be marked, dated, and timed in ink on the patient's skin at the affected level. The practice of marking the sensory level on the skin can avoid much uncertainty when a number of examiners are involved. A known challenge of CCC is adequate hand-off or transfer of notes between the levels of care. When available, permanent markers can be used on the injured soldier's skin to aid the documentation process.

## Spinal Shock

Spinal shock is defined as the loss of spinal reflexes after injury to the spinal cord, which affects the muscles innervated by the cord segments situated below the site of the lesion.[25] The loss of reflex function is most severe closest to the site of spinal cord injury. Patients with high-level cervical cord injuries may retain some distal sacral reflex function (bulbocavernosus reflex and anal wink) despite loss of more proximal reflex function.[26,27] The documentation of the bulbocavernosus reflex is a key early determinant of whether spinal shock has resolved in patients that had initially lost distal sacral reflex function. Return of spinal reflex function occurs in a caudal to rostral direction. The return of the bulbocavernosus reflex marking the end of spinal shock is variable but often occurs within 24 hours of cord injury.[26,27,28,29,30] The bulbocavernosus reflex is elicited by simultaneous digital rectal exam and lightly squeezing the glans penis (males) or by gently tugging on a placed Foley catheter in female or male patients. An involuntary increase in tone around the examiner's digit with these maneuvers indicates the presence of an intact bulbocavernosus reflex (normal). The absence of a bulbocavernosus reflex implies the patient is still in spinal shock. When the bulbocavernosus reflex is absent, the prognostic value of the motor exam following a spinal injury is inconclusive. The prognosis of a spinal injury patient with a complete cord syndrome, following the return of the bulbocavernosus reflex, is poor. Complete cord syndrome patients have a less than 5 percent chance of functional recovery if no motor function improvement is documented at 24 hours following return of the bulbocavernosus reflex.[29,31] Spinal shock following spine trauma should be differentiated from neurogenic shock, an injury syndrome characterized by flaccid paralysis, moderate hypotension, and varying degrees of bradycardia.[32]

> The absence of a bulbocavernosus reflex implies the patient is still in spinal shock, and the prognostic value of the motor exam following a spinal injury is inconclusive. The return of the bulbocavernosus reflex marking the end of spinal shock is variable but often occurs within 24 hours of cord injury.

## Spinal Immobilization

If following the initial patient evaluation suspicion exists for a spinal cord injury, strict spinal cord injury precautions must be observed until spinal injury has been ruled out (provided battlefield conditions allow). Civilian studies have suggested that neurologic deficits progress as a result of inadequate spinal immobilization in up to 5 percent of hospitalized patients during their initial stay.[2,33] Keeping the combat casualty immobilized on a full-length backboard during the initial resuscitation often facilitates patient care. This method of stabilization facilitates patient transportation and allows for rapid logrolling of the patient to prevent aspiration in case of vomiting.

Upon identifying a potentially unstable spinal injury on standard radiography, CT imaging is often the next step in defining the injury. The most conservative management style is to maintain spinal immobilization until a CT scan is performed to better delineate the mechanical stability of the injured spine. Aggressive pain management will often be necessary to alleviate the discomfort resulting from immobilization on a hard backboard. Special care (e.g., padding hard surfaces) will need to be taken to avoid pressure necrosis of the skin and underlying tissue that can develop within hours of immobilization on a hard surface.[34,35]

> Pressure necrosis of the skin and underlying tissue can develop within hours of immobilization on a hard surface.

The most effective method of initial cervical immobilization is the use of bilateral neck supports (e.g., sandbags or rolled towels) and taping of the patient across the forehead to a spine board, along with the use of a rigid cervical collar (which serves to limit extension) (Fig. 6).[36,37] In unstable cervical spine injuries, a soft collar, extrication collar, hard collar, or Philadelphia collar alone is not sufficient for immobilization.[36] A poster brace (e.g., four-poster brace) or sternal occipital mandibular immobilizer (SOMI brace) is not utilized on the battlefield. Securing a patient to a standard long spine board is also standard practice for immobilization of the thoracolumbar spine. This enables rotating of the patient (e.g., if they need to clear their airway and vomit) while providing maximal support to the thoracolumbar spine.[36] Cadaveric studies of recreated unstable spinal injuries suggest that significant translational and rotational spinal movement still occurs, despite in-line traction and backboard immobilization during logrolling maneuvers.[38,39,40] Hence, rotational movement of suspected spinal injury patients should be minimized. Spinal immobilization is discontinued only after radiographic and clinical evaluation have excluded unstable spinal injury. This usually occurs at the CSH where trauma surgeons and radiologists are available to interpret radiographic imaging and further assess patients.

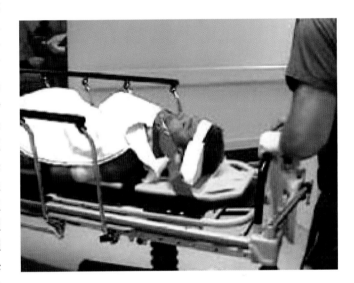

Figure 6. *Image demonstrating appropriate initial cervical immobilization with the use of bilateral neck supports, taping of the patient's forehead to a spine board, and use of a rigid cervical collar.*

> The most effective method of initial cervical immobilization is the use of bilateral neck supports (e.g., sandbags) and taping of the patient across the forehead to a spine board (stretcher or litter), along with the use of a rigid cervical collar.

## Tactical Combat Casualty Care

Care-under-fire or at the point of injury is dictated by the tactical situation. The combat casualty may have to be moved to a safer location before an assessment can be accomplished. In battlefield conditions, rapid casualty evacuation is often a life-threatening process. When only one person is available to assist the combat casualty, the casualty is carried or often dragged to a safer location. Patients with suspected spine injuries should undergo spinal immobilization as soon as it is feasible. Strict spinal cord injury precautions are ideally observed until spinal injury has been ruled out.

In care-under-fire tactical situations without direct confirmation of spinal injury, the presence or absence of associated risk factors should be identified. Associated risk factors for spinal injuries include bullet, fragmentation, and stab wounds, and direct trauma to the face, neck, head, or back. One may also include extreme twisting of the trunk and major blows to the head or chest that may occur from large blast injuries or body impact from landing following the blast wave (tertiary blast injury). Along with documented neurologic deficits, a Glasgow Coma Scale (GCS) score of 8 or below is associated with a higher risk (odds ratio = 2.77) of cervical spine injuries when associated with traumatic brain injuries.[41]

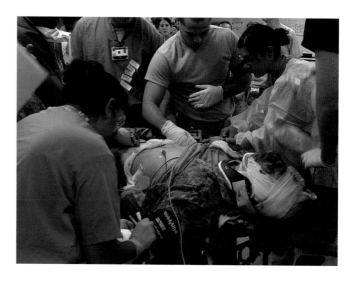

Figure 7. *Example of a rigid cervical collar applied to a combat casualty with head trauma.*

The standard battlefield cervical collar is the Vertebrace® Extrication Collar (VEC) (Fig. 7). Many Level I careproviders not only carry the VEC, but also have access to long spineboards that can be attached to the military litter prior to transport. Medical and rescue personnel should make every attempt to control the spine during initial extrication and evacuation until proper cervical and thoracolumbar spine precautions can be provided. Documentation of known injuries and neurological deficits must occur during the stabilization and resuscitative phases of treatment, often taking place prior to the injured combatant reaching a Level III care facility.

## Spinal Resuscitation

Once spinal injury is recognized, it is important to begin resuscitative efforts as soon as possible. The ATLS guidelines have been designed to ensure full body resuscitation of the traumatized patient.[1] It is important to note that the injured spinal cord itself needs to be carefully resuscitated. In general terms, resuscitation of the spinal cord implies that perfusion with oxygenated blood to the injured area is restored to begin the process of healing and prevent further injury.[42,43]

Resuscitation of the spinal cord involves minimizing secondary injury due to hypoxemia, hypoperfusion, and mass effect.

Definitive evidence of discrete hemodynamic resuscitation parameters leading to improved clinical outcomes following spinal injury does not exist. A series of animal and human studies do support the concept of optimizing spinal cord perfusion following spinal cord injury.[44,45] Suggested treatment options include ensuring hemodynamic stability and maintaining mean arterial pressures greater than or equal to 80 mm Hg to optimize spinal cord perfusion.[30,42,43,46,47,48,49,50,51] Similarly, ensuring adequate oxygen delivery to the spinal cord is important. This often requires supplemental oxygenation via breathing apparatus and the application of pulse oximetry. Likewise, airway, breathing, and circulatory compromises need to be corrected to ensure optimal resuscitation of the injured spine. Maintaining a minimum hemoglobin value of 7 grams per deciliter in trauma patients is recommended, and the timing of blood transfusion (triggers) should be based on bedside clinical findings rather than absolute hemoglobin values.[52]

## Neurogenic Shock

Spine trauma may result in neurogenic shock, a syndrome characterized by flaccid paralysis, moderate hypotension, and varying degrees of bradycardia.[32,53] The typical neurogenic shock patient will have suffered a traumatic spinal cord injury, resulting in disruption of T1 to L2 sympathetic outflow.[54] Vagal tone is unopposed, and moderate hypotension and bradycardia ensue. Bradycardia is a distinguishing sign in neurogenic shock as opposed to other shock states where tachycardia is often observed.

Neurogenic shock is a diagnosis of exclusion and should be made only after life-threatening hemorrhage has been excluded, as hypovolemic shock is the most common shock state observed after battlefield trauma. Recognition of neurogenic shock will minimize excessive use of crystalloid fluids and resultant dilutional coagulopathy and pulmonary edema. Vasopressors may be used following the restoration of intravascular volume to maintain normal blood pressures and minimize excessive fluid administration.[55]

> Neurogenic shock, a syndrome characterized by flaccid paralysis, moderate hypotension, and varying degrees of bradycardia, is a diagnosis of exclusion and should be made only after life-threatening hemorrhage has been excluded.

## Restoring Spinal Alignment

An immediate initial treatment priority is to realign the spine. Subluxed or dislocated spinal segments often result in additional mechanical stress and ischemic injury to the spinal cord. Alignment of the spine is accomplished through a variety of interventions ranging from traction devices to operative interventions. Spinal realignment requires specialized equipment, spine surgeons, and support staff. Hence, attempts at spinal realignment must typically await transfer of the spinal injury patient to Level III or higher facilities.

## Role of Glucocorticosteroids

The use of steroids in the battlefield for treatment of spinal injury is not recommended.[56,57,58,59] The role of glucocorticosteroids in the treatment of the acute spinal cord injury has long been controversial. The purported mechanisms through which steroids exert their effects following spinal cord injury are unclear. There is no evidence to suggest administration of glucocorticosteroids results in neurologic improvement following penetrating spinal trauma, and some studies suggest increased harm.[58,60,61,62] Inconsistency in study methodology and reporting has largely discredited any pre-existing civilian data, such as the National Acute Spinal Cord Injury Studies (NASCIS), suggesting benefit to the administration of glucocorticosteroids following blunt spinal trauma.[56,57,58,62,63,64,65,66,67,68]

> The use of steroids following penetrating spinal injury is not recommended as there is no evidence to suggest improved neurologic outcomes, and some studies suggest increased harm.

# Detailed Assessment of Spinal Injury

A complete and thorough understanding of spinal anatomy and spinal cord function is integral to the appropriate recognition and subsequent management of spinal injuries. In-depth assessments of spinal injuries are performed after patients are removed from immediate danger, immobilized, hemodynamically stabilized, and transferred to appropriate levels of care. This level of assessment and evaluation is typically performed in Level III and higher facilities. Computed tomography evaluation and serial neurological evaluations constitute the critical elements that help careproviders further assess and subsequently manage spinal injuries.

## *Spinal Anatomy*

Due in large part to its flexibility and exposure, the cervical segment is the most commonly injured part of the spinal cord.[69] In contrast, the thoracic spine (T1 to T10 vertebral bodies) is a rigid and fixed structure. This results from ribs attaching to their respective transverse processes and forming articulations anteriorly with the sternum. Cervical nerve roots exit the spinal canal above their respective vertebral bodies. Thoracolumbar nerve roots exit the spinal canal below their respective vertebral bodies. The neural canal is narrower in the thoracic spine than in the cervical or lumbar spine. These anatomic characteristics and the fact that great force is required to damage the thoracic spine probably account for the high incidence of significant neurologic injuries following fractures of the thoracic spine.[69,70] Because of its unique anatomy, the thoracolumbar junction is the second most injured area of the spine.[69,70] Unlike the other ribs, the 11th and 12th ribs do not articulate with the sternum, nor do they attach to their respective transverse processes.

> Due in large part to its flexibility and exposure, the cervical segment is the most commonly injured part of the spinal cord, while the thoracolumbar junction is the second most injured area.

The orientation of lumbar vertebral body articulating facets and thicker lumbar intervertebral discs allow for more flexion, extension, and lateral bending of the lumbar spine. Thus, the rigidly fixed thoracic spine abruptly transitions to a less rigidly supported lumbar spine. This abrupt transition likely explains the susceptibility of the thoracolumbar junction (T11 to L2 vertebral bodies) spinal segment to injury.[69] The spinal canal is relatively wide at this region. Hence, thoracolumbar junction injuries often result in incomplete cord lesions. The spinal cord's terminal segment is called the conus medullaris. It terminates at the first lumbar (L1 vertebral body) level in adults and at the L2 or L3 vertebral body level in pediatric patients. Individual nerve roots extending distal to this segment constitute the cauda equina. The lower lumbar and sacral segments are less prone to spinal cord injury, and the neurologic sequelae are usually less severe.[69,71]

The blood supply to the spinal cord consists of the anterior and posterior spinal arteries and radicular arteries (Fig. 8). The anterior spinal artery perfuses the anterior and central cord, and the posterior spinal artery supplies the posterior one-third of the spinal cord. The anterior and posterior spinal arteries ascend from the vertebral arteries and travel downward along the anterior and posterior aspects of the spinal cord. With the exception of the cervical region, these small arteries inadequately maintain the viability of the spinal cord. Radicular arteries serve to augment the blood supply to the spinal cord in areas where the anterior

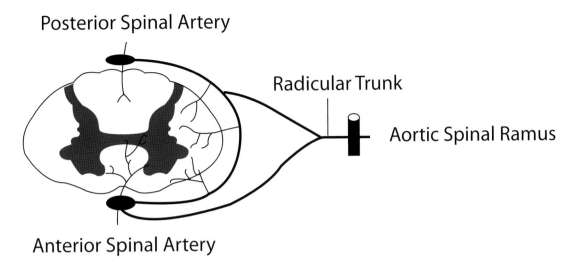

**Posterior Spinal Artery**

**Radicular Trunk**

**Aortic Spinal Ramus**

**Anterior Spinal Artery**

Figure 8. *Cross-section illustration of spinal cord anatomy demonstrating its vascular supply.*

and posterior arteries alone are insufficient. The radicular arteries arise from the thoracoabdominal aorta, among other sources. They form anastomotic tracts with the spinal arteries. The midthoracic region of the spinal cord is described as a watershed area. This region has limited blood flow and is located between the well-perfused superior and inferior segments of the spinal cord. One of the larger radicular arteries is the great radicular artery of Adamkiewicz. It enters the spinal canal between the T10 and L2 vertebral bodies. Injury to this artery explains how neurologic deficits resulting from spinal cord ischemia may extend cephalad from a more caudal vertebral body fracture or dislocation.[29,72]

## *Radiographic Considerations*

Plain radiography, CT imaging, and MRI are used in the evaluation of spinal injuries. In civilian studies, up to 5 percent of trauma patients who are unable to give a reliable history or have a painful distracting injury have a spinal injury.[73,74,75] Conversely, the patient who has neither spinal pain or midline tenderness on palpation nor neurologic signs or symptoms and is awake, alert, and without major distracting injuries does not require routine spinal radiographs.[76] While indications for plain radiography of the thoracolumbar spine have not been clearly defined, the application of criteria developed for cervical spine radiography appears reasonable.[77,78]

A standard trauma spinal series should include a cross-table lateral and an anterior-posterior (AP) view radiograph. An open-mouth odontoid view is needed for cervical spine evaluation. While the

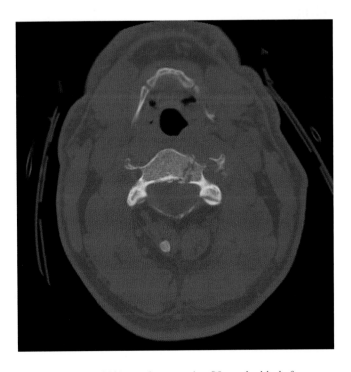

Figure 9. *Axial CT image demonstrating C3 vertebral body fracture.*

sensitivity and specificity of these views are controversial, a normal and technically optimal study is widely considered adequate to exclude major fractures and dislocations. The primary exceptions include patients with unexplained neurologic deficits or underlying musculoskeletal conditions (e.g., severe spondylosis). Patients with unexplained neurologic deficits or a major fracture or dislocation identified on plain radiographs should undergo CT scan to further define the extent of injury. Patients with inadequate plain films or areas of suspicion on plain radiographs typically undergo CT scanning.[76,79]

> Patients with inadequate plain films, unexplained neurologic deficits or a major fracture or dislocation identified on plain radiographs should undergo CT imaging to further define the extent of injury.

Computed tomography imaging is more accurate than plain radiography in delineating the extent of fractures and bone fragment displacement.[76,79,80] A CT scan is also useful in identifying minor fractures, many of which are missed on plain radiography. Standard axial CT images are adequate to delineate most injuries (Fig. 9). Chance fractures and odontoid fractures are exceptions.[18,81,82,83,84] Their detection often requires sagittal reconstruction of CT or MRI images and concurrent plain radiographs (Fig. 10).[83,84] Computed tomography imaging fails to adequately visualize the spinal cord, hence it cannot give direct evidence of spinal cord injury. The excellent bone visualization, wide accessibility, and speed of CT imaging make it the primary supplementary method of imaging the spine.

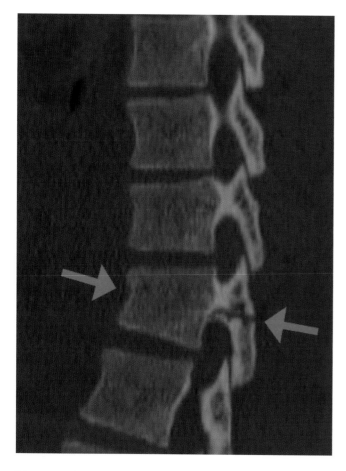

Figure 10. *Sagittal reconstruction of CT images demonstrating a Chance fracture. Adapted image courtesy of LearningRadiology.com.*

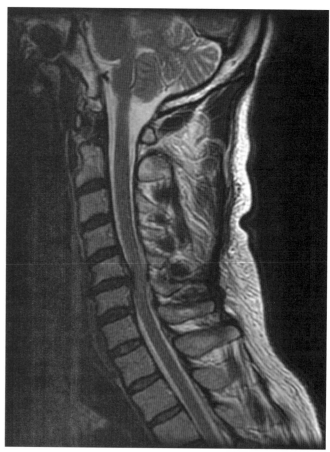

Figure 11. *MRI, available at Level IV or V facilities, allows precise visualization of the spinal cord. MRI imaging is more sensitive than CT imaging for ligamentous and soft-tissue injury.*

Magnetic resonance imaging plays a vital role in spinal cord injury evaluation (Fig. 11). More sensitive than CT scan for ligamentous and soft-tissue injury, MRI also allows precise visualization of the spinal cord.[85,86] Logistical difficulties, including limited accessibility, limited ability to monitor the patient while in the scanner, and prolonged imaging time, currently prevent routine use of MRI in the evaluation of acute spinal injury patients. MRI is not available until Level IV or V care for combat casualties.

## Determining Spinal Stability

Determining the stability of the spinal column is an important initial step in the evaluation of spinal injuries. White and Panjabi provided a widely accepted definition of spinal stability.[87,88] They defined spinal stability as the ability of the spine, under physiologic loads, to limit patterns of displacement, to preclude damage and irritation to the neural elements, and to prevent incapacitating deformity or pain due to structural changes.

While White and Panjabi's definition lends itself to the subjectivity of the examiner, the use of CT allows for a much more objective approach to determining mechanical stability. The advent of CT led to an evolution of theory regarding the determinants of spinal column stability. In 1983, Denis devised an anatomic three-column theory of stability based on a retrospective review of 412 spinal injuries and their CT features (Fig. 12).[89] Denis divided the spinal column into anterior, middle, and posterior columns. The anterior column consists of the anterior longitudinal ligament, anterior half of the vertebral body, and the annulus fibrosus. The middle column consists of the posterior half of the vertebral body, posterior longitudinal ligament, and posterior part of the annulus fibrosus. The posterior column consists of the neural arch, ligamentum flavum, facet joint capsules, and the supraspinous and interspinous ligaments. Denis concluded that the integrity of the middle column determines the stability of the spine. Experience over subsequent years has generally supported this concept. Therefore, a definitive assessment of the integrity of the middle column is made at a facility where CT imaging is available, typically at a Level III CSH.

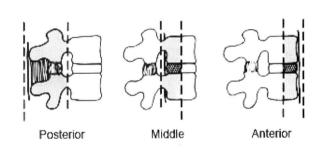

Figure 12. *Three-column Denis classification of the spine. The posterior column consists of the posterior ligamentous complex. The middle column includes the posterior longitudinal ligament, posterior annulus fibrosus, and posterior wall of the vertebral body. The anterior column consists of the anterior vertebral body, anterior annulus fibrosus, and anterior longitudinal ligament.*

> Spinal stability is defined as the ability of the spine, under physiologic loads, to limit patterns of displacement, preclude damage and irritation to neural elements, and prevent incapacitating deformity or pain due to structural changes.

## Spinal Cord Injury Patterns

### Complete Cord Syndrome

A complete spinal cord syndrome is characterized by flaccid paralysis and loss of sensation below the level of spinal cord injury.[78] Deep tendon reflexes and the bulbocavernosus reflex are absent in the acute phase. This reflex is useful in assessing the integrity of the lower sacral cord segments. The return of the bulbocavernosus reflex marking the end of spinal shock is variable but often occurs within 24 hours of cord injury.[26,27,30,90] The development of spasticity, clonus, hyperreflexia, and Babinski reflexes is more variable. These findings develop days to months after injury. Functional motor recovery following a complete cord syndrome injury is extremely poor. Complete injuries have a less than 5 percent chance of functional motor recovery if no improvement occurs within 24 hours of injury, and virtually no chance of recovery after 48 hours.[29,31,90] Therefore, intervening surgically on a complete injury typically is futile if the goal is neurologic recovery. The restoration of mechanical stability following a complete cord syndrome injury can be delayed until the combat casualty reaches Level IV and V facilities.

> Restoration of mechanical stability following a complete cord syndrome injury can be delayed until the combat casualty reaches Level IV or V facilities. With incomplete cord syndromes, a delay in decompression and stabilization is tolerated until the evacuee arrives at Level IV or V facilities, unless the combatant's neurologic condition is deteriorating.

## Incomplete Cord Syndromes

A spinal cord injury is termed incomplete if there is some sparing of motor or sensory function below the level of injury. Incomplete spinal cord syndrome patients usually improve from their presenting condition, with some patients regaining the ability to ambulate.[28,78,91,92,93,94] The decision of where and when to surgically intervene remains a challenge for battlefield surgeons. Unless the combatant's neurologic condition is deteriorating, a delay in decompression and stabilization is tolerated until the evacuee arrives at Level IV and V facilities. In an unpublished analysis of combat-related spine injuries, zero of 52 patients evacuated from OEF/OIF had deterioration in neurologic status (Bellabarba, personal communication, 2009). Therefore, it stands to reason that if a combat casualty has tolerated evacuation from the point of injury to a Level III facility without neurologic deterioration, decompression with or without spinal fusion can often be delayed until evacuation to Level IV and V centers. In the presence of neurologic deterioration, the judgment of whether to proceed with surgery in-theater rests with the careprovider at that given level.

### Anterior Cord Syndrome

The anterior cord syndrome is the result of an injury to the anterior two-thirds of the spinal cord (Fig. 13). The syndrome typically results from anterior spinal cord compression by adjacent bone or disc fragments following a hyperflexion injury.[93] Hyperextension is a less common mechanism of injury. Anterior cord syndrome is characterized by immediate, complete paralysis with hypesthesia to the level of the lesion, with preservation of light touch, motion, position, and part of vibration sense. This syndrome has a better prognosis for recovery than a complete spinal cord syndrome.[92,93] In one of the earliest descriptions of anterior cord syndrome, Schneider reported that five of 11 patients in his case series regained the ability to ambulate.[92] This potential for recovery underscores the importance of a careful neurologic examination aimed at detecting any residual neurologic function in spinal cord injury patients.[95]

### Central Cord Syndrome

The central cord syndrome commonly occurs in the cervical region and typically occurs in the setting of preexisting degenerative spine disease. The spinal cord is thought to be compressed between the ligamentum flavum posteriorly and osteophytes anteriorly during hyperextension. As a result, centrally located spinal tract fibers are injured. Weakness is greater distally than proximally and worse in the upper extremities than

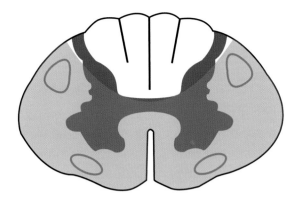

Anterior Cord Syndrome

Figure 13. *The anterior cord syndrome is typically the result of anterior spinal cord compression following a hyperflexion injury. It is characterized by immediate, complete paralysis with hypesthesia to the level of the lesion, with preservation of light touch, motion, position, and part of vibration sense.*

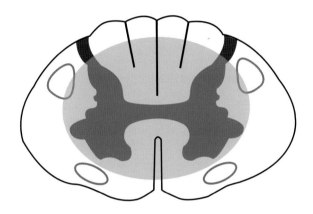

Central Cord Syndrome

Figure 14. *The central cord syndrome is typically seen following a hyperextension injury. Weakness is greater distally than proximally and worse in the upper extremities than in the lower extremities. Sensory loss is variable.*

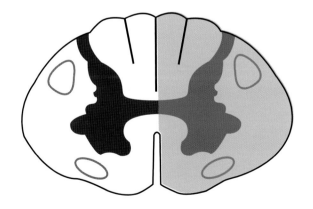

Brown Séquard-Syndrome

Figure 15. *The Brown-Séquard syndrome is characterized by ipsilateral proprioceptive and motor loss and contralateral loss of pain and temperature sensation.*

in the lower extremities. Sensory loss is variable. In severe cases, upper extremity paralysis, loss of sensation, and urinary retention may occur.[96] The lower extremities are relatively spared. The recovery potential with this syndrome is favorable.[70] Previous studies of central cord syndrome patients have revealed that more than 50 percent become ambulatory and regain functional use of their hands (Fig. 14).[94,97,98]

### *Brown-Séquard Syndrome*

The Brown-Séquard syndrome is characterized by ipsilateral proprioceptive and motor loss and contralateral loss of pain and temperature sensation (Fig. 15).[99] Anatomically, only one-half of the spinal cord is damaged. This results in spinothalamic tract, corticospinal tract, and dorsal column injury. This syndrome, which was previously thought to occur only in penetrating trauma, is increasingly described following blunt trauma. The prognosis for recovery in this syndrome is good. Several case series have documented functional recovery in up to 75 percent of patients with Brown-Séquard syndrome.[91,94,98]

## Cauda Equina Syndrome

The cauda equina syndrome results from injury to the lumbosacral nerve roots within the neural canal. The clinical manifestations vary and include sensorimotor deficits of the lower limbs and bowel and bladder areflexia. The prognosis for recovery is similar to peripheral nerve injuries and is significantly better than that for spinal cord injuries.

## Spinal Nerve Root Syndromes

Nerve root syndromes deserve special mention because they often occur in the setting of spinal fractures and facet dislocations. The spinal nerve root can be injured along with the spinal cord, or an isolated nerve root injury can occur. Motor and sometimes sensory deficits will be found in the distribution of one or several contiguous nerve roots. The prognosis for recovery from these lesions is good, provided adequate reduction and anatomic restoration of the vertebral column occurs.[100,101,102] Given that nerve root injuries have a good prognosis for recovery, nerve root decompression may be delayed until patients reach Level IV and V facilities, unless a progressive loss of neurologic function occurs.

---

Nerve root decompression may be delayed until patients reach Level IV or V facilities unless a progressive loss of neurologic function occurs.

---

## Spinal Cord Injury Without Radiographic Abnormality

Spinal cord injury without radiographic abnormality (SCIWORA) is a post-traumatic myelopathy with no radiographic evidence of fracture or dislocation on plain radiography and CT scan evaluation.[86,103,104,105] Although the syndrome was initially described in children, it can occur in the adult population as well.[106] Anatomic differences of the pediatric spine allow for significant intersegmental movement without bony column disruption. The spinal cord does not share the same degree of elasticity, thus contusions, transections, infarctions, and stretch injuries result. While the exact mechanism for SCIWORA in adults is varied, patients with underlying stenosis, either congenitally or degeneratively, are at considerably much higher risk.[106]

# Spinal Injury Management Considerations

## *Spinal Immobilization and Transport Considerations*

Once an unstable spinal injury is identified at a Level III facility, full spinal immobilization pending definitive stabilization is indicated. The medical evacuation network in the theater of operation has greatly reduced the evacuation and transport time for injured combatants. If a prolonged delay in definitive care exists, moving the patient to a bed using strict spinal cord injury precautions is often attempted. The risk of worsening the patient's neurologic status must be weighed against the risk of pressure necrosis of the skin and degree of patient discomfort resulting from the backboard.[34,35,107] Level I care is often limited to hard cervical collars, Kendrick Extrication Device (K.E.D.®) short boards, and long spineboards placed on a military stretcher. Due to the space limitations inherent in casualty evacuation (ground ambulance and helicopter), the equipment used on the battlefield for spine immobilization is limited.

> When a prolonged delay in definitive care of unstable spinal injuries exists, the risk of worsening the patient's neurologic status during transfer to a bed must be weighed against the risk of pressure necrosis of the skin, and degree of patient discomfort, resulting from full spinal immobilization on a backboard.

Patients at greatest risk for pressure sores are those who remain on the spine board for more than two hours without being repositioned.[34,35] Careproviders must use their discretion. If enough manpower is not present to move the patient safely, or there is any doubt about the patient's ability to cooperate with spinal injury precautions, the patient should be kept immobilized on the backboard. The patient should be moved as little as possible as even minimal movement may worsen the neurologic deficit in an unstable spinal injury. If a spine injury is excluded or deemed to be a stable injury, prompt removal of the patient from the backboard to a more comfortable setting is indicated.

## *Timing of Surgical Interventions*

The role and timing of operative intervention in patients with acute spinal cord injury are controversial.[108,109,110,111,112] The paucity of prospective randomized trials defining operative indications for acute spinal injury results in a disparate approach to these injuries among spine specialists. Issues germane to CCC providers may be addressed by using three clinical categories: (1) patients with complete spinal cord syndromes; (2) patients with incomplete but progressive spinal cord syndromes; and (3) patients with incomplete but nonprogressive spinal cord syndromes.

> Emergency spine surgery for penetrating or closed injuries of the spinal cord is indicated only in the presence of neurologic deterioration.

If a spinal cord neurologic injury can be determined to be a complete injury (i.e., the bulbocavernosus reflex is intact and complete loss of sensorimotor function, including proprioception exists), spinal segment realignment may proceed at a less urgent pace. There does not seem to be any evidence to indicate that early surgical treatment can alter the prognosis of patients who present with complete cord syndromes.[113] Although this subset of patients may need subsequent stabilization of the spine, they do not require emergency surgery. An exception may be in the cervical spine, where urgent reduction may improve the rate of "root-sparing" recovery.[114,115]

There is broad support for emergency surgery for patients with incomplete but progressive spinal cord syndromes. This syndrome is rare, but may result from progressive spinal cord injury via fracture displacement, bone fragment compression, expanding hematoma, spinal cord edema, or infarction.[116] Animal studies have indicated that immediate decompression of neural elements is associated with reduction of permanent neurologic sequelae.[117,118] In combat environments, transport times and access to Level III, IV, and V care must be weighed by CCC providers when considering the timing of surgical interventions.

> While there does not seem to be any evidence to indicate that early surgical treatment can alter the prognosis of patients who present with complete cord syndromes, there is broad support for emergency surgery for patients with incomplete but progressive spinal cord syndromes.

Management of incomplete and nonprogressive spinal cord syndromes involves rapid spinal segment reduction and stabilization to minimize neurologic injury. In the cervical spine, such management frequently involves the application of skull traction devices at Level III or higher facilities. In the thoracolumbar spine, traction is less successful, so if neutral supine body positioning does not restore anatomic alignment, definitive correction of the malalignment will typically be performed at the time of stabilization surgery (typically at Levels IV and V).

## Spinal Reduction Interventions

### Axial Traction

Prior to any attempt at reduction of a malaligned cervical spine, the entity of atlanto-occipital disassociation must be excluded (Fig. 16). When severe hyperflexion or hyperextension combined with distraction occurs in the upper cervical spine, atlanto-occipital disassociation may occur. Atlanto-occipital disassociation (dislocation) is characterized by complete disruption of ligamentous attachments between the occiput and the atlas.[119,120] Death commonly occurs due to concurrent injury to the brainstem.[119,121,122] Radiographically, pathologic separation between the base of the occiput and the arch of atlas is noted.[120] Cervical traction is absolutely contraindicated with atlanto-occipital disassociation since further stretching of the brainstem can occur. Atlanto-occipital disassociation may initially be evaluated with lateral plain radiographs, but it is most reliably detected with CT imaging.

An unstable or malaligned cervical spine requires either more stable immobilization or axial traction to achieve reduction.[123,124,125] Two types of axial

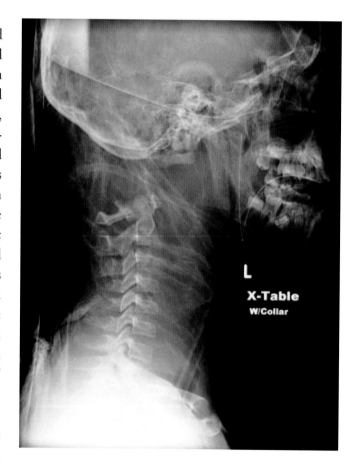

Figure 16. *Atlanto-occipital disassociation.*

traction devices are available: Gardner-Wells tongs and the halo ring apparatus (Tables 4 and 5).[126,127,128] Gardner-Wells tongs are a simple, effective means of applying axial traction for reduction, but they do not significantly limit voluntary rotation, flexion, or extension in an uncooperative patient (Figs. 17 and 18). Gardner-Wells tongs can be applied with minimal skin preparation and without assistance. In contrast, the halo ring allows axial traction for reduction and provides rather stable immobilization with the application of a vest but its application requires an assistant, and it takes longer to apply than Gardner-Wells tongs. Traction devices are typically utilized at the Level III CSH where appropriate radiographic support and a more secure setting are found.

## GARDNER-WELLS TONG APPLICATION

- After the patient is placed in a supine position, the provider identifies the external auditory meatus, bilaterally
- A position on the skin is marked one centimeter (cm) superior and one cm anterior to the external auditory meatus
- The skin is infiltrated with lidocaine with epinephrine to assist with pain control and bleeding from the scalp
- The tongs are placed over the crown of the head with the pins positioned on the skin prepared area
- The pins are inserted into the skull by symmetrically tightening the knobs
- Weights are then applied to the tongs such that the traction vector is directed superiorly
- Traction should be initiated at 10 pounds (lbs) and increased by five- to 10-lb increments (5 lb weight added for each spinal level)
- Reduction should be performed in awake patients with administration of intravenous sedation and analgesia, as necessary
- Fluoroscopy or serial radiographs and serial neurologic examinations should be performed to detect excessive distraction of spinal segments
- In patients with neurologic symptoms or signs or one centimeter distraction of a disk space, closed reduction should be stopped and further images taken

Table 4. *Gardner-Wells Tong application.*

## HALO RING APPLICATION

- The correct ring size is selected according to head circumference
- The ring is placed around the head, at a level one centimeter above the eyebrows and is held temporarily with plastic pod attachments
- After the patient's eyelids are closed, the skin is prepared, and local anesthetic is infiltrated through the ring holes
- Pins are then placed through the ring holes and are torqued down in an opposing fashion to 8 inch-pounds in adults and 4 inch-pounds in pediatric patients 8 years or younger
- After 24 hours, these pins will require reevaluation of proper torque as they often loosen early on

Table 5. *Halo Ring application.*

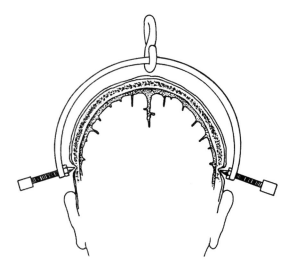

Figure 17. *Gardner-Wells tongs are applied when cervical spine traction is desired. Image courtesy of the Borden Institute, Office of The Surgeon General, Washington, DC.*

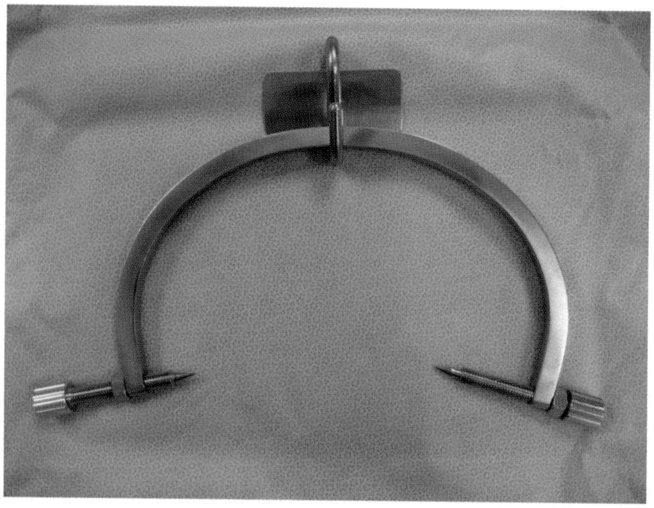

Figure 18. *Atlanto-occiptal disassociation must be ruled out prior to application of cervical traction with Gardner-Wells tongs. Image courtesy of Jonathan Martin, MD, Connecticut Children's Medical Center.*

> If traction is applied, radiographs must be obtained to ascertain that no undiagnosed ligamentous injury has been exacerbated by the added weight.

A halo ring can be applied when definitive treatment is anticipated to be in a halo or in cases in which distraction cannot be achieved with Gardner-Wells tongs. Placing a halo vest underneath the patient, prior to or during transfer to the bed, can help attach the ring to the vest while the patient is in traction after reduction. Open halo rings offer the advantage over previous whole rings in their ability to be placed without putting the patient's head on a head holder off the stretcher.

## *Penetrating Injury to the Spine*

### Management
#### *Mechanical Stability*

The majority of gunshot wounds to the spine in patients with normal neurological exams are mechanically stable.[14,15,16] In assessing the stability of the cervical spine, it has been noted that 36 percent of the weight of the head is carried by the anterior vertebral bodies and disks and 32 percent by each of the two posterolateral columns, which are composed of facet joints and lateral masses.[129] In the vast majority of cases, the projectile does not destabilize the spine, and collars or any other type of bracing are not necessary. However, the cervical collar does have the benefit of maintaining a neutral neck position that may be important in the setting of head injuries.

> The majority of gunshot wounds to the spine are mechanically stable in patients with normal neurological exams. Unlike closed spinal cord injuries, it is rarely necessary to operate on gunshot wounds to the spine for purposes of establishing mechanical spinal stability.

In the thoracic and lumbar spine, the three-column concept of Denis can be applied, but the careprovider

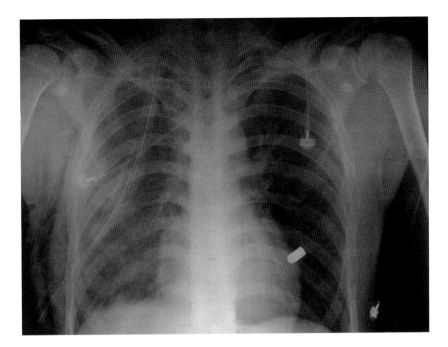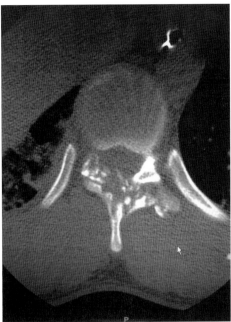

Figure 19. *The majority of gunshot wounds to the spine are mechanically stable in patients with normal neurologic exams:* (Left) *This patient sustained a transthoracic gunshot wound. Right-sided hemothorax is noted and the missile is resting in the subcutaneous space of the posterior thorax.* (Right) *Mechanical stability was determined when CT images demonstrated isolated injury to the posterior column.*

should understand that the mechanism of destruction is considerably different from that in the closed injuries for which this classification was designed.[129] When destruction is limited to one of the three columns, then no particular immobilization is needed (Fig. 19). If two or three columns are compromised by the gunshot wound, then use of spine precautions and immobilization are recommended until definitive management occurs at Level IV and V facilities.

Unlike closed spinal cord injuries, it is rarely necessary to operate on gunshot wounds of the spine for purposes of establishing stability. The length of immobilization for mechanically unstable injuries of the cervical, thoracic, or lumbar spine is normally six to eight weeks. At that time, further radiographic imaging of the affected region is performed to establish whether the spine has adequately healed and is stable.

### Infection Control

Disruption of the dura (e.g., open spinal injury) is associated with a significant risk of central nervous system infection.[130] Reports from combat settings (i.e., Iran-Iraq, Vietnam, and Lebanese conflicts) have documented infection rates of 4 to 11 percent following penetrating brain injuries.[131,132,133] The benefits of administering prophylactic antibiotics prior to elective neurosurgical procedures have been used to justify the administration of prophylactic antibiotics following penetrating injuries to the spine.[134]

Prophylactic antibiotics may be of benefit following open spinal injury given the significant risk of central nervous system infection.

If a hollow viscus is not violated with penetrating spine injuries, the administration of three to five days of prophylactic parenteral antibiotics has been recommended.[135] Cefazolin, one gram intravenously every 8 hours, is often given in these situations.[136] If a concern for meningitis exists, as in the case of persistent cerebrospinal fluid (CSF) leakage after dural violation by a projectile, ceftriaxone (one gram intravenously every 12 hours) is often prescribed.[137] Better defining the role (e.g., optimal duration of therapy, choice of antibiotic) of these treatment regimens requires future study.

It is also important to consider associated hollow viscus injuries in patients with penetrating projectile injury to the spine. If the projectile has potentially penetrated the pharynx, esophagus, or colon, then extra precautions should be taken to prevent spine infection.[129] This is essential only when the bullet has first penetrated the viscus and then penetrated the spine, and it does not seem to be clinically important if the bullet first traversed the spine before perforating the viscus. In contrast to prior recommendations, which promoted radical spine debridement, the best results have been reported by Roffi and coworkers, who recommended minimal spine debridement and one to two weeks of prophylactic parenteral antibiotics.[138] The parenteral antibiotics should be broad-spectrum agents directed at the particular bacteria normally associated with hollow viscus injury.[139]

> In contrast to prior recommendations that advocated radical spine debridement for cases of penetrating spinal injury with associated hollow viscus violation, current evidence supports minimal spinal debridement in conjunction with parenteral antibiotics.

## Complications: Penetrating Spine Trauma

Complications from penetrating injuries to the spine are a concern for CCC providers. Even in the face of proper initial triage and management, these complications may present either early in the treatment course or up to several weeks later. It is absolutely critical that CCC providers promptly recognize and treat these complications as they can have devastating effects on patients. Cerebrospinal fluid fistulae, infection, and vascular injuries are some of the more common situations that may be faced by the battlefield medical team.[3,4,5,131,132,133]

### *Cerebrospinal Fluid Fistulae*

Cerebrospinal fluid fistulae have been recognized after penetrating injuries, and they are defined as an abnormal CSF conduit within either the skin or body cavities.[4,31] Stauffer et al. studied bullet removal following penetrating spinal injury and found that CSF fistulae commonly occurred after surgical treatment with laminectomy.[140] The incidence of CSF fistulae was 6 percent in patients treated with laminectomy, debridement, irrigation and bullet removal.[140] As previously stated, routine surgical intervention following spine injuries with stable neurological exams does not change neurologic outcomes.[141] The fact that most CSF fistulae occur following surgical interventions is yet another reason to reserve surgical intervention for later in the treatment course, unless emergent decompression due to neurological deterioration is indicated.

> If emergency spinal surgery is performed (e.g., due to neurologic deterioration), it is imperative that meticulous dural repair occurs. Augmentation of dural repair with tight closure of the paraspinal muscles, fascia, and skin will minimize the occurrence of postoperative CSF fistulae.

Meningitis is a devastating complication of persistent CSF leakage and it is imperative to avoid this dreaded complication.[4,142] When spinal surgery is performed, meticulous dural repair is essential. Augmentation of dural repair with tight closure of the paraspinal muscles, fascia, and skin will minimize the occurrence of postoperative CSF fistulae (Fig. 20). Likewise, it is advised that an intraoperative valsalva

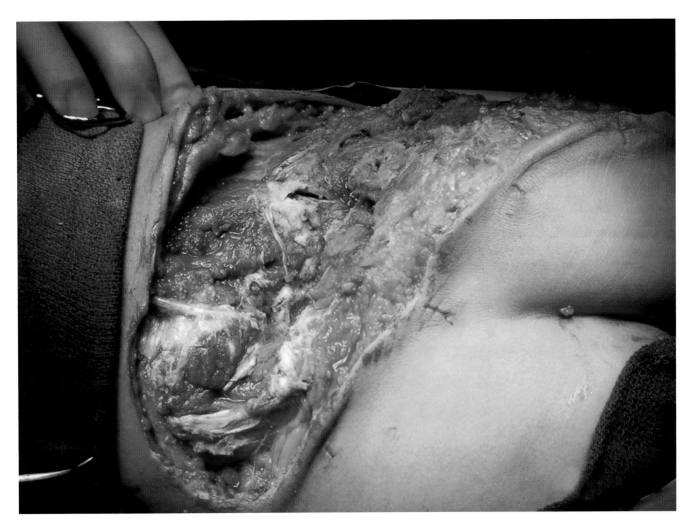

Figure 20. *Pediatric host nation patient with penetrating spinal injury (patient's lumbar region). After wound debridement, a gluteal flap was created and rotated over the spinal canal to prevent CSF leakage and infection. Image courtesy of the Borden Institute, Office of The Surgeon General, Washington, DC.*

maneuver should be performed after the dural leak is repaired to ensure the seal is watertight, and if persistence of the leakage occurs, a lumbar drain should be placed. Most Level II and III facilities will not have subarachnoid (lumbar) drains on-hand, thus providing another reason to delay elective surgical interventions.

CSF fistulae can either track cutaneously (externally) or into other body cavities (internally). The cutaneous variety typically are easily identifiable. However, fistulae emptying into a deep body cavity can be overlooked. When a penetrating spinal injury patient has persistent postural headaches, the existence of a CSF fistulae with a course that tracks to an internal cavity should be suspected. Radionucleotide studies can be effective in confirming the diagnosis and localizing the tract.[143] However, these studies require introduction of the radionucleotide into the subarachnoid space and are not available to Level II and III CCC providers. When a CSF fistula is suspected, the placement of a lumbar (subarachnoid) drain is recommended followed by supine patient body positioning pending resolution of the leak.

### Spinal Infections
Spinal infections following penetrating spinal injury are often accompanied by perforation of a hollow

viscus.[138] Postoperative spine infections can be another common scenario in association with penetrating spinal injury. Stauffer found the rate to be 4 percent after decompressive laminectomy with projectile removal.[140] For these reasons, perioperative antibiotic prophylaxis and the administration of antibiotics for up to 14 days post-injury have been recommended when a dural tear is in communication with a hollow viscus injury.[144] In such patients, an internal fistula may also be present in association with the spine infection. It is virtually impossible to resolve a spine infection unless the fistula is corrected. General surgery techniques such as diversion of the drainage with nutritional hyperalimentation may be necessary when a deep space CSF fistula is present.

> Local surgical exploration, debridement, or diversion may be required in cases of penetrating spinal injury associated with hollow viscus involvement, given the risk of infection.

In the face of progressive paralysis or deformity in association with spine infection, the necessity to identify an organism, problematic foreign body, or failure of nonoperative management are all indications to proceed with exploratory surgery. In most cases, spine infections may not be readily apparent until later in the evacuation of the battlefield trauma patient, and CT-guided biopsy with abscess drainage along with parenteral antibiotic administration is the typical management strategy. Routinely, the Level V facility has this capability.

### Vascular Injuries

Vascular injury must be considered in all patients with penetrating injury to the spine. The vertebral arteries within the transverse foramina of the cervical spine, the thoracic aorta associated with the thoracic spine, and the iliac vessels anterior to the lumbar spine are vulnerable to injury following penetrating spine trauma. Suspicion for vascular injury should be further heightened in the face of progressive anemia or persistent hypotension in the spine trauma patient. Current recommendations advise that wounds should be explored when significant warning signs for vascular injury are present.[145,146] Hard signs such as pulsatile bleeding, neurovascular compromise, an expanding hematoma, and a palpable thrill are obvious warning signs for vascular injury.

### Projectile in the Disc Space

Several factors have traditionally been considered in deciding whether surgery is indicated when projectiles are located in the disk space. The first consideration is whether lead poisoning (plumbism) or other projectile-associated toxicity will develop. Reports in the literature suggest that the lead is leached out of a bullet that is bathed in synovial fluid, and lead poisoning can subsequently occur.[129] Plumbism is a late complication and is typically not an immediate concern for CCC providers. Second, the careprovider should determine whether mechanical disruption of physiologic spinal segment movement has resulted from the presence of a projectile within the disk. Mechanical stability is an issue when the patient is placed upright and typically can be dealt with at higher levels of care outside of the battlefield. Lastly, it must be determined whether disk extrusion has resulted from a penetration of the disk space by the projectile. If disk extrusion leading to symptomatic neural compression occurs, neural decompression and removal of the disk fragments are indicated. This occurrence is extremely uncommon, but it has been reported in the literature.[129]

The need to remove a projectile resting in the disk space is rare. If this operative intervention is required, it should be performed at Level IV or V facilities, unless progressive neurologic deterioration is noted at a Level III facility and skilled spine surgeons are available to operatively intervene.

## *Projectile in the Spinal Canal*

Many anecdotal articles have been written concerning removal of bullets (projectiles) from the spinal canal.[97,140,147,148,149,150] Prior to the 1990's, this topic had not been studied in a methodologically rigorous manner. For study conclusions to be robust, the two study groups must have equivalent pathology, with one group having bullets removed and the other group having bullets left in place. It is also important that this study be done on a prospective basis, recording adequate neurologic information as well as quantitative assessment of clinical variables (e.g., pain). A well-designed study of the removal of bullets from within the spinal canal was performed by Waters et al.[31] The study reviewed 90 cases of patients with bullets lodged within their spinal canals, of whom 32 had bullets removed and 58 had bullets left in place. They concluded that between the T12 (thoracic) to L5 (lumbar) spinal levels statistically significant neurologic motor improvement occurred with removal of the bullet from the spinal canal. There was no difference, however, in sensation or in pain experienced by the patients. In thoracic spine injuries, from T1 to T11, no statistical difference was seen for either complete or incomplete injuries, whether or not the bullet was removed. Similarly, no difference was seen with bullet removal in the cervical spine; however, the authors suggest that the patient numbers were too small to be able to draw statistical conclusions about the cervical spine.

The medical literature does not support the routine removal of projectiles resting in the spinal canal when located between T1 to T12 vertebral bodies. For projectiles in the canal inferior to T12 vertebral body, removal of the projectile in-theater should only be attempted if the neurological exam is deteriorating. If the exam remains unchanged or improves, then removal may occur at Level IV or V facilities. There is insufficient data to provide more definitive recommendations regarding cervical spinal canal bullet fragment removal.

Elective removal of projectiles from within the spinal canal should ideally be performed seven to 10 days following the injury. This time lag will minimize many cases of CSF leakage and considerably simplify dural tear management.

Once the decision has been made to surgically remove the projectile from the spinal canal, it is essential that a scout radiograph be taken in the operating room before the incision is made. The reason for this is that the projectile can occasionally migrate within the spinal canal, depending on the position of the patient.[129] This is especially true for patients with large spinal canals and relatively small embedded projectiles. Elective removal of projectiles from within the spinal canal should ideally be performed seven to 10 days following the injury. This time lag will minimize many cases of CSF leakage and considerably simplify dural tear management.[129]

# Summary

Spinal injuries cause significant morbidity. Spinal injury patients often have multiple coexisting, life-threatening injuries. Knowledge of spinal anatomy is necessary to accurately evaluate and manage spinal injury patients. Combat casualty care providers must have an accurate understanding of the emergency management, diagnostic evaluation (e.g., radiological studies), transport considerations, and therapeutic management of spinal injury patients.

# References

1. American College of Surgeons Committee on Trauma. Advanced trauma life support program for doctors. 7th ed. Chicago, IL: American College of Surgeons; 2004.

2. Marshall LF, Knowlton S, Garfin SR, et al. Deterioration following spinal cord injury. A multicenter study. J Neurosurg 1987;66(3):400-404.

3. Hammoud MA, Haddad FS, Moufarrij NA. Spinal cord missile injuries during the Lebanese civil war. Surg Neurol 1995;43(5):432-437; discussion 437-442.

4. Kahraman S, Gonul E, Kayali H, et al. Retrospective analysis of spinal missile injuries. Neurosurg Rev 2004;27(1):42-45.

5. Splavski B, Vrankovic D, Saric G, et al. Early management of war missile spine and spinal cord injuries: experience with 21 cases. Injury 1996;27(10):699-702.

6. Weaver FM, Burns SP, Evans CT, et al. Provider perspectives on soldiers with new spinal cord injuries returning from Iraq and Afghanistan. Arch Phys Med Rehabil 2009;90(3):517-521.

7. Kraus JF, Franti CE, Riggins RS, et al. Incidence of traumatic spinal cord lesions. J Chronic Dis 1975;28(9):471-492.

8. Ergas Z. Spinal cord injury in the United States: a statistical update. Cent Nerv Sys Trauma 1985;2(1):19-32.

9. Price C, Makintubee S, Hemdon W, et al. Epidemiology of traumatic spinal cord injury and acute hospitalization and rehabilitation charges for spinal cord injuries in Oklahoma, 1988-1990. Am J Epidemiol 1994;139:37-47.

10. Eastridge BJ, Jenkins D, Flaherty S, et al. Trauma system development in a theater of war: experiences from Operation Iraqi Freedom and Operation Enduring Freedom. J Trauma 2006;61(6):1366-1372; discussion 1372-1373.

11. Carlton PK Jr, Jenkins DH. The mobile patient. Crit Care Med 2008;36(7 Suppl):S255-257.

12. Ling GS, Rhee P, Ecklund JM. Surgical innovations arising from the Iraq and Afghanistan wars. Annu Rev Med 2010;61:457-468.

13. Harman DR, Hooper TI, Gackstetter GD. Aeromedical evacuations from Operation Iraqi Freedom: a descriptive study. Mil Med 2005;170(6):521-527.

14. Arishita GI, Vayer JS, Bellamy RF. Cervical spine immobilization of penetrating neck wounds in a hostile environment. J Trauma 1989;29(3):332-337.

15. Ramasamy A, Midwinter M, Mahoney P, et al. Learning the lessons from conflict: pre-hospital cervical spine stabilisation following ballistic neck trauma. Injury 2009;40(12):1342-1345.

16. Barkana Y, Stein M, Scope A, et al. Prehospital stabilization of the cervical spine for penetrating injuries of the neck—is it necessary? Injury 2000;31(5):305-309.

17. Saboe LA, Reid DC, Davis LA, et al. Spine trauma and associated injuries. J Trauma 1991;31(1):43-48.

18. Anderson PA, Rivara FP, Maier RV, et al. The epidemiology of seatbelt-associated injuries. J Trauma 1991;31(1):60-67.

19. American Spinal Injury Association. Standard neurological classification of spinal cord injury. 2006 [cited 2010 May 12]. Available from: URL: http://www.asia-spinalinjury.org/publications/2006_Classif_worksheet.pdf.

20. Gupta A, el Masri WS. Multilevel spinal injuries. Incidence, distribution and neurological patterns. J Bone Joint Surg Br 1989;71(4):692-695.

21. Hadden WA, Gillespie WJ. Multiple level injuries of the cervical spine. Injury 1985;16(9):628-633.

22. Henderson RL, Reid DC, Saboe LA. Multiple noncontiguous spine fractures. Spine 1991;16(2):128-131.

23. Korres DS, Katsaros A, Pantazopoulos T, et al. Double or multiple level fractures of the spine. Injury 1981;13(2):147-152.

24. Vaccaro AR, An HS, Lin S, et al. Noncontiguous injuries of the spine. J Spinal Disord 1992;5(3):320-329.

25. Dorland's Illustrated Medical Dictionary. 29th ed. Philadelphia, PA: W.B. Saunders; 1980. p. 1633.

26. Atkinson PP, Atkinson JL. Spinal shock. Mayo Clin Proc 1996;71(4):384-389.

27. Abdel-Azim M, Sullivan M, Yalla SV. Disorders of bladder function in spinal cord disease. Neurol Cin 1991;9(3):727-740.

28. Stauffer ES. Neurologic recovery following injuries to the cervical spinal cord and nerve roots. Spine 1984;9(5):532-534.

29. Schneider RC, Crosby ED, Russo RH, et al. Chapter 32. Traumatic spinal cord syndromes and their management. Clin Neurosurg 1973;20:424-492.

30. Stevens RD, Bhardwaj A, Kirsch JR, et al. Critical care and perioperative management in traumatic spinal cord injury. J Neurosurg Anesthesiol 2003;15(3):215-229.

31. Waters RL, Adkins RH. The effects of removal of bullet fragments retained in the spinal canal. Spine 1991;16(8):934-939.

32. Zipnick RI, Scalea TM, Trooskin SZ, et al. Hemodynamic responses to penetrating spinal cord injuries. J Trauma 1993;35(4):578-582; discussion 582-583.

33. Colterjohn NR, Bednar DA. Identifiable risk factors for secondary neurologic deterioration in the cervical spine-injured patient. Spine 1995;21:2293-2297.

34. Curry K, Cassidy L. The relationship between extended periods of immobility and decubitus ulcer formation in the acutely spinal cord-injured patient. J Neurosci Nurs 1992;24(4):185-189.

35. Linares HA, Mawson AR, Suarez E, et al. Association between pressure sores and immobilisation in the immediate post-injury period. Orthopedics 1987;10(4):571-573.

36. Gupta MC, Benson DR, Keenen TL. Initial evaluation and emergency treatment of the spine-injured patient. In: Browner BD, Green NE, editors. Skeletal trauma. 4th ed. WB Saunders Co; 2008. p. 730-778.

37. Podolsky S, Baraff LJ, Simon RR. Efficacy of cervical spine immobilization methods. J Trauma 1983;23(6):461-465.

38. Conrad BP, Horodyski M, Wright J, et al. Log-rolling technique producing unacceptable motion during body position changes in patients with traumatic spinal cord injury. J Neurosurg Spine 2007;6(6):540-543.

39. DiPaola CP, DiPaola MJ, Conrad BP, et al. Comparison of thoracolumbar motion produced by manual and Jackson-table-turning methods. Study of a cadaveric instability model. J Bone Joint Surg Am 2008;90(8):1698-1704.

40. McGuire RA, Neville S, Green BA, et al. Spinal instability and the log-rolling maneuver. J Trauma 1987;27(5):525-531.

41. Holly LT, Kelly DF, Counelis GJ, et al. Cervical spine trauma associated with moderate and severe head injury: incidence, risk factors, and injury characteristics. J Neurosurg 2002;96(3 Suppl):285-291.

42. Tator CH. Hemodynamic issues and vascular factors in acute experimental spinal cord injury. J Neurotrauma 1992;9(2):139-140; discussion 141.

43. Rengachary SS, Alton SM. Resuscitation and early medical management of the spinal cord injury patient. In: Tator CH, Benzel EC, editors. Contemporary management of spinal cord injury: from impact to rehabilitation. 2nd ed. Park Ridge, IL: American Academy of Neurologic Surgeons Publishing; 2000. p. 61-73.

44. Dolan EJ, Tator CH. The effect of blood transfusion, dopamine, and gamma hydroxybutyrate on

posttraumatic ischemia of the spinal cord. J Neurosurg 1982;56(3):350-358.

45. Ducker TB, Saleman M, Perot PL, et al. Experimental spinal cord trauma, I: correlation of blood flow, tissue oxygen and neurologic status in the dog. Surg Neurol 1978;10(1):60-63.

46. Kobrine AI, Doyle TF, Rizzoli HV. Spinal cord blood flow as affected by changes in systemic arterial blood pressure. J Neurosurg 1976;44(1):12-15.

47. Tator CH, Fehlings MG. Review of the secondary injury theory of acute spinal cord trauma with emphasis on vascular mechanisms. J Neurosurg 1991;75(1):15-26.

48. Levi L, Wolf A, Belzberg H. Hemodynamic parameters in patients with acute cervical cord trauma: description, intervention, and prediction of outcome. Neurosurgery 1993;33(6):1007-1016; discussion 1016-1017.

49. Zach GA, Seiler W, Dollfus P. Treatment results of spinal cord injuries in the Swiss Paraplegic Centre of Basel. Paraplegia 1976;14(1):58-65.

50. Stratman RC, Wiesner AM, Smith KM, et al. Hemodynamic management after spinal cord injury. Orthopedics 2008;31(3):252-255.

51. Vale FL, Burns J, Jackson AB, et al. Combined medical and surgical treatment after spinal cord injury: result of a prospective pilot study to assess the merits of aggressive medical resuscitation and blood pressure management. J Neurosurg 1997;87(2):329-246.

52. Napolitano LM, Kurek S, Luchette FA, et al. Clinical practice guideline: red blood cell transfusion in adult trauma and critical care. Crit Care Med 2009;37(12):3124-3157.

53. Piepmeier JM, Lehmann KB, Lane JG. Cardiovascular instability following acute cervical spinal cord trauma. Cent Nerv Sys Trauma 1985;2(3):153-160.

54. Albuquerque F, Wolf A, Dunham CM, et al. Frequency of intraabdominal injury in cases of blunt trauma to the cervical spinal cord. J Spinal Disord 1992;5(4):476-480.

55. Grundy D, Swain A, Russell J. ABC of spinal cord injury: early management and complication—I. Br Med J (Clin Res Ed) 1986;292(6512):44-47.

56. Short DJ, Masry WS, Jones PW. High dose methylprednisolone in the management of acute spinal cord injury—a systematic review from a clinical perspective. Spinal Cord 2000;38(5):273-286.

57. Hugenholtz H. Methylprednisolone for acute spinal cord injury: not a standard of care. CMAJ 2003;168(9):1145-1146.

58. Nesathurai S. Steroids and spinal cord injury: revisiting the NASCIS 2 and NASCIS 3 trials. J Trauma 1998;45(6):1088-1093.

59. Eck JC, Nachtigall D, Humphreys SC, et al. Questionnaire survey of spine surgeons on the use of methylprednisolone for acute spinal cord injury. Spine 2006;31(9):E250-253.

60. Prendergast MR, Saxe JM, Ledgerwood AM, et al. Massive steroids do not reduce the zone of injury after penetrating spinal cord injury. J Trauma 1994;37(4):576-579; discussion 579-580.

61. Bracken MB, Shepard MJ, Collins WF, et al. A randomized controlled trial of methylprednisolone or naloxone in the treatment of acute spinal cord injury: the results of the National Acute Spinal Cord Injury Study. N Engl J Med 1990;322(20):1405-1411.

62. Pharmacological therapy after acute spinal cord injury. Neurosurgery 2002;50(3 Suppl):S63-72.

63. Bracken MB, Shepard MJ, Collins WF Jr, et al. Methylprednisolone or naloxone treatment after acute spinal cord injury: 1 year follow-up data. Results of the Second National Acute Spinal Cord Injury Study. J Neurosurg 1992;76(1):23-31.

64. Bracken MB. Pharmacological treatment of acute spinal cord injury: current status and future projects. J Emerg Med 1993;11 (Suppl 1):43-48.

65. Bracken MB, Shepard MJ, Holford TR, et al. Administration of methylprednisolone for 24 and 48 hours or tirilazad mesylate for 48 hours in the treatment of acute spinal cord injury: results of the third National Acute Spinal Cord Injury Randomized Controlled Trial. JAMA 1997;277(20):1597-1604.

66. Bracken MB, Collins WF, Freeman D, et al. Efficacy of methylprednisolone in acute spinal cord injury. JAMA 1984;251(1):45-52.

67. Ducker TB, Zeidman SM. Spinal cord injury: role of steroid therapy. Spine 1994;19(20):2281-2287.

68. Hall ED. The neuroprotective pharmacology of methylprednisolone. J Neurosurg 1992;76(1):13-22.

69. Fife D, Kraus J. Anatomic location of spinal cord injury relationship to cause of injury. Spine 1986;11(1):2-5.

70. Meyer PR Jr, Cybulski GR, Rusin JJ, et al. Spinal cord injury. Neurol Clin 1991;9(3):625-61.

71. Riggins RS, Kraus JF. The risk of neurologic damage with fractures of the vertebrae. J Trauma 1977;17(2):126-133.

72. Wagner FC Jr. Management of acute spinal cord injury. Surg Neurol 1977;7(6):346-350.

73. Terregino CA, Ross SE, Lipinski MF, et al. Selective indications for thoracic and lumbar radiography in blunt trauma. Ann Emerg Med 1995;26(2):126-129.

74. Samuels LE, Kerstein MD. 'Routine' radiologic evaluation of the thoracolumbar spine in blunt trauma patients: a reappraisal. J Trauma 1993;34(1):85-89.

75. Reid DC, Henderson R, Saboe L, et al. Etiology and clinical course of missed spine fractures. J Trauma 1987;27(9):980-986.

76. Hoffman JR, Mower WR, Wolfson AB, et al. Validity of a set of clinical criteria to rule out injury to the cervical spine in patients with blunt trauma. National Emergency X-Radiography Utilization Study Group. N Engl J Med 2000;343(2):94-99.

77. Winslow JE III, Hensberry R, Bozeman WP, et al. Risk of thoracolumbar fractures doubled in victims of motor vehicle collisions with cervical spine fractures. J Trauma 2006;61(3):686-687.

78. Savitsky E, Votey S. Emergency department approach to acute thoracolumbar spine injury. J Emerg Med 1997;15(1):49-60.

79. Holmes JF, Akkinepalli R. Computed tomography versus plain radiography to screen cervical spine injury: a meta-analysis. J Trauma 2005;58(5):902-905.

80. Ross SE, Schwab CW, David ET, et al. Clearing the cervical spine: initial radiographic evaluation. J Trauma 1987;27(9):1055-1060.

81. Groves CJ, Cassar-Pullicino VN, Tins BJ, et al. Chance-type flexion-distraction injuries in the thoracolumbar spine: MR imaging characteristics. Radiology 2005;236(2):601-608.

82. Pepin JW, Bourne RB, Hawkins RJ. Odontoid fracture, with special reference to the elderly patient. Clin Orthop 1985;193:178-183.

83. Lin JT, Lee JL, Lee ST. Evaluation of occult cervical spine fractures on radiographs and CT. Emerg Radiol 2003;10(3):128-134.

84. O'Callaghan JP, Ullrich CG, Yuan HA, et al. CT of facet distraction in flexion injuries of the thoracolumbar spine: the "naked" facet. AJR Am J Roentgenol 1990;134(3)563-568.

85. Qaiyum M, Tyrrell PNM, McCall IW, et al. MRI detection of unsuspected vertebral injury in acute spinal trauma: incidence and significance. Skeletal Radiol 2001;30(6):299-304.

86. Grabb PA, Pang D. Magnetic resonance imaging in the evaluation of spinal cord imaging without radiographic abnormality in children. Neurosurgery 1994;35(3):406-414.

87. White AA, Panjabi MM. Clinical biomechanics of the spine. 2nd ed. Philadelphia, PA: JB Lippincott; 1990.

88. White AA III, Johnson RM, Panjabi MM, et al. Biomechanical analysis of clinical stability in the cervical spine. Clin Orthop 1975;109:85–96.

89. Denis F. The three-column spine and its significance in the classification of acute thoracolumbar spinal injuries. Spine 1983;8(8):817-831.

90. Stauffer ES. Diagnosis and prognosis of acute cervical spinal cord injury. Clin Orthop Relat Res 1975;112:9-15.

91. Roth EJ, Park T, Pang T, et al. Traumatic cervical Brown-Sequard and Brown-Sequard-plus syndromes: the spectrum of presentations and outcomes. Paraplegia 1991;29(9):582-589.

92. Schneider RS, Thompson JM, Bebin J. The syndrome of acute anterior cervical spinal cord injury. J Neurosurg 1958;21:216.

93. Foo D, Subrahmanyan TS, Rossier AB. Post-traumatic acute anterior spinal cord syndrome. Paraplegia 1981;19(4):201-205.

94. Bosch A, Stauffer ES, Nickel VL. Incomplete traumatic quadriplegia: a ten-year review. JAMA 1971;216(3):473-478.

95. Schrader SC, Sloan TB, Toleikis R. Detection of sacral sparing in acute spinal cord injury. Spine 1987;12(6):533-535.

96. Scheider RC, Cheery G, Pantek H. The syndrome of acute central cervical spinal cord injury; with special reference to the mechanisms involved in hyperextension injuries of cervical spine. J Neurosurg 1954;11(6):546-577.

97. Heiden JS, Wess MH, Rosenberg AW, et al. Management of cervical spine cord trauma in Southern California. J Neurosurg 1975;43(6):732-736.

98. Mortara RW, Flanagan M. Acute central cervical spinal cord syndrome caused by a missile injury: case report and brief review of syndrome. Neurosurgery 1980;6(2):176-180.

99. Gentleman D, Harrington M. Penetrating injury to the spinal cord. Injury 1984;16(1):7-8.

100. Nissen SJ, Laskowski ER, Rizzo TD Jr. Burner syndrome: recognition and rehabilitation. Phys Sportsmed 1996;24(6):57-64.

101. Robertson WC Jr, Eichman PL, Clancy WG. Upper trunk brachial plexopathy in football players. JAMA 1979;241(14):1480-1482.

102. Poindexter DP, Johnson EW. Football shoulder and neck injury: a study of the "stinger." Arch Phys Med Rehabil 1984;65(10):601-602.

103. Pang D, Wilberger JE Jr. Spinal cord injury without radiographic abnormalities in children. J Neurosurg 1982;57(1):114-129.

104. Pollack IF, Pang D, Sclabassi R. Recurrent spinal cord injury without radiographic abnormalities in children. J Neurosurg 1988;69(2):177-182.

105. Hayashi K, Yone K, Ito H, et al. MRI findings in patients with a cervical spinal cord injury who do not show radiographic evidence of a fracture or dislocation. Paraplegia 1995;33(4):212-215.

106. Hendey GW, Wolfson AM, Mower WR, et al. Spinal cord injury without radiographic abnormality: results of the National Emergency X-Radiography Utilization Study in blunt cervical trauma. J Trauma 2002;53(1):1-4.

107. Chan D, Goldberg R, Tascone A, et al. The effect of spinal immobilization on healthy volunteers. Ann Emerg Med 1994;23(1):48-51.

108. Burke DC, Murray DD. The management of thoracic and thoraco-lumbar injuries of the spine with neurological involvement. J Bone Joint Surg Br 1976;58:72-78.

109. Tator CH, Rowed DW. Current concepts in the immediate management of acute spinal cord injuries. Can Med Assoc J 1979;121(11):1453-1464.

110. Wilmot CB, Hall KN. Evaluation of acute surgical intervention in traumatic paraplegia. Paraplegia 1986;24(2):71-76.

111. Tator CH, Duncan EG, Edmonds VE, et al. Comparison of surgical and conservative management in 208 patients with acute spinal cord injury. Can J Neurol Sci 1987;14(1):60-69.

112. Krompinger WJ, Frederickson BE, Mino DE, et al. Conservative treatment of fracture of the thoracic and lumbar spine. Orthoped Clin North Am 1986;17(1):161-170.

113. Bohlman HH, Freehafer A, Dejak J. The results of treatment of acute injuries of the upper thoracic spine with paralysis. J Bone Joint Surg 1985;67:360-369.

114. Yablon IG, Palumbo M, Spatz E, et al. Nerve root recovery in complete injuries of the cervical spine. Spine 1991;16(10 Suppl):S518-521.

115. McQueen JD, Khan MI. Evaluation of patients with cervical spine lesions. In: Cervical Spine Research Society, Editorial Subcommittee, editors. The cervical spine. Philadelphia: JB Lippincott; 1983.

116. Chapman JR, Anderson PA. Thoracolumbar spine fracture with neurologic deficit. Orthoped Clin North Am 1994;25(4):595-612.

117. Dolan EJ, Tator CH, Endrenyi L. The value of decompression for acute experimental spinal cord compression injury. J Neurosurg 1980;53(6):749-755.

118. Rivlin AS, Tator CH. Effect of duration of acute spinal cord compression in a new acute cord injury model in the rat. Surg Neurol 1978;10(1):38-43.

119. Harmanli O, Koyfman Y. Traumatic atlanto-occipital dislocation with survival: a case report and review of the literature. Surg Neurol 1993;39(4):324-330.

120. Govender S, Vlok GJ, Fisher-Jeffes N, et al. Traumatic dislocation of the atlanto-occipital joint. J Bone Joint Surg Br 2003;85(6):875-878.

121. Papadopoulos SM, Dickman CA, Sonntag VK, et al. Traumatic atlantooccipital dislocation with survival. Neurosurgery 1991;28(4):574-579.

122. Matava MJ, Whitesides TE Jr, Davis PC. Traumatic atlanto-occipital dislocation with survival. Serial computerized tomography as an aid to diagnosis and reduction: a report of three cases. Spine 1993;18(13):1897-1903.

123. Star AM, Jones AA, Cotler JM, et al. Immediate closed reduction of cervical spine dislocation using traction. Spine 1990;15(10):1068-1072.

124. Cotler JM, Herbison GJ, Nasuti JF, et al. Closed reduction of traumatic cervical spine dislocations using traction weights up to 140 pounds. Spine 1993;18(3):386-390.

125. Crutchfield WG. Skeletal traction for dislocation of the cervical spine: report of a case. South Surg 1933;2:156-159.

126. Botte MJ, Byrne TP, Garfin SR. Application of the halo device for immobilization of the cervical spine utilizing an increased torque pressure. J Bone Joint Surg Am 1987;69(5):750-752.

127. Gardner W. The principle of spring-loaded points for cervical traction. Technical note. J Neurosurg 1973;39(4):543-544.

128. Garfin SR, Botte MJ, Centeno RS, et al. Osteology of the skull as it affects halo pin placement. Spine 1985;10(8):696-698.

129. Eismont F, Roper JG. Gunshot wounds of the spine. In: Browner BD, Green NE, editors. Skeletal trauma. 4th ed. Edinburgh: WB Saunders Co; 2008. p. 431-452.

130. Al-Haddad SA, Kirollos R. A 5-year study of the outcome of surgically treated depressed skull fractures. Ann R Coll Surg Engl 2002;84(3):196-200.

131. Aarabi B, Taghipour M, Alibaii E, et al. Central nervous system infections after military missile head wounds. Neurosurgery 1998;42(3):500-507; discussion 507-509.

132. Rish BL, Caveness WF, Dillon JD, et al. Analysis of brain abscess after penetrating craniocerebral injuries in Vietnam. Neurosurgery 1981;9(5):535-541.

133. Taha JM, Haddad FS, Brown JA. Intracranial infection after missile injuries to the brain: report of 30 cases from the Lebanese conflict. Neurosurgery 1991;29(6):864-868.

134. Haines SJ. Efficacy of antibiotic prophylaxis in clean neurosurgical operations. J Neurosurg 1989;24(3):401-405.

135. Bayston R, de Louvois J, Brown EM, et al. Use of antibiotics in penetrating craniocerebral injuries. "Infection in Neurosurgery" Working Party of British Society for Antimicrobial Chemotherapy. Lancet 2000;355(9217):1813-1817.

136. Klekner A, Ga'spa'r A, Kardos S, et al. Cefazolin prophylaxis in neurosurgery monitored by capillary electrophoresis. J Neurosurg Anesthesiol 2003;15(3):249-254.

137. Velanovich V. A meta-analysis of prophylactic antibiotics in head and neck surgery. Plast Reconstr Surg 1991;87(3):429-434.

138. Roffi RP, Watera RL, Adkins RH. Gunshot wounds to the spine associated with a perforated viscus. Spine 1989;14(8):808-811.

139. Lin SS, Vaccaro AR, Reisch S. Low-velocity gunshot wounds to the spine with an associated transperitoneal injury. J Spinal Disord 1995;8(2):136-144.

140. Stauffer ES, Wood RW, Kelly EG. Gunshot wounds of the spine: the effects of laminectomy. J Bone Joint Surg Am 1979;61(3):389-392.

141. Bowen TE, Bellamy RF. Emergency war surgery. Second US revision of the Emergency War Surgery NATO Handbook. Washington, DC: US Government Printing Office; 1988.

142. Kitchell S, Eismont FJ, Green BA. Closed subarachnoid drainage for management of cerebrospinal fluid leakage after an operation on the spine. J Bone Joint Surg Am 1989;71(7):984-987.

143. Gellad FE, Paul KS, Geisler FH. Early sequelae of gunshot wounds to the spine: radiologic diagnosis. Radiology 1988;167(2):523-526.

144. Buxton N. The military medical management of missile injury to the spine: a review of the literature and proposal of guidelines. J R Army Med Corps 2001;147(2):168-172.

145. Sheely CH 2nd, Mattox KL, Reul GJ Jr. Current concepts in the management of penetrating neck trauma. J Trauma 1975;15(10):895-900.

146. Bishop M, Shoemaker WC, Avakian S. Evaluation of a comprehensive algorithm for blunt and penetrating thoracic and abdominal trauma. Am Surg 1991;57(12):737-746.

147. Cybulski GR, Stone JL, Kant R. Outcome of laminectomy for civilian gunshot injuries of the terminal spinal cord and cauda equina: review of 88 cases. Neurosurgery 1989;24(3):392-397.

148. Kupcha PC, An HS, Colter JM. Gunshot wounds to the cervical spine. Spine 1990;15(10):1058-1063.

149. Simpson RK Jr, Venger BH, Narayan RK. Treatment of acute penetrating injuries to the spine: a retrospective analysis. J Trauma 1989;29(1):42-46.

150. Yashon D, Jane JA, White RJ. Prognosis and management of spinal cord and cauda equina bullet injuries in sixty-five civilians. J Neurosurg 1970;32(2):163-170.

# PEDIATRIC TRAUMA

*Chapter 11*

**Contributing Authors**
Philip C. Spinella, MD
Jonathan Martin, MD
Kenneth S. Azarow, MD, FACS, FAAP, COL (Ret), MC, US Army

All figures and tables included in this chapter have been used with permission from Pelagique, LLC, the UCLA Center for International Medicine, and/or the authors, unless otherwise noted.

**Disclaimer**
The opinions and views expressed herein belong solely to those of the authors. They are not nor should they be implied as being endorsed by the United States Uniformed Services University of the Health Sciences, Department of the Army, Department of the Navy, Department of the Air Force, Department of Defense, or any other branch of the federal government.

# Table of Contents

# Introduction

The care of injured children from combat-related injuries is an unfortunate but consistent consequence of all conflicts. The ability to provide care to injured children is complicated by unfamiliarity with treating severely injured children by most deployed United States (US) combat casualty care (CCC) providers. In addition, lack of pediatric-sized equipment and medications to care for severely injured children increases the difficulty in caring for these patients. The anxiety and emotion that are invoked by an injured child further complicates their management. United States military doctrine clearly states that during combat operations health careproviders are to resuscitate all patients with injuries that threaten life, limb, or eyesight. The care of children injured during combat is an opportunity for military personnel to show compassion and to strengthen relationships with the civilian population. Appropriate care and attention towards wounded children are critical and provide opportunities to strengthen mutual respect and understanding.

# Epidemiology

Multiple publications have described the epidemiology of injuries suffered by children (patients less than 18 years of age) treated at US military medical facilities in both Iraq and Afghanistan.[1,2,3,4,5] These reports indicate that CCC providers will frequently treat children. These children often sustain severe injuries that are associated with increased mortality compared to adults.

The relative distribution of pediatric admissions to Level III care facilities between Operation Enduring Freedom (OEF) in Afghanistan (53 percent) and Operation Iraqi Freedom (OIF) in Iraq (47 percent) is similar, as is the mean age of pediatric patients (10 years, ± 5) in both locations.[6] Children account for 4 to 7 percent of all admissions to US military hospitals in OEF and OIF, and they account for 10 to 12 percent of all hospital bed days.[1,5] In Afghanistan, these proportions are increased with children comprising 15 percent of all admissions and 25 percent of all hospital bed days. The mean hospital length of stay, 7 days, is similar in both locations.[6] In both Iraq and Afghanistan, penetrating trauma accounts for approximately 75 percent of pediatric traumatic injuries. In Iraq, gunshot wounds are the mechanism of injury for 57 percent of pediatric admissions compared to 21 percent in Afghanistan. In Afghanistan, burn and landmine explosive injuries account for 15 percent of admissions each, while in Iraq they are the mechanism of injury for 6 percent and 1 percent of pediatric admissions, respectively.[6]

Combat casualty careproviders will frequently treat children who often sustain severe injuries that are associated with increased mortality compared to adults. Children account for 4 to 7 percent of all admissions to US military hospitals in OEF and OIF, and 10 to 12 percent of all hospital bed days.

When data from Iraq and Afghanistan are combined, the overall primary causes of death are traumatic brain injury (29 percent) and burns (27 percent) (Fig. 1).[6] Death as a result of infection was more common in Afghanistan (12 percent) than Iraq (2 percent), whereas death from penetrating abdominal and thoracic injuries was more common in Iraq (13 percent) than Afghanistan (5 percent).[6] In a review of children treated at a Combat Support Hospital (CSH) in Iraq, children less than eight years of age, as compared to older children and adults, had an increased severity of injury according to the Injury Severity Score (ISS) and an increased incidence of death after adjusting for increased severity of injury.[7]

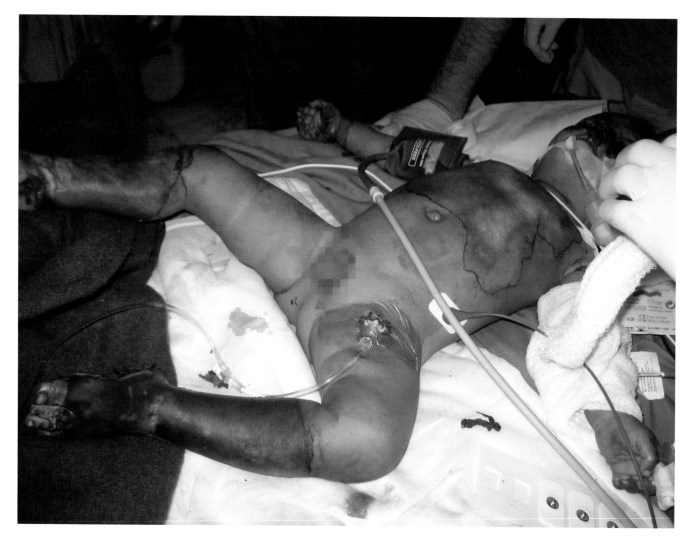

Figure 1. *Resuscitative efforts in progress at a CSH. This host nation toddler was injured in a civilian motor vehicle accident and sustained 30% TBSA second- and third-degree burn wounds and severe inhalation injury.*

## Anatomic Considerations

### Airway

The pediatric airway is significantly different than an adult airway. In addition to the obvious size differences in airway anatomy, the infant and young child's (less than eight years of age) oropharyngeal cavity is relatively smaller due to a larger tongue-to-cavity ratio in the child. The larger head in relation to body size also makes visualization of the larynx with laryngoscopy more difficult and often requires elevating the shoulders and upper thorax to allow for a more direct line of site of the larynx. The epiglottis in a child is typically omega-shaped (long and narrow) and attached at the vocal cords at an acute angle. The vocal cords are more cephalad and anterior compared to those in an adult. The subglottic area is narrower and cone-shaped, rather than more cylindrical in shape. An endotracheal tube (ETT) that passes easily through the vocal cords may encounter resistance in the subglottic area. Furthermore, children less than 12 years of age have a small, pliable, mobile larynx and cricoid cartilage making a surgical cricothyrotomy difficult to perform.[8]

| Age | Preterm | Newborn | Infant | 1 Yr | 3 Yrs | 6 Yrs | 10 Yrs | 14 Yrs |
|---|---|---|---|---|---|---|---|---|
| Laryngoscope Blade Size | 0 | 1 | 1 | 1 to 2 | 2 | 2 | 2 to 3 | 3 |
| ETT Size | 2.5 to 3.0 | 3.0 to 3.5 | 3.5 to 4.0 | 4.0 to 4.5 | 4.5 to 5.0 | 5.0 to 5.5 | 6.0 to 6.5 | 6.5 to 7.0 |
| Suction Catheter (Fr) | 5 | 6 | 8 | 8 | 8 to 10 | 10 | 10 | 10 to 14 |
| Chest Tube | 8 to 10 | 10 to 12 | 10 to 12 | 16 to 20 | 16 to 20 | 20 to 28 | 28 to 32 | 32 to 40 |
| NG Tube or Foley Catheter (Fr) | 5 | 5 to 8 | 5 to 8 | 8 | 8 to 10 | 10 to 12 | 12 to 14 | 14 to 18 |

Table 1. *Equipment size according to the age of the patient.*

The pediatric airway differs significantly compared to an adult airway. The larynx is more difficult to visualize during laryngoscopy, and the subglottic area is narrow and cone-shaped. An ETT that readily passes through the vocal cords may still encounter resistance in the subglottic area. Furthermore, children less than 12 years of age have a small, pliable, mobile larynx and cricoid cartilage making a surgical cricothyrotomy difficult to perform.

Selecting an appropriately sized ETT is a crucial first step when preparing to intubate a pediatric trauma victim. A number of methods intended to assist physicians with selecting the optimal ETT have been published. Using the internal diameter of the external nasal nares or nailbeds of the fifth digits of the child has been reported to facilitate the selection of an appropriately sized ETT.[9] While these approaches may provide reasonable approximations of ETT sizing, they require the physical presence of the patient. This precludes the ability of careproviders to have this equipment prepared prior to patient arrival. Using the age (in years) added to 16 divided by 4 to represent the internal tube diameter in millimeters has also been recommended.[9] Irrespective of the initially selected tube size, the physician should always be prepared to use either smaller or larger diameter tubes if the patient's airway dictates it (Table 1). The Broselow® tape is a commonly used and helpful method to standardize the approach to the resuscitation of children.[10] It provides a valuable reference source for the appropriate sizing of pediatric airway equipment and dosing of medications.

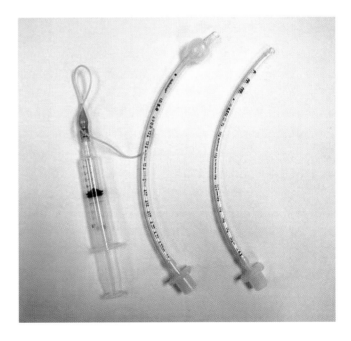

Figure 2. *Cuffed versus uncuffed endotracheal tubes. With an uncuffed ETT, the narrowed subglottic space should provide an adequate seal around an appropriately selected ETT. Cuffed tubes are likely just as safe as uncuffed tubes, and may protect against tube dislodgment and gastric content aspiration by creating tighter seals.*

The issue of whether or not to use cuffed or uncuffed ETT in younger children often arises (Fig. 2). Advocates for using uncuffed tubes contend there is no need for a cuffed tube in children less than eight years of age.[11,12] Their rationale is that the narrowest part of a young child's airway is subglottic in location. The narrowed subglottic space should provide an adequate seal around an appropriately selected ETT. Cuffed tube critics also believe these tubes decrease tracheal mucosal blood flow and increase the incidence of post-extubation laryngeal edema and tracheal stenosis.[13] Proponents of using cuffed tubes believe that modern day low pressure (less than 25 cm $H_2O$), high-volume ETT cuffs are safer than the older models. They claim appropriately used, cuffed endotracheal tubes are just as safe as uncuffed endotracheal tubes.[14] They believe cuffed tubes provide added protection against tube dislodgment and gastric content aspiration by creating tighter seals. Special caution must be exercised to avoid overinflating ETT cuffs. Monitors are now available that will measure cuff pressures and should be used to maintain cuff pressures less than or equal to 25 cm $H_2O$ to minimize the incidence of cuff-related tracheal injury.[14]

---

Selecting an appropriately sized ETT is crucial; (age + 16)/4 may help in selecting ETT diameter. Current pediatric standards taught in the Pediatric Advanced Life Support (PALS) course recommend the use of cuffed endotracheal tubes to optimize oxygenation and ventilation in all children.

---

One method of providing an immediate surgical airway for a child less than 12 years of age is to perform a needle cricothyrotomy and initiate percutaneous transtracheal ventilation (PTTV) (Fig. 3).[15,16] Percutaneous transtracheal ventilation is performed by having a 14- or 16-gauge angiocatheter inserted through the cricothyroid membrane, positioned intratracheally, and attached to a high-flow oxygen source.[17] Regular oxygen tubing may be attached to a three-way stopcock, which is attached to the angiocatheter. Alternatively, a 14- or 16-gauge angiocatheter may be attached to one prong of a dual-pronged nasal cannulae, while the other end of the nasal cannulae is attached to a high-flow oxygen source. A one-second inspiratory and three-second expiratory cycle will allow time for adequate oxygenation and ventilation. The oxygen source should provide at least 50 pounds per square inch of air pressure (i.e., deliver flow rates of 15

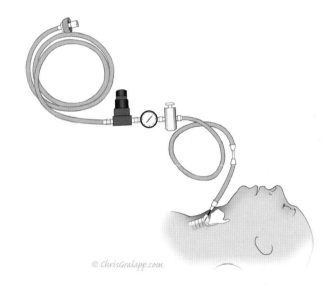

Figure 3. *Percutaneous transtracheal ventilation (PTTV). Illustrator: Chris Gralapp.*

liters per minute). Unfortunately, PTTV will not protect the airway from aspiration of gastric contents. In addition, this technique may eventually fail to provide adequate ventilation. Over time, progressive hypercarbia and acidemia may ensue. Percutaneous transtracheal ventilation technique should be viewed as a temporizing measure until a definitive airway in the form of a tracheostomy is established. If high-oxygen flow (jet) ventilation is not possible, an adapter from a 2.5 millimeter or 3.0 millimeter-sized ETT can be used to attach the angiocatheter to bag-valve-mask, thus enabling manual ventilation.

One method of providing an immediate surgical airway for a child less than 12 years of age is to perform a needle cricothyrotomy and initiate PTTV. Percutaneous transtracheal ventilation should be viewed as a temporizing measure until a definitive airway in the form of a tracheostomy is established. Percutaneous transtracheal ventilation will not protect the airway from aspiration of gastric contents, and the technique may eventually fail to provide adequate ventilation.

It is the opinion of the authors and many experienced pediatric surgery and otolaryngology specialists that when a surgical airway is emergently needed in a child less than six years of age, a tracheotomy should be performed. At this age, cricoid cartilage versus tracheal anatomy is difficult to discern. Extra care needs to be exercised to stay well below the cricoid cartilage in order to avoid subglottic stenosis during the healing phase after the surgical airway. In younger children (e.g., less than three years of age), the concern with performing a needle cricothyrotomy is that it will be very difficult to place the needle in the airway. This is due to the laxity of the airway, and since the diameter of the airway is so small the risk of going through its posterior wall is high. The neck anatomy is better defined in older children (i.e., over six years of age), and it is easier to perform a needle cricothyrotomy. The choice of performing a surgical airway versus needle cricothyrotomy in children of all ages is dependent upon the comfort and experience of the provider in performing these procedures. If tracheostomy is attempted, the use of a cuffed ETT will be required. Accessing the correctly sized tracheostomy tube (lengthwise) will be nearly impossible in a combat environment where supplies are limited. Cuffed ETT of all sizes are not always available. As a result, advanced planning will be required regardless of the type of airway intervention.

## Head and Spinal Cord

The risk of head injury is higher in children compared to adults, while the risk of spinal cord injury is lower.[18,19,20] This is a result of the relative increase in head-to-body size and more flexible cervical ligaments of children compared to adults. There is also less subarachnoid space and fluid in children compared to adults. The anatomy of an infant's head with an open fontanelle and mobile cranial sutures allows for significant isolated intracranial bleeding. In addition, extracranial bleeding such as caput succedaneum, cephalohematoma, or subgaleal hematoma can cause severe anemia and hyperkalemia secondary to bleeding and eventual thrombolysis.[19,20,21,22,23] The incidence of spinal cord injury in children is low and is likely related to flexible vertebral interspinous ligaments and anteriorly wedged vertebrae. As a result, with flexion injuries vertebral bodies slide forward minimizing the risk of spinal cord injury. However, spinal cord injury without radiographic abnormality (SCIWORA) does exist, and children injured by way of blast mechanisms are at risk. Diagnosis is difficult. Attention needs to be given to the presence of pain, tenderness on palpation of the spine, and the neurologic examination.

The risk of head injury is higher in children compared to adults. The anatomy of an infant's head with an open fontanelle and mobile cranial sutures allows for significant isolated intracranial bleeding. Extracranial bleeding such as caput succedaneum, cephalohematoma, or subgaleal hematoma can cause severe anemia and hyperkalemia secondary to bleeding and eventual thrombolysis.

There are several important radiographic variations in the pediatric cervical spine that warrant mentioning. Being aware of these variations is necessary in order to avoid misinterpreting these normal findings as injured spinal segments. The prevertebral soft-tissue of the pediatric cervical spine is prone to great variation. Emergency radiologic evaluation of the pediatric cervical spine can be challenging because of the confusing appearance of synchondroses, normal anatomic variants, and injuries that are unique to children.[24] Cervical spine injuries in children are usually seen in the upper cervical region owing to the unique biomechanics and anatomy of the pediatric cervical spine. Knowledge of the normal embryologic development and anatomy of the cervical spine is important to avoid mistaking synchondroses for fractures in the trauma setting. Familiarity with anatomic variants is also important for correct image interpretation.[24] These variants include pseudosubluxation, absence of cervical lordosis, wedging of the cervical vertebra, widening of the predental space, prevertebral soft-tissue widening, intervertebral widening, and "pseudo Jefferson fracture" (normal C1 vertebra variant in young children).[24] In addition, familiarity with mechanisms of injury and appropriate imaging modalities will aid in the correct interpretation of radiologic images of the pediatric cervical spine.[24] Using prevertebral soft-tissue swelling to detect injury is neither a sensitive nor specific indicator of acute injury in pediatric patients. In adults, a predental space of greater than three millimeters is regarded as abnormal. Children have more laxity of their spinal segments, and a predental space of up to five millimeters in children age 13 or younger is deemed within normal limits.[25]

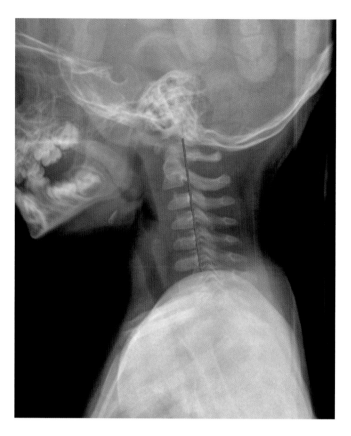

Figure 4. *Physiological pseudosubluxation on pediatric cervical spine radiograph. Normal displacement of C2 on C3 may be so pronounced as to be mistaken for a pathologic condition. Image courtesy of Swaminatha V. Mahadevan, MD, Stanford University.*

The most prominent abnormality in pediatric cervical spine films is the physiologic pseudosubluxation of the C2 on C3 vertebral body (Fig. 4).[25] Physiologic pseudosubluxation may occur at several levels between C2 to C5. There may be up to four millimeters of subluxation at the C2 to C3 junction as part of normal variation in children up to the age of 16 years.[25] This pseudosubluxation pattern is unusual beyond the age of 16. Use of the spinolaminar line (also known as the posterior cervical line) as a reference may be helpful in differentiating acute injuries from normal anatomical variants. The spinolaminar line junction of the C2 vertebral segment should be within two millimeters of a line drawn between the C1 and C3 spinolaminar line junction.[26] If the C2 spinolaminar line junction is offset by two or more millimeters, the radiograph should be interpreted as abnormal and suspicious for an injury.[26,27] The spinolaminar line should only be applied in cases where anterior displacement of the C2 on C3 vertebral body exists. When the C2 and C3 vertebral bodies are in a neutral or extended position, an offset of two millimeters or more of the C2 spinolaminar line may be a normal finding.

Emergency radiologic evaluation of the pediatric cervical spine can be challenging because of the confusing appearance of synchondroses, normal anatomic variants, and injuries that are unique to children. Due to unique pediatric anatomy, cervical spine injuries are usually seen in the upper cervical spine. The synchondrosis at the junction of the dens and body of C2 is often the site of injury. The most prominent abnormality in pediatric cervical spine films is the physiologic pseudosubluxation of the C2 on C3 vertebral body, which may be mistaken for pathologic motion.

The synchondrosis at the junction of the dens and body of C2 is often the site of injury.[28,29] The dens and body of the axis synchondrosis may remain unfused up to the age of seven, mimicking a dens fracture. Any anterior angulation of the dens should be viewed as suspicious for injury.[27] The anterior vertebral bodies of C3, C4, and C5 will often have a wedged appearance mimicking wedge compression fractures (Fig. 5). As their ossification sites fully calcify, they will take on the appearance of adult vertebral bodies. Small calcifications may sometimes be seen inferior to the cervical vertebral bodies. These represent normal ring epiphyses. Looking for any subluxation, soft-tissue swelling, or any clinical evidence of injury at those levels is helpful in deciding whether any radiographic abnormalities in those regions represent acute injuries. Children suffer a disproportionate number of high cervical spine injuries.[18] Children are also still vulnerable to lower cervical spine injuries, although injury in this location is not as common.[18]

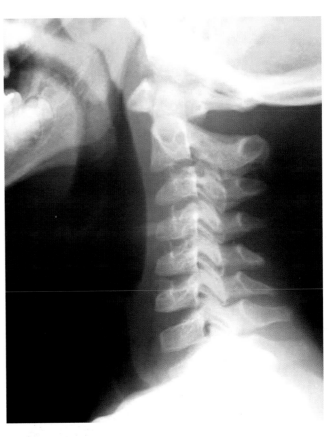

Figure 5. *Wedge-shaped appearance of vertebral bodies, most prominent at C3, should not be confused with compression fractures. The vertebrae take on a more rectangular appearance with age. Image courtesy of Swaminatha V. Mahadevan, MD, Stanford University.*

Spinal cord injury without radiographic abnormality (SCIWORA) is a post-traumatic myelopathy that results from acute spinal cord or nerve root injury and results in some combination of sensory and motor deficit.[30] Spinal cord injury without radiographic abnormality is defined as a post-traumatic myelopathy that occurs without radiographic evidence of fracture or dislocation on plain radiography and computed tomography (CT) scan evaluation. Anatomic differences of the pediatric spine allow for significant intersegmental spinal movement without bony column disruption. The spinal cord does not share the same degree of elasticity as the spinal column. This explains why, despite the lack of radiographic evidence of spinal column disruption, spinal cord injury may still occur. In a recent meta-analysis of pediatric studies describing SCIWORA syndrome, 27 percent of patients (24/88) experienced delayed onset of symptoms.[30] Paralysis developed hours to days after patients' initial injuries. The prognosis of patients with SCIWORA syndrome is better than patients with similar neurologic deficits who exhibit radiographic evidence of bony column disruption. Nevertheless, patients with complete cord syndromes or severe deficits on initial examination generally do not recover.[31] In more recent studies, SCIWORA syndrome has been documented in adult patients as well.[30]

> Spinal cord injury without radiographic abnormality is defined as a post-traumatic myelopathy that occurs without radiographic evidence of fracture or dislocation on plain radiography and CT scan evaluation.

Trauma victims who complain of either transient or persistent symptoms potentially attributable to a spinal cord injury should be assumed to have an unstable spinal column until proven otherwise. Radiographic evaluation often involves plain radiography and CT. High-dose glucocorticosteroid (i.e., methylprednisolone) therapy was the standard of care in adult patients with blunt trauma and clinical evidence of spinal cord injury. That was largely based on the results of the National Acute Spinal Cord Injury Study (NASCIS) II trial, which have since been called into question.[32] This trial did not include any patient age 12 or younger. There are no published trials that support administering high-dose methylprednisolone in children age 12 and younger with spinal cord injuries. The benefits of administering high-dose glucocorticosteroids following blunt spinal cord injury has been refuted by many experts who feel the practice is of no value and possibly harmful.[33]

> There are no published trials that support administration of high-dose methylprednisolone in children age 12 and younger with spinal cord injuries.

## Skeletal and Body Surface Area

Due to incomplete calcification and multiple unfused growth plates, the skeleton of a child is more pliable than an adult skeleton. As a result, significant internal organ injury can occur in children without notable overlying skeletal findings.[34,35] For example, pulmonary contusions commonly occur in children, without associated rib fractures. Conversely, rib fractures denote significant trauma and are commonly associated with underlying injuries.[34,35] Thus, when a rib or central bony structure is fractured, a diligent search for underlying internal organ injuries should follow, irrespective of how hemodynamically stable the child initially appears. The head is another area where a skull fracture may not occur, but there can be significant underlying cerebral pathology.[36] Skin surface-area-to-body-volume ratio is highest at birth and decreases with age.[37] As a result, heat transfer occurs much more rapidly in smaller children. Therefore, injured children are prone to hypothermia and must be evaluated and monitored vigilantly.

> The skeleton of a child is more pliable than an adult skeleton. As a result, significant internal organ injury can occur without notable overlying skeletal injuries.

| AGE (YEARS) | WEIGHT (KG) | RESPIRATORY RATE | PULSE |
|:---:|:---:|:---:|:---:|
| Less than 1 | 3 | 40 to 60 | 130 to 150 |
| 1 to 5 | 10 to 20 | 20 to 40 | 110 to 130 |
| 6 to 10 | 20 to 35 | 12 to 20 | 75 to 100 |
| 11 to 18 | 35 to 70 | 12 to 20 | 70 |

Table 2. *Physiologic parameters for respiratory rate and pulse rates in children.*

## Physiology

### Vital Signs and Other Physiologic Parameters

Normal respiratory and pulse rates vary with age as is described in Table 2. The definition of hypotension (less than fifth percentile) according to systolic blood pressure is less than 70 mm Hg for infants, less than 70 mm Hg + 2 x (age in years) for children one to 10 years of age, and for children older than 10 years of age, it is less than 90 mm Hg.[38] Children also have a smaller circulating blood volume than adults. Using 80 milliliters of blood volume per kilogram of body weight will allow for an accurate estimation of a child's intravascular blood volume. For example, the calculated intravascular blood volume for a five-kilogram infant would be 400 milliliters.

> The definition of hypotension according to systolic blood pressure for infants is less than 70 mm Hg, for children one to 10 years of age is less than 70 mm Hg + 2 x (age in years), and for children older than 10 years of age is less than 90 mm Hg.

Normal intracranial pressure (ICP) in a child is similar to an adult and ranges between five to 15 mm Hg in the supine position with the exception of infants with an open fontanel where the ICP will be slightly lower. Similar to adults, the standard goal is to maintain ICP less than 20 mm Hg.[39] The threshold to treat low cerebral perfusion pressure (CPP), defined by mean arterial pressure minus ICP, in children is dependent upon their age. In general, CPP should be maintained greater than 40 mm Hg for children under two years of age, greater than 50 mm Hg for those two to six years of age, greater than 60 mm Hg for those six to 12, and greater than 70 mm Hg for patients older than 13 years of age.[39]

Normal central venous pressures in children range between three to five mm Hg. Since children rarely have diastolic dysfunction, the central venous pressure is a relatively accurate measure of intravascular volume. For patients requiring positive-pressure mechanical ventilation, the intrapulmonary pressure that is transmitted to the intrapleural space will elevate the measured central venous pressure.[40] The amount of central venous pressure elevation will be dependent upon the degree of compliance of the lungs, with increased lung compliance causing less transmission of pressure and therefore less effect on the measured central venous pressure.[41] Intraabdominal pressure in children can be approximated with any device that measures urinary bladder pressure or intragastric pressure as is done in adults. Normal intraabdominal pressure in children is less than 10 mm Hg and typically three to five mm Hg, which is similar to adults, and in critically ill children requiring mechanical ventilation without signs of abdominal compartment syndrome, normal intraabdominal pressures were reported to be seven ± three mm Hg.[42]

Abdominal compartment syndrome has been loosely defined in children, as in adults, by an intraabdominal pressure greater than 20 mm Hg.[43] Children may develop abdominal compartment syndrome at lower pressures compared to adults.[43] Splanchnic perfusion pressure, defined as mean arterial pressure minus intraabdominal pressure, may also be calculated. Splanchnic perfusion pressure is as a more accurate marker of splanchnic blood flow, and a decrease in splanchnic perfusion pressure may be the most sensitive early finding of abdominal compartment syndrome.[44] Aggressive volume resuscitation in combination with inflammatory processes that promote capillary leak syndrome increases the risk of abdominal compartment syndrome, which can manifest as renal failure, decreased pulmonary compliance, and multiorgan failure.[43]

> Aggressive volume resuscitation in combination with inflammatory processes that promote capillary leak syndrome increases the risk of abdominal compartment syndrome, which can manifest as renal failure, decreased pulmonary compliance, and multiple organ system failure.

Due to higher metabolic rates, oxygen consumption is increased in infants and younger children compared to adolescents and adults.[45] A significant related consequence is that younger children will become hypoxemic more rapidly during rapid sequence intubation. Methods to monitor the relationship between oxygen delivery and consumption in children are similar to what is practiced in adults. Blood gas analysis of arterial partial pressure of oxygen, base deficit or lactate concentrations, central venous oxygen saturations, and systemic arterial and cerebral tissue oxygen saturation monitoring are all used to directly or indirectly measure oxygen delivery, consumption, and cardiac output.

| WEIGHT (KG) | HOURLY RATE OF FLUIDS |
|---|---|
| 3 to 10 | 4 milliliters (ml) per kilogram per hour |
| 11 to 20 | 40 ml per hour + 2 ml per kilogram per hour |
| 20 to 70 | 60 ml per hour + 1 ml per kilogram per hour |

e.g., for weight of 13 kg, maintenance fluid requirement is 40 ml/hr + 2(3) ml/hr = 46 ml/hr
e.g., for weight of 37 kg, maintenance fluid requirement is 60 ml/hr + 1(17) ml/hr = 77 ml/hr

The exception is day 1 to day 2 of life in full-term neonates. Day 1 use = 60 to 80 ml per kilogram per day. Day 2 use = 80 to 100 ml per kilogram per day.

Table 3. *Daily maintenance fluid requirement for pediatric patients, based on weight.*

> Higher oxygen consumption in infants and young children combined with decreased functional residual capacity compared to adults causes children to become hypoxemic more rapidly during rapid sequence intubation.

Fluids, Electrolytes, Nutrition, and Glucose Metabolism
Daily fluid requirements in children are dependent upon their weight (Table 3).[46] For children who present with intravascular volume depletion due to fluid losses, these deficits should be replaced with non-dextrose containing isotonic saline rapidly if the child is hemodynamically compromised and more gradually (e.g., over 24 hours) if the losses have been subacute and the child is hemodynamically stable.

Determining intravascular volume in pediatric patients is difficult since there is no direct method to measure it. Patient vital signs, physical exam findings, urine output, hemodynamic parameters, and laboratory values must be collectively evaluated to estimate the patient's intravascular volume status. When intravenous fluids are used, close attention needs to be paid to the child's electrolyte status. Critical illness in children increases antidiuretic hormone production, which increases free water retention. The risk of hyponatremic seizures increases with the use of hypotonic saline such as one-quarter normal saline (0.22 percent NaCl).[47] Therefore, one-half normal saline (0.45 percent NaCl) to isotonic fluids such as normal saline (0.9 percent NaCl) or lactated Ringer's solution should be used to provide maintenance fluids in critically ill children. This is a change from classical teaching that stressed the use of hypotonic fluids. Recent literature shows that the use of hypotonic fluids provides too much free water and should be abandoned.[47]

> Intravascular volume depletion should be rapidly reversed with non-dextrose containing isotonic saline if the child is hemodynamically unstable, and more gradually reversed if the fluid deficit is subacute and the child is hemodynamically stable.

Potassium daily requirements are 1 to 2 milliequivalents (mEq) per kilogram per day.[48] In children less than one month of age this can be achieved with the addition of 10 mEq per liter of potassium chloride and in children greater than three months of age by adding 20 mEq per liter of potassium chloride to their intravenous fluid solution. The standard maximum potassium chloride concentrations suggested for peripheral intravenous (IV) solution is 80 mEq per liter and is 200 mEq per liter for central line administration.[48] In non-immediately life-threatening scenarios, the maximum IV rate of potassium-containing solutions is 0.5 mEq per kilogram per hour with a maximum of 40 mEq per hour for children weighing greater than 40 kilograms.[49] To minimize the risk of significant electrolyte disturbances, serum electrolytes should be monitored at least daily in all children requiring intravascular fluids.

Children in areas of combat operations are often malnourished. Consequently, nutritional deficiencies are common, which increases the risk of many nutritional comorbid disorders such as sepsis and poor wound healing.[50,51] A major difference between children and adults is caloric requirements. Daily caloric resting energy requirements decrease with age (Table 4). The standard caloric requirement or resting energy expenditure for an infant is 90 to 120 kilocalories (kcal) per kilogram per day compared to 25 to 30 kcal per kilogram per day in adults.[46] There is no one simple formula that can

| AGE (YEARS) | KCAL/KG |
|---|---|
| 0 to 1 | 90 to 120 |
| 1 to 7 | 75 to 90 |
| 7 to 12 | 60 to 75 |
| 12 to 18 | 30 to 60 |
| Greater than 18 | 25 to 30 |

Table 4. *Daily maintenance caloric requirements in children. Note the decrease of caloric requirements associated with age.*

be used to calculate critically ill patients' total caloric requirements. This requires direct calorimetry, which will not typically be available at Combat Support Hospitals. Alterations in energy expenditure as a result of critical illness in children cannot be estimated accurately, therefore nutritional support should be provided according to measurement of resting energy expenditure to avoid the consequences of overfeeding or malnutrition.[52]

Enteral feeding compared to parenteral is preferred since it preserves gastrointestinal function and has been associated with decreased infections and length of hospital stay in critically ill children.[53] Enteral feeds are indicated early in the course of critical illness as soon as enteric peristalsis is established, unless there is a medical or surgical contraindication. Post-pyloric feeds are advantageous due to less gastric distention and decreased risk of gastroesophageal reflux compared to gastric feeding.[53] Nasoduodenal tubes can often be placed blindly 30 minutes after the administration of a prokinetic agent with the child in the right lateral decubitus position. Promotility agents can be used to improve gastric motility, and non-narcotic agents can be used for sedation to decrease the risk of ileus.[54]

Children in areas of combat operations are often malnourished, which increases the risk of many comorbid disorders such as sepsis and poor wound healing. Enteral feeding is preferred to parenteral feeding since it preserves gastrointestinal function and has been associated with decreased infections and length of hospital stay in critically ill children.

Hypoglycemia is a significant risk in young children if glucose is not provided (in some form) early after initial resuscitation. This is due to decreased hepatic stores of glycogen and increased metabolism in children.[55] For neonates it is standard to provide 10 percent dextrose (D10) when parenteral fluids are required and 5 percent dextrose (D5) for all other ages until adolescence.[48] Clinical signs and symptoms of hypoglycemia may not be easily recognized in sedated and mechanically ventilated children. The risk of hypoglycemia makes it necessary to evaluate serum glucose values at least once a day if not more frequently in these critically ill children. Adolescent age children have larger glucose stores and are able to temporarily tolerate maintenance fluids without dextrose, similar to adults. Table 5 summarizes the range of acceptable choices of solutions, with dextrose concentrations and additives. For the treatment of symptomatic hypoglycemia in neonates and infants, it is preferred to give 4 ml per kilogram of D10 solution by intravenous bolus infusion and to check the glucose concentration within 15 to 30 minutes. The use of D25 and D50 solutions should be avoided in neonates and infants due to the theoretical risk of intraventricular hemorrhage following the rapid infusion of a hyperosmotic agent and the risk of infiltration and tissue injury when administered into a peripheral vein.[48]

| AGE | DEXTROSE (PERCENT) | SOLUTION | POTASSIUM CHLORIDE (KCl) |
|---|---|---|---|
| 0 to 2 Days | 10 | Water + 2 mEq/kg NaCl + 1 mEq/kg KCl | |
| 3 Days to 1 Month | 5 or 10 | 0.45 Normal Saline | 10 mEq per liter |
| 1 Month to 1 Year | 5 | 0.45 to 0.9 Normal Saline or LR | 20 mEq per liter* |
| 1 to 8 Years | 5 | 0.45 to 0.9 Normal Saline or LR | 20 mEq per liter* |
| 8 to 18 Years | 0 or 5 | 0.45 to 0.9 Normal Saline or LR | 20 mEq per liter* |

*Potassium chloride should not empirically be added to lactated Ringer's (LR) solution if not required.

Table 5. *Appropriate range of fluid solutions and additives in children.*

Hypoglycemia is a significant risk in young children if glucose is not provided in some form early after initial resuscitation. The use of D25 and D50 solutions should be avoided in neonates and infants due to the theoretical risk of intraventricular hemorrhage with the rapid use of a hyperosmotic agent and the risk of infiltration and tissue injury when used within a peripheral vein.

Respiratory System

While there are age-dependent changes in pulmonary compliance and resistance and chest wall compliance, in children as compared to adults, these differences have minimal effect on the treatment of respiratory failure once it has occurred in children.[56] Increased resistance due to smaller airways and increased metabolic rates and lower functional residual capacities may increase the risk of respiratory failure in young children. Once a child is intubated, the same open-lung or low-lung tidal volume strategies that are applied in adults should also be applied in children (e.g., 5 ml per kilogram as an initial tidal volume). Principles of permissive hypercapnia and permissive hypoxemia to prevent ventilator-associated lung injury are also practiced in children.[57] Complications of hypercapnia are minimal as long as the pH of the blood is medically controlled at a pH of 7.1 or above.

> Once a child is intubated, the same open-lung or low-lung tidal volume strategies that are applied in adults should also be applied. Principles of permissive hypercapnia and permissive hypoxemia to prevent ventilator-associated lung injury are also applied to children.

## Pharmacology

The dosing of most, if not all, medications for children is weight-based. Multiple references for appropriate dosing and how to adjust for renal and hepatic impairment in addition to contraindications and adverse reactions are available and must be used for the safe and appropriate use of medications in children. The Harriet Lane Handbook is a small soft-cover book that is an invaluable resource for pediatric medication dosing and adjustment.[58] All Combat Support Hospitals should have this reference available.

> The Harriet Lane Handbook is a small soft-cover book that is an invaluable resource for pediatric medication dosing and adjustment.[58] Level III care facilities should have this reference available.

Succinylcholine and propofol are two pharmaceutical agents that are commonly used for patients with traumatic injuries that have added risks or considerations in children compared to adults.[59] Succinylcholine has historically been the paralytic of choice for true rapid sequence induction due to its rapid onset of action (30 seconds) and brief duration of action (five to six minutes).[8] This was undoubtedly true, especially when there were no other similar profile agents. The increased risks associated with succinylcholine in children must be recognized and alternative choices should at least be considered. The major risk associated with its use is life-threatening hyperkalemia, which is increased when used in children with undiagnosed neuromuscular disorders, massive multiorgan trauma, widespread intestinal ischemia, and subacute burn injuries.[59] In addition, risks associated with succinylcholine use include malignant hyperthermia, masseter spasm, increased intracranial, intraocular, and gastric pressure, sinus bradycardia with hypotension, and pulmonary edema.[59] Several methods of blunting the transient rise of ICP directly resulting from succinylcholine administrations have been studied. The use of lidocaine (1 to 1.5 milligrams [mg] per kilogram) IV has shown mixed results in the literature; the studies demonstrating benefit required a minimum of three minutes of time to pass prior to administering succinylcholine.[60] The administration of a defasciculating dose (0.01 mg per kilogram) of a nondepolarizing paralytic agent such as pancuronium has been shown to decrease succinylcholine-associated rises in ICP.[59] Administration of atropine will eliminate the risk of bradycardia with laryngoscopy.[59] The use of these premedication agents often negates the rapid onset of action of succinylcholine since it takes time for these agents to be administered and take effect. If succinylcholine is used in pediatric patients, infants may require 2 to 3 mg per kilogram and children 1 to 2 mg per kilogram of succinylcholine compared to the adult intravenous dose of 1 to 1.5 mg per kilogram.[59]

An alternative agent that has near similar onset of action that should be considered in children is rocuronium. Rocuronium at a dose of 0.6 mg per kilogram typically produces paralysis at 50 to 80 seconds, and using an increased dose of 0.8 mg per kilogram will decrease the average time to 30 seconds.[59] The duration of action in children is typically 30 to 40 minutes, which is much longer than succinylcholine since it is an intermediate-acting nondepolarizing paralytic.[59] Hence, careproviders will need to provide airway and breathing support for this extended period of time if endotracheal intubation is unsuccessful. Hemodynamic effects include mild increase in heart rate. It is metabolized primarily by the liver and excreted by the kidneys. Since there are now suitable alternatives to succinylcholine, many in the pediatric emergency medicine and critical care communities discourage its use and support the alternative use of agents such as rocuronium.[59]

> Succinylcholine has historically been the paralytic of choice for true rapid sequence induction due to its rapid onset of action and brief duration of action. An alternative agent that has near similar onset of action that should be considered in children is rocuronium.

Propofol is an intravenous anesthetic agent that gained wide acceptance for long-term sedation in adult intensive care units as a result of its potent anesthetic properties, fast-onset, and short duration of action. Propofol's attractive rapid-onset and rapid-offset pharmacologic profile has resulted in extending its use to critically ill pediatric patients (e.g., enabling near-term neurologic exams in patients with head injuries). Short-term use of propofol for procedural sedation and operative cases has not been shown to be a problem, but the use of propofol for prolonged sedation in the critical care setting has raised concerns. A fatal metabolic acidosis syndrome associated with prolonged use of propofol has been described. The mechanism is unclear, but duration of therapy and higher doses are the most commonly cited factors associated with the syndrome. Notably, children have been reported to develop a rapidly fatal metabolic acidosis syndrome when higher doses of propofol have been used for sedation for more than two to three days.[61,62,63,64] While this has also been reported in adults, it has been more commonly associated with pediatric use (specifically in brain injury and burn patients), hence the black box warning for long-term use in children.[65]

> Propofol has an attractive rapid-onset and rapid-offset pharmacologic profile, which has resulted in extending its use to critically ill pediatric patients. The use of propofol for prolonged sedation in the critical care setting has raised concerns. With prolonged sedation of more than two to three days, a fatal metabolic acidosis syndrome, also known as propofol infusion syndrome, can occur.

Fatal metabolic acidosis, also known as propofol infusion syndrome, can present with the following signs and symptoms: lactic acidosis, rhabdomyolysis, elevated hepatic enzymes, and fatal dysrhythmias. Discontinuation of propofol and supportive care is the only treatment.[61,62,63,64] Since there are alternative agents that can produce adequate deep sedation such as fentanyl, remifentanil, midazolam, ketamine, barbiturates, and dexmedetomidine, the use of propofol for greater than 24 hours must be carefully considered. If propofol is used for long-term sedation, patients should be carefully monitored for the development of propofol infusion syndrome.

## Patient Monitoring Considerations

Standard monitoring of vital signs in children includes continuous end-tidal carbon dioxide monitoring for children who are intubated.[66] A main benefit of continuous end-tidal carbon dioxide monitoring is the rapid recognition that the ETT has been displaced out of the airway. Children, due to their shorter tracheas and difficulty in maintaining adequate sedation, are at increased risk of accidental extubations (Fig. 6). Immediate recognition of ETT displacement before the child becomes hypoxemic will minimize adverse outcomes. Continuous end-tidal carbon dioxide waveform analysis monitoring improves the recognition

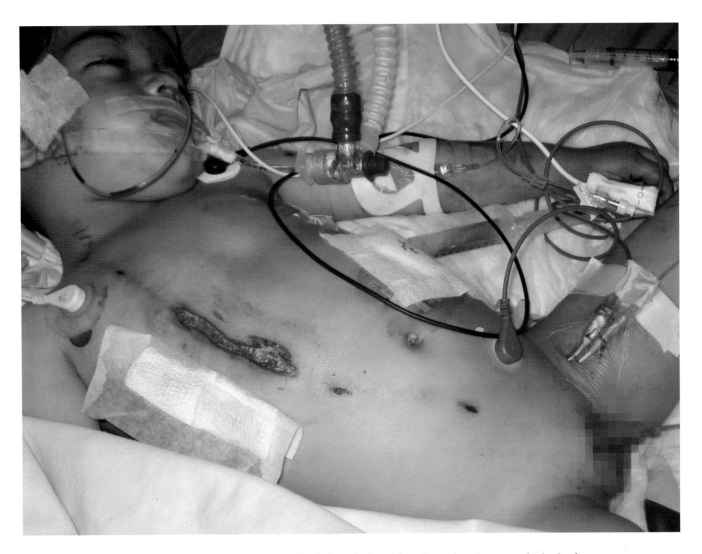

Figure 6. *A pediatric victim of an IED blast undergoing mechanical ventilation with cardiac and respiratory monitoring in place.*

of obstructive airway disease, whether it is from reactive airways or mucus plugging.[66] It is also beneficial for the child with severe traumatic brain injury where the goal is to keep the arterial partial pressure of carbon dioxide ($PCO_2$) within a certain range and can also be used to estimate pulmonary dead space.[66] Once correlated with the arterial $PCO_2$, the end-tidal carbon dioxide can be used to titrate ventilation and has the potential to minimize phlebotomy.

Because children are at increased risk of accidental extubations, standard monitoring should include continuous end-tidal carbon dioxide monitoring, which may aid in rapid recognition of a displaced ETT.

The use of intracranial ventriculostomy catheters for patients with severe traumatic brain injury is standard practice in children.[39] Diagnostic benefits include the monitoring of ICP, while therapeutic benefits include the ability to drain cerebrospinal fluid (CSF) via the catheters when intracranial pressures become elevated. Compared to intraparenchymal pressure monitoring devices, there is an increased infection risk with the use of ventriculostomy catheters, but this risk is still very low and the therapeutic benefits outweigh the risks.[39]

# Resuscitation

## General Considerations

Advanced Trauma Life Support (ATLS) course principles all apply for children. The Broselow® tape is a commonly used and helpful method to standardize the approach to the resuscitation of children (Fig. 7).[10] It provides a valuable reference source for the appropriate sizing of pediatric resuscitation equipment and dosing of medications.

## Airway and Breathing

For the conscious child with an obstructed airway, back blows or the Heimlich maneuver should be performed to dislodge any foreign body.[38] Attempts

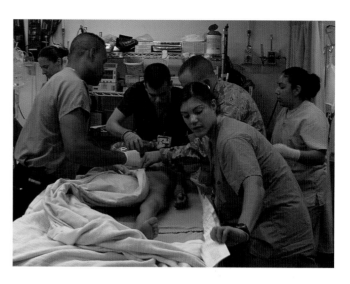

Figure 7. *Pediatric resuscitation of a host nation casualty cared for at a Level III facility. By measuring the patient's body length, the Broselow® tape allows careproviders to rapidly determine appropriate resuscitation equipment and medication dosing.*

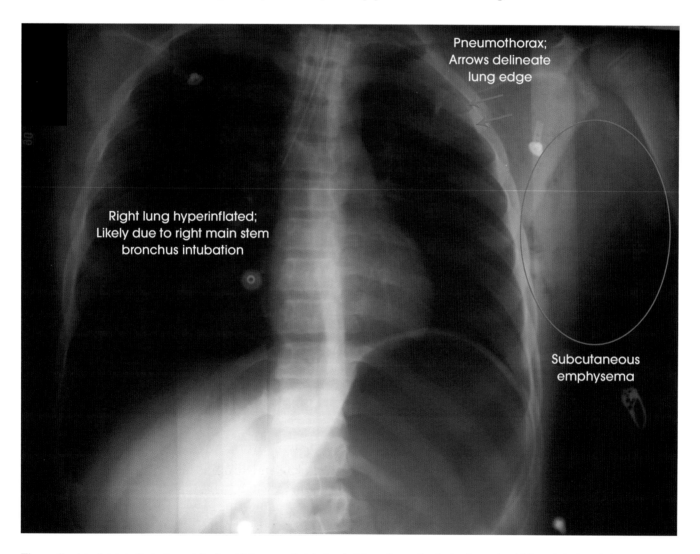

Figure 8. *A pediatric patient who sustained multiple traumatic injuries. A right mainstem intubation is noted, with hyperinflation of the right lung.*

to manually remove the obstruction should only occur if a foreign body is visible.[38] In cases where positive-pressure ventilation is indicated, the use of an oral airway will greatly improve the ability to bag-valve-mask ventilate a young child since the tongue often obstructs a child's airway. The use of a Miller blade and the Sellick maneuver will often improve your ability to visualize the larynx in a young child.

Always consider ETT misplacement (e.g., right mainstem bronchus intubation) if it is difficult to increase a child's arterial oxygen saturations or if the peak inspiratory pressures are higher than expected. The trachea of a child is much shorter than it is in an adult and it is easy to mistakenly advance the ETT into the right mainstem bronchus (Fig. 8). The proximal airways in an intubated child obstruct very easily due to their small size. Nebulized hypertonic saline, respiratory vibratory and percussive therapy, and the use of mucolytics (nebulized or instilled) can be considered and have been used with mixed results to minimize airway obstruction in a variety of conditions.[67,68,69]

> The trachea of a child is much shorter than it is in an adult, and it is easy to mistakenly advance the ETT into the right mainstem bronchus. Always consider ETT misplacement (e.g., right mainstem bronchus intubation) if it is difficult to increase a child's arterial oxygen saturations or if the peak inspiratory pressures are higher than expected.

Current pediatric standards taught in the Pediatric Advanced Life Support (PALS) course advise the use of cuffed endotracheal tubes to optimize oxygenation and ventilation in all children. The primary benefit is to secure the tube and prevent significant air leaks around the ETT. With the use of cuffed ETT tubes comes the responsibility of maintaining the appropriate ETT cuff pressure (less than 25 cm $H_2O$). This will minimize the risk of subglottic stenosis that may occur from ischemic injury to this area from over inflated endotracheal cuffs.[70] The short length of the trachea especially in infants can make it very difficult to keep the ETT in proper midtracheal position. To minimize the risk of accidental extubations it is wise to: (1) keep the infant and young child well-sedated; (2) ensure the ETT is securely taped; (3) immediately change the tape if it loosens (e.g., due to oropharyngeal secretions); (4) obtain daily chest radiographs to determine the position of the ETT; and (5) always use continuous end-tidal carbon dioxide monitoring to enable immediate recognition of ETT dislodgment. In circumstances where it is difficult to maintain an orally-placed ETT in proper position, considerations should be given to performing nasotracheal intubation.

## Rapid Sequence Intubation
Careproviders need to consider multiple important factors when performing rapid sequence intubation in young children. Atropine should be strongly considered as a premedication prior to intubation in infants and young children. Infants have a strong vagal response to laryngoscopy and can develop significant bradycardia as a result.[70] Oropharyngeal secretions in young children can make airway visualization difficult during laryngoscopy. This is especially true with the use of ketamine, which is a potent sialogogue. Atropine has been shown to decrease oral secretions and may also reduce the risk of vomiting during recovery from ketamine use.[71] Interestingly, while glycopyrrolate and atropine have been traditionally used to minimize secretions, recent studies have found that neither drug has been shown to decrease serious adverse respiratory events associated with ketamine use.[72,73]

Infants and young children have a strong vagal response to laryngoscopy and can develop significant bradycardia as a result. Atropine should be strongly considered as a premedication prior to intubation of infants and young children.

Due to increased metabolic rates and decreased functional residual capacity compared to adults, children will undergo arterial oxygen desaturation more quickly with rapid sequence intubation.[74] This is especially true for children with nutritional deficiencies and decreased muscular strength and those with distended abdomens either from malnutrition or hepatic enlargement. For children who require bag-valve-mask ventilation prior to intubation, intragastric air can increase intraabdominal pressure significantly enough to decrease pulmonary compliance and make it more difficult to maintain adequate oxygenation (Fig. 9). To minimize increased intragastric air accumulation, the Sellick maneuver should be used during bag-valve-mask ventilation once the child is sedated. If gastric distension still occurs, the placement of a nasogastric tube to decompress the stomach should also be considered.

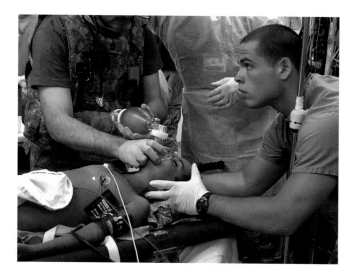

Figure 9. *For children who require bag-valve-mask ventilation prior to intubation, intragastric air can increase intraabdominal pressure significantly enough to decrease pulmonary compliance and make it more difficult to maintain adequate oxygenation. In such cases, prompt nasogastric tube decompression is warranted.*

## Vascular Access

Rapid resuscitation of a child is best accomplished through the largest peripheral intravascular access that can be obtained. If a child is in need of immediate intravascular access and standard peripheral or central intravenous access cannot be rapidly established, an intraosseous (IO) needle should be inserted.[70]

Intraosseous needles can be inserted by hand or with the use of a tool such as the EZ-IO® (Fig. 10).[75] The preferred landmark for IO line placement is two centimeters inferior to the tibial tuberosity and perpendicular to the medial flat surface of the tibia. Local anesthetic (e.g., lidocaine) injected at the site of needle insertion several minutes prior to needle insertion will minimize procedural discomfort. Alternative sites include the distal tibia, distal femur, and proximal humerus (Fig. 11). All resuscitative medications and blood products that can be given intravenously can be administered via an IO needle.[70] Marrow sinusoids drain into venous channels, which lead into nutrient and emissary veins, which in turn, drain into the systemic venous system. Medications infused via intraosseous lines can reach the central circulation rapidly and in a similar timeframe compared to peripheral injections, even in hypoperfused states. Pressure bags or manual syringe infusion are the recommended methods for attaining adequate infusion rates. Passive flow rates (i.e., gravity infusion of hanging saline bags) are suboptimal. Blood can also be sampled from an IO needle for laboratory analysis.[76]

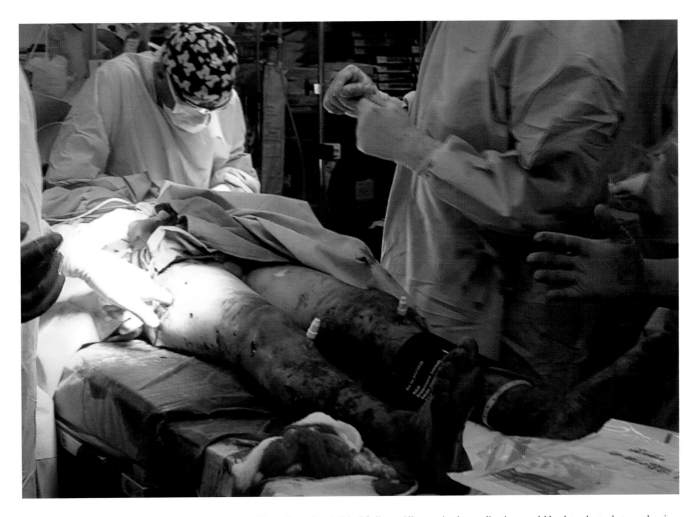

Figure 10. *Vascular access in this patient includes bilateral proximal tibia IO lines. All resuscitative medications and blood products that can be given intravenously can be administered via an IO needle.*

> If a child is in need of immediate intravascular access and standard peripheral or central intravenous access cannot be rapidly established, an IO needle should be inserted. All resuscitative medications and blood products that can be given intravenously can be administered via an IO needle. Pressure bags or manual syringe infusion are the recommended methods for attaining adequate flow rates, as passive flow rates are suboptimal.

Complications of IO lines include subcutaneous extravasation of infusate, extremity compartment syndrome, tibial fracture, and osteomyelitis.[75] Intraosseus line utilization should be regarded as temporary vascular access and should be replaced with traditional IV access within 24 hours. This is due to the concern that there is an increased risk of osteomyelitis with prolonged IO access.[77] Close monitoring for extravasation of fluid is crucial. Early recognition of a malfunctioning IO line will minimize the risk of compartment syndromes at IO infusion sites.

## *Circulation*

Damage control or hemostatic resuscitation principles can be applied to children in hemorrhagic shock.[78] There is no contraindication to the use of appropriately cross-matched whole blood for children who

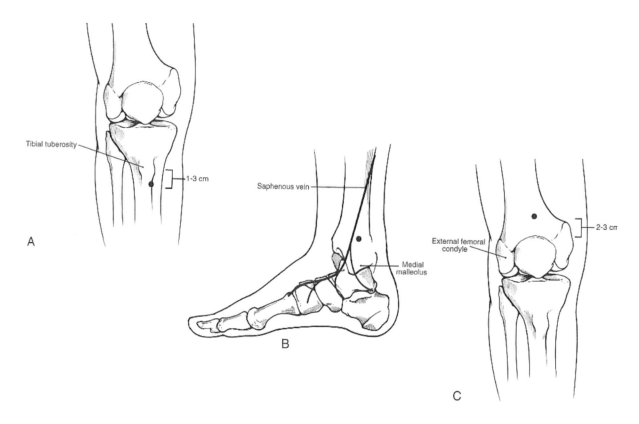

Figure 11. *Sites for IO line placement. The preferred landmark for IO line placement is two centimeters inferior to the tibial tuberosity and perpendicular to the medial flat surface of the tibia. Alternative sites include the distal tibia, distal femur, and proximal humerus. Image courtesy of Elsevier. In: Roberts JR and Hedges JR. Clinical Procedures in Emergency Medicine. 4th ed. Philadelphia (PA): WB Saunders; 1998.*

present in hemorrhagic shock. In fact, the only randomized controlled trial of whole blood was performed in children after cardiac surgery.[79] In this study, whole blood was transfused in both the operating room and intensive care unit, and outcomes were statistically adjusted. The results indicated that whole blood transfusion compared to blood product components decreased postoperative blood loss.[79] This study is often compared to another that reported increased length of stay with the use of whole blood compared to components.[80] It is important to realize that in this study by Mou et al., whole blood was only transfused in the operating room, and the analysis did not adjust for other factors associated with length of stay.[80] The use of type O whole blood should only be considered when there is no other alternative, and the child is in immediate risk of death. Every effort should be made to use type-specific whole blood when it is indicated. All vasoactive agents used in adults to increase cardiac output can be used in children, including vasopressin.[81,82] Relative adrenal insufficiency is common in critically ill children.[83] Hydrocortisone is used for its treatment with reported dosing that varies from 2 mg per kilogram IV every 4 hours to a 50 mg per day continuous infusion.[84] Of note, the benefit of low-dose hydrocortisone in critically ill children in septic shock remains poorly defined. The recognition of low ionized calcium concentrations and its treatment in hypotensive children is important since correction improves myocardial contractility and vasomotor tone.[81]

Damage control or hemostatic resuscitation principles can be applied to children in hemorrhagic shock, as in adults. Standard volumes for red blood cell, fresh frozen plasma, and platelet transfusions range from 10 to 15 ml per kilogram. For children requiring massive transfusion, which is typically defined as more than one blood volume (70 to 80 ml per kilogram) in 24 hours, hypothermia, hyperkalemia, and hypocalcemia are all risks.

## Blood Product Transfusion

Standard volumes for red blood cell, fresh frozen plasma (FFP), and platelet transfusions range from 10 to 15 ml per kilogram. Cryoprecipitate dose is 1 to 2 units per 10 kilograms bodyweight.[85] For children requiring massive transfusion, which is typically defined as more than one blood volume (70 to 80 ml per kilogram) in 24 hours, hypothermia, hyperkalemia, and hypocalcemia are all risks.[86] As a result, the use of a blood warmer should be strongly considered, and frequent electrolyte monitoring is required. The treatment of hypocalcemia is important for patients with coagulopathy since calcium is required for optimal coagulation factor function.[86] This is critical in the patient requiring massive transfusion. The large citrate load in packed red blood cells binds calcium, increasing the risk of hypocalcemia.[86] If left uncorrected, this will lead to decreased cardiac function.[87] In addition, for children requiring massive transfusion, the treatment of acidosis with alkaline solutions with either sodium bicarbonate or THAM (tromethamine) can be considered.[86] Adjunctive pro-hemostatic agents such as recombinant factor VIIa (rFVIIa) and antifibrinolytics can also be considered.[78,86] If rFVIIa is given, anecdotal experience and preliminary data indicate that it works best when used in conjunction with cryoprecipitate.[88] If thromboelastography is available, it can be used to direct hemostatic resuscitation and specifically determine if rFVIIa or antifibrinolytics are indicated.[78] For children who are hemodynamically stable without active bleeding, a hemoglobin concentration below 7 grams per deciliter is an appropriate red blood cell transfusion trigger.[89]

# Specific Medical Condition Management

## *Acute Respiratory Distress Syndrome (ARDS)*

Acute respiratory distress syndrome (ARDS) in children is defined as it is in adults: (1) Partial pressure of oxygen in arterial blood ($PaO_2$)/fraction of inspired oxygen ($FiO_2$) ratio less than 200 mm Hg; (2) presence of bilateral lung infiltrates on the chest radiograph; (3) no clinical evidence of heart failure; and (4) absence of COPD or other chronic pulmonary disorders. Principles practiced in adults regarding ventilator (e.g., permissive hypercapnia) and fluid management are also used for children.[57] Goals include keeping peak inspiratory pressures less than 30 cm $H_2O$ with the use of tidal volumes between 4 to 6 ml per kilogram bodyweight.[57] In addition, judicious fluid administration is recommended to prevent an excessive fluid balance since it has been associated with worse outcomes in adults with ARDS.[90] There is no limit to the amount of positive end-expiratory pressure that can be used to support oxygenation, and the prone position is also commonly used to attempt to improve oxygenation indices.[57] Nonconventional modes of ventilation, such as alternating pressure release ventilation (APRV) and high-frequency oscillation ventilation (HFOV), and alternative therapies, such as nitric oxide and surfactant therapy, are not currently available at Combat Support Hospitals.

> Acute respiratory distress syndrome in children is defined as it is in adults. Principles practiced in adults regarding ventilator (e.g., permissive hypercapnia) and fluid management are also used for children. Nonconventional modes of ventilation are not currently available at Combat Support Hospitals.

## *Severe Sepsis and Septic Shock*

Children respond differently hemodynamically to sepsis than adults.[81] Children typically have decreased

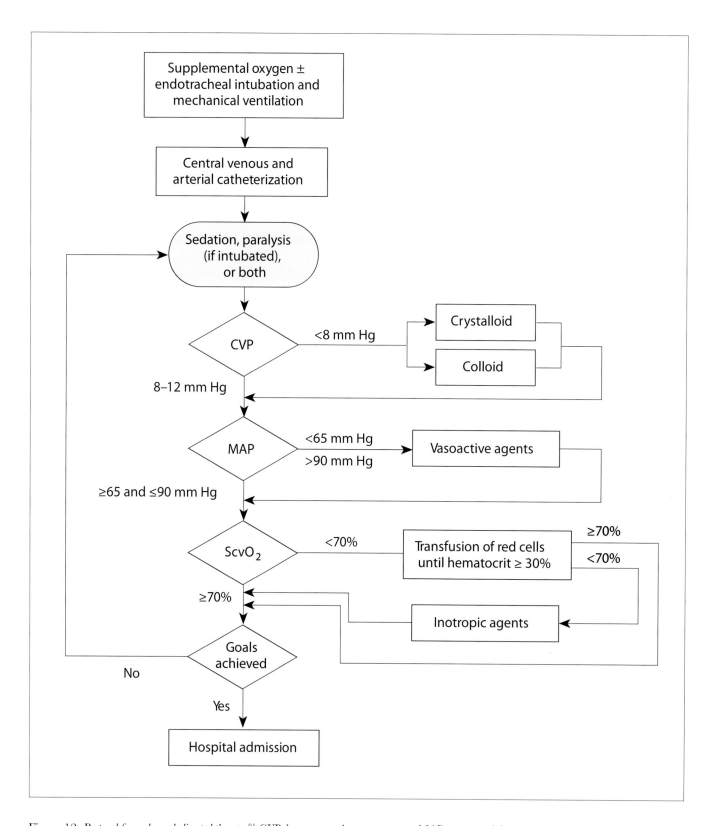

Figure 12. *Protocol for early goal-directed therapy.*[91] *CVP denotes central venous pressure, MAP mean arterial pressure, and ScvO₂ central venous oxygen saturation. Image courtesy of Massachusetts Medical Society.*

myocardial function and compensate with increased systemic vascular resistance commonly referred to as "cold shock." This is in contrast to adults who conversely first develop loss of vasomotor tone and compensate with increased cardiac function or what has been termed "warm shock."[81]

Adhering to principles of goal-directed therapy for treatment of patients with severe sepsis and septic shock is warranted (Fig. 12).[91,92] Therefore, the standard approach to septic shock in children is early administration of antibiotics and volume resuscitation, while correcting hypoglycemia and low ionized calcium concentrations. Correcting hypocalcemia is important since cardiac contractility is dependent upon normal serum ionized calcium concentrations. These interventions are coupled with infection source control (e.g., debridement of infected tissue). Either dopamine or epinephrine is appropriate as the initial inotrope.[82] If cold shock persists and intravascular volume is adequate (determined primarily by a central venous pressure of greater than 8 mm Hg), the use of an afterload reducing agent, either dobutamine or milrinone, is appropriate. If warm shock develops, norepinephrine, phenylephrine, or vasopressin is appropriate. Hydrocortisone should be used for patients with catecholamine-resistant shock.[82] Pulmonary artery catheters and other methods of determining cardiac output are not usually available at Combat Support Hospitals.

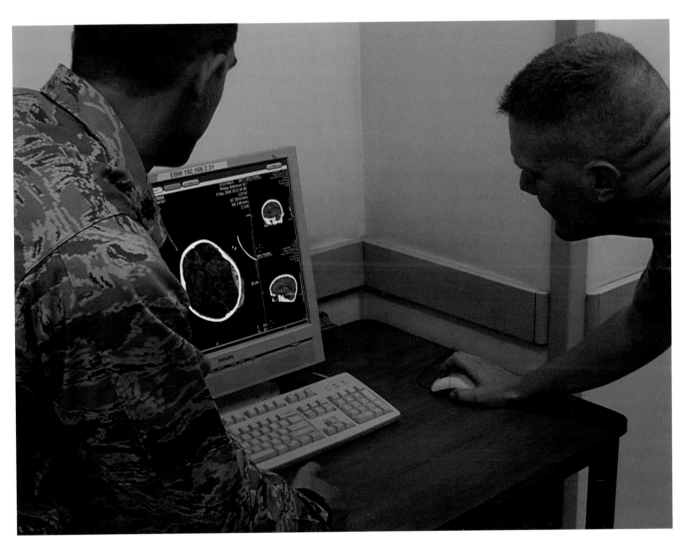

Figure 13. *Careproviders reviewing a CT scan of the brain demonstrating an epidural hematoma.*

Adhering to principles of goal-directed therapy for treatment of patients with severe sepsis and septic shock is warranted. The standard approach to septic shock in children is early administration of antibiotics and volume resuscitation while correcting hypoglycemia and low ionized calcium concentrations.

## Cerebral Herniation Syndromes

Several immediate interventions are indicated when a child has signs and symptoms of impending cerebral herniation (hypertension, bradycardia, abnormal breathing pattern, and posturing). These include hyperventilation by manual bag-valve-mask as a temporizing measure while initiating additional interventions. Additional measures include elevation of the head of the bed to approximately 30 degrees, and the rapid administration of an osmotic agent. Mannitol or hypertonic saline can be used as osmotic agents.[39] If the patient is hypovolemic and volume resuscitation is problematic, mannitol should not be used since it will often have a diuretic effect several hours after infusion. The decrease in mean arterial pressure from diuresis will translate into decreased cerebral perfusion pressure.[93] Hypertonic saline may be a better choice in hypovolemic pediatric patients. The dose of 3% hypertonic saline is 10 ml per kilogram IV (maximum dose 250 ml per bolus) and should be given as a fast intravenous push for impending herniation. Pediatric dosage handbooks mention it is preferable to use a central line with hypertonic saline since there is a risk of thrombophlebitis when used peripherally.[49] This risk has also been noted with mannitol.[94] Therefore, the safest approach may be to use either agent with a central line.

If a child displays evidence of impending cerebral herniation, hyperventilation, elevation of the head of the bed, and infusion of mannitol or hypertonic saline are indicated.

Concurrent efforts (cranial computed tomography scanning) should be made to determine whether a neurosurgically treatable intracranial lesion exists (e.g., epidural hematoma) (Fig. 13). Prompt neurosurgical consultation will also enable placement of intracranial ventriculostomy tubes, which can real-time monitor intracranial pressures and provide a method to decrease intracranial pressure through the removal of CSF.[39]

## Seizure Management

The etiology of seizures in children that are evacuated to a Combat Support Hospital after an acute injury is likely to be related to traumatic brain injury or a consequence of hypoxic ischemic injury (Fig. 14). Hypoglycemia, hyponatremia, and other electrolyte disturbances should always be immediately ruled out as the cause of seizure. The differential diagnosis should also include meningitis, epilepsy, hypertension, and drug ingestion.

After determining that the patient's airway is patent and breathing and circulation are adequate, oxygen should be applied and vascular access obtained. A rapid-acting benzodiazepine such as lorazepam (0.1 mg per kilogram) or diazepam (0.2 mg per kilogram) should be administered intravenously as a first-line therapeutic agent if continued tonic-clonic seizure activity persists beyond one minute. If the seizure persists beyond several minutes, repeat dosing of rapid-onset benzodiazepines is indicated. Alternative routes of benzodiazepine administration include intraosseous, intranasal, buccal, and rectal administrations. If seizures recur or persist in the minutes that follow infusion of first-line agents (benzodiazepines), second-line therapy is indicated. Second-line agents include intravenous administration of phenytoin (18 to 20

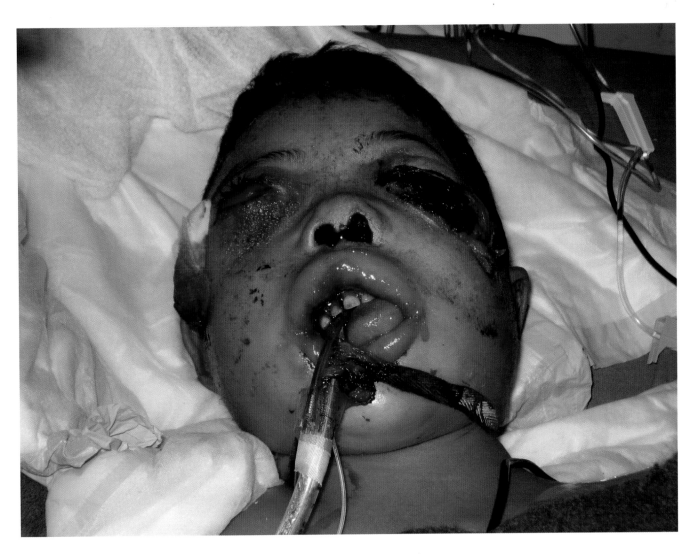

Figure 14. *A critically ill head-injured child at high risk for seizure activity.*

mg per kilogram) or fosphenytoin (15 to 20 mg phenytoin equivalents per kilogram).[95] If phenytoin is administered, the rate should not exceed 1 mg per kilogram per minute (maximum infusion rate 50 mg per minute) due to the risk of fatal dysrhythmias.[95] Fosphenytoin has become the preferred second-line agent for the acute management of seizures in children for several reasons. While fosphenytoin will not work any faster than phenytoin and is more expensive, it does not have the serious risk of tissue necrosis that phenytoin possesses upon extravasation into soft tissues and can be administered intramuscularly or intravenously.[96] Phenobarbital (15 to 20 mg per kilogram) can be used in children instead of phenytoin or fosphenytoin as a second-line antiepileptic agent. Phenobarbital carries a profound respiratory depressant effect and can also cause hypotension upon intravenous administration.[95] Careproviders must be prepared to treat hypotension and/or apnea subsequent to infusion of barbiturates or multiple doses of benzodiazepines to control seizure activity.

The etiology of seizures in children that are evacuated to a Combat Support Hospital after an acute injury is likely to be related to traumatic brain injury or hypoxic ischemic injury. A rapid-acting benzodiazepine such as lorazepam (0.1 mg per kilogram) or diazepam (0.2 mg per kilogram) should be administered intravenously as a first-line therapeutic agent if continued tonic-clonic seizure activity persists beyond one minute.

## Pediatric Advanced Life Support (PALS)

The Pediatric Advanced Life Support (PALS) course concepts have been developed to improve the recognition and treatment of cardiopulmonary failure in children. Early recognition of respiratory or cardiac failure and its reversal is obviously optimal. However, if a child arrests and cardiopulmonary resuscitation (CPR) is initiated, the following principles should be applied: the rate of cardiac compression should be 100 per minute, and full elastic recoil should occur with compressions to improve venous return into the thoracic cavity. Efficacy of CPR can be most effectively assessed by evaluating the diastolic pressure on the invasive arterial blood pressure monitor. The respiratory rate should not exceed 12 breaths per minute as hyperventilation will decrease venous return.[70] The differential diagnosis for all nonperfusing, bradycardic, and tachycardic rhythms include: hypoxemia, hypovolemia, hypothermia, hyper/hypokalemia, acidosis, tamponade physiology, tension pneumothorax, drug overdose, trauma, and thromboembolism.

> For a pediatric cardiac arrest, the cardiac compression rate should be 100 compressions per minute. Full elastic recoil of the chest should occur between compressions to improve venous return to the thoracic cavity. The respiratory rate should not exceed 12 breaths per minute as hyperventilation will decrease venous return.

## Cardiac Rhythm Disturbances

Treatment of cardiac rhythm disturbances must occur with the clinical context of the patient in mind. The treatment of pulseless electrical activity in the setting of hypovolemic shock due to traumatic hemorrhage will be futile unless concurrent efforts to restore blood volume and stop ongoing hemorrhage are undertaken. However, CCC providers should be familiar with standard therapies for the more commonly encountered cardiac rhythm

| Age (years) | Time |
|---|---|
| Infants to 3 | ≥ 80 milliseconds |
| 4 to 9 | > 80 milliseconds |
| 9 to 11 | > 90 milliseconds |
| 12 and above | > 100 milliseconds |

Table 6. *Definition of wide QRS complex based on patient's age.*

disturbances encountered in critically ill children. In reality, many cases will involve immediately initiating cardiac rhythm disturbance treatments while identifying and treating concurrent contributory medical conditions. It is important to note that the QRS complex is age-dependent. A wide QRS complex is defined as greater than or equal to 80 milliseconds in infants and young children up to age three years; greater than 80 milliseconds in children ages four to nine years; greater than 90 millseconds between ages nine and 11 years; and greater than 100 milliseconds in children age 12 and above (Table 6).[97,98]

> Combat casualty careproviders should be familiar with standard therapies for the more commonly encountered cardiac rhythm disturbances encountered in critically ill children.

### Asystole and Pulseless Electrical Activity

Rapid initiation of CPR should occur followed by 0.1 ml per kilogram of epinephrine (1:10,000) or 0.01 mg per kilogram of epinephrine IV injection every three to five minutes while attempting to reverse the cause of the arrest.[70]

## Pulseless Ventricular Tachycardia and Ventricular Fibrillation

Standard treatment includes the rapid initiation of CPR, then defibrillation at 2 joules per kilogram, another five cycles of CPR, defibrillation at 4 joules per kilogram, then epinephrine (1:10,000) 0.1 ml per kilogram IV, five cycles of CPR, defibrillate at 4 joules per kilogram, then amiodarone (5 mg per kilogram) IV, while attempting to identify and reverse the cause of the arrest.[70]

## Bradycardia with Poor Perfusion

Cardiopulmonary resuscitation should be initiated for a pulse rate less than 60 with poor perfusion, then epinephrine, atropine, and cardiac pacing should be considered while attempting to identify and reverse the cause of the arrest. Keep in mind that bradycardia is a very common manifestation of hypoxemia in children.[70] Conversely, bradycardia with good perfusion occurs with severe traumatic brain injury and herniation syndrome.

Bradycardia is a very common manifestation of hypoxemia in children.

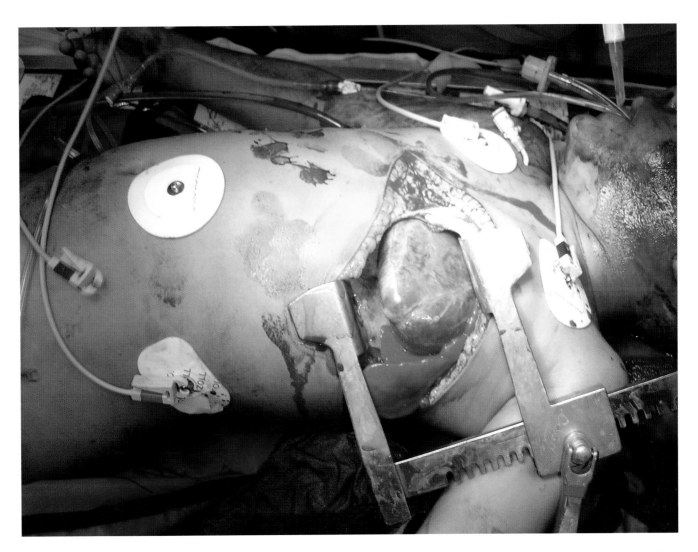

Figure 15. *The left anterior fifth intercostal space is used as the standard approach for resuscitative thoracotomies in pediatric patients, as in adults. Image courtesy of J. Christian Fox, MD, University of California, Irvine.*

## Narrow Complex (Supraventricular) Tachycardia

If good perfusion is noted, administer adenosine 0.1 mg per kilogram IV as a fast-push infusion. Since the half-life of adenosine is five seconds, the use of a three-way stopcock with another syringe in-line for a flush allows for rapid bolus administration. A repeat dose of adenosine at 0.2 mg per kilogram IV can be given if needed.[70] Amiodarone 5 mg per kilogram over 20 to 60 minutes can be used as a second-line agent in refractory cases. If poor perfusion is noted, synchronized cardioversion with 0.5 to 1 joules per kilogram is indicated followed by adenosine and amiodarone administration as indicated.[70]

## Wide Complex (Ventricular) Tachycardia

If good perfusion is noted, amiodarone, 5 mg per kilogram IV over 20 minutes should be administered. Administration of adenosine, 0.1 mg per kilogram IV fast-push can be considered in patients with adequate perfusion who are suspected of having supraventricular dysrhythmias with associated bundle branch block(s) resulting in wide complex QRS rhythms. If poor perfusion is noted, synchronized cardioversion of the patient with 0.5 to 1 joules per kilogram is indicated. This is followed by administration of amiodarone, and then adenosine as indicated.[70]

## *Surgical Considerations*

### Thoracic Interventions

Resuscitative thoracotomies are best done for penetrating trauma when vital signs have been present within minutes of patient arrival to the trauma suite (Fig. 15).[99] Resuscitative thoracotomies for blunt trauma are almost uniformly unsuccessful when vital signs have been lost prior to arrival in the trauma suite.[100] A left anterior fifth intercostal space is the approach most commonly employed during emergency resuscitative thoracotomy. Advantages of this approach include ease of access to the heart and great vessels. The disadvantage is that access to the lower lobes of the lung becomes more difficult. Regardless of the approach, Rummel tourniquets should be available on all resuscitative thoracotomy trays for children and infants (Fig. 16). This obviates the concern about the appropriate-sized vascular clamp. The other point unique to children is that pneumonectomies in the very young will lead to scoliosis and lack of chest wall development on that side (post-pneumonectomy syndrome).[101] Thus, trauma pneumonectomy should be considered only as a last resort. As in adults, the vast majority of chest trauma can be managed with either observation or tube thoracostomy alone.[102]

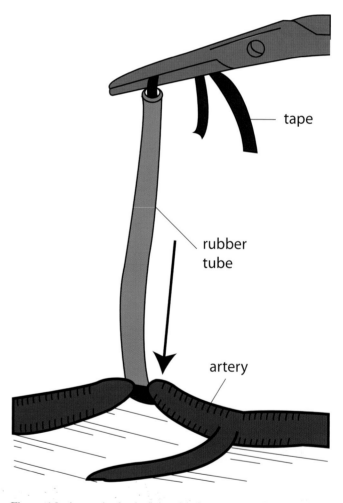

tape

rubber tube

artery

Figure 16. *Appropriately-sized vascular clamps are not always available in combat settings. As an alternative, Rummel tourniquets may be used for vascular control. A tourniquet is fashioned by passing umbilical tape around a vessel, threading both ends through a short rubber catheter, and securing with a perpendicularly placed hemostat.*

Resuscitative thoracotomies for penetrating trauma are most successful when vital signs have been present within minutes of patient arrival to the trauma suite. Resuscitative thoracotomies for blunt trauma are almost uniformly unsuccessful in patients arriving without signs of life.

## Abdominal Interventions

For children less than two years of age, a transverse laparotomy is thought to provide adequate exposure to the entire abdomen, has a lower dehiscence rate, and is generally the accepted approach for elective operations.[103] While this is true for elective operative cases, many surgeons would argue for an alternative incisional approach in the case of traumatic injury.[104] A midline laparotomy allows for supraceliac aortic control as well as iliac control with minimal changes in retraction (Fig. 17).[104] The approach should be dependent upon the mechanism and severity of the injury, as well as the hemodynamic instability of the patient.

Pediatric surgeons favor splenic salvage whenever possible. An important point in splenic preservation is complete mobilization of the spleen prior to addressing the hilum. The goal is to spare at least 30 percent of the spleen for immunologic function, as less than that will not yield a benefit.[105] Also, it is important to

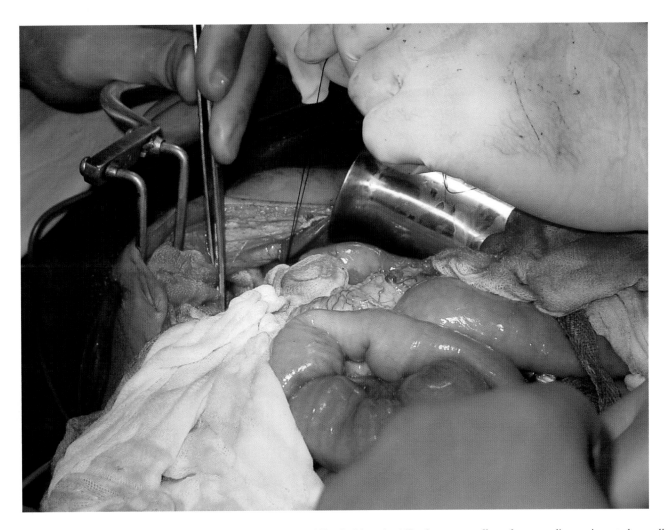

Figure 17. *Laparotomy in a 5-year-old male performed through a midline incision. A midline laparotomy allows for supraceliac aortic control as well as iliac control with minimal changes in retraction. Image courtesy of the Borden Institute, Office of The Surgeon General, Washington, DC.*

remember that associated injuries (especially head) represent relative contraindications to attempting nonoperative splenic preservation.

When dealing with a liver injury, the decision whether to pack or repair the injury is critical. Some advocate that this decision should be delayed until the liver has been fully mobilized. This requires division of both triangular ligaments as well as the falciform ligament from their respective diaphragmatic attachments. Only then can adequate compression be applied and the decision to pack versus repair be made. However, others are in favor of preserving ligamentous attachments to achieve more effective packing. If repair is attempted, blood flow to the liver needs to be temporarily controlled in order to prevent overwhelming blood loss.[106] The correct size of vascular clamps is not always available in the pediatric-aged population, thus Rummel tourniquets are extremely helpful to control the portal hilum as well as the hepatic veins, retrohepatic cava, and inferior vena cava in order to achieve complete vascular isolation of the liver.

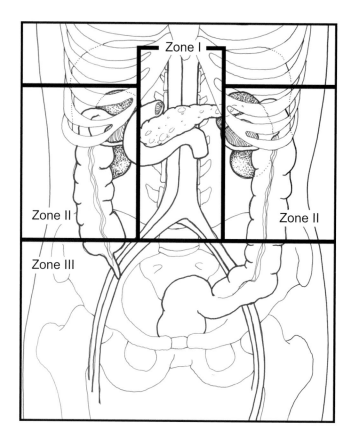

Figure 18. *Zones of the retroperitoneum. Image courtesy of the Borden Institute, Office of The Surgeon General, Washington, DC.*

While the surgical approach to retroperitoneal injuries (pancreas, duodenum, aorta) represents a chapter in and of itself, the following principles hold true. Prior to entering a zone I (central) retroperitoneal hematoma, vascular control of the aorta and vena cava, respectively, needs to be achieved (Fig. 18). For any central hematoma involving the duodenum or pancreas, a full Kocher maneuver to elevate the head of the pancreas and to inspect the posterior duodenum needs to be performed. This will assist in vascular control and allow for complete inspection of the head of the pancreas and duodenum. Finally, for all injuries requiring surgery for the pancreas and/or duodenum, wide drainage should be employed before closing the abdomen.

For traumatic injuries of the pancreas involving ductal disruption, there has been support for a nonoperative approach.[107] Operative intervention will necessitate full hospital and ancillary support (e.g., parenteral nutrition), prolonged hospitalization, and interventional radiology support to address complications.[108] If resources are at a premium, major pancreatic ductal disruptions need to be surgically corrected either with distal pancreatectomy or a Whipple procedure depending upon injury location. There has been a recent case report of a minimally invasive splenic preserving approach to pancreatic injury.[109] It is the authors' opinion that splenic preservation and a minimally invasive approach are not part of the algorithm for the operative management of severe pancreatic traumatic disruptions in a combat environment. The limited resources in most CCC environments make nonoperative management of such injuries difficult.

In the case of major penetrating duodenal injury, there is paucity in the literature of long-term outcomes or even large series in children. It is generally accepted that children tolerate primary duodenal repair better than their adult counterparts, and this needs to be considered if the head of the pancreas is spared in the face of a duodenal injury. This approach will decrease the operative time and eliminate the need for future intervention. However in the authors' opinion, when in a combat theater where total parenteral nutrition, intensive unit care, blood products, and preoperative factors such as the nutritional status and immunologic status of the patients are questionable, primary repair should either be avoided or performed in carefully selected patients. In the event of significant additional injuries (e.g., burns) that may affect healing, primary repair may give way to a more complex approach that involves isolation, exclusion, and drainage maneuvers that are well developed in adults.[110] These include pyloric exclusion proximal to a duodenal repair and gastrojejunostomy or tube externalization of the duodenum, t-tube decompression of the biliary system, gastrostomy, and jejunostomy with or without antrectomy and establishment of gastrointestinal continuity.[111]

When encountering intestinal perforations, the decision to exteriorize the injury or primarily repair it has its evidence-based background embedded in military history. Once again, there is a lack of evidence-based literature in children, so our practice relies on the adult experience. The state of the art has gone from initial primary repair, to exteriorization of all colon injuries, to a physiologic basis for our operative decisions.[112] The decision to perform colostomies or small intestinal stomas should be based upon the degree of hemodynamic instability, shock, and the presence of other injuries, rather than the degree of destruction of the colon or small intestine.[113]

Finally, the single most important decision when performing a trauma laparotomy is when and how to close. Deciding that any procedure is only for "damage control" is best done within the first 20 minutes of the procedure.[114,115] Children, like adults, do not tolerate abdominal compartment syndrome. Unlike adults, the physiologic response in children is not one of gradual and progressive hemodynamic compromise (i.e., decreased urine output, development of hypotension, response to volume and pressors, and then continued deterioration). Children often develop increased intraabdominal pressure with less overt signs and symptoms and then unexpectedly suffer a major cardiorespiratory event.[116] This may be due to the fact that abdominal compartment syndrome is underrecognized in children.

Monitoring of intraabdominal pressure and following a calculated splanchnic perfusion pressure has been useful in managing other models of abdominal compartment syndrome, specifically gastroschisis.[44] The placement of silon sheeting has been the traditional approach to this problem in congenital anomalies.[117] This is suboptimal in a traumatic situation where drainage and monitoring of the intraabdominal fluid has both diagnostic and therapeutic value. The development and use of the wound vacuum-assisted closure (V.A.C.®) devices or "trauma vac" have become a useful adjunct to control fascial contraction, allow for abdominal wall expansion, monitor for bleeding, manage fluids, and allow instant access for reoperation (Fig. 19).[118] In addition, the concern of increased morbidity

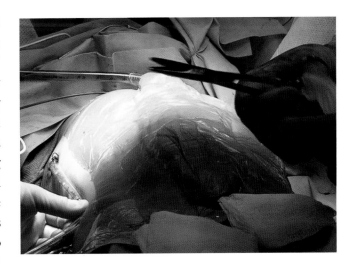

Figure 19. *Pediatric damage control laparotomy following fragmentation injuries from an IED blast. Given the susceptibility of children to abdominal compartment syndrome, the abdominal wall was left open and covered with a wound V.A.C.®*

from bowel fistulization has not been born out in the recent literature.[119] In the authors' opinion, use of this system alleviates the need for constant intraabdominal pressure monitoring and should be employed liberally as part of the damage control procedure in children. In addition, one can achieve a V.A.C.®-like closure with any sterile adhesive plastic drape, sponges, sterile plastic sheets, and a suction apparatus. These materials are typically available in a Combat Support Hospital.

> The single most important decision when performing a trauma laparotomy is when and how to close the abdomen. Deciding that any procedure is only for damage control is best done within the first 20 minutes of the procedure.

## Burn Care

Differences in burn care for children versus adults are minimal and predominantly involve fluid and nutritional management (Fig. 20). For children less than 30 kg, glucose should be added to the intravenous maintenance fluids that are in addition to the amount of fluid replacement calculated based upon the Parkland or any other formula that is used.[120] The body surface area burned is based upon second- and third-degree burns and can be estimated according to age-based charts.[120] In general, the size of the child's palm is equal to one percent of body surface area.[121]

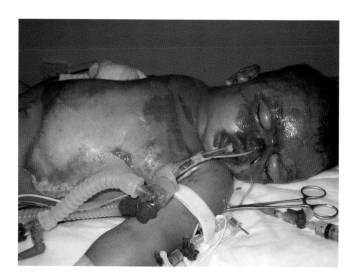

Figure 20. *Pediatric burn patient with injuries sustained from a civilian motor vehicle accident. The patient developed capillary leak syndrome, acute respiratory distress syndrome, and abdominal compartment syndrome.*

Both hyper- and hypoglycemia should be avoided. There is always a risk of over-resuscitating a patient with burn injuries when algorithmic fluid infusion and urine output alone are used to guide fluid replacement. Vital signs and hemodynamic parameters should also be utilized to determine the patient's intravascular volume status. The development of conditions associated with over-resuscitation such as acute respiratory distress syndrome or abdominal compartment syndrome should be closely monitored. It is critical to avoid over-resuscitation in a combat environment while remembering that most burns encountered in a combat environment are almost always associated with blast injuries. Thus underlying muscle damage causing myolysis and eventual renal failure are accentuated with low urine output states. Early excision and grafting for all nonviable skin are recommended. When dealing with large volume surface area burns, care must be taken to preserve all viable skin surface. The availability of artificial skin barriers and temporary skin coverage may be limited and the only viable grafting material may be the patient's surviving skin. Finally, transfer to a burn unit, while always the first option, may not be possible or available; thus, a clean environment needs to be established for the acute and chronic care of these patients.

> Differences in burn care for children versus adults are minimal and predominantly involve fluid and nutritional management. There is always a risk of over-resuscitating a patient with burn injuries when algorithmic fluid infusion and urine output alone are used to guide fluid replacement. Vital signs and hemodynamic parameters should also be utilized to determine the patient's intravascular volume status.

## Neurosurgical Interventions

### Forward Neurosurgical Care by Non-Neurosurgical Careproviders

Non-neurosurgical providers are increasingly tasked with the care of neurotrauma patients in a CCC environment. Unconventional warfare places children in harm's way, where the combination of their natural curiosity, disproportionate head size, and lack of protective equipment can lead to tragic results. Local geography, weather, tactical considerations, medical rules of engagement, and limited subspecialty availability often conspire to bring these casualties to the door of facilities staffed with non-neurosurgical careproviders. Caring for these patients is resource intensive and emotionally taxing for all members of the health care team. It requires both a clear understanding of coalition and host nation medical capabilities and advanced preparation on the part of providers and facilities.

While a complete review of forward neurosurgical care is beyond the scope of this chapter, careproviders should acquire technical and decision-making skills in neurotrauma prior to deployment. The training of non-neurosurgical personnel for this task is not a new concept, but surprisingly little progress has been made in this area since World War I.[122] However, past successes in civilian settings both in the United States and elsewhere speak to the potential of this approach.[123,124] Resources include formal courses, informal courses by local neurosurgical providers, and self-education through literature review.[125,126] While deployment may require a careprovider to reach into the periphery of clinical comfort zones, some lines are better not crossed. Each careprovider should carefully assess his or her ability to perform select critical neurosurgical interventions in a forward environment. Critical interventions include: (1) scalp closure; (2) ICP monitoring; and (3) limited craniectomy for extradural hemorrhage. Individual non-neurosurgical careproviders will need to decide whether they are competent to perform such procedures when clinically indicated in a forward environment. Palliative care remains a viable option for patients with devastating neurological injuries and is often the prudent course of action in a CCC environment with limited resources.

> Non-neurosurgical providers are increasingly tasked with the care of neurotrauma patients in a CCC environment. Careproviders should acquire technical and decision-making skills in neurotrauma prior to deployment. Critical interventions include: (1) scalp closure; (2) ICP monitoring; and (3) limited craniectomy for extradural hemorrhage.

| Additional Instruments | Suggested Disposables |
| --- | --- |
| • Raney clip applier | • Raney clips |
| • Hudson brace | • Gelfoam® |
| • Disposable perforator bit (Codman®) | • Thrombin™ |
| • Penfield dissectors #1, #4 | • Surgicel® |
| • Leksell rongeur, large | • Bone wax |
| • Kerrison rongeur, 3 mm or greater | • 35 cm-ventricular catheter with trochar |
| • Adson cerebellar retractor | • Lumbar drain catheter |
| • Bipolar cautery unit (if available) | • ICP monitor system |

Table 7. *Instruments typically available for neurosurgical interventions at a Level III facility.*

Local facility considerations are of paramount importance (Table 7). Medical rules of engagement, equipment availability, careprovider skill sets, imaging capabilities, and coalition and host nation medical assets all influence medical decision making in a deployed environment. Pediatric neurotrauma patients are particularly problematic from a disposition standpoint, as many resource-constrained nations are not equipped to provide supportive care for patients whose needs exceed the limited holding capabilities of deployed medical facilities. It is the responsibility of facility leadership to address these issues, prospectively if possible, and to ensure that care delivery does not place unsustainable burdens on host nation medical facilities. This may involve difficult ethical decisions that are among the most challenging aspects of deployment medical care.

### Surgical Management of Head Injuries

The principles of caring for adult and pediatric neurotrauma patients are more similar than different. However, the assessment and management of pediatric neurotrauma patients do provide unique challenges in the delivery of care.

### Triage and Initial Assessment

Good triage requires the timely consideration of pertinent clinical information about multiple casualties within the framework of resources available. In a deployed environment, this may result in decisions to delay or even withhold treatment that would be readily offered in a civilian environment. As host nation citizens, pediatric casualties must be treated with the intention to return them to host nation medical facilities within a timeframe that is compatible with the treating facility's holding capacity and mission.

Presenting neurologic status is consistently cited as a valuable tool in predicting outcome from both closed and penetrating head injuries.[127,128] A complete, concise neurologic assessment is therefore invaluable to the triage officer in evaluating salvageability of casualties in a deployed environment. In the authors' opinion, the presenting exam is the most valuable information available for determining prognosis of a casualty. For the exam to be valid, it must be obtained following appropriate resuscitation and in the absence of confounding medications including sedatives, hypnotics, analgesics, and muscle relaxants. This requires resuscitation to normotension, normothermia, and restoration of physiologic arterial oxygen and carbon dioxide pressures.

> Presenting neurologic status is consistently cited as a valuable tool in predicting outcomes following head injuries. For the exam to be valid, it must be obtained following appropriate resuscitation and in the absence of confounding medications including sedatives, hypnotics, analgesics, and muscle relaxants.

On occasion, some patients may require administration of appropriate weight-based medication reversal agents and twitch-monitor assessment to ensure pre-facility medications do not interfere with a baseline exam (Table 8). Reversal of medications with antiepileptic properties (e.g., benzodiazepines) in the setting of head injury may precipitate seizure activity, which would further secondary brain injury. Alternative approaches include providing supportive care pending metabolism and elimination of confounding medications.

Pupillary exam is an important indicator of outcome in civilian closed and penetrating head injuries. In the setting of epidural hematoma, latency to treatment exceeding 90 minutes after the development of

- Neostigmine (50 micrograms [mcg] per kilogram)
- Glycopyrrolate (10 mcg per kilogram)
- Naloxone (0.1 mg per kilogram)
- Flumazenil (10 mcg per kilogram)

Table 8. *Weight-based dosing of agents to assist with pharmacologic reversal of sedation/paralysis.*

| | GCS | PEDIATRIC GCS | INFANT FACE SCALE |
|---|---|---|---|
| **Eyes** | | | |
| 1 | No opening | No opening | No opening |
| 2 | Open to pain | Open to pain | Open to pain |
| 3 | Open to voice | Open to voice | Open to voice |
| 4 | Spontaneous | Spontaneous | Spontaneous |
| **Verbal** | | | |
| 1 | No response | No response | No facial expression to pain |
| 2 | Incomplete sounds | Inconsolable, agitated | Grimaces to pain |
| 3 | Inappropriate words | Inconsistently inconsolable | Cries to deep pain only |
| 4 | Confused | Cries, consolable | Cries to minor pain, alternating with sleep |
| 5 | Oriented | Smiles, tracks appropriately | Cries to minor pain, alternating with wakefulness |
| **Motor** | | | |
| 1 | No response | No response | Flaccid |
| 2 | Decerebrate | Decerebrate | Decerebrate |
| 3 | Decorticate | Decorticate | Abnormal rhythmic movements (seizure-like) |
| 4 | Flexion withdrawal | Withdraws to pain | Nonspecific movements to deep pain |
| 5 | Localization | Withdraws to touch | Hypoactive spontaneous movements |
| 6 | Follows commands | Purposeful | Normal spontaneous movements |

Table 9. *Modified scales of neurologic assessment in pediatric patients.*

anisocoria has been shown to correlate with dramatic increase in mortality.[129] In penetrating injury, bilaterally fixed and dilated pupils have been shown to be highly predictive of mortality.[130] Pupil responsiveness is an objective finding that is easily assessed regardless of patient age. A common misconception by careproviders is that muscle relaxants and paralytic medications (e.g., pancuronium) impair pupil responsiveness. They do not. Among medications frequently used during resuscitation in children, atropine and epinephrine are likely to impair pupillary responsiveness, with effects varying from minutes to several hours.[131]

Pupillary responsiveness is an objective finding that is easily assessed regardless of patient age and is an important indicator of outcome. Muscle relaxants and paralytic medications (e.g., pancuronium) do not impair pupillary responsiveness.

The Glasgow Coma Scale (GCS) is a highly effective tool in the assessment of neurotrauma patients. Developed to improve communication about the neurologic state of comatose patients, the GCS is an excellent predictor of neurologic outcome in head-injured patients.[132,133] Glasgow Coma Scale scores in preverbal children are more problematic due to immature motor pathways and limited or absent verbal skills on an age-related continuum. Alternative grading scales such as the pediatric GCS or Infant FACE Scale should be utilized in these patients (Table 9).[134]

Glasgow Coma Scale scores in pre-verbal children are problematic due to immature motor pathways and limited verbal skills. Alternative grading scales include the pediatric GCS or Infant FACE scales.

Neuroimaging, when available, is another valuable tool for patient triage. Computed tomography (CT) scanners are currently available at Level III facilities in both Afghanistan and Iraq (Fig. 21). Reliable forward imaging technology has been a major advance of the past decade. The Traumatic Data Coma Bank Classification Scale identified two findings that were consistently predictive of worsened neurologic outcome: compression or absence of patent basal cisterns and degree of midline shift (Fig. 22).[135] Additional anatomic information regarding relative distribution (lateralized versus diffuse pathology), location (intradural versus extradural and frontal/temporal/parietal), and reversibility of injuries can also be determined for both adult and

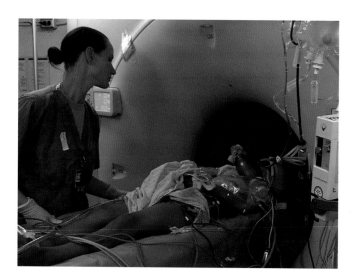

Figure 21. *CT scanners are currently available at Level III facilities in both Afghanistan and Iraq.*

pediatric patients by cranial CT. In the clinically unstable patient, ICP monitoring can also be used as a triage tool. Uncontrolled intracranial hypertension has been associated with a high rate of mortality and poor neurologic outcome.[136] Unstable patients undergoing emergent laparotomy/thoracotomy with suspected severe head injuries can undergo simultaneous ICP monitor placement, facilitating decisions on cessation of clinical efforts for overwhelming injuries. The authors employed the following algorithm in the management of pediatric head trauma patients in 2007 at a Level III facility with neurosurgical support and a two-week patient holding capacity (Table 10).

### Repair of Scalp Injuries

Early and aggressive treatment of scalp injuries is perhaps the most important technical skill for careproviders to acquire in the management of the forward head-injured patient (Fig. 23). Adequate exposure of injuries is essential, and aggressive shaving of the scalp is often required to fully identify what are frequently multiple injuries (Fig. 24). The value of routine practice of shaving scalp wounds has been questioned, and civilian studies have linked routine preoperative skin shaving with increased infection

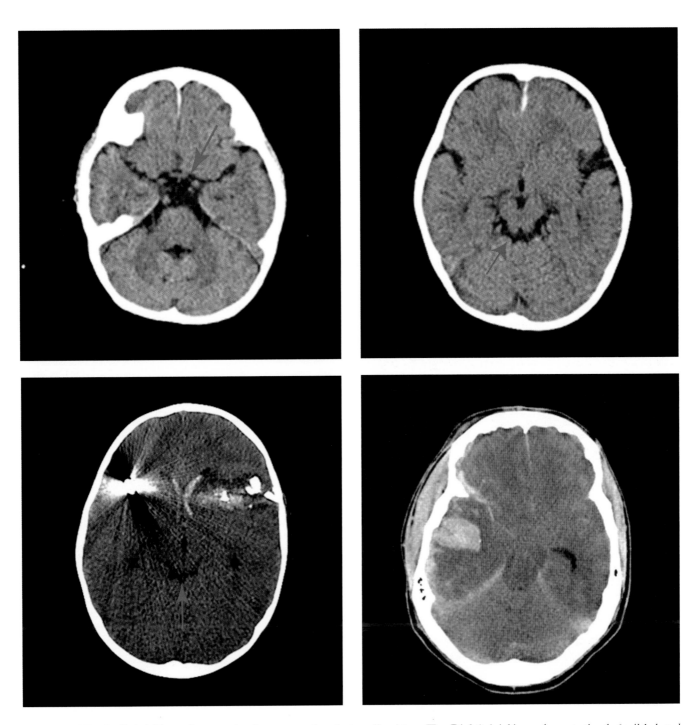

Figure 22. (Top Left) *Axial image demonstrating the pentagon-shaped suprasellar cistern.* (Top Right) *Axial image demonstrating the 'smile'-shaped quadrageminal plate cistern. Normal head CT demonstrating patency of basal cisterns in the setting of normal ICP. These small-volume spinal fluid spaces are excellent indirect markers of ICP.* (Bottom Left) *Despite trajectory of fragment across the midline and ventricular system, no midline shift is present and the basal cisterns remain patent. The patient required limited debridement only and was discharged from the hospital on post-injury day four.* (Bottom Right) *In this patient who suffered a blast-related injury, marked midline shift is present with effaced basal cisterns. Palliative care was elected, and the patient expired.*

1. **Assess Pupils**
   - Palliative care if *bilateral fixed and dilated pupils* or *unilateral fixed and dilated pupils* documented for greater than 90 minutes without signs of direct trauma to the globe

2. **Perform GCS Score or Age-Equivalent Assessment**
   - GCS scores 9 to 15 mandate aggressive intervention
   - GCS scores 6 to 8 consider intervention based on available resources. Imaging helpful in identifying favorable prognosis
   - GCS scores 3 to 5 indicate palliative care

3. **Review imaging if available**
   - Favorable prognosis: Basal cisterns patent, less than 1 centimeter midline shift, focal extraaxial mass lesion
   - Unfavorable prognosis: Basal cisterns effaced, greater than 1 centimeter midline shift, intraaxial hemorrhage, diffuse injury pattern

Table 10. *Suggested algorithm for neurosurgical triage at Level III facilities.*

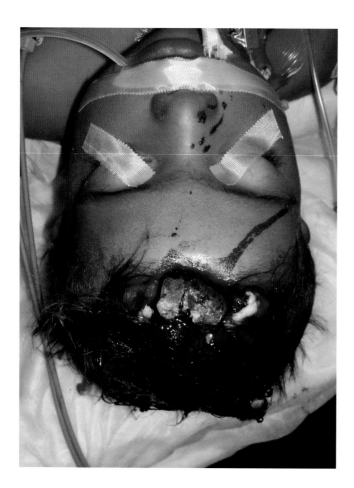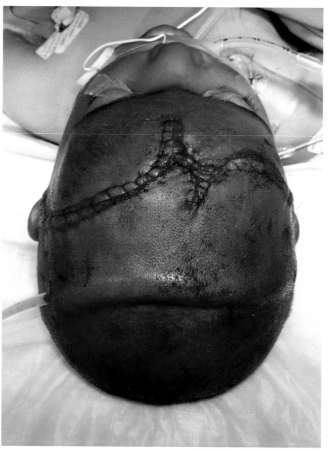

Figure 23. *Local advancement flaps to address scalp defect:* (Left) *One-year-old female with midfrontal penetrating fragment head injury.* (Right) *Opposing advancement flap closure of scalp defect performed after wide local shaving, exposure, and management of intracranial injury.*

rates.[137,138,139,140,141] In civilian practice, routine scalp shaving has given way to clipping, cutting hair with scissors, or using lubricant gel to congeal and move hair away from wound margins. The complex wound patterns seen in combat and difficulty identifying multiple scalp injuries are cited as reasons for shaving of the scalp to enable better wound bed visualization.

> Early and aggressive treatment of scalp injuries is perhaps the most important technical skill for careproviders to acquire in the management of the forward head-injured patient.

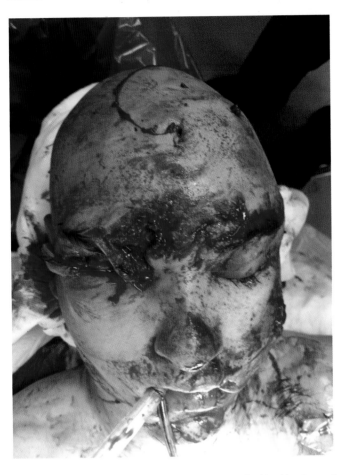

Figure 24. *Aggressive shaving of the scalp allows for identification and exposure of all injuries and is essential in the management of wartime penetrating head injuries.*

Judicious debridement techniques, identifying vascular pedicles, simple rotational and advancement flap techniques, and two-layer closure techniques (galea and skin) can be rapidly learned by all clinicians with even limited surgical skill. Excellent reviews of these techniques are readily available in the literature.[142] Scalp closure alone, as opposed to more extensive cranial operative intervention, is often the primary surgical intervention required to manage patients with low-velocity, fragmentary (e.g., shrapnel) penetrating head injuries.[143] For example, Taha et al. found that 32 such patients with a GCS score of 10 or higher, entry wounds less than two centimeters in size, and treated within six hours of injury who had negative CT scans for intracranial bleeding, did well with scalp wound closure alone in the emergency department.[143]

Pediatric patients with limited circulating blood volume are highly susceptible to hypovolemic shock from scalp injuries. Beyond common-sense measures such as the application of pressure, management of scalp lacerations associated with closed head injuries can be facilitated by the use of local vasoconstricting agents such as Xylocaine® (0.5% lidocaine with epinephrine 1:100,000), with weight-based lidocaine with epinephrine dosing not to exceed 7.5 mg per kilogram. Use of lidocaine in penetrating head injuries should be tempered by the potential for subarachnoid infusion with seizure induction. Simple hemostatic devices can also be utilized. Raney clips are widely available within surgical sets at Level III facilities (Fig. 25). They are of lower utility in infants and toddlers due to limited scalp thickness in these patients. Another technique is the application of Dandy clamps (hemostats) along the galea with the application of upward traction or reflection of the clamps outward.

> With smaller circulating blood volumes, pediatric patients are highly susceptible to hypovolemic shock from scalp injuries.

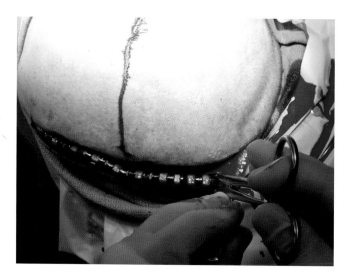

Figure 25. *Application of Raney clips to the scalp and galea is a valuable technique for hemostasis in the surgical management of head injuries.*

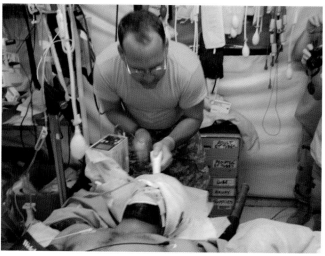

Figure 26. *Intracranial pressure monitoring systems can readily be inserted in an austere environment to assist with the diagnosis and management of the head-injured patient.*

## *Intracranial Pressure Monitoring*

Intracranial pressure monitors and intraventricular drainage catheters are powerful tools that provide valuable diagnostic information and therapeutic benefits for head-injured patients. Both parenchymal and fluid-coupled systems are currently available in the US military medical supply system (Fig. 26). The Codman® ICP EXPRESS (Codman, USA) is the standard intraparenchymal monitoring system utilized, while several vendors have 35-centimeter ventricular catheters with trochars available. Insertion techniques for these systems are easily taught to careproviders with basic surgical skills, and relative complication rates for insertion are low.[144] In the authors' experience, infection rates for intraventricular catheters placed in a field environment are high, and the choice for insertion of these catheters over parenchymal monitors should be weighed carefully. Appropriate indications for intraventricular catheter placement include management of refractory intracranial hypertension and spinal fluid leak.[39]

Intracranial pressure monitors and intraventricular drainage catheters are powerful tools that provide valuable diagnostic information and therapeutic benefits for head-injured patients. Insertion techniques for these systems are easily taught to careproviders with basic surgical skills, and relative complication rates for insertion are low.

While anatomic landmarks for insertion are identical to those used for adult patients, differences in scale between the two populations can lead to errors in the choice of insertion site resulting in preventable complications. The coronal suture is readily palpable in infants and toddlers. It is essential that the monitor or catheter be placed at or in front of this landmark and a minimum of two centimeters off of the midline to avoid the motor cortex and superior sagittal sinus, respectively (Fig. 27). The lateral edge of the anterior fontanelle is an acceptable point of entry in very young children. Regardless of patient age, parenchymal monitors should be placed to a depth of one to two centimeters. Ventricular catheters are inserted to depths along an age-based continuum: three to four centimeters in infants, four to five centimeters in toddlers, and five to six centimeters in older children and adults. When used for CSF drainage, replacing the volume removed (5 to 10 ml per hour on average) with 0.9% NaCl + 20 mEq KCl per liter to avoid hyponatremia and hypokalemia from solute loss in CSF has been recommended.[145]

# Landmarks for ICP monitor placement

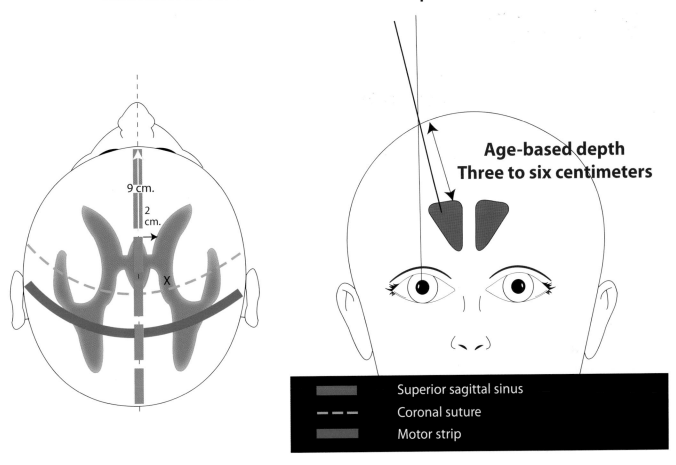

Figure 27. *Landmarks for insertion of intracranial monitoring systems. The drill hole should be placed two centimeters off of midline, just anterior to the coronal suture, to avoid the superior sagittal sinus and motor strip. In children over the age of five, the average distance posterior to the nasion is nine centimeters.*

## Management of Skull Fractures

Treatment of fractures along the skull convexity in a forward environment is limited to the care of associated injuries. Closed skull fractures without significant neurologic impairment such as so called ping-pong fractures in infants or minimally depressed fractures do not require specific treatment in a CCC environment (Fig. 28). Closed fractures are often encountered in combination with underlying intradural and extradural hemorrhage. Under those circumstances, surgical management may be appropriate as discussed later (see Management of Intradural and Extradural Hemorrhage).

Open skull fractures require irrigation and judicious debridement to remove devitalized tissue and reduce risks of infection. In the current environment of counterinsurgency warfare (OEF and OIF), most of these injuries are the result of low-velocity projectiles. Aggressive debridement and watertight dural closure were advocated in the past.[146] This form of management is unnecessary for most low-velocity projectile injuries encountered in OEF and OIF. Long-term follow-up of patients who underwent wide margin, aggressive debridement of embedded bone fragments has not been demonstrated to reduce infection and is technically more challenging for non-neurosurgical providers.[147] Attempts at watertight

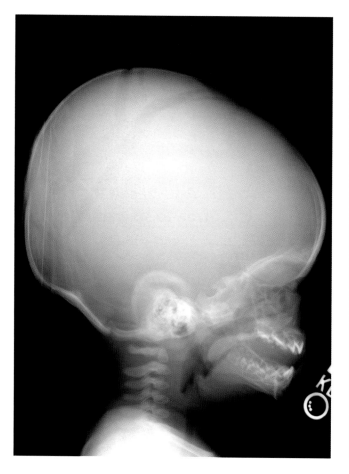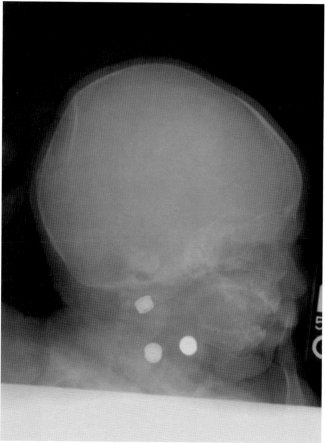

Figure 28. (Left) *Linear skull fracture.* (Right) *Ping-pong fracture.*

dural closure can add significant time to the surgical intervention, and in the authors' opinion, is not required for supratentorial injuries. Onlay dural substitutes (DuraGen® Dural Graft Matrix, Integra Neurosciences) are widely available for the coverage of these injuries. Complete coverage of any dural defect with this material followed by meticulous scalp closure is acceptable in such patients.

> Open skull fractures require irrigation and judicious debridement to remove devitalized tissue and reduce infection risk. Antibiotic administration following open fractures with embedded fragments is controversial, and no standard guidelines regarding either choice or duration of antibiotic therapy exist.

Antibiotic coverage for open fractures with embedded fragments is controversial. No standard guidelines regarding either choice or duration of antibiotic therapy exist.[130] The presence of both gram-positive and gram-negative organisms in abscesses resulting from penetrating head injuries has resulted in widespread use of broad-spectrum coverage for three days to two weeks by some practitioners.[148] Single agent gram-positive antibiotic therapy has been shown to be effective in reducing wound infection rates following open skull fractures.[143] In the authors' experience, patients receiving prompt care with debridement and layered closure without subsequent CSF leakage did well with a single dose of an appropriately selected antibiotic (based on local resistance patterns) against skin flora.

Fractures or penetration of the anterior or lateral skull base carry additional risks of spinal fluid leakage and subsequent infection (Fig. 29).[149] Pediatric patients harbor a lower risk of spinal fluid leakage from

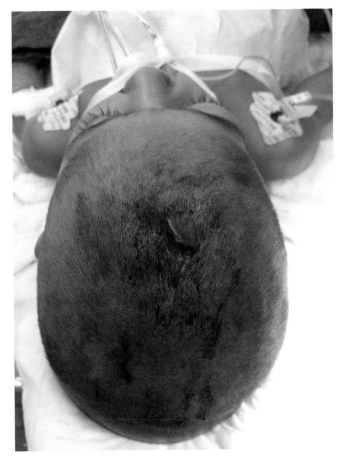

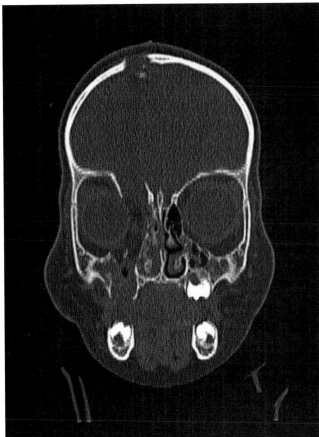

Figure 29. *Penetrating injuries involving the anterior skull base:* (Top Left) *Vertex view of the scalp in a child impaled with rebar rod. Note the site of penetration and mild proptosis of the right eye.* (Top Right) *Coronal CT reconstruction demonstrating penetrating injury extending through the right frontal bone, orbital roof, and maxilla.* (Bottom Right) *Intraoperative photograph following right frontal craniotomy demonstrating penetration of the floor of the anterior cranial fossa.*

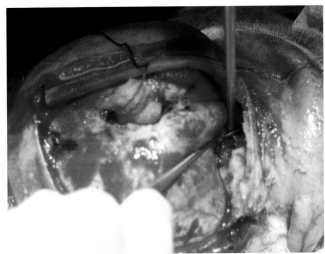

injuries to the anterior cranial fossa due to age-related pneumatization of the paranasal sinuses, which is complete by the mid-teens.[150] When CSF leaks do occur, conservative management through head elevation is advocated. Inflammation following the initial injury may result in closure of a persistent CSF fistula; therefore, time may be all that is needed in this circumstance. In the authors' opinion, prophylactic antibiotics for spinal leaks should be avoided, since it may increase the risk of selecting out resistant organisms without any known benefit. Refractory spinal fluid leaks in pediatric patients are not acute medical issues and require subspecialty consultation for management with a trial of lumbar drainage or surgical management by craniotomy and/or sinus exenteration. While leptomeningeal cysts or growing skull fractures can result from open fractures with dural disruption in infants and toddlers, they are a more chronic concern that is beyond the scope of deployed medical elements.[151]

Fracture or penetration of the anterior or lateral skull base carries an additional risk of CSF leakage and subsequent infection. Cerebrospinal fluid leaks are conservatively managed. Refractory CSF leaks in pediatric patients are not acute medical issues and require subspecialty consultation for management with a trial of lumbar drainage or surgical management by craniotomy and/or sinus exenteration.

### Management of Intradural and Extradural Hemorrhage

Indications for performance of a limited craniotomy or craniectomy by a non-neurosurgical provider on a pediatric patient in a deployed environment are limited. The treatment of intradural injuries (e.g., subdural hematoma and intraparenchymal hemorrhage) requires advanced surgical training and clinical experience (Fig. 30). The surgical management of such injuries is beyond the scope of practice of forward non-neurosurgical CCC providers. On occasion, events may conspire to place a well-prepared careprovider in the presence of an acutely deteriorating patient with clinical or radiologic findings supportive of an underlying epidural hematoma (Fig. 31). A clinically significant extradural hemorrhage is one form of injury likely to benefit from surgical intervention by non-neurosurgical careproviders under these circumstances.[152]

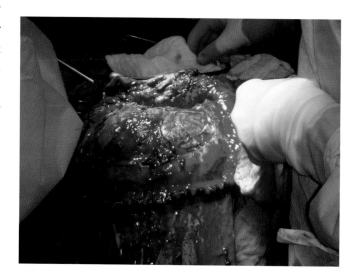

Figure 30. *Intradural neurotrauma surgery poses significant operative challenges to the inexperienced careprovider.*

Techniques for expedient craniotomy/craniectomy are similar between pediatric and adult patients. Patients are positioned supine with a bolster under the ipsilateral shoulder and hip with the head in a gel roll or equivalent. Generous hair removal assists with visualization of landmarks. Scalp opening should be well controlled and minimized to reduce blood loss. In the case of image confirmed epidural hemorrhage, placement of a burr hole over the site of injury followed by enlargement with rongeurs is both technically easier to accomplish and more expedient than turning a bone flap (Fig. 32). Exploratory burr holes can be performed with enlargement if a bloodclot is identified at the operative site. Complete removal of the hemorrhage is not essential; decompression of the hemorrhage is usually sufficient to resolve acute neurologic changes. Use of a Hemovac® or Jackson-Pratt® drain under the scalp is useful to prevent blood reaccumulation.

## Spinal Injuries

### Closed Injuries

Management of closed pediatric spinal injuries in a deployed environment is primarily nonoperative. While spinal instrumentation and intraoperative fluoroscopy are available at select deployed facilities,

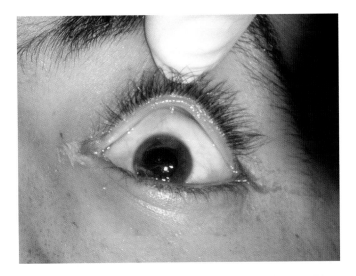

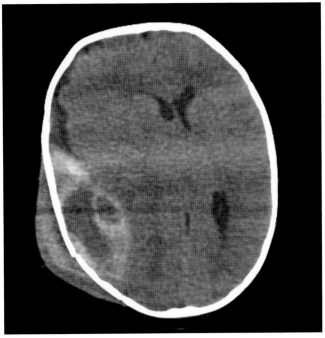

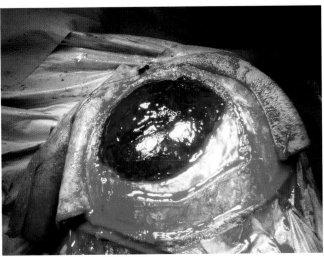

Figure 31. *Epidural hematoma:* (Top Left) *In the patient harboring an epidural hematoma, impaired neurologic examination including pupillary asymmetry and GCS of 9 or less are independent predictors of poor outcomes.* (Top Right) *CT scan demonstrating a large right parietal epidural hematoma in a toddler. Note the mixed density of the collection indicative of active hemorrhage and marked midline shift.* (Bottom Left) *Intraoperative image demonstrating a large epidural hematoma following removal of the overlying calvarial bone.*

most injuries can be managed locally with more modest resources. The majority of closed spinal column injuries are biomechanically stable. In a neurologically intact patient, upright and weight-bearing films can establish the stable nature of these injuries. For the patient with neurologic impairment or unstable fracture, forward facilities are poorly equipped to deal with short- or long-term issues faced by these patients. Realistic goals include restoration of anatomic alignment and immobilization.

Management of closed pediatric spinal injuries in a deployed environment is primarily nonoperative. Forward facilities are poorly equipped to deal with short- or long-term issues faced by patients with neurologic impairment or unstable fractures. Realistic goals include restoration of anatomic alignment and immobilization.

Gardner-Wells tongs are available in surgical sets for Level III facilities; they are a low-cost means of obtaining or maintaining alignment in the cervical spine (Fig. 33). In children older than two years of age, application is identical to adult patients. When utilized appropriately, torque application should not result in penetration of the skull in these patients.[153] In the authors' experience, less weight is generally required to achieve reduction: two pounds (lbs) per level compared to five to 10 lbs in adult patients. Immobilization can be achieved with bedrest for thoracolumbar fractures, or with appropriately-sized commercial collars for cervical spine fractures. In the absence of appropriate collar sizes, field-expedient

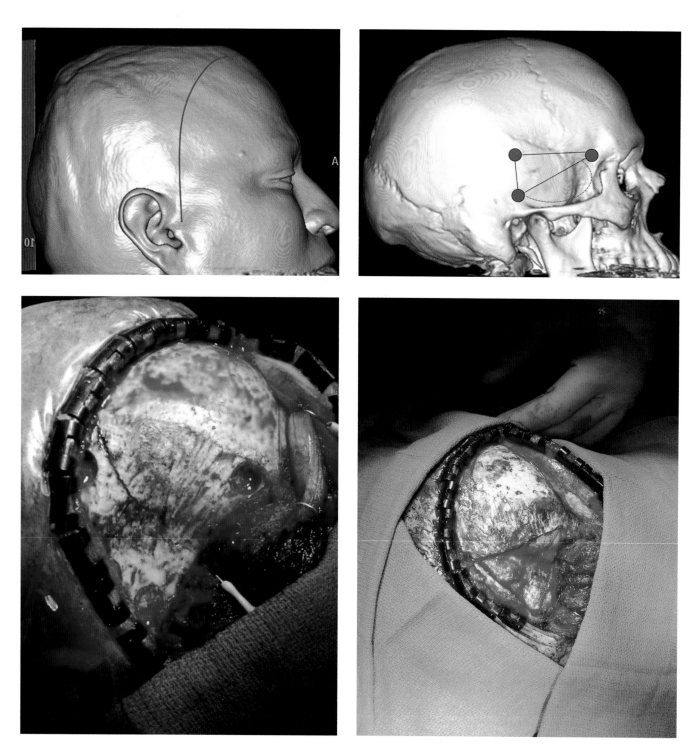

Figure 32. *Damage control craniectomy. Extradural hemorrhage localized or extending into the middle cranial fossa is an ideal indication for this procedure.* (Top Left) *The scalp incision extends from the root of the zygoma toward the frontal hairline. The incision extends through the underlying temporalis fascia to expose the lateral surface of the middle cranial fossa.* (Top Right) *Schematic of burr hole sites for middle fossa craniectomy. Note location of posterior-inferior burr hole immediately above the zygomatic root. Craniectomy proceeds between burr holes and extends anteriorly along the greater wing of the sphenoid as indicated.* (Bottom Left) *Burr hole placed by a non-neurosurgical provider. Note fracture line that resulted in underlying intracranial injury.* (Bottom Right) *Image following completion of craniectomy and evacuation of local epidural hemorrhage. This craniectomy is ideally located low in the middle cranial fossa resulting in relief of brainstem compression along the medial aspect of the affected temporal lobe.*

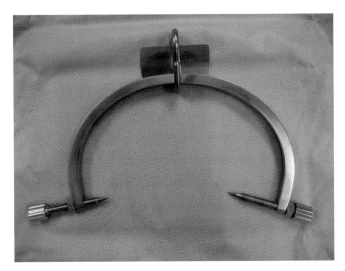

Figure 33. (Left) *Gardner-Wells tongs are a simple device capable of assisting with the stabilization and reduction of cervical spinal column injuries.*

Figure 34. (Below) *Thecal sac ligation following penetrating injuries to the spine. Blast injuries can result in massive tissue loss with devastating injuries to the spinal axis and thecal sac. In this case, an IED blast caused extensive destruction of the dorsal elements of the lumbar spine and dura. The ventral surface of the dura is indicated by the arrow. A staged, collaborative surgical approach allowed for ligation of the thecal sac to prevent spinal fluid leak, staged debridement, and spinal stabilization and flap-assisted wound closure.*

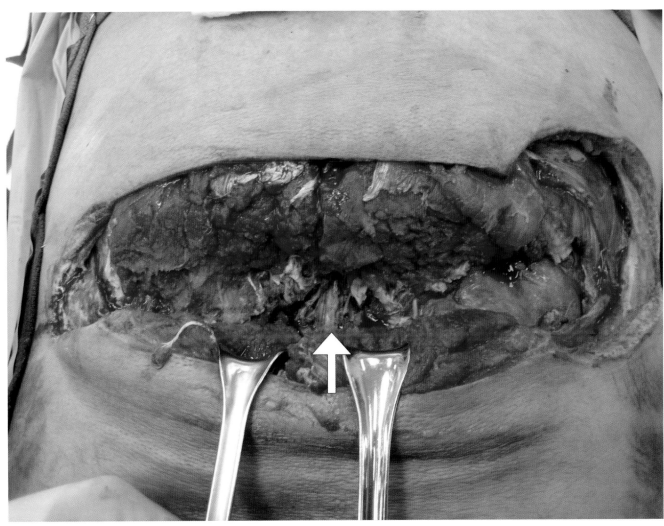

collars can be custom contoured with SAM® SPLINTS or other materials. Pediatric-sized halo vests are rarely available in a deployed environment. In the exceptional case that an appropriately-sized vest is available, application differs from adult patients in the number of pins used and torque applied.[154] Six to eight pins with an applied torque of four inch-pounds (in-lbs) are sufficient to secure the halo ring in children aged two through eight years of age. Adult application guidelines can be used in children age nine and above.

## Penetrating (Open) Injuries

The acute management of penetrating injuries of the spine mirrors that of adult patients with these injuries. Depending on the trajectory of the projectile, abdominal and thoracic injuries are addressed first. Antibiotic therapy is tailored to the individual needs of injuries in these adjacent compartments. Penetrating injuries rarely produce acute spinal instability; however, children with neurologic impairment are at high risk for developing late spinal deformity.[155,156] Such concerns are beyond the capabilities of forward CCC providers.

> The acute management of penetrating injuries of the spine mirrors that of adult patients with similar injuries. Depending on the trajectory of the projectile, abdominal and thoracic injuries are addressed first. Penetrating injuries rarely produce acute spinal instability. Local debridement and wound closure are appropriate at the time of presentation. Massive injuries with extensive tissue loss and spinal cord avulsion are best managed through ligation of the thecal sac.

Local debridement and wound closure are appropriate at the time of presentation. Cerebrospinal fluid fistulae, either externally or into adjacent cavities such as the thorax, are infrequent but challenging problems. Massive injuries with extensive tissue loss and spinal cord avulsion are best managed through ligation of the thecal sac (Fig. 34). In injuries with less tissue destruction, visualization of the leak is more limited. It is the authors' opinion and experience that local tissue patch with external spinal fluid diversion is a rapid and technically less demanding option for these patients. Lumbar drainage systems are available through the military supply system and are an invaluable adjunct for such patients. Catheters can be placed at the time of exploration, or percutaneously by anesthesia providers at the L4 to L5 interspace when the fistula is recognized in patients as young as two years of age. It is the authors' opinion and experience that height-controlled drainage of 10 to 15 ml per hour is usually sufficient to stop the flow of spinal fluid with closure of the fistula within 72 hours in most cases.

## End-of-Life Care

While children are very resilient, there are times when enough is enough and it is more appropriate to halt the resuscitation or to recognize that certain wounds are not treatable and further care is futile. In these circumstances, treatment should be focused on providing the appropriate level of pain relief and comfort. It is often very hard for practitioners to recognize when care is futile in children since the death of a child is a very emotional event. The medical team needs to remain objective and truly balance the benefits and risks of treating certain injuries with providing comfort care if the wounds are lethal or severely neurologically debilitating. Balancing what you can do for a child with what can be handled medically in the host nation is a very difficult task, but this dichotomy must be recognized.

# References

1. Burnett MW, Spinella PC, Azarow KS, et al. Pediatric care as part of the US Army medical mission in the global war on terrorism in Afghanistan and Iraq, December 2001 to December 2004. Pediatrics 2008;121(2):261-265.

2. Coppola CP, Leininger BE, Rasmussen TE, et al. Children treated at an expeditionary military hospital in Iraq. Arch Pediatr Adolesc Med 2006;160(9):972-976.

3. McGuigan R, Spinella PC, Beekley A, et al. Pediatric trauma: experience of a combat support hospital in Iraq. J Pediatr Surg 2007;42(1):207-210.

4. Patel TH, Wenner KA, Price SA, et al. A U.S. Army Forward Surgical Team's experience in Operation Iraqi Freedom. J Trauma 2004;57(2):201-207.

5. Spinella PC, Borgman MA, Azarow KS. Pediatric trauma in an austere combat environment. Crit Care Med 2008;36(7 Suppl):S293-296.

6. Creamer KM, Edwards MJ, Shields CH, et al. Pediatric wartime admissions to US military combat support hospitals in Afghanistan and Iraq: learning from the first 2000 admissions. J Trauma 2009;67(4):762-768.

7. Matos RI, Holcomb JB, Callahan C, et al. Increased mortality of young children with traumatic injuries at a US Army combat support hospital in Baghdad, Iraq, 2004. Pediatrics 2008;122(5):e959-966.

8. Wheeler M, Cote CJ, Todres D. A Practice of Anesthesia for Infants and Children. 3rd ed: W.B. Saunders; 2001.

9. Antosia RE, Cahill JD. Evaluation and management of pediatric disaster victims. In: Weiner D, Nigrovic Manzi S, Shannon MW, editors. Handbook of bioterrorism and disaster medicine. New York, NY: Springer US; 2006. p. 369-374.

10. Luten RC, Zaritsky A, Wears R, et al. The use of the Broselow tape in pediatric resuscitation. Acad Emerg Med 2007;14(5):500-501.

11. Weber T. Uncuffed tubes should continue to be used in pediatric anesthesia. Pediatr Anesth 2009;19(S1):46-49.

12. Deakers TW, Reynolds G, Stretton M, et al. Cuffed endotracheal tubes in pediatric intensive care. J Pediatr 1994;125(1):57-62.

13. Silva MJ, Aparício J, Mota T, et al. Ischemic subglottic damage following a short-time intubation. Eur J Emerg Med 2008;15(6):351-353.

14. Weiss M, Dullenkopf A, Fischer JE, et al. Prospective randomized controlled multi-centre trial of cuffed or uncuffed endotracheal tubes in small children. Br J Anaesth 2009;103(6):867-873.

15. Ravussin P, Bayer-Berger M, Monnier P, et al. Percutaneous transtracheal ventilation for laser endoscopic procedures in infants and small children with laryngeal obstruction: report of two cases. Can J Anaesth 1987;34(1):83-86.

16. Smith RB, Myers EN, Sherman H. Transtracheal ventilation in paediatric patients; case reports. Br J Anaesth 1974; 46(4):313-314.

17. Patel RG. Percutaneous transtracheal jet ventilation: a safe, quick, and temporary way to provide oxygenation and ventilation when conventional methods are unsuccessful. Chest 1999;116(6):1689-1694.

18. Eleraky MA, Theodore N, Adams M, et al. Pediatric cervical spine injuries: report of 102 cases and review of the literature. J Neurosurg 2000;92:(1 Suppl)12-17.

19. Plauche WC. Subgaleal hematoma: a complication of instrumental delivery. JAMA 1980;244(14):1597-1598.

20. Kendall N, Woloshin H. Cephalhematoma associated with fracture of the skull. J Pediatr 1952;41(2):125-132.

21. Kozinn PJ, Ritz ND, Moss AH, et al. Massive hemorrhage-scalps of newborn infants. Am J Dis Child. 1964;108(4):413-417.

22. Benaron DA. Subgaleal hematoma causing hypovolemic shock during delivery after failed vacuum extraction: a case report. J Perinatol 1993;13(3):228-231.

23. Kırımi E, Tuncer O, Atas B, et al. Hyperkalemia most likely associated with massive cephalhematoma in a newborn infant who was treated with urgent peritoneal dialysis: case report. J Emerg Med 2003;24(3):277-279.

24. Lustrin ES, Karakas SP, Ortiz AO, et al. Pediatric cervical spine: normal anatomy, variants, and trauma. Radiographics 2003;23(3):539-560.

25. Menezes AH, Traynelis VC. Anatomy and biomechanics of normal craniovertebral juntion (a) and biomechanics of stabilization (b). Childs Nerv Syst 2008;24(10):1091-1100.

26. Lovelock JE, Schuster JA. The normal posterior atlantoaxial relationship. Skeletal Radiol 1991;20(2): 121-123.

27. Swischuk LE. Anterior displacement of C2 in children: physiologic or pathologic. Radiology 1977;122(3):759-763.

28. Sanderson SP, Houten JK. Fracture through the C2 synchondrosis in a young child. Pediatr Neurosurg 2002;36(5):277-278.

29. Hill SA, Miller CA, Kosnik EJ, et al. Pediatric neck injuries. A clinical study. J Neurosurg 1984;60(4): 700-706.

30. Launay F, Leet AI, Sponseller PD. Pediatric spinal cord injury without radiographic abnormality: a meta-analysis. Clin Orthop Relat Res 2005;433:166-170.

31. Pang D. Spinal cord injury without radiographic abnormality in children, 2 decades later. Neurosurgery 2004;55(6):1325-1342; discussion 1342-1343.

32. Bracken MB, Shepard MJ, Collins WF et al. A randomized, controlled trial of methylprednisolone or naloxone in the treatment of acute spinal cord injury. Results of the Second National Acute Spinal Cord Injury Study. N Engl J Med 1990;322(20):1405-1411.

33. Nesathurai S. Steroids and spinal cord injury: revisiting the NASCIS 2 and NASCIS 3 trials. J Trauma 1998;45(6):1088-1093.

34. Sartorellia KH, Vane DW. The diagnosis and management of children with blunt injury of the chest. Semin Pediatr Surg 2004;13(2):98-105.

35. Dykes EH. Paediatric trauma. Br J Anaesth 1999;83(1):130-138.

36. Lloyd DA, Carty H, Patterson M, et al. Predictive value of skull radiography for intracranial injury in children with blunt head injury. Lancet 1997;349(9055):821-824.

37. Boniol M, Verriest JP, Pedeux R, et al. Proportion of skin surface area of children and young adults from 2 to 18 years old. J Invest Dermatol 2008;128(2):461-464.

38. 2005 American Heart Association Guidelines for Cardiopulmonary Resuscitation and Emergency Cardiovascular Care. Part 11: Pediatric Basic Life Support. Circulation 2005;112:IV-156-166.

39. Adelson PD, Bratton SL, Carney NA, et al. Guidelines for the acute medical management of severe traumatic brain injury in infants, children, and adolescents. Chapter 10. The role of cerebrospinal fluid drainage in the treatment of severe pediatric traumatic brain injury. Pediatr Crit Care Med 2003;4(3 Suppl):S38-39.

40. Falke KJ, Pontoppidan H, Kumar A, et al. Ventilation with end-expiratory pressure in acute lung disease. J Clin Invest 1972;51(9):2315-2323.

41. Marini JJ, Ravenscraft SA. Mean airway pressure: physiologic determinants and clinical importance—Part 2: Clinical implications. Crit Care Med 1992;20(11):1604-1616.

42. Ejike JC, Bahjri K, Mathur M. What is the normal intra-abdominal pressure in critically ill children and how should we measure it? Crit Care Med 2008;36(7):2157-2162.

43. Jensen AR, Hughes WB, Grewal H. Secondary abdominal compartment syndrome in children with

burns and trauma: a potentially lethal complication. J Burn Care Res 2006;27(2):242-246.

44. McGuigan RM, Mullenix PS, Vegunta R, et al. Splanchnic perfusion pressure: a better predictor of safe primary closure than intraabdominal pressure in neonatal gastroschisis. J Pediatr Surg 2006;41(5):901-904.

45. Roberts JD, Cronin JH, Todres DI. A practice of anesthesia for infants and children. In: Cote CJ, editor. Neonatal emergencies. New York: McGraw-Hill; 2010. p. 294.

46. US Department of Defense (US DoD). Pediatric Care. In: Emergency War Surgery. Third United States Revision. Washington, DC: Department of the Army, Office of the Surgeon General, Borden Institute; 2004. p. 33.1-33.8.

47. Choong K, Kho ME, Menon K, et al. Hypotonic versus isotonic saline in hospitalised children: a systematic review. Arch Dis Child 2006;91(10):828-835.

48. Gunn VL, Nechyba C. Fluids and electrolytes. In: The Harriet Lane handbook. 16th ed. Philadelphia, PA: Elsevier Mosby; 2002. p.233-253.

49. Taketomor CK, Hodding JH, Kraus DM. Lexi-Comp's Pediatric Dosage Handbook. 13th ed. Hudson, OH: Lexi-Comp; 2006-2007.

50. Deitch EA, Ma WJ, Ma L, et al. Protein malnutrition predisposes to inflammatory-induced gut-origin septic states. Ann Surg 1990;211(5):560–567; discussion 567-568.

51. Albina JE. Nutrition and wound healing. J Parenter Enteral Nutr 1994;18(4):367-376.

52. Havalad S, Quaid MA, Sapiega V. Energy expenditure in children with severe head injury: lack of agreement between measured and estimated energy expenditure. Nutr Clin Pract 2006;21(2):175-181.

53. Mehta N, Leticia C. Nutrition in the critically ill child. In: Fuhrman BP, Zimmerman JJ, editors. Pediatric critical care. 3rd ed. Philadelphia, PA: Elsevier Mosby; 2006. p. 1076.

54. Diaz SM, Rodarte A, Foley J, et al. Pharmacokinetics of dexmedetomidine in postsurgical pediatric intensive care unit patients: preliminary study. Pediatr Crit Care Med 2007;8(5):419-424.

55. Losek JD. Hypoglycemia and the ABC'S (sugar) of pediatric resuscitation. Ann Emerg Med 2000;35(1):43-46.

56. Papastamelos C, Panitch HB, England SE, et al. Developmental changes in chest wall compliance in infancy and early childhood. J Appl Physiol 1995;78(1):179-184.

57. Spinella PC, Priestley MA. Damage control mechanical ventilation: ventilator induced lung injury and lung protective strategies in children. J Trauma 2007;62(6 Suppl):S82-83.

58. Gunn VL, Nechyba C. The Harriet Lane handbook. 16th ed. Philadelphia, PA: Elsevier Mosby; 2002.

59. Cook RD. Neuromuscular blocking agents. In: Fuhrman BP, Zimmerman JJ, editors. Pediatric critical care. 3rd ed. Philadelphia, PA: Elsevier Mosby; 2006. p. 1729-1747.

60. Lev R, Rosen P. Prophylactic lidocaine use preintubation: a review. J Emerg Med 1994;12(4):499-506.

61. Wysowski DK, Pollock ML. Reports of death with the use of propofol (Diprivan) for nonprocedural (long-term) sedation and literature review. Anesthesiology 2005;105(5):1047-1051.

62. Corbett SM, Montoya ID, Moore FA. Propofol-related infusion syndrome in intensive care patients. Pharmacotherapy 2008;28(2):250-258.

63. Bray RJ. Propofol infusion syndrome in children. Pediatr Anaesth 1998;8(6):491-499.

64. Murdoch SD, Cohen AT. Propofol-infusion syndrome in children. Lancet 1999;353(9169):2074-2075.

65. Okamoto MP, Kawaguchi DL, Amin AN. Evaluation of propofol infusion syndrome in pediatric intensive care. Am J Health Syst Pharm 2003;60(19):2007-2014.

66. Wratney AT, Cheifetz IM. Gases and drugs used in support of the respiratory system. In: Slonim AD, Pollack MM, editors. Pediatric Critical Care Medicine. Philadelphia, PA: Lippincott Williams & Wilkins; 2006. p. 717-729.

67. Pryor JA. Physiotherapy for airway clearance in adults. Eur Respir J 1999;14(6):1418-1424.

68. Rossman CM, Waldes R, Sampson D, et al. Effect of chest physiotherapy on the removal of mucus in patients with cystic fibrosis. Am Rev Respir Dis 1982;126(1):131-135.

69. Robinson M, Regnis JA, Bailey DL, et al. Effect of hypertonic saline, amiloride and cough on mucociliary clearance in patients with cystic fibrosis. Am J Respir Crit Care Med 1996;153(5):1503-1509.

70. 2005 American Heart Association Guidelines for Cardiopulmonary Resuscitation and Emergency Cardiovascular Care. Part 12: Pediatric Advanced Life Support. Circulation 2005;112:IV-167-187.

71. Heinz P, Geelhoed GC, Wee C, et al. Is atropine needed with ketamine sedation? A prospective, randomised, double blind study. Emerg Med J 2006;23(3):206–209.

72. Green SM, Roback MG, Krauss B. Anticholinergics and ketamine sedation in children: a secondary analysis of atropine versus glycopyrrolate. Acad Emerg Med 2010;17(2):157-162.

73. Brown L, Christian-Kopp S, Sherwin TS, et al. Adjunctive atropine is unnecessary during ketamine sedation in children. Acad Emerg Med 2008;15(4):314-318.

74. Walls RM. Rapid Sequence Intubation. In: Walls RM, Murphy MF, editors. Manual of emergency airway management. 3rd ed. Philadelphia, PA: Lippincott Williams & Wilkins; 2008. p. 23-35.

75. Buck ML, Wiggins BS, Sesler JM. Intraosseous drug administration in children and adults during cardiopulmonary resuscitation. Ann Pharmacother 2007;41(10):1679-1686.

76. Johnson L, Kissoon N, Fiallos M, et al. Use of intraosseous blood to assess blood chemistries and hemoglobin during cardiopulmonary resuscitation with drug infusions. Crit Care Med 1999;27(6):1147-1152.

77. Peutrell JM. Intrasosseous cannulation. Anaesth Intensive Care Med 2006;7(1):28-30.

78. Nylund CM, Borgman MA, Holcomb JB, et al. Thromboelastography to direct the administration of recombinant activated factor VII in a child with traumatic injury requiring massive transfusion. Pediatr Crit Care Med 2009;10(2):e22-26.

79. Manno CS, Hedberg KW. Kim HC, et al. Comparison of the hemostatic effects of fresh whole blood, stored whole blood, and components after open heart surgery in children. Blood 1991;77(5):930-936.

80. Mou SS, Giroir BP, Molitor-Kirsch EA, et al. Fresh whole blood versus reconstituted blood for pump priming in heart surgery in Infants. N Engl J Med 2004;351(16):1635-1644.

81. Carcillo JA, Fields AI. Clinical practice parameters for hemodynamic support of pediatric and neonatal patients in septic shock. Crit Care Med 2002;30(6):1365-1378.

82. Brierley J, Carcillo JA, Choong K, et al. Clinical practice parameters for hemodynamic support of pediatric and neonatal septic shock: 2007 update from the American College of Critical Care Medicine. Crit Care Med 2009;37(2):666-688.

83. Pizarro CF, Troster EJ, Damiani D, et al. Absolute and relative adrenal insufficiency in children with septic shock. Crit Care Med 2005;33(4):855-859.

84. Gunn VL, Nechyba C. Oncology. In: The Harriet Lane handbook. 16th ed. Philadelphia, PA: Elsevier Mosby; 2002. p. 507-508.

85. Gunn VL, Nechyba C. Hematology. In: The Harriet Lane handbook. 16th ed. Philadelphia, PA: Elsevier Mosby; 2002. p. 283-306.

86. Perkins JG, Cap AP, Weiss BM, et al. Massive transfusion and nonsurgical hemostatic agents. Crit Care Med 2008;36(7 Suppl):S325-339.

87. Lang RM, Fellner SK, Neumann A, et al. Left ventricular contractility varies directly with blood ionized calcium. Ann Intern Med 1988;108(4):524-529.

88. Spinella PC, Perkins JG, McLaughlin DF, et al. The effect of recombinant activated factor VII on

mortality in combat-related casualties with severe trauma and massive transfusion. J Trauma 2008;64(2):286-293; discussion 293-294.

89. Lacroix J, Hebert PC, Hutchison JS, et al. Transfusion strategies for patients in pediatric intensive care units. N Engl J Med 2007;356(16):1609-1619.

90. Sakr Y, Vincent JL, Reinhart K, et al. High tidal volume and positive fluid balance are associated with worse outcome in acute lung injury. Chest 2005;128(5):3098-3108.

91. Rivers E, Nguyen B, Havstad S, et al. Early goal-directed therapy in the treatment of severe sepsis and septic shock. N Engl J Med 2001;345(19):1368-1377.

92. Arnal LE, Stein F. Pediatric septic shock: why has mortality decreased?—the utility of goal-directed therapy. Semin Pediatr Infect Dis 2003;14(2):165-72.

93. Francony G, Fauvage B, Falcon D, et al. Equimolar doses of mannitol and hypertonic saline in the treatment of increased intracranial pressure. Crit Care Med 2008;36(3):795-800.

94. Edwards, JJ, Samuels D, Fu ES. Forearm compartment syndrome from intravenous mannitol extravasation during general anesthesia. Anesth Analg 2003;96(1):245-246.

95. Hanhan UA, Fiallos MR, Orlowski JR. Status epilepticus. Pediatr Clin North Am 2001;48(3):683-694.

96. Curry WJ, Kulling DL. Newer antiepileptic drugs: gabapentin, lamotrigine, felbamate, topiramate and fosphenytoin. Am Fam Physician 1998;57(3):513-520.

97. Park MK. Pediatric cardiology for practitioners. 3rd ed. St Louis, MO: Mosby; 1996.

98. Davignon A, Rautaharju P, Boiselle E, et al. Normal ECG standards for infants and children. Pediatr Cardiol 1979;1:123-131.

99. Karmy-Jones R, Nathens A, Jurkovich GJ, et al. Urgent and emergent thoracotomy for penetrating chest trauma. J Trauma 2004;56(3):664-668.

100. Calkins CM, Bensard DD, Partrick DA, et al. A critical analysis of outcome for children sustaining cardiac arrest after blunt trauma. J Pediatr Surg 2002;37(2):180-184.

101. Langer M, Chiu PP, Kim PC. Congenital and acquired single-lung patients: long-term follow-up reveals high mortality risk. J Pediatr Surg 2009;44(1):100-105.

102. Tovar JA. The lung and pediatric trauma. Semin Pediatr Surg 2008;17(1):53-59.

103. Waldhausen JH, Davies L. Pediatric abdominal wound dehiscence: transverse versus vertical incisions. J Am Coll Surg 2000;190(6):688-691.

104. Harris BH, Stylianos S. Operative management of abdominal injuries in children. Semin Pediatr Surgery 2001;10(1):20-22.

105. Resende V, Petroianu A. Functions of the splenic remnant after subtotal splenectomy for treatment of severe splenic injuries. Am J Surg 2003;185(4):311-315.

106. Khaneja SC, Pizzi WF, Barie PS, et al. Management of penetrating juxtahepatic inferior vena cava injuries under total vascular occlusion. J Am Coll Surg 1997;184(5):469-474.

107. Wales PW, Shuckett B, Kim PC. Long-term outcome after nonoperative management of complete traumatic pancreatic transection in children. J Pediatr Surg 2001;36(5):823-827.

108. Meier DE, Coln CD, Hicks BA, et al. Early operation in children with pancreas transection. J Pediatr Surg 2001;36(2):341-344.

109. Nikfarjam M, Rosen M, Ponsky T. Early management of traumatic pancreatic transection by spleen-preserving laparoscopic distal pancreatectomy. J Pediatr Surg 2009;44(2):455-458.

110. Bozkurt B, Ozdemir BA, Kocer B, et al. Operative approach in traumatic injuries of the duodenum. Acta Chir Belg 2006;106(4):405-408.

111. Weigelt JA. Duodenal injuries. Surg Clin North Am 1990;70(3):529-539.

112. Steele SR, Wolcott KE, Mullenix PS, et al. Colon and rectal injuries during Operation Iraqi Freedom: are there any changing trends in management or outcome? Dis Colon Rectum 2007;50(6):870-877.

113. Vertrees A, Wakefield M, Pickett C, et al. Outcomes of primary repair and primary anastomosis in war-related colon injuries. J Trauma 2009;66(5):1286-1291; discussion 1291-1293.

114. Beekley AC. Damage control resuscitation: a sensible approach to the exsanguinating surgical patient. Crit Care Med 2008;36(7 Suppl):S267-274.

115. Blackbourne LH. Combat damage control surgery. Crit Care Med 2008;36(7 Suppl):S304-310.

116. Carlotti AP, Carvalho WB. Abdominal compartment syndrome: a review. Pediatr Crit Care Med 2009;10(1):115-120.

117. Shermeta DW. Simplified treatement of large congenital ventral wall defects. Am J Surg 1977;133(1):78-80.

118. Boele van Hensbroek P, Wind J, Dijkgraaf MG, et al. Temporary closure of the open abdomen: a systemic review on delayed primary fascial closure in patients with an open abdomen. World J Surg 2009;33(2):199-207.

119. Shaikh IA, Ballard-Wilson A, Yalamarthi S, et al. Use of topical negative pressure 'TNP' in assisted

abdominal closure does not lead to high incidence of enteric fistulae. Colorectal Dis 2009. [Epub ahead of print]

120. Gunn VL, Nechyba C. Trauma and burns. In: The Harriet Lane handbook. 16th ed. Philadelphia, PA: Elsevier Mosby; 2002. p. 89-94.

121. Malic CC, Karoo RO, Austin O, et al. Resuscitation burn card—a useful tool for burn injury assessment. Burns 2007;33(2):195-199.

122. Hanigan WC. Surgery of the head and 70-day brain surgeons. Neurosurgery 2003;53(3):713-721; discussion 721-722.

123. Rinker CF, McMurry FG, Groeneweg VR, et al. Emergency craniotomy in a rural level III trauma center. J Trauma 1988;44(6):984-989; discussion 989-990.

124. Newcombe R, Merry G. The management of acute neurotrauma in rural and remote locations: a set of guidelines for the care of head and spinal injuries. J Clin Neurosc 1999;6(1):85-93.

125. Defense Medical Readiness Institute. Emergency War Surgery Course. San Antonio, TX.

126. The International Association for Trauma Surgery and Intensive Care. Definitive Surgical Trauma Care Course. San Antonio, TX.

127. Aldrich EF, Eisenberg HM, Saydjari C, et al. Predictors of mortality in severely head-injured patients with civilian gunshot wound: a report from the NIH Traumatic Coma Data Bank. Surg Neurol 1992;38(6):418-423.

128. Ducrocq SC, Meyer PG, Orliaquet GA, et al. Epidemiology and early predictive factors of mortality and outcome in children with traumatic severe brain injury: experience of a French pediatric trauma center. Pediatr Crit Care Med 2006;7(5):461-467.

129. Cohen JE, Montero A, Israel ZH. Prognosis and clinical relevance of anisocoria-craniotomy latency for epidural hematoma in comatose patients. J Trauma 1996;41(1):120-122.

130. Guidelines for the management of penetrating brain injury. Antibiotic prophylaxis for penetrating brain injury. J Trauma 2001;51(2 Suppl):S34-40.

131. Cullumbine H, McKee HE, Creasey NH. The effects of atropine sulphate upon healthy male subjects. Q J Exp Physiol Cogn Med Sci 1955;40(4):309-319.

132. Teasdale G, Jennett B. Assessment of coma and impaired consciousness. A practical scale. Lancet 1974;2(7872):81-84.

133. Levy ML, Masri LS, Lavine S, et al. Outcome prediction after penetrating craniocerebral injury in a civilian population: aggressive surgical management in patients with admission Glasgow Coma Scale

scores of 3, 4, or 5. Neurosurgery 1994;35(1):77-85.

134. Durham SR, Clancy RR, Leuthardt E, et al. CHOP Infant Coma Scale ("Infant Face Scale"): a novel coma scale for children less than two years of age. J Neurotrauma 2000;17(9):729-737.

135. Vos PE, van Voskuilen AC, Beems T, et al. Evaluation of the traumatic coma data bank computed tomography classification for severe head injury. J Neurotrauma 2001;18(7):649-655.

136. Miner ME, Ewing-Cobbs L, Kopaniky DR, et al. The results of treatment of gunshot wounds to the brain in children. Neurosurgery 1990;26(1):20-24; discussion 24-25.

137. Alexander JW, Fischer JE, Boyajian M, et al. The influence of hair-removal methods on wound infections. Arch Surg 1983;118(3):347-352.

138. Cruse PJE. Classification of operations and audit of infection. In: Taylor EW, editor. Infection in surgical practice. 1st ed. Oxford, England: Oxford University Press; 1992. p. 1-7.

139. Cruse PJ, Foord R. The epidemiology of wound infection. A 10-year prospective study of 62,939 wounds. Surg Clin North Am 1980;60(1):27-40.

140. Siddique MS, Matai V, Sutcliffe JC. The preoperative skin shave in neurosurgery: is it justified? Br J Neurosurg 1998;12(2):131-135.

141. Kretschmer T, Braun V, Richter HP. Neurosurgery without shaving: indications and results. Br J Neurosurg 2000;14(4):341-344.

142. Leedy JE, Janis JE, Rohrich RJ. Reconstruction of acquired scalp defects: an algorithmic approach. Plast Reconstr Surg 2005;116(4):54e-72e.

143. Taha JM, Saba MI, Brown JA. Missile injuries to the brain treated by simple wound closure: results of a protocol during the Lebanese conflict. Neurosurgery 1991;29(3):380-383.

144. Rickert K, Sinson G. Intracranial pressure monitoring. Operative Techn Gen Surg 2003;5(3):170-175.

145. Simpson S, Yung M, Slater A. Severe dehydration and acute renal failure associated with external ventricular drainage of cerebrospinal fluid in children. Anaesth Intensive Care 2006;34(5): 659-663.

146. Mathews WE. The early treatment of craniocerebral missile injuries: experience with 92 cases. J Trauma 1972;12(11):939-954.

147. Amirjamshidi A, Abbassioun K, Rahmat H. Minimal debridement of simple wound closure as the only surgical treatment in war victims with low-velocity penetrating head injuries: indications and management protocol based upon more than 8 years follow-up of 99 cases from Iran-Iraq conflict. Surg

Neurol 2003;60(2):105-111.

148. Carey ME, Young H, Mathis JL, et al. A bacteriological study of craniocerebral missile wounds from Vietnam. J Neurosurg 1971;34(2 pt 1):145-154.

149. Arendall RE, Meirowsky AM. Air sinus wounds: an analysis of 163 consecutive cases incurred in the Korean War, 1950-1952. Neurosurgery 1983;13(4):377-380.

150. Fatu C, Puisoru M, Rotaru M, et al. Morphometric evaluation of the frontal sinus in relation to age. Ann Anat 2006;188(3):275-280.

151. Singhal A, Steinbok P. Operative management of growing skull fractures: a technical note. Childs Nerv Syst 2008;24(5):605-607.

152. Rosenfeld JV. Damage control neurosurgery. Injury 2004;35(7):655-660.

153. Lerman JA, Dickman CA, Haynes RJ. Penetration of cranial inner table with Gardner-Wells tongs. J Spinal Disord 2001;14(3):211-213.

154. Arkader A, Hosalkar HS, Drummond DS, et al. Analysis of halo-orthoses application in children less than three years old. J Child Orthop 2007;1(6):337-344.

155. Waters RL, Sie IH. Spinal cord injuries from gunshot wounds to the spine. Clin Orthop Relat Res 2003;408:120-125.

156. Lancourt JE, Dickson JH, Carter RE. Paralytic spinal deformity following traumatic spinal-cord injury in children and adolescents. J Bone Joint Surg Am 1981;63(1):47-53.

# ACUTE BURN CARE

*Chapter 12*

**Contributing Authors**
Evan M. Renz, MD, FACS, LTC(P), MC, US Army
Leopoldo C. Cancio, MD, FACS, COL, MC, US Army

All figures and tables included in this chapter have been used with permission from Pelagique, LLC, the UCLA Center for International Medicine, and/or the authors, unless otherwise noted.

Use of imagery from the Defense Imagery Management Operations Center (DIMOC) does not imply or constitute Department of Defense (DOD) endorsement of this company, its products, or services.

**Disclaimer**

The opinions and views expressed herein belong solely to those of the authors. They are not nor should they be implied as being endorsed by the United States Uniformed Services University of the Health Sciences, Department of the Army, Department of the Navy, Department of the Air Force, Department of Defense, or any other branch of the federal government.

# Table of Contents

# Introduction

The harsh cruelty of war, as witnessed by those who treat the wounded, would be intolerable if it were not for the belief that the art of medicine is advanced with each lesson learned. In order to pay proper respect to those who have suffered from their wounds, physicians must be dedicated to advancing and applying these lessons of combat casualty care (CCC) (Fig. 1).

Many of the lessons learned from Operation Enduring Freedom (OEF) in Afghanistan and Operation Iraqi Freedom (OIF) relate to problems that have existed as long as wars have been waged. Problems include: the remote and often austere environment in which the battle occurs; the presence, experience, and capability of CCC providers at each level of care; access to necessary supplies and

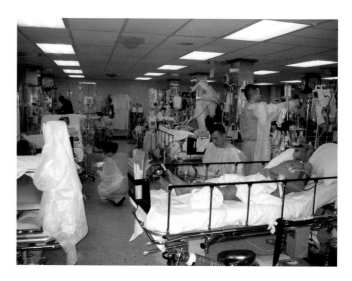

Figure 1. *Burn patients are frequently encountered in combat. This photograph demonstrates Iraqi burn patients on board the USNS Comfort hospital ship in 2003 in the Persian Gulf.*

equipment to implement care; the need to transport casualties expeditiously across dangerous terrain to a safe environment for further recovery; and the inevitability that innocents, too often children, will present among the wounded and require care.[1]

> Children with severe burns are part of the reality of war, and their arrival at field hospitals should come as no surprise to anyone, least of all the surgeon. Care of pediatric burn patients should be anticipated.

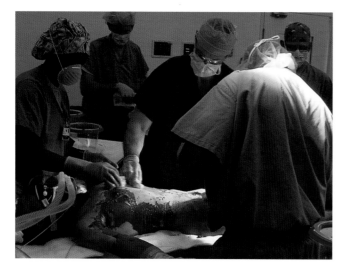

Figure 2. *A host nation burn victim undergoing wound care at Balad AB, Iraq.*

The ultimate hope of all those associated with providing burn care is that prevention and safety programs will mitigate, if not minimize, thermal injury as a cause of mortality and morbidity. Unfortunately, military operations are often accompanied by sophisticated means of destroying the enemy, and explosives are often part of this equation. Despite methods of protection nearly as advanced as the weaponry, combatants on both sides are subject to the thermal effects of the tools of war. Such has been true for many decades, and recent events in Iraq and Afghanistan have proved to be no exception (Fig. 2).

# Combat versus Civilian Burns

Analysis of burn injuries sustained in the civilian United States (US) population compared to those observed in combat zones reveals both similarities and differences. Severe burn injury occurs in approximately 5 to 10 percent of combat casualties.[2] Casualties may sustain thermal injuries from a variety of mechanisms, including the explosion of incendiary devices, as well as the secondary fires that occur as nearby combustible materials ignite. However, in the austere environment of the overseas military post, the hazards associated with everyday life, such as burning refuse or refueling operations, also contribute to injury.[3]

Whether the injury occurs in a combat or civilian environment, the severity of burn is generally determined by the intensity of the thermal energy to which the patient is exposed, the duration of exposure, and the total body surface area (TBSA) burned. The pattern of injury for military casualties is also related to the protective equipment worn at the time of burn. Unless specifically working in an environment associated with high-risk thermal or chemical exposure, such as firefighting, most civilians are wearing everyday clothing at the time of burn. By contrast, military personnel routinely wear durable uniforms; body armor provides additional protection to the torso. Despite efforts to improve protection against burn injury for combatants, the face and hands continue to be the least protected, resulting in significant numbers of burns to these areas (Fig. 3).[4]

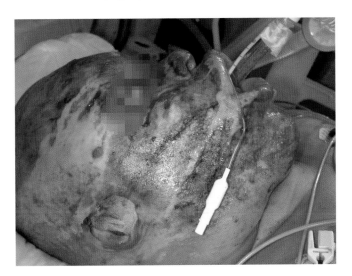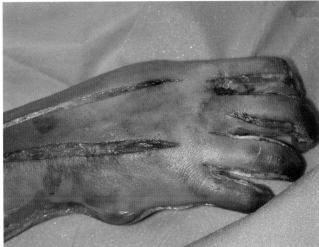

Figure 3. *US soldier injured by a vehicle-borne improvised explosive device (IED) with fragmentation and burn injury to the face, torso, and extremities (following escharotomies). Note the escharotomy incision along the ulnar aspect of the hand has extended slightly deeper than intended through the fascia with protrusion of muscle.*

> Burns involving the hands are common on the battlefield and are associated with devastating disability, making fire-resistant gloves essential gear for at-risk military personnel.

The civilian burn patient is generally assessed and treated near the place of injury by emergency medical services personnel. The patient is rapidly transferred by ground or air ambulance to the closest available medical facility, which may then transfer the patient to a regional burn center. The civilian patient is typically admitted to no more than two medical facilities during his or her hospital course. Although transport distances may be considerable for persons living in remote regions within the US, most civilian burn patients can be transported from the site of injury to a definitive care facility within a few hours. In contrast, US military casualties are often transported to one or more intermediary facilities prior to final air evacuation over thousands of miles back to the US for definitive care.[5,6]

Triage is an important consideration in military burn care. North American Treaty Organization (NATO) triage criteria define the expectant category as including patients in whom there are signs of impending death, or in whom there are injuries requiring an expenditure of resources exceeding those available.[7] The latter subset of expectant category triaged patients may include patients with burns of greater than 85% TBSA.[8] Sound clinical judgment is required to appropriately allocate resources during times of excessive patient influx.

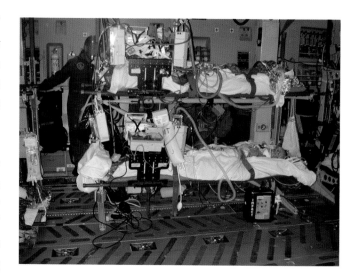

Figure 4. *US Army Burn Flight Team assists in rapid evacuation of severely burned combat casualties back to the US.*

Of note, young casualties with severe burns, even those with greater than 90% TBSA involvement may now survive to leave the hospital, provided rapid resuscitation and evacuation are available.[9] Even the most severely burned combat casualty will likely tolerate evacuation back to the US to receive care, with the support of family and friends at his or her bedside (Fig. 4). Providers are encouraged to contact US Army Institute of Surgical Research (USAISR) Burn Center staff at Brooke Army Medical Center for advice and assistance should survivability become a factor in decisions concerning continuation of care or evacuation. Providers are encouraged to call (210) 916-2876 or DSN (312) 429-2876 to contact the burn center attending surgeon. Consultation may also be initiated by sending an email message (burntrauma.consult@us.army.mil) to US Army Medical Department (AMEDD) burn consultants.

> Young casualties with severe burns, even those with greater than 90% TBSA involvement, will usually tolerate long-range evacuation provided adequate resuscitative support is available, making expectant status rare for US casualties.

The process of caring for burn patients in a combat zone can also be complicated by the presence of multiple open wounds sustained in a dirty environment, combined with hemorrhage related to the injury. Operative intervention for lifesaving treatment or stabilization of concurrent injuries is not uncommon before the combat casualty is evacuated out of the theater of operations. Associated nonthermal trauma is more common in combat than in non-combat burn injury patients.[6]

## Initial Evaluation and Management

Perhaps the single most important lesson to learn when providing acute care for the burn casualty is to remember that burn patients are trauma patients. The visible nature of burn injury should not distract CCC

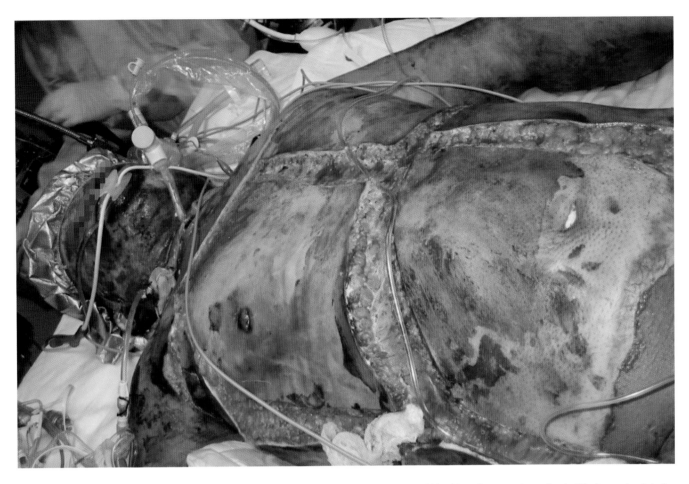

Figure 5. *Combat casualty care providers must resist becoming distracted by burn injuries and identify and manage immediately life-threatening injuries, which are often less visually graphic in nature (e.g., airway edema and obstruction).*

providers from the fact that the patient may have several other life-threatening injuries. This is particularly true when managing blast injury casualties (Fig. 5).[6,10,11]

> Burn casualties are trauma patients, and as such deserve a complete evaluation for associated injuries beyond burn. Treat the patient, not the burn.

## Primary and Secondary Survey

Successful treatment of burn patients starts with a thorough primary and secondary survey of the patient. In a combat zone this often requires a combined strategy of airway and breathing evaluation and protection and hemorrhage control. It is very easy for the careprovider unaccustomed to severe burns to become fixated on the horrendous tissue damage, particularly that involving the face (Fig. 6). Combat casualty care providers must resist becoming distracted by burn injuries and identify and manage immediately life-threatening injuries, which are often less visually graphic in nature (e.g., airway edema and obstruction or internal hemorrhage from concurrent solid organ injury).

The initial management of the combat burn casualty proceeds in a stepwise process as outlined by the Advanced Trauma Life Support (ATLS) guidelines of the American College of Surgeons Committee on Trauma, modified for the special needs of the burn patient. The principles described in the Advanced

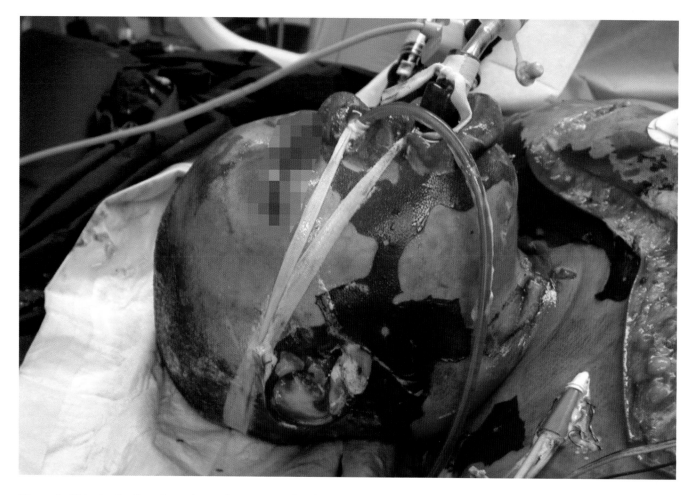

Figure 6. *This visually distracting and severe burn to a casualty's head and neck region poses a significant immediate risk to the airway.*

Burn Life Support (ABLS) curriculum sponsored by the American Burn Association (ABA) reflect these modifications.[12] As an important example, the two-liter bolus of lactated Ringer's solution described in ATLS is contraindicated in the hemodynamically stable burn patient, as this likely contributes to edema formation with no lasting benefit.

## Patient Inspection and Decontamination
Despite many improvements in military clothing and equipment, including fire-resistant uniforms, military burn casualties need to be disrobed just like any other trauma patient in order to fully examine them and ensure that thermal or chemical tissue injury is stopped. Chemical burn injury can occur when a patient comes in contact with an acid, base, or toxic organic compound. The incidence of chemical burn injury in OEF and OIF has been very low.[11] Petroleum-based products are best removed with soap and water. Brush off any debris on a patient prior to irrigation.

White phosphorous is an incendiary munition that is also found in civilian products such as fertilizers, fireworks, and pesticides. While rarely encountered in OEF and OIF, white phosphorous exposure can result in severe, combined thermal and chemical injuries. White phosphorous is extremely volatile and can ignite spontaneously upon exposure to air. In addition, phosphoric acids form during combustion and cause further tissue injury.[13,14,15]

A Woods lamp can be used to identify embedded white phosphorous particles, which fluoresce under ultraviolet light. Treatment of patients with these embedded particles involves: (1) immediate debridement of visible debris; (2) copious irrigation; (3) coverage of exposed areas with saline or liquid-soaked gauze pads that must be kept wet; and (4) cardiac monitoring and serial measurement of serum electrolytes and calcium correction.[13,14] Profound hypocalcemia, hyperphosphatemia, and sudden death have been associated with white phosphorous chemical injury.[15]

Careproviders must take precautions to ensure that they do not sustain injuries in their attempt to clean and treat the casualty. Standard universal precautions (i.e., face mask, gloves, and gown protection) should be routinely practiced. The location in which patient decontamination is performed needs to be individualized based on the nature of the chemical exposure and characteristics of the care facility. Providers need to minimize secondary contamination of patient care areas. In the authors' experience, the combined thermal and chemical burn injuries most commonly encountered in OEF and OIF have not (thus far) routinely necessitated a separate area for patient decontamination.

> Identify the cause of the burn and ensure that the thermal or chemical tissue injury process is stopped. Careproviders should use standard universal precautions when caring for patients with possible chemical agent injury, and prevent secondary contamination of patient care areas.

Electrical injuries deserve special mention as they typically cause a disproportionate degree of underlying deep tissue injury relative to visible burn injury to the skin.[16,17] Electrical burns are most severe at the source of electrical contact (e.g., hands) and ground contact points (e.g., feet).[18] As such, careproviders should carefully evaluate electrical burn patients for systemic complications and specifically for rhabdomyolysis and compartment syndromes.[18]

### Airway and Breathing Interventions

Patients with facial burns or large surface area burns who receive a large volume of resuscitation often develop progressive upper airway edema in the first 48 hours following injury. This makes delayed intubation difficult, if not impossible. This distortion of upper airway anatomy is a consequence of massive anasarca and occurs even in the absence of inhalation injury.[19] Early prophylactic intubation of patients with greater than 40% TBSA involvement or deep facial burns is recommended. Burn casualties, at risk for upper airway edema, who require long-range transport should have a definitive airway established prior to

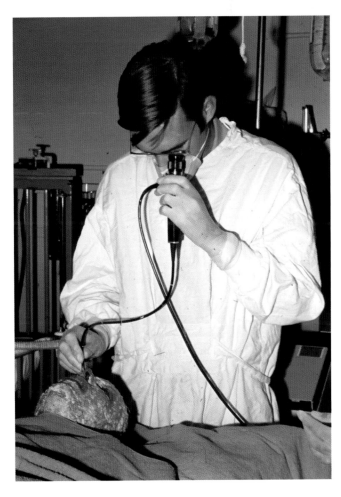

Figure 7. *Fiberoptic laryngoscopy can be used to assess the upper airway for evidence of burn injury or edema.*

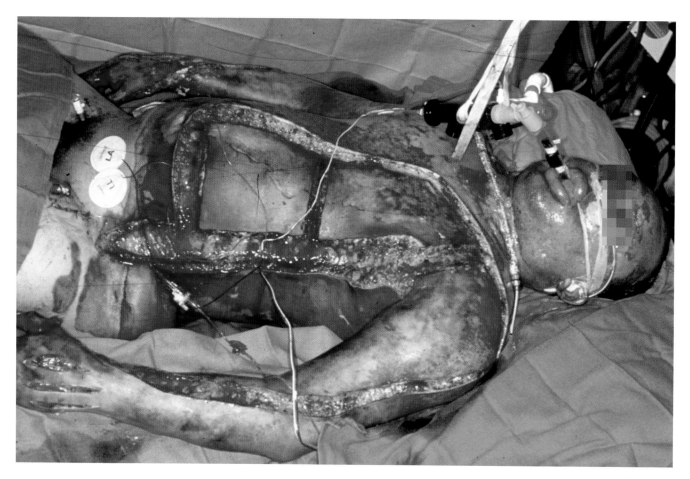

Figure 8. (Above) *Circumferential burns to the chest may impair effective ventilation and should be treated with thoracic escharotomy.*

Figure 9. (Right) *Effective chest excursion was achieved after thoracic escharotomy in this pediatric burn patient.*

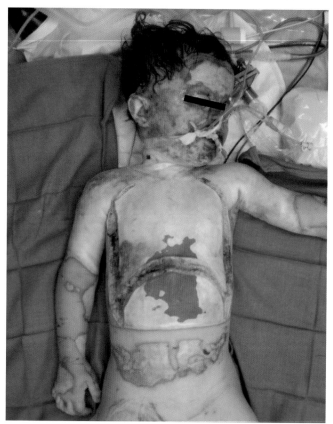

movement between medical treatment facilities.[20] Inhalation injury is relatively uncommon, being diagnosed in approximately 10 percent of burn injuries.[21] Casualties with facial burns, large TBSA burn size, and those who are trapped within a burning vehicle or structure are those most at risk for inhalation injury.[21] Clinical findings such as stridor or production of carbonaceous sputum should increase suspicion of inhalation injury, but are by no means definitively diagnostic.[22] Fiberoptic laryngoscopy (if available) can be used to assess the upper airway for evidence of burn injury or edema in equivocal cases (Fig. 7). Patients suspected of suffering significant inhalation injury benefit from early airway protection by endotracheal intubation and subsequent support with mechanical ventilation.

As in the case of large burn size, the authors' experience is that it is better to err on the side of earlier rather than later intubation of patients with inhalation injury.[23]

---

Treatment of life-threatening airway or breathing compromise and bleeding wounds takes priority over initial burn wound care. Prophylactic intubation of the patient with extensive burns or inhalation injury is advisable, especially if ongoing resuscitation is required. Protect the burn patient's airway and establish effective ventilation in preparation for aeromedical evacuation.

---

Patients with inhalation injury should be intubated with the largest size endotracheal tube possible. Sloughing of tissue from the friable airway following inhalation injury, coupled with blood and secretions, may quickly occlude an endotracheal or tracheostomy tube. Larger-sized endotracheal tubes will mitigate this process and facilitate subsequent interventions (e.g., bronchoscopy). Interval suctioning of the airway is important. The use of aerosolized heparin alternating with aerosolized $N$-acetylcysteine in burn patients with inhalational injury requiring ventilatory support has been shown to decrease the incidence of reintubation for progressive respiratory failure, decrease atelectasis, and reduce mortality in adults and children with massive burn and inhalation injury.[24,25] Fiberoptic bronchoscopy is also recommended to document extent of injury, as well as to remove large plugs under direct visualization.[20]

Patients who sustain circumferential burns of the chest, especially full-thickness burns resulting in a tight eschar, are at risk of respiratory impairment (Fig. 8). Effective chest excursion can be markedly impeded by thoracic eschar, resulting in hypercapnia, hypoxia, and respiratory arrest.[26] Such patients require thoracic escharotomy (Fig. 9).

---

Circumferential burns involving the chest can impair ventilation and/or oxygenation due to reduced thoracic excursion. Thoracic escharotomy, performed at the bedside, can be a lifesaving intervention.

---

### Comorbid Life-Threatening Injury Care

The purpose of the primary and secondary trauma survey is to rapidly assess a combat casualty and identify and mitigate imminent threats to life. Combat casualties, including those with burns, are most likely to die within the first 24 hours from exsanguination related to a penetrating wound.[27] Airway, breathing, and hemorrhage control must be addressed immediately in all casualties. Treatment of life-threatening airway or breathing compromise and bleeding wounds takes priority over initial burn wound care.

In addition to burn wounds, primary and secondary surveys of the casualty may reveal intraabdominal injuries as well as significant soft-tissue wounds and long-bone fractures, an observation noted among a large percentage of military burn casualties injured from explosions.[28] Military personnel may also sustain burn injuries while traveling in moving vehicles attacked with improvised explosive devices (IEDs), mandating evaluation for blunt trauma, as well as for penetrating injuries.

## Burn Wound Evaluation and Patient Resuscitation

In a deployed environment, burn patients are routinely transported to the operating room not only for treatment of associated injuries, but also for debridement and dressing of all wounds. The operating room provides the most sterile environment available for such interventions (Fig. 10). The presence of anesthesia staff to provide pain control and sedation during debridement and dressing changes makes the operating room an optimal location for these procedures.[10]

## Estimating Depth of Burns

Burns are classically described as first-degree, second-degree (partial-thickness), or third-degree (full-thickness) in depth. First-degree burns affect a variable portion of the epidermis, feature erythema without extensive blistering, and heal within a few days. An example is a mild sunburn. For purposes of CCC (to include calculation of total burn size and fluid resuscitation needs), first-degree burns are

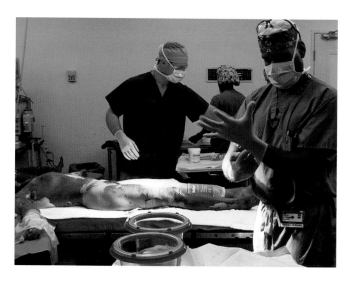

Figure 10. *The operating room provides the most sterile environment for debridement and dressing of burn wounds.*

of no consequence. Second-degree (partial-thickness) burns affect the entire thickness of the epidermis and a variable portion of the dermis. An example is a blistered scald burn. Because these burns spare the hair follicles and other epidermal analogs, they are capable of spontaneous healing. However, the healing time is highly variable. For this reason, second-degree burns are further subdivided into superficial second-degree burns (those that will heal with rapid reepithelialization and minimal scarring within 14 days) and deep second-degree burns (those that will heal after 14 days or more). Finally, third-degree (full-thickness) burns destroy the entire depth of the epidermis, dermis, and epidermal analogs. An example is a flame burn from gasoline, a house fire, or an IED. The burned skin may appear leathery, pale, or charred. These wounds are incapable of healing spontaneously, except by wound contraction, and almost always merit excision and

| DEGREE OF BURN | DEPTH OF WOUND | WOUND DESCRIPTION |
|---|---|---|
| First | Epidermis | Pink or red, without blister formation; capillary refill and sensation intact |
| Second (partial-thickness) | | |
| • Superficial partial-thickness | Epidermis, papillary layer of dermis | Blistering of skin, exposed dermis is red and moist; capillary refill and sensation intact, painful |
| • Deep partial-thickness | Epidermis, papillary and reticular layers of dermis | Blistering of skin, exposed dermis is pale, white to yellow; capillary refill is absent, pain sensation is diminished |
| Third (full-thickness) | All epidermal and dermal structures are destroyed | Charred, pearly white, or leathery appearance; capillary refill absent, insensate |
| Fourth | Epidermis, dermis, fat/muscle/bone | Variable appearance; thrombosed blood vessels, insensate |

Table 1. *Classification of burn depth.*

grafting. The term fourth-degree burns is sometimes used to describe burns that affect even deeper layers, such as fat, muscle, and/or bone (Table 1 and Fig. 11).

Accurate burn classification is needed to identify which burns require skin grafting to accelerate healing, improve cosmetic results, and prevent contractures. Time to healing and scar development is retrospectively used to grade burns that were not initially excised and grafted. Partial-thickness burns that heal prior to 14 days are unlikely to scar, while those that take over 21 days to heal will likely scar and/or result in contractures (Fig. 12).

> Accurate estimation of a patient's burn size, expressed as the percentage of the TBSA burned, is the most important component in determining the severity of burn injury, and should be done in collaboration with consulting burn surgeons.

Clinical assessment of burn depth is fairly accurate for distinguishing first- and third-degree burns. Unfortunately, it is less accurate for determining which second-degree burns would benefit from immediate excision and grafting, and which will heal spontaneously within 14 days.[29,30] Expert burn surgeons are only 60 to 75 percent accurate in correctly classifying partial-thickness burn depth and recovery potential at time of initial injury.[30] To address this problem, a variety of standard (e.g., biopsy and histology) and advanced technologies (e.g., thermography, dye studies, laser Doppler imaging, noncontact high-frequency ultrasonography) have been used to assess tissue characteristics and/or perfusion as methods for determining burn depth.

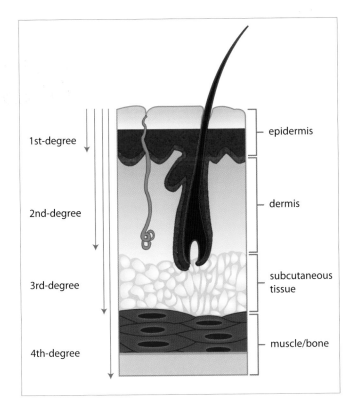

Figure 11. (Left) *Schematic cross section of skin anatomy demonstrating layers involved with differing burn depths.*

Figure 12. (Below) *A severe hand burn, now with scarring and contractures. Early excision and grafting, followed by timely splinting and rehabilitation, are essential to prevent outcomes like this in the treatment of burns of the hands and across major joints.*

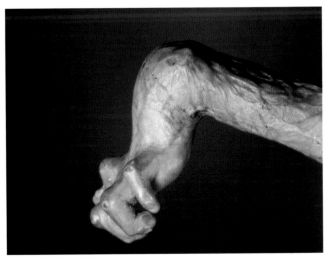

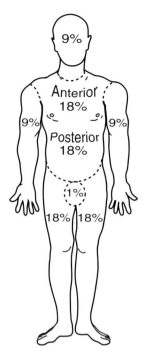

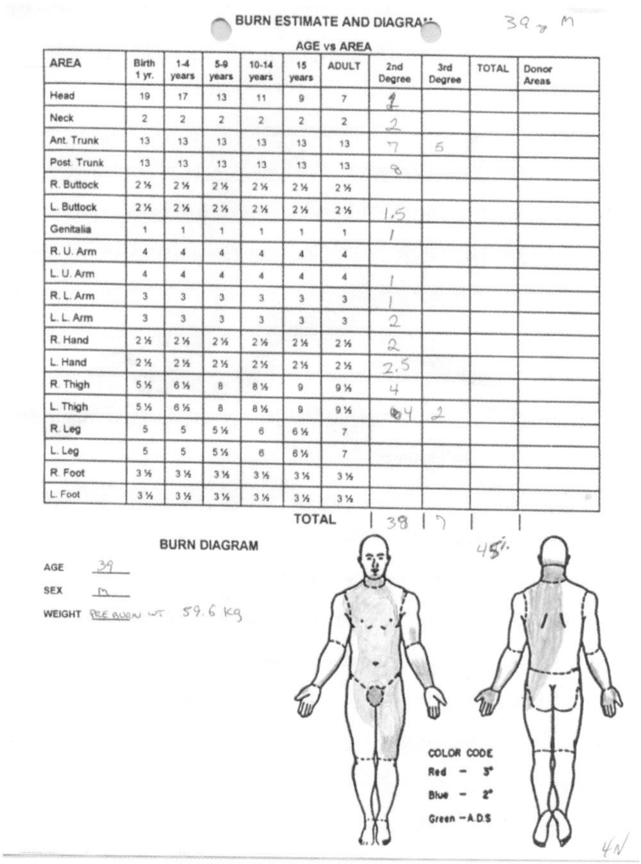

| AREA | Birth 1 yr. | 1-4 years | 5-9 years | 10-14 years | 15 years | ADULT | 2nd Degree | 3rd Degree | TOTAL | Donor Areas |
|---|---|---|---|---|---|---|---|---|---|---|
| Head | 19 | 17 | 13 | 11 | 9 | 7 | 4 | | | |
| Neck | 2 | 2 | 2 | 2 | 2 | 2 | 2 | | | |
| Ant. Trunk | 13 | 13 | 13 | 13 | 13 | 13 | 7 | 5 | | |
| Post. Trunk | 13 | 13 | 13 | 13 | 13 | 13 | 8 | | | |
| R. Buttock | 2½ | 2½ | 2½ | 2½ | 2½ | 2½ | | | | |
| L. Buttock | 2½ | 2½ | 2½ | 2½ | 2½ | 2½ | 1.5 | | | |
| Genitalia | 1 | 1 | 1 | 1 | 1 | 1 | 1 | | | |
| R. U. Arm | 4 | 4 | 4 | 4 | 4 | 4 | | | | |
| L. U. Arm | 4 | 4 | 4 | 4 | 4 | 4 | 1 | | | |
| R. L. Arm | 3 | 3 | 3 | 3 | 3 | 3 | 1 | | | |
| L. L. Arm | 3 | 3 | 3 | 3 | 3 | 3 | 2 | | | |
| R. Hand | 2½ | 2½ | 2½ | 2½ | 2½ | 2½ | 2 | | | |
| L. Hand | 2½ | 2½ | 2½ | 2½ | 2½ | 2½ | 2.5 | | | |
| R. Thigh | 5½ | 6½ | 8 | 8½ | 9 | 9½ | 4 | | | |
| L. Thigh | 5½ | 6½ | 8 | 8½ | 9 | 9½ | 4 | 2 | | |
| R. Leg | 5 | 5 | 5½ | 6 | 6½ | 7 | | | | |
| L. Leg | 5 | 5 | 5½ | 6 | 6½ | 7 | | | | |
| R. Foot | 3½ | 3½ | 3½ | 3½ | 3½ | 3½ | | | | |
| L. Foot | 3½ | 3½ | 3½ | 3½ | 3½ | 3½ | | | | |

TOTAL | 38 | 7

**BURN DIAGRAM**

AGE    39

SEX    M

WEIGHT  PRE BURN WT   59.6 kg

COLOR CODE
Red — 3°
Blue — 2°
Green — A.D.S

45°

Figure 13. (Above) *Estimation of body surface area using the Rule of Nines is relatively inaccurate. Image courtesy of the Borden Institute, Office of The Surgeon General, Washington, DC.*

Figure 14. (Right) *Estimation of body surface area using a Lund-Browder chart is an accurate tool for assessing extent of burn injury.*

Combat casualty careproviders in OEF and OIF will need to make clinical assessments of burn depth in collaboration with consulting burn surgeons. Burns that do not heal within 14 days following injury are likely to benefit from excision and grafting, as well as from advanced rehabilitation, to ensure optimal cosmetic and functional outcomes.

## Estimation of Burn Severity

Accurate estimation of a patient's burn size, expressed as the percentage of the TBSA burned, is the most important component in determining the severity of burn injury. Total body surface area burned is an important predictor of mortality (along with other factors including age, inhalation injury, and concurrent injuries). Total body surface area burned is the most important factor to consider when initiating burn resuscitation. The "Rule of Nines" is a commonly used, but relatively inaccurate, tool for estimating TBSA (Fig. 13).[31] The Lund-Browder chart is a more accurate (but more time-consuming) tool for assessing and documenting the extent of burn injury that takes into account differences in patient age (Fig. 14).[31]

## Burn Location

As previously noted, circumferential burns (e.g., thorax and extremities) are at high risk for compromising tissue perfusion. Full-thickness and partial-thickness burns to critical areas such as the face, ears, hands, feet, perineum, and genitalia are also considered high-risk injuries and require burn specialist consultation. In addition, full-thickness or partial-thickness burns over joint areas need careful follow-up evaluation and management to prevent contractures.

## Initial Fluid Resuscitation

Intravenous (IV) fluid resuscitation is typically required for all burn patients with greater than 20% TBSA involvement, and for some with greater than 10% TBSA involvement. Before any resuscitative fluids can be administered, IV access is required. Thermal burns often increase the difficulty of establishing and maintaining IV access. Problems include loss of normal landmarks, loss of skin pliability, and difficulty in penetrating the eschar with the catheter. Although it is preferable to establish IV access through unburned skin, access through burned skin is acceptable. When a peripheral IV catheter cannot be placed, central venous or intraosseous access should be obtained without delay.[32]

It is acceptable to establish IV access through burned skin, if necessary. When a peripheral IV catheter cannot be placed, central venous or intraosseous access should be obtained without delay.

Once adequate IV access is established, the catheter must be secured. The routine use of adhesive tape or transparent dressings does not work over burned skin. Securing the IV catheter to skin (or eschar) with sutures or surgical staples is a very effective method (Fig. 15). Redundant access (i.e., at least two IV catheters) is essential prior to transporting the patient, especially during the critical phase of burn resuscitation.

Placement of a urinary catheter should be performed early during patient resuscitation, as urine output is an important indicator of the adequacy of resuscitative efforts. Burns to the genitalia and/or the perineal region are not contraindications to Foley catheter placement. The CCC provider may need to remove eschar on the glans penis to visualize the urethral meatus to enable placing the catheter. This simple intervention is far superior to placement of a suprapubic catheter and the complications associated with inadvertent violation of the peritoneal cavity.

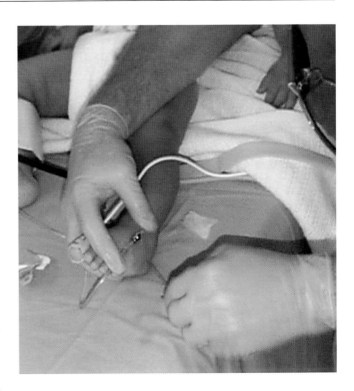

Figure 15. *An IV catheter is secured to the skin using sutures.*

One of the most challenging and controversial aspects of burn care continues to be providing optimal resuscitation during the initial 24 to 48 hours following injury.[33] Severe burns lead to massive fluid shifts from the intravascular space to the interstitium in both burned and nonburned tissues. The hypovolemia caused by this shift and an increase in systemic vascular resistance leads to a reduction in cardiac output and decreased end-organ perfusion. Early volume replacement with crystalloid solutions to maintain adequate perfusion of vital organs reverses burn shock and can be lifesaving. Excessive fluid resuscitation, beyond the minimum required to maintain end-organ perfusion, exacerbates tissue edema, contributes to devastating complications such as abdominal compartment syndrome, and leads to increased mortality.[34]

# Burn Flow Sheet Documentation

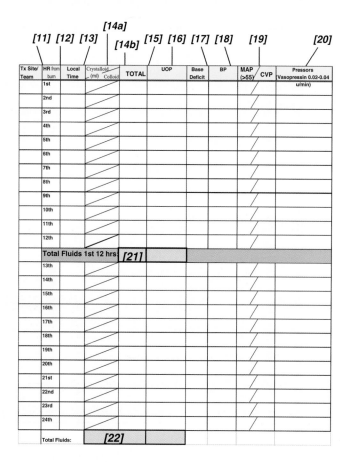

[1] **Date**: Today's date

[2] **Initial Treatment Facility**: Where this form is initiated

[3] **Name**: Patient's name

[4] **SSN**: Patient's social security number

[5] **Weight (Kg)**: Estimated weight PRE-BURN "dry weight"

[6] **% TBSA**: Total body surface area burned

[7] **1st 8 Hrs**: ½ total calculated fluids per burn resuscitation formula (ABLS), given over 1st 8 hrs post-burn

[8] **2nd 16 Hrs**: Remaining ½ of the calculated fluids over the next 16 hrs

[9] **Estimated Total Fluids**: Total fluids calculated for the first 24 hrs post-burn injury

[10] **Time of Injury**: Time the patient burned, **NOT** the time patient arrived at the facility

[11] **Treatment (Tx) Site/Team**: Facility, CCATT or care team providing care at specified hour

[12] **Hour From Burn**: "1st" hour is the first hour post burn. For example: pt arrives @ facility 3 hrs post-burn. Clinicians will start their charting for the "4th" hour. Enter IVF & UOP totals from level I & II care, prior to arrival at the current facility, in the "3rd" hour row.

[13] **Local Time**: Current time being used by recorder

[14a] **Crystalloid (mL)**: Total crystalloid volume given over last hour (LR, NS, etc.)

[14b] **Colloid (mL)**: Total colloid volume given over the last hour (Albumin 5%-25%, blood products, Hespan, etc.) **Note when using Albumin**: With large resuscitations, start 5% Albumin at the 12 hour mark; with normal resuscitations, start at the 24 hour mark.

[15] **Total**: Total volume (crystalloid + colloid) for the hour

[16] **UOP**: Urine output for last hour

[17] **Base Deficit**: enter lab value, if avail. (indicates acidemia)

[18] **BP**: Systolic BP / Diastolic BP

[19] **MAP/CVP**: MAP and/or CVP if available.

[20] **Pressors**: Vasopressin, Levophed, etc., and rate/dose

[21] **12-hr Total**: Total IVF & UOP for 1st 12 hours post-burn

[22] **24-hr Total**: Total IVF & UOP for 1st 24 hours post-burn

| Pre-burn Est. Wt (kg) | %TBSA | Fluid Volume ACTUALLY received | | |
|---|---|---|---|---|
| | | 1st 8 hrs | 2nd 16th hrs | 24 hr Total |
| | | [a] | [b] | [c] |

**Page 2 (24-48 hrs)**

The guidelines for page 2 remain the same as for page 1, with the exception of the calculation table. On page 2, the values in [a] and [c] are the **actual** volumes delivered and recorded from page 1, blocks 21 & 22. [b] is the **actual** volume delivered from the 9th hour through the 24th hour. These values allow caregivers to re-calculate the mL/kg/% TBSA, and evaluate for over-resuscitation

| Pre-burn Est. Wt (kg) | %TBSA | Fluid Volume ACTUALLY received | | |
|---|---|---|---|---|
| | | 1st 24 hrs | 2nd 24 hrs | 48 hr Total |
| | | [d] | [e] | [f] |

**Page 3 (48-72 hrs)**

The guidelines for page 3 remain the same as for pages 1 & 2, with the exception of the calculation table. On page 3, the values in [d] and [e] are the **actual** 24 hour fluid totals recorded from pages 1 & 2. [f] is the **total** volume delivered over the first 48 hrs ([d] + [e]). Once again, these values allow caregivers to re-calculate the mL/kg/% TBSA, and evaluate for over-resuscitation

Figure 16. *The standardized Burn Flow Sheet has improved documentation, communication, and outcomes following battlefield burn resuscitation. Image courtesy of the Borden Institute, Office of The Surgeon General, Washington, DC.*

Excessive fluid administration (over-resuscitation), beyond the minimum required to maintain end-organ perfusion, produces its own constellation of complications termed resuscitation morbidity. Resuscitation morbidity includes upper airway obstruction, pulmonary or cerebral edema, and compartment syndromes affecting the extremities and abdomen.

Patients presenting with concurrent injuries, which require fluid administration unrelated to burn treatment, complicate resuscitation of military burn casualties. Resuscitation is also made complex by virtue of multiple careproviders with varying backgrounds providing burn care during the patient's initial management and subsequent aeromedical evacuation and care. The implementation of a standardized Burn Resuscitation Flowsheet and Burn Resuscitation Guidelines (Fig. 16), by improving documentation and inter-echelon communication, has improved outcomes following battlefield burn resuscitation.[35,36]

## Modified Brooke Formula

The current clinical practice guideline for resuscitation of the military burn casualty recommends initiating fluid resuscitation utilizing the modified Brooke Formula: lactated Ringer's solution totaling (2 ml x %TBSA burned x kilogram weight) divided over 24 hours, with half of the total amount administered during the first 8 hours following injury.[37] An abbreviated method of calculating the initial fluid resuscitation rate (only applicable to adults weighing over 40 kilograms) is to multiply the estimated %TBSA burned x 10. Coined the "Rule of Ten" at the USAISR (Chung KC, unpublished data 2009), this simple equation provides the initial hourly infusion rate for lactated Ringer's solution (Fig. 17).

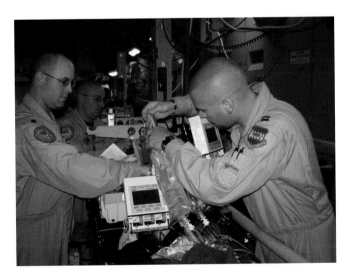

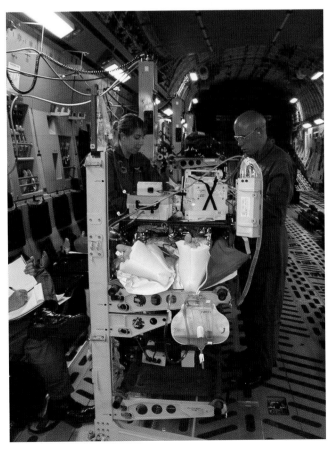

Figure 17. (Above) *Ongoing resuscitation of a burn victim with lactated Ringer's infusion during critical care transport.*

Figure 18. (Right) *Patient monitoring during air evacuation.*

For children, body weight remains a critical consideration, and the modified Brooke Formula for children is used: (3 ml x %TBSA burned x kilogram weight) divided over 24 hours, with half of the total amount programmed for administration during the first eight hours following injury.[38] In addition, children require a maintenance fluid, which is not adjusted during resuscitation.

*Modified Brooke Formula:*
Lactated Ringer's total (2 ml x %TBSA burned x kilogram weight); first half infused in first eight hours

*Modified Brooke Formula for Children:*
Lactated Ringer's total (3 ml x %TBSA burned x kilogram weight); first half infused in first eight hours

These estimates, or any other burn resuscitation formulas, simply provide a point at which to start the resuscitation. Burn resuscitation must be closely monitored and adjusted based on clinical response and endpoints. Administer no more fluid than is necessary for end-organ perfusion as observed by adequate urine output, generally accepted as 30 to 50 ml per hour in adults, and 1 to 2 ml per kilogram per hour in children.[39] Intravenous fluid rates should be adjusted hourly, avoiding boluses of fluid and making incremental adjustments by 20 to 25 percent up or down, based on urine output. Current research and development efforts are underway to improve this process though the development of decision-assist software.[40]

Optimal Burn Resuscitation:
  Estimate → Initiate → Monitor → Adjust → Document
  Repeat monitoring and adjustment process at hourly intervals to optimize resuscitation

Inadequate resuscitation can lead to ischemia of renal and mesenteric vascular beds and can worsen end-organ injury.[41,42] Excessive fluid administration (over-resuscitation) produces its own constellation of complications termed resuscitation morbidity. Resuscitation morbidity includes upper airway obstruction, pulmonary or cerebral edema, and compartment syndromes affecting the extremities and abdomen.[43]

Patient monitoring becomes more advanced as the patient is transported to better-resourced facilities (Fig. 18). Vital sign monitoring (assessment of pulses and manual measurement of blood pressure) rapidly advances as the patient is evacuated to higher levels of care, to include continuous electrocardiographic monitoring, pulse oximetry, and interval automated blood pressure measurements. Placement of arterial and central venous catheters provides continuous measurements of arterial and central venous pressures. An improving base deficit has also been identified as a helpful indicator of resuscitation efficacy.[44]

While central venous pressure, central venous saturation, and arterial base deficit are often followed during resuscitation, there are no accepted guidelines with respect to use of these variables as endpoints.[45] Adequate end-organ perfusion, manifested by a urine output of 30 to 50 ml per hour in adults (1 ml per kilogram per hour in children less than 30 kilograms), is the primary index of resuscitation adequacy used in burn patients.

While hemodynamic variables (e.g., hypotension) are helpful in identifying uncompensated shock, they inadequately detect hypoperfusion in compensated shock states. Patients with compensated shock may appear normotensive, yet still suffer from regional hypoperfusion, as evidenced by progressive metabolic acidosis. Current methods for assessing the adequacy of fluid resuscitation in critically ill patients are suboptimal. While much emphasis has been placed on defining markers of global perfusion adequacy (e.g., base deficits), future efforts will likely involve better defining markers of regional perfusion adequacy (e.g., gastric intramucosal pH monitoring) and endpoints for resuscitation.

---

Adequate end-organ perfusion, manifested by a urine output of 30 to 50 ml per hour in adults (1 ml per kilogram per hour in children less than 30 kilograms), is the primary index of resuscitation adequacy used in burn patients.

---

## Complications of Burn Injury

### Abdominal Compartment Syndrome

Patients with significant burns are at risk for developing abdominal compartment syndrome. This risk increases with the volume of fluid infused over the first 24 hours following burn injury. Infusion of fluid volumes exceeding 250 ml per kilogram within the first 24 hours following injury is particularly hazardous.[46] Thus, initiation of serial measurements of the bladder pressure may be prudent as soon as a patient, during the first 24 hours post-burn, receives greater than 200 ml per kilogram of fluid infusion. Other risk factors for abdominal compartment syndrome include extensive TBSA involvement and full-thickness burn size, aggressive fluid resuscitation in the early resuscitative period, and deep or circumferential burns to the abdomen and thorax.[47]

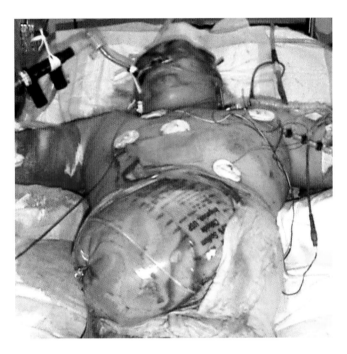

Figure 19. *This image illustrates an open abdomen following decompressive laparotomy for abdominal compartment syndrome.*

---

If abdominal compartment syndrome develops, a decompressive laparotomy will likely be required.

---

If intraabdominal hypertension occurs (i.e., bladder pressure greater than 25 mm Hg): (1) escharotomies of any eschar involving the abdominal wall are warranted; (2) every effort should be made to reduce the fluid infusion rate; and (3) bedside placement of a peritoneal drain should be considered to remove ascites.[46,48,49] If these methods fail to reduce bladder pressure and if the patient develops abdominal compartment syndrome (e.g., intraabdominal hypertension with rising airway pressures, cardiovascular collapse, and/or oliguria despite adequate preload), a decompressive laparotomy will likely be required (Fig. 19).[50] Because the open abdomen becomes heavily contaminated and may be impossible to close, decompressive laparotomy is a high-risk procedure in burn patients.[46,49,50] In the authors' experience, such an intervention is associated with a mortality exceeding 80 percent. Techniques proposed to reduce the fluid infusion rate in patients with intraabdominal hypertension include early use of colloid and use of hypertonic crystalloid solutions.[51,52,53]

> Both over-resuscitation and under-resuscitation of burn patients must be avoided; each invokes unique morbidity.

## Traumatic Rhabdomyolysis

Patients with traumatic rhabdomyolysis are at risk of acute kidney injury and acute tubular necrosis.[54] These patients present with gross myoglobinuria, which can be distinguished from hematuria by a urinalysis that is dipstick positive for blood but microscopically negative for red blood cells. The diagnosis is further supported by documenting elevated levels of serum creatine phosphokinase (CPK). Once diagnosed, rhabdomyolysis is treated with an increase in the intravenous fluid rate in order to achieve a target urine output of 1 ml per kilogram per hour (i.e., commonly 75 to 100 ml per hour in adults), to clear the tubules of myoglobin. In addition, urgent fasciotomy and/or debridement of necrotic muscles may be required to eliminate sources of ongoing pigment release (tissue injury). If these measures fail to produce a gradual clearing of pigment from the urine (as determined by visual inspection over several hours) or a decline in the serum CPK level, then infusion of mannitol and/or administration of bicarbonate to alkalinize the urine should be considered.[18,54,55] The efficacy of mannitol and bicarbonate therapy for rhabdomyolysis remains controversial.[56,57,58,59]

## Electrolyte Disturbances

Burn patients may present with a variety of electrolyte disturbances. Patients with massive tissue destruction, such as those with traumatic rhabdomyolysis, are at risk for hyperkalemia. Loss of the evaporative barrier to water loss leads to very large insensible water losses and thus to hypernatremia. This mandates intravascular volume replacement with hypotonic intravenous (such as D5W) and/or oral solutions, beginning about 48 hours post-burn.[60] The amount of these losses can be roughly estimated by the formula, daily water requirement = (1 ml x TBSA burned x weight in kilograms). However, patients are also at risk of hyponatremia because of abnormalities in the thirst mechanism and in some cases the syndrome of inappropriate secretion of antidiuretic hormone (SIADH).[61]

The rate of serum sodium correction depends on the severity of symptoms and rate at which the derangement developed (acute versus chronic).[62] The treatment of acute (less than 48 hours duration) hyper- and hyponatremia associated with burn injury involves correcting intravascular volume deficits and correcting hyper- or hypotonicity. The serum sodium should be corrected at an initial rate of 1 mEq per liter per hour. Serial serum electrolyte measurements should be performed every one to two hours during initial treatment phases. The correction of chronic sodium disturbances (greater than 48 hours duration) should be at a rate not to exceed 0.5 mEq per liter per hour.[63] Serum sodium correction is performed more rapidly if a neurological complication, such as ongoing seizure activity, is attributed to sodium derangement.

The predictive accuracy of formulas for serum sodium and intravascular volume repletion is limited.[64] Lindner et al. studied the predictive accuracy of formulaic approaches to serum sodium correction and found that individual patient variability of response to treatment dictates such formulas should only be used as a guide. Serial measurements of serum sodium are recommended to ensure appropriate treatment. Finally, burn patients may develop severe hypophosphatemia during the first three to five days post-burn, most likely reflecting the tremendous increase in metabolic demand that occurs during this period.[65] Thus, serum electrolytes must be monitored frequently (minimum of twice daily) in patients with major burns.

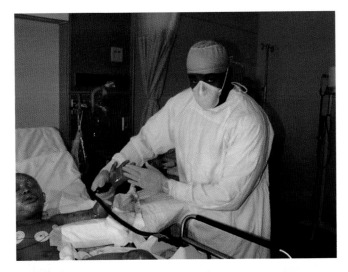

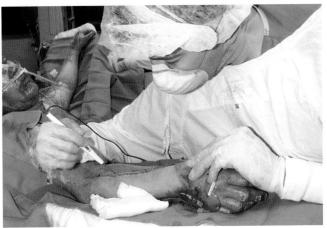

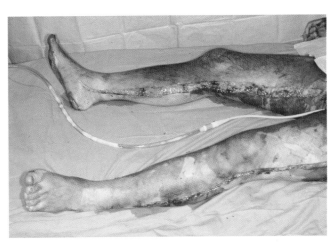

Figure 20. (Left) *With circumferential burns, elevation of the burned extremity and frequent evaluation are extremely important.*

Figure 21. (Bottom Left and Bottom Right) *Extremity escharotomies following circumferential burns.*

## Escharotomy and Fasciotomy

Circumferential burns of the extremities and torso are prone to the compressive effect of eschar. Fluid resuscitation can rapidly exacerbate such compression through increased tissue edema, with resultant vascular obstruction, ischemia, and limb loss.[26] This most commonly occurs in the setting of circumferential full-thickness burns, but does on occasion occur with deep partial-thickness burns, or noncircumferential burns. Elevation of burned extremities well above the level of the heart is a simple but critically important intervention that will minimize tissue edema in the initial 48 hours following burn injury. Elevate burned limbs and evaluate them hourly during patient resuscitation (Fig. 20). This can be done with pillows and blankets, or better yet, with slings constructed of surgical netting hung from IV poles. When this fails to maintain adequate distal blood flow, escharotomy (a longitudinal incision through the burned skin) is required (Fig. 21).

> Elevation of burned extremities well above the level of the heart is a simple but critically important intervention that will minimize tissue edema in the initial 48 hours following burn injury.

Progressive diminution of pulsatile arterial flow by Doppler flowmetry is the primary indication for escharotomy. Other indications include cyanosis of distal unburned skin, impaired capillary refill, or progressive neurological deficits.[66] Such neurologic deficits include paresthesias progressing to hypesthesia or loss of motor function. In addition, early escharotomy should be considered for any patient with deep,

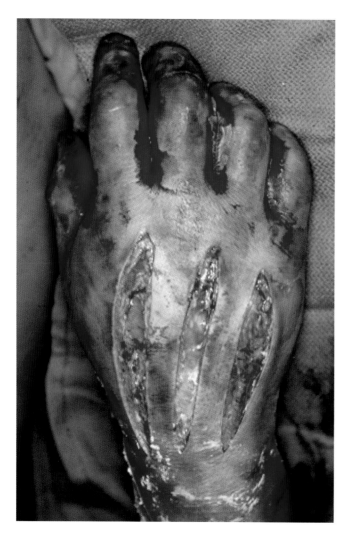

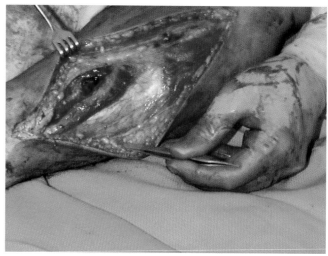

Figure 22. (Left) *Hand escharotomies. Burned skin is incised to the subcutaneous level, providing decompression while avoiding deeper structures.*

Figure 23. (Below) *Compartment syndrome is unusual following thermal injury. Unlike circumferential eschar, which is treated with escharotomy, a true compartment syndrome requires fasciotomy as demonstrated here.*

circumferential extremity burns who is being evacuated between military medical treatment facilities on the battlefield.

Escharotomy is considered to be a relatively urgent procedure and can be performed at the bedside, using sharp incision with a knife or electrocautery device. Regardless of the technique used, escharotomies should be performed in the most sterile environment possible. The burned skin is incised down to the subcutaneous level, providing decompression through the incision sites.[26] Escharotomies are generally performed on the lateral and medial aspects of the limbs, avoiding any underlying neurovascular structures, and without entering the deep (investing) fascia (Fig. 22). Pain control during this procedure should be managed with titrated doses of intravenous narcotics or ketamine. Once the escharotomy has been completed, neurovascular examination is serially repeated to verify effectiveness.

Early escharotomy should be considered for patients with circumferential, deep burns involving the extremities, especially in anticipation of long-range aeromedical transport.

Except in cases involving high-voltage electrical injury, fractures deep to the burn, or vascular injury to the limb, fasciotomies of burned extremities are rarely required.[2,67] If compartment syndrome is suspected in a circumferentially burned limb, escharotomies should be performed, and the patient reevaluated (to include neurovascular exam and measurement of intracompartmental pressures).

> Fasciotomies are performed only when clinical findings indicate intracompartmental hypertension (compartment syndrome). They should not be performed prophylactically, solely on the basis of circumferential burns.

A delay in performing a clinically indicated escharotomy, or an inadequately performed escharotomy, may lead to a true compartment syndrome mandating fasciotomy (Fig. 23).[67] In addition, massive fluid resuscitation can result in a compartment syndrome in a normal (unburned) limb.[68] In the authors' experience, the regions most sensitive to post-burn compartment syndrome are the anterior lower leg and the forearm. Fasciotomies of the thigh and upper arm as part of post-burn management are rarely indicated. Post-burn compartment syndromes of the hand do occur, and are best managed by a surgeon with appropriate expertise (e.g., hand plastic surgeon).[69,70]

External fixation is generally the preferred treatment option for combat casualties with major burns and underlying extremity fractures, as these wounds are assumed to be contaminated.[71] Although the presence of nonviable tissue at the pin sites is far from ideal, alternative treatment options are even less attractive. The use of external fixation does not contribute to an increase in compartment pressures and it allows for ease of monitoring of tissue edema and viability during burn resuscitation.[72] Internal fixation may be considered in selected cases, provided there are clear advantages over external fixation and the operation can be performed before the wound becomes heavily colonized (i.e., within the first one to two days post-burn).[72]

> External fixation is generally the preferred treatment option for combat casualties with major burns and underlying extremity fractures, as these wounds are assumed to be contaminated.

### Initial Wound Care

When considering the acute management of the burn wound, it is crucial to remember that the skin is intimately linked at a physiologic level to the function of every other organ system. Generally speaking, the larger the burn wound, the greater the adverse effect on each of those systems. The sooner the burn wound is addressed, the sooner the patient can commence recovery. A thorough and continuous assessment of the burn and its healing status are paramount.

The term 'wound care' includes multiple activities often performed in a progressive manner from point of injury through initial hospital resuscitation, wound management, and rehabilitation. From the perspective of the first responder, the primary activities related to wound care involve halting the burning process and protecting the skin from further injury. In some cases, this may mean quite literally extinguishing the fire, or more often, simply removing any residual clothing or equipment that may be retaining heat, thereby furthering the insult to the tissue.

Cleansing and debridement of the burned skin follow as the next logical step in care of the burn wound. This action may include cleaning of the patient's skin with a disinfectant soap and warm water. For patients with burns related to possible chemical exposure, irrigating the skin with copious amounts of water is crucial. Brush off debris before irrigation as the damaging effects of certain chemical agents can be compounded with irrigation.

Initial debridement of patients with large surface area burns is best performed in a clean, warm operating room with anesthesia support, resuscitation capability, adequate lighting, and appropriate dressing materials. In the combat environment, this means formal debridement may have to be delayed until the patient is evacuated to a Level III Combat Support Hospital (CSH). Casualties with partial-thickness burns often demonstrate blisters as the epidermis separates from the dermis and fluid (similar in composition to plasma) fills the void (Fig. 24). In the field, it is recommended that blisters be left intact until such time as formal wound care, in a clean environment, can be performed.[73] A clean, dry bed sheet will usually provide adequate protection of the blistered skin.

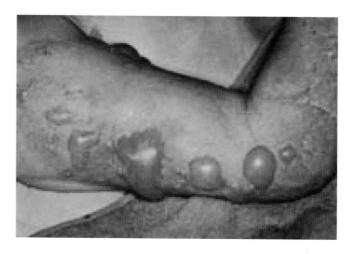

Figure 24. *Partial-thickness burns demonstrate fluid-filled blisters that should be left intact until formal wound care is performed. Image courtesy of Robert H. Demling, MD, Harvard Medical School.*

The choice of topical burn dressings and when to apply them is based on several factors: materials on-hand, provider preference, adjacent wounds, and the anticipated time and distance between successive medical facilities. Providers in the field should simply cover burns with a clean, dry dressing and avoid applying any topical ointments, including burn creams, to the wounds.[73] This approach eliminates the need for careproviders to later have to remove creams when patients present at the next facility in the evacuation chain. The use of a silver-impregnated dressing such as Silverlon®, Acticoat®, or SilverSeal® as the initial dressing is a reasonable alternative, since these materials are relatively easy to apply, provide a topical antimicrobial effect, and do not impede the subsequent examination and debridement process.[74]

> Providers in the field should simply cover burns with a clean, dry dressing and avoid applying any topical ointments, including burn creams, to the wounds.

Once the burns have been formally cleansed and debrided, dressing the wound in a silver-impregnated dressing covered by layer of gauze provides a clean, protective milieu that utilizes the silver ion as the antimicrobial agent.[74] This dressing is effective for many hours to several days. This eliminates the need for twice daily reapplication of topical creams such as Silvadene® or Sulfamylon®.[75,76] However, we caution that silver dressings do not take the place of meticulous care when wounds are contaminated or infected. Thus, burn patients with such wounds will continue to require once or twice daily dressing changes, cleansing with chlorhexidene gluconate, and reapplication of topical antimicrobial creams.

Burns sustained in combat often involve adjacent areas of open soft-tissue wounds that result from direct tissue loss, degloving injuries, or surgical debridement. Wounds of this nature are left open for serial debridement and until definitive coverage or closure can be performed.

## Patient Exposure and Hypothermia

Just as it is very important to completely expose the burn patient during the initial assessment, it is also crucial to remember that burn casualties are predisposed to hypothermia. Burn patients with large surface area burns can quickly become hypothermic due to loss of normal skin thermoregulatory function.[77] Hypothermia is even more likely in the burn patient who also has severe trauma and blood loss. Burn patients are prone to hypothermia during multiple phases of care, including operating room wound debridement, routine dressing changes, and transport.

> Burn patients with large surface area burns, especially those with traumatic injuries resulting in blood loss, can quickly become hypothermic due to loss of normal skin thermoregulatory function.

Because of this high risk of hypothermia, the burn casualty in the prehospital setting should be kept warm and dry (e.g., covered with a clean sheet and a warm blanket). Use of hypothermia prevention kits is recommended during all phases of transport. Do not wet the patient and do not apply wet sheets. The operating room should be kept as warm as possible for the casualty. Warmed intravenous fluids should be used during the resuscitation process. Research is ongoing to further evaluate the feasibility of internal warming using specialized venous catheters during the early phases of resuscitation of the military casualty.

## Pain Control

The severity of pain reported by burn casualties varies greatly. This variability is due, in part, to the extent that pain receptors are affected, the presence of concurrent injuries, and subjective components related to pain.

> The judicious administration of intravenous narcotics is generally effective in controlling pain for the burn patient. Indiscriminate dosing of narcotics may cause adverse consequences such as hypotension and respiratory depression.

Intermittent dosing of intravenous morphine or fentanyl is effective for controlling background burn injury pain. The addition of IV ketamine (0.25 to 1.0 mg per kilogram) provides very effective analgesia (disassociative sedation at higher doses) during dressing changes and other painful procedures.[78] More recently, the use of oral transmucosal fentanyl citrate (Actiq®, Cephalon Inc., Fraser, PA) has been used for acute pain management in combat.[79] Sedation using a benzodiazepine in small doses decreases anxiety and is an important adjunct to pain control. The routine use of continuous infusions of these drugs in CCC settings is discouraged unless the patient can be closely monitored to ensure optimal pain control, sedation, and immediate detection of adverse effects (e.g., respiratory depression and hypotension).

## *Advanced Burn Wound Care*

## Wound Excision

The surgical process of sharply excising burned skin (excision) and replacing it with autologous skin (grafting) is based on sound principles of general surgical wound management. Expediting this process has been shown to decrease mortality and morbidity in US burn centers.[80,81] The process of excision and grafting requires a substantial commitment of resources (personnel, supplies, and hospital support services). Excision and grafting are ideally postponed until the casualty arrives at a Level V care facility such as a burn center that is fully staffed and equipped to complete all phases of care, including rehabilitation.

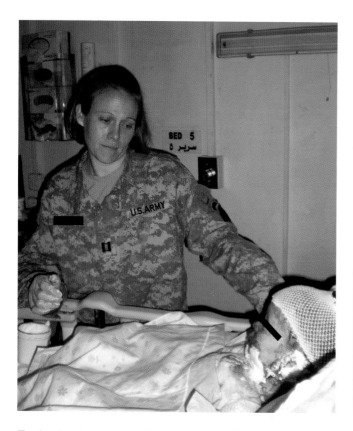

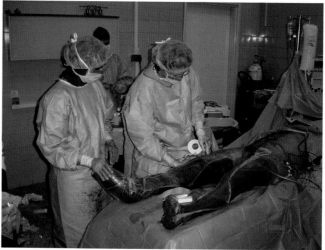

Figure 25. (Left) *Treatment of host nation patients may require surgeons to provide definitive burn care with excision and grafting.*

Figure 26. (Below) *Placement of a negative-pressure wound dressing on the lower extremities following excision and grafting is one way to achieve postoperative splinting of freshly grafted wounds.*

Early (in-theater) excision and grafting are not recommended for any patient who can be evacuated to a designated burn center within one to two weeks of burn injury. To intentionally excise the burned skin, without a means of covering the exposed tissue bed, invites unnecessary contamination and may ultimately impede definitive wound closure. Similarly, to proceed with skin grafting prior to arrival at the burn center would place the fresh grafts at undue risk for shear force injury and loss during the transport process.

On the other hand, experiences in the current conflicts in Afghanistan and Iraq have provided numerous examples of the need for forward-deployed surgeons to perform excision and grafting of burn patients who cannot be evacuated.[1] This primarily involves host nation patients whose only hope of recovery often rests with the facility at which they initially present (Fig. 25). As a consequence, staff at deployed military hospitals should be prepared to provide definitive burn care.

> Early (in-theater) excision and grafting are not recommended for any patient who can be evacuated to a designated burn center within one to two weeks of burn injury. However, forward-deployed surgeons should be familiar with this procedure for treatment of those who cannot be evacuated or host nationals.

Unlike US military casualties who are usually evacuated to medical treatment facilities within hours of injury, host nation casualties often present several days to weeks after injury. The surgeon must assess such patients with respect to wound contamination, determine whether an infection is present, and decide whether autografting would be prudent. Host nation patients presenting in a delayed fashion with invasive burn wound infections pose special management challenges (see Infection Control). A viable option for treatment of dirty or contaminated burns is to excise the wound to healthy-appearing tissue and to perform scheduled dressing changes using negative-pressure wound therapy (NPWT) until the bed appears optimal for grafting (Fig. 26).[82] Placement of allograft (cadaver skin, with or without NPWT) as a temporary

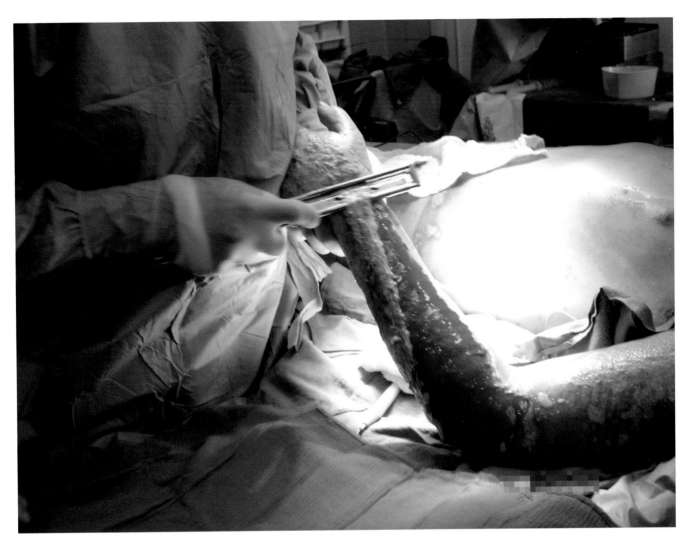

Figure 27. *The technique of tangential excision can be rapidly accomplished with a large hand dermatome. Note the potential for massive blood loss associated with this operation.*

measure to prime the wound bed is an option, if available.[83] Gammagraft® (Promethean LifeSciences, Inc., Pittsburgh, PA), an irradiated allograft product with a long shelf-life, may be considered when no other source of allograft exists.[1]

### Tangential Excision
Dermal burns are excised with multiple tangential passes of a manual dermatome (such as a Blair, Humby, Brown, Braithewaite, Watson, or Goulian-Weck instrument) until viable tissue is reached (Fig. 27). This method of tangential excision allows maximum preservation of viable dermis and subcutaneous fat. This leads to better long-term results in the quality of the healed grafts and improved mobility and range of motion for the patient. Regardless of the instrument used, the key is to remove only that which is deemed nonviable and to preserve that which may heal. Areas requiring intricate or delicate work, such as the hand and fingers, are best approached using small instruments like the Goulian dermatome, with shallow penetration and multiple passes.[84]

### Fascial Excision
Subdermal burns extending well into the subcutaneous tissue, and those that are heavily colonized or

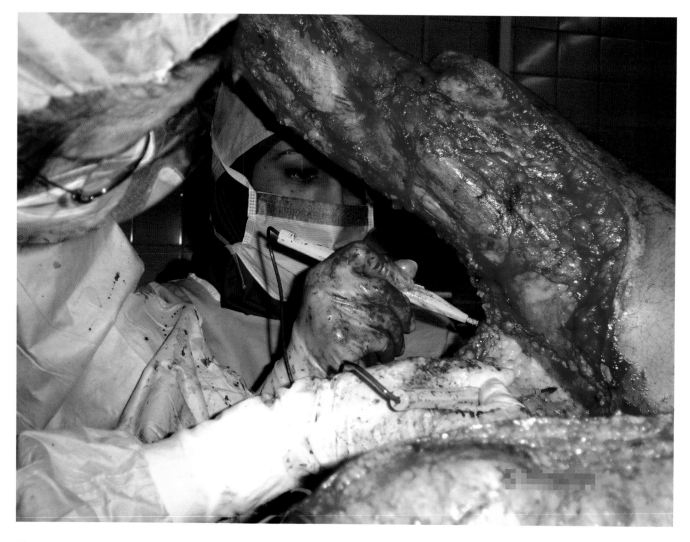

Figure 28. *Excision to fascia of deep burns of the lower extremity at a Level III facility. Excision to fascia is indicated for deep third-degree burns and infected burns. A marked step-off will be created by this soft-tissue defect.*

infected, are often best excised primarily to the level of the investing fascia (Fig. 28). Excision to this level can proceed rapidly using a knife, scissors, or electrocautery device. Fascial excision often results in less overall blood loss compared to tangential excision, as excision proceeds in a rapid manner along the fascial planes, removing all eschar with the underlying subcutaneous tissue. This process can result in the removal of a significant amount of tissue, especially in obese patients, with marked step-offs and associated soft-tissue defects.[85]

Engraftment of autograft onto fascia is often better than when grafting onto subcutaneous tissue, thereby speeding wound closure. The undesirable aspects of fascial excision and grafting include: (1) inferior cosmetic appearance, (2) increased edema in distal extremities due to the loss of venous and lymph vessels, and (3) decreased sensation and inferior functional results.[86] Each of these factors must be considered when deciding which technique to use when removing burned tissue.

Areas that have been adequately debrided show brisk punctate bleeding in healthy-appearing dermis. Poor bleeding in grayish-colored dermis indicates inadequate debridement, requiring deeper excision. As debridement progresses deeper into and through the dermis, more fat appears and capillary bleeding gives way to flow from larger arterioles and veins. The total amount of blood loss from extensive excision may be massive, and the surgical team must endeavor to monitor the wound bed for excessive bleeding and temper the pace of excision to address hemostasis.[85]

> Effective excision of burned skin uncovers the underlying vascular bed. The surgeon must monitor the pace and extent of surgical excision to ensure hemostasis is achieved.

Hemostasis in the debrided wound bed is routinely obtained using pinpoint electrocautery. Repetitive dabbing of the excised wound bed with a dry gauze sponge is an effort in futility. Instead, a bulb syringe can be used to irrigate blood off of the field during electrocautery. Compressive dressings soaked in dilute (1:100,000 or 0.01 mg per milliliter) epinephrine placed on the exposed capillary bed are effective adjunctive methods of achieving hemostasis (Fig. 29).[85] A nonadherent, perforated, polyester-film material such as TELFA™ (Kendall Brands, Covidien Inc., Mansfield, MA) can be used with the epinephrine-soaked gauze to help prevent clot dislodgment from the wound surface when the gauze is removed. Local pressure and the use of temporary elastic bandages can improve hemostasis. Recombinant human thrombin or fibrin sealants can also be used.[87,88]

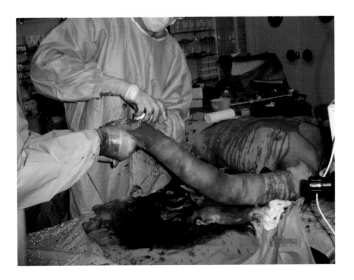

Figure 29. *Compressive dressings soaked in dilute epinephrine placed on the exposed capillary bed are effective hemostatic adjuncts.*

Whether utilizing tangential or fascial techniques to excise burned skin, blood loss can be significantly reduced with the use of pneumatic tourniquets in conjunction with temporary exanguination of the extremity. Since bleeding from the wound bed cannot be utilized as an indicator of tissue viability when using tourniquets, the operating surgeon must possess experiential knowledge of the desired appearance of the wound bed to avoid unnecessary or inadequate depth of excision. Regardless of which debridement option the surgeon chooses, he or she must be prepared for the blood loss associated with excision of burns. Two to six units of packed red blood cells should be typed and crossed for the patient in anticipation of excisions involving greater than 10% TBSA. Estimation of blood loss is difficult even for experienced burn care teams. It is recommended that less experienced teams limit their excisions to less than 10% TBSA at a time, or two hours in duration.

> Two to six units of packed red blood cells should be typed and crossed for the patient in anticipation of excisions involving greater than 10% TBSA.

## Skin Grafting
Coverage of open wounds, following either excision of burns or debridement of injured soft-tissue, can be accomplished using autograft, allograft, or biosynthetic products. Ultimate wound closure involves use of

autologous tissue, either in the form of split- or full-thickness grafts or flaps.

### Harvesting of Skin

An autograft in the form of a split-thickness skin graft (STSG) is routinely harvested at a depth of between 0.006 to 0.012 inches using either a manual, or more commonly, a powered dermatome. The advantages of using powered dermatomes are uniformity and speed in the harvesting process. Use of dilute (1:1,000,000) epinephrine in lactated Ringer's solution injected by clysis into the subcutaneous space aids in hemostasis and assists in "leveling" of the operative field prior to harvesting (Fig. 30).[89] The use of a 60-ml syringe coupled to a 18- to 16-gauge needle works satisfactorily for the clysis procedure, and can be performed fairly rapidly even for a large surface area.

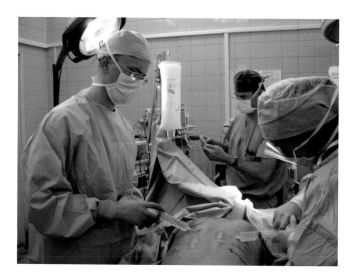

Figure 30. *Subdermal clysis aids in hemostasis and "leveling" of the operative field prior to skin harvesting.*

The selection of donor site dressing is largely a matter of operator preference.[85] Xeroform® gauze is commonly available, even in the deployed military environment, and has proven to be effective. Donor sites generally heal in about 10 to 14 days and may be reharvested multiple times once healed.

> Survival of the combat burn casualty is linked to wound closure, and the surgeon must exploit all possible donor sites to facilitate coverage. The scalp is an excellent donor site and should not be overlooked.

A STSG may be placed on the wound bed as either a sheet graft or meshed graft (Figs. 31 and 32). Typically, a properly placed STSG is adherent to the wound bed in three to five days and is durable enough for fairly aggressive cleansing after about seven days. Cleansing of the healing graft is important, especially when debris fills the interstices, impeding wound closure.

Excellent functional outcomes with STSG coverage can be achieved with early and progressive rehabilitation and through close communication between the surgeon, wound care team, and rehabilitation team to determine a safe and effective rehabilitation plan. Rehabilitation efforts involving grafted areas should be minimized during the first three days following graft placement. Mobilization activities such as transfers can be performed during this time if the area of grafting can be safely protected from shear forces. As the STSG matures, rehabilitation activities may be advanced, but every consideration must be given to protection of the healing graft until durable adherence is confirmed, usually around postoperative day seven.

Areas of burn graft in which an optimal functional or cosmetic result is desirable should be covered with thick unmeshed STSGs (Fig. 33).[90] Examples of areas best served by sheet grafting versus meshed skin grafting include the face, neck, and dorsum of the hand. Availability of adequate donor sites affects how much grafting can be accomplished using sheet grafts.[91]

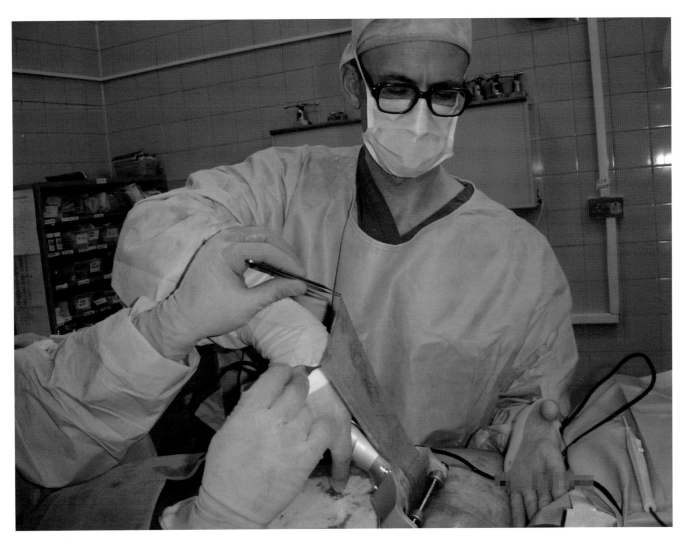

Figure 31. *Harvesting of a split-thickness skin graft at a depth of 10/1,000 inch is facilitated by subdermal clysis with a solution of epinephrine (concentration 1:1,000,000) in lactated Ringer's, injected using a 60-milliliter syringe and an 18-gauge needle. Harvesting is performed by use of an air or electric-powered dermatome. Xeroform gauze is stapled into place, followed by a dry gauze dressing and a compressive wrap such as an Ace® bandage or surgical netting (depending on location).*

## Meshed Skin Grafts

Meshing of skin allows for greater graft coverage from available donor sites, improves conformity of the graft, and provides a route of escape for serous fluid beneath the graft. Instrumentation used to reproducibly mesh skin comprises a mechanical device that allows the surgeon to expand the skin in ratios between 1:1 and 6:1. As the expansion ratio increases, the cosmetic quality of the skin decreases, and the healing time increases. A meshing ratio of 3:1 or less is employed for most circumstances due to the friability and prolonged healing associated with wider expansion.[91] There are times, however, when donor sites are so limited as to demand that ratios of 4:1 or higher are used. Using a "sandwich" technique in which widely meshed autograft is covered with sheet allograft serves to protect the underlying tissue bed during prolonged healing.[91]

There are several different types of meshing devices available to the surgeon (Fig. 34). Some devices utilize a flat carrier upon which the skin is placed prior to being passed through the cutting blades. Another version of this device utilizes carriers with fine ridges, which work with the mesher blades to create the desired

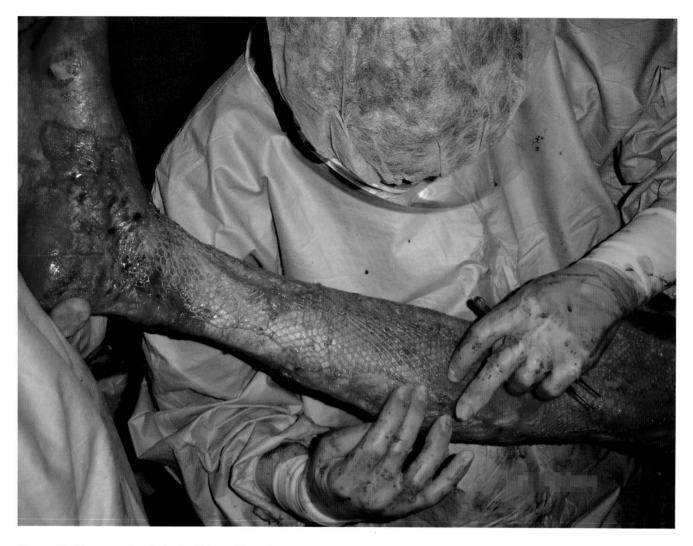

Figure 32. *Placement of meshed split-thickness skin graft on the lower extremity following excision to fascia, performed at a Level III facility. Excision and grafting at hospitals in the combat zone are generally not performed, except in cases of host national casualties who do not have other treatment options.*

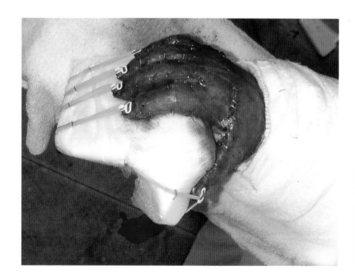

Figure 33. *Unmeshed split-thickness skin grafts should be used in areas where optimal function or cosmetic result is desirable.*

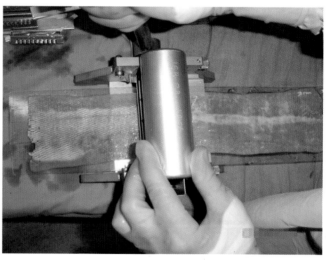

Figure 34. *Meshing of the skin allows for greater graft coverage, improved conformity of the graft, and drainage of serous fluid.*

pattern. A third type uses no carrier, requiring only that the skin be fed through the cutting rollers in a uniform manner.

> Regardless of the type of mesher utilized, it is imperative that both the surgeon and the operating room technician know how to use the meshing device prior to starting the case to avoid wasting any valuable donor autograft.

### Full-Thickness Skin Grafts

The most common alternative to the STSG is a full-thickness skin graft (FTSG). The main advantages of using the FTSG are durability of the healed wound, minimal contracture, and cosmesis.[90] The disadvantages of using a FTSG include loss of valuable donor site and necessity for excellent vascularization for graft survival. The technique of harvesting a FTSG involves sharply incising the skin into the subcutaneous layer, then preparing the FTSG by removing as much of the subcutaneous tissue as possible from the dermis. Donor sites for a FTSG may be closed primarily or covered with a STSG. Most FTSGs heal in 10 to 14 days.[91]

Regardless of the type of graft used, protection of the graft with proper limb splinting and positioning is essential.[85] Mobilization activities such as transfers and ambulation can be performed within the first few days after grafting, provided that the graft site can be safely protected. Excellent functional outcomes with FTSG coverage can be achieved with early and progressive rehabilitation and through close communication between the surgeon, wound care team, and rehabilitation therapists.

### Engraftment

Meticulous wound management during the immediate postoperative period is vital to graft viability and patient survival due to the importance of burn wound closure. Movement of the graft or shear is the principal cause of graft failure; infection is the second.[92,93] Securing the graft to the wound bed is important because unintended motion disrupts neovascularization, leading to death of the graft.

> Movement of the graft or shear is the principal cause of graft failure; infection is the second.

To minimize the possibility of movement, grafts are typically secured with staples or sutures. Surgical staples are quickly applied and relatively easy to remove. Advantages of sewing the grafts in place include more precise placement and the ability to use absorbable suture, eliminating the need for later removal. Suturing generally takes considerably longer than stapling. Adhesives such as fibrin glue may be used to supplement adherence, especially in areas with irregular contours.[87] When using biological glue, it is important to ensure that any dressing applied over the graft does not adhere to wound.

Splints incorporated into the final dressing help maintain the desired limb position and help prevent graft loss due to shear, especially over joints. The use of negative-pressure wound dressings has increased in popularity due to their effectiveness in promoting engraftment and protection against shear, provided that negative pressure is maintained. At the first dressing change, the nonadherent dressing can be left in place, provided there are no signs of infection. This layer is removed over the course of the next two to three days as the graft interstices close. Removal of the dressing in contact with the graft is facilitated by soaking the dressing with 5% solution of Sulfamyalon® or saline prior to removal.

## Infection Control

Despite many advances in burn care, local infection related to unhealed burn wounds can lead to systemic illness and death.[94] Measures to prevent burn wound infection include meticulous wound care. This includes effective topical antimicrobial therapy, removing all nonviable tissue (tissue debridement), and timely excision and grafting when indicated. Contact precautions, including isolation in private rooms, should be liberally employed in the treatment of burn patients. The use of gloves and gowns when in contact with the burn patient assists in minimizing nosocomial spread of infection. Meticulous and regular use of antimicrobial hand cleanser should be the rule for all providers caring for burn patients.[95]

> Measures to prevent burn wound infection include topical antimicrobial therapy, tissue debridement, and timely excision and grafting when indicated. The use of prophylactic antibiotics in burn patients is not recommended except perioperatively.

Burns should be considered contaminated wounds, and casualties should have their tetanus immunization status updated accordingly. The use of prophylactic antibiotics in burn patients is not recommended except perioperatively (in association with excision and grafting procedures).[96] A rim of mildly erythematous tissue often surrounds healing burns, but extension of the erythema more than two centimeters past the wound margin implies cellulitis, which should be treated with antibiotics aimed at beta-hemolytic streptococcal and staphylococcal infections (Fig. 35).[97] Such gram-positive infections are highly responsive to therapy.[95]

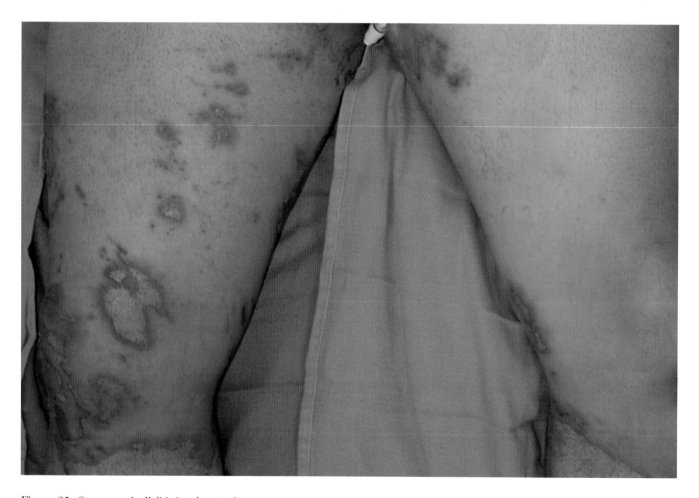

Figure 35. *Streptococcal cellulitis in a burn patient.*

By contrast, when burn patients demonstrate systemic evidence of sepsis, particularly when coupled with color changes in the wound, an invasive gram-negative burn wound infection should be suspected and treated aggressively (Fig. 36). In the absence of effective topical antimicrobial therapy, the risk of gram-negative wound infection is a function of burn size (i.e., patients with larger burns are more likely to present with and die from such infections).[98] These patients require: (1) aggressive resuscitation (early goal-directed therapy treatment for sepsis); (2) topical therapy with mafenide acetate cream (Sulfamylon®); (3) treatment with antibiotics effective against gram-negative organisms (the authors currently use imipenem-cilastatin, and amikacin, to cover multiple-drug-resistant *Pseudomonas* spp. and *Klebsiella pneumoniae*); (4) prompt infection source control by excision to fascia; (5) a scheduled second-look operation; and (6) subsequent grafting.[95] In addition, post-excision topical use of 5% Sulfamylon® solution, or of dilute Dakin's solution (0.025% sodium hypochlorite), may be used to combat gram-negative colonization.[99]

## Metabolic and Nutritional Considerations

Burn patients demonstrate extraordinary increases in metabolic rate, as a function of burn size.[100,101] There are several important consequences of this. Patients demonstrate a persistent tachycardia that makes heart

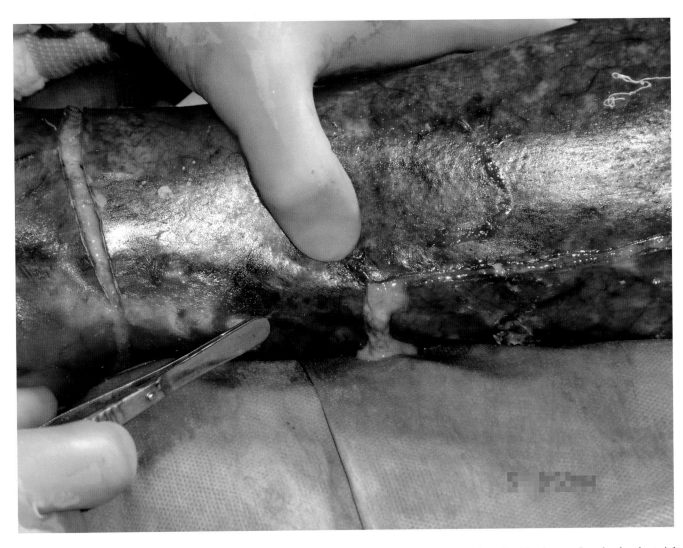

Figure 36. *Host nationals may present with sepsis due to infected burn wounds several days after injury. In this photograph, subeschar bacterial proliferation and suppuration have occurred. After resuscitation, this patient's burns were excised primarily to fascia.*

rate a poor indicator of both effective resuscitation and suspected sepsis. Elevated core temperature is also common. Therefore, the usual definitions of fever need to be adjusted upwards, accepting core temperature values of up to 38.5°C before antipyretics are given.[102,103] The massive caloric requirements engendered by this hypermetabolic state cannot be met by oral alimentation alone. Therefore, patients with burns totaling greater than 30% TBSA require Dobhoff or nasogastric tube feeding. Early enteral nutrition is encouraged, provided the patient is not hemodynamically unstable or requiring pharmacological support with vasopressor agents.[104] Immediate post-burn administration of acid-suppressive medications (proton-pump inhibitors, $H_2$-blockers, or antacids) is critical for preventing gastroduodenal ulceration (Curling's ulcer).[105,106,107,108]

## *Aeromedical Transport and Definitive Care*

All military burn casualties who require the level of care offered by a burn center are transferred to the USAISR Burn Center at Brooke Army Medical Center in San Antonio, Texas (Fig. 37). The ability to safely transport burn casualties across long distances, while continuing resuscitation, allows rapid transfer of patients to facilities capable of providing definitive care. This capability facilitates the overall process of burn care for combat casualties as it enables early excision and grafting and early rehabilitation therapy. Evacuation policies regarding burn casualties are similar to guidelines published by the American Burn Association (ABA) for burn center admission criteria. Both are based on the severity of burn injury, the presence of inhalation injury, and other associated injuries (Table 2).[109]

Critically injured burn casualties, typically those with large surface area burns and/or inhalation injury, are transported to the burn center by one of the US Army's Burn Flight Teams. Each team consists of a general surgeon, a registered nurse, a licensed vocational nurse, a respiratory therapist, and an operations officer, each of whom work daily in the intensive care units of the burn center.[110] Burn casualties not requiring Burn Flight Team support, but with one or more other critical problems of lesser severity, are transported by a US Air Force Critical Care Air Transport Team (CCATT). The CCATT crews consist of a physician, registered nurse, and respiratory technician, each trained in the management of critically ill patients in flight.[111,112,113]

For patients requiring mechanical ventilation during flight, the choice of ventilator and ventilator mode during transport is based on the patient's severity of injury, pulmonary status, and response to ventilatory support. Patients with inhalation injury may require significant ventilatory support beyond the capabilities of conventional ventilators

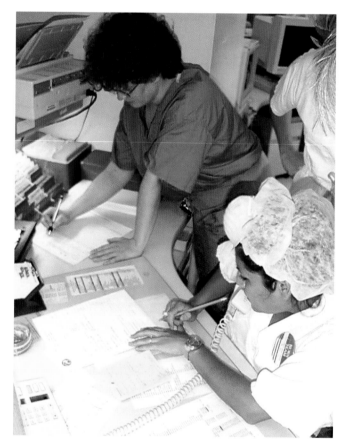

Figure 37. *Staff at the USAISR Burn Center take a call from a referring hospital. Early and frequent communication between the referring medical treatment facility and the burn center are absolutely essential to successful transfer of a patient with severe thermal injury.*

Table 2. *Evacuation policies surrounding burn casualties mirror ABA burn center admission criteria.*[109]

used for evacuation. Extensive use of the Volumetric Diffusive Respiration ventilator (VDR-4®) by the USAISR Burn Center to treat patients with inhalation injury and other severe pulmonary problems led to extensive use of the VDR-4® in patient transport.[20] The TXP® pressure-controlled ventilator is also used in the evacuation of patients because of its simplicity, compact size, and effectiveness in this patient population.[114] Both the VDR® and TXP® are powered by compressed air or oxygen, have no electrical requirements, and are approved for use on all military aircraft.

As with the interfacility transfer of any critically ill or injured patient, communication between the sending and accepting physician is essential for optimal continuity of care. Staff at the USAISR Burn Center is available 24 hours per day, seven days per week, to respond to questions and to facilitate evacuation of seriously injured burn casualties.

Providers are encouraged to call (210) 916-2876 to contact the burn center attending surgeon, or DSN (312) 429-2876 if commercial access is not available. Consultation may also be initiated by sending an email message to US Army Medical Department burn consultants (burntrauma.consult@us.army.mil).

## *Summary*

Critical elements of caring for burn patients in a combat environment are: (1) careful titration of fluid resuscitation (neither too much, nor too little) during a burn shock period that lasts at least 48 hours; (2) awareness of the risks of over-resuscitation and prompt recognition and management of such complications (e.g., abdominal and extremity compartment syndromes); (3) strategically-timed aeromedical evacuation, which balances the need for close monitoring and hemodynamic stability during the burn shock period against the need for early excision of large burns in a dedicated burn center; and (4) recognition of the scope and burden of civilian burn care during combat (e.g., definitive surgical care that includes excision and grafting of burned children and adults).

# References

1. Cancio LC, Horvath EE, Barillo DJ, et al. Burn support for Operation Iraqi Freedom and related operations, 2003 to 2004. J Burn Care Rehabil 2005;26(2):151-161.

2. Pruitt BA, Mason AD Jr. Epidemiological, demographic and outcome characteristics of burn injury. In: Herndon DN, editor. Total burn care. 3rd ed. London: W.B. Saunders; 1996. p. 5-15.

3. Kauvar DS, Wade CE, Baer DG. Burn hazards of the deployed environment in wartime: epidemiology of noncombat burns from ongoing United States military operations. J Am Coll Surg 2009;209(4):453-460.

4. Chapman TT, Richard RL, Hedman TL, et al. Combat casualty hand burns: evaluating impairment and disability during recovery. J Hand Ther 2008;21(2):150-158; quiz 159.

5. Renz EM, Cancio LC, Barillo DJ, et al. Long range transport of war-related burn casualties. J Trauma 2008;64(2 Suppl):S136-144; discussion S144-145.

6. Wolf SE, Kauvar DS, Wade CE, et al. Comparison between civilian burns and combat burns from Operation Iraqi Freedom and Operation Enduring Freedom. Ann Surg 2006;243(6):786-792; discussion 792-792.

7. US Department of Defense (US DoD). Triage. In: Emergency War Surgery, Third United States Revision. Washington, DC: Department of the Army, Office of the Surgeon General, Borden Institute; 2004. p. 3.1-3.17.

8. Burkle FM Jr, Orebaugh S, Barendse BR. Emergency medicine in the Persian Gulf War-Part 1: Preparations for triage and combat casualty care. Ann Emerg Med 1994;23(4):742-747.

9. Wolf SE, Rose JK, Desai MH, et al. Mortality determinants in massive pediatric burns. An analysis of 103 children with > or = 80% TBSA burns (> or = 70% full-thickness). Ann Surg 1997;225(5):554-565; discussion 565-569.

10. White CE, Renz EM. Advances in surgical care: management of severe burn injury. Crit Care 2008;36(7 Suppl):S318-324.

11. Kauvar DS, Wolf SE, Wade CE, et al. Burns sustained in combat explosions in Operations Iraqi and Enduring Freedom (OIF/OEF explosion burns). Burns 2006;32(7):853-857.

12. Advanced Burn Life Support Course Instructor's Manual. Chicago, IL: American Burn Association, 2001.

13. Barillo DJ, Cancio LC, Goodwin CW. Treatment of white phosphorus and other chemical burn injuries at one burn center over a 51-year period. Burns 2004;30(5):448-452.

14. Davis KG. Acute management of white phosphorus burn. Mil Med 2002;167(1):83-84.

15. Bowen TE, Whelan TJ Jr, Nelson TG. Sudden death after phosphorus burns: experimental observations of hypocalcemia, hyperphosphatemia and electrocardiographic abnormalities following production of a standard white phosphorus burn. Ann Surg 1971;174(5):779-784.

16. Lee RC. Injury by electrical forces: pathophysiology, manifestations, and therapy. Curr Probl Surg 1997;34(9):677-764.

17. Lee RC, Zhang D, Hannig J. Biophysical injury mechanisms in electrical shock trauma. Annu Rev Biomed Eng 2000;2:477-509.

18. Cancio LC, Jimenez-Reyna JF, Barillo DJ, et al. One hundred ninety-five cases of high-voltage electric injury. J Burn Care Rehabil 2005;26(4):331-340.

19. Zak AL, Harrington DT, Barillo DJ, et al. Acute respiratory failure that complicates the resuscitation of pediatric patients with scald injuries. J Burn Care Rehabil 1999;20(5):391-399.

20. Cancio LC. Airway management and smoke inhalation injury in the burn patient. Clin Plastic Surg 2009;36(4):555-567.

21. Shirani KZ, Moylan JA Jr, Pruitt BA Jr. Diagnosis and treatment of inhalation injury in burn patients. In: Loke J, editor. Pathophysiology and treatment of inhalation injuries. New York: Marcel Dekker; 1988. p. 239-280.

22. Clark WR, Bonaventura M, Myers W. Smoke inhalation and airway management at a regional burn unit: 1974-1983. Part I: Diagnosis and consequences of smoke inhalation. J Burn Care Rehabil 1989;10(1):52-62.

23. Clark WR, Bonaventura M, Myers W, et al. Smoke inhalation and airway management at a regional burn unit: 1974 to 1983. II. Airway management. J Burn Care Rehabil 1990;11(2):121-134.

24. Desai MH, Mlcak R, Richardson J, et al. Reduction in mortality in pediatric patients with inhalation injury with aerosolized heparin/N-acetylcystine [correction of acetylcystine] therapy. J Burn Care Rehabil 1998;19(3):210-212.

25. Miller AC, Rivero A, Ziad S, et al. Influence of nebulized unfractionated heparin and N-acetylcysteine in acute lung injury after smoke inhalation injury. J Burn Care Res 2009;30(2):249-256.

26. Orgill DP, Piccolo N. Escharotomy and decompressive therapies in burns. J Burn Care Res 2009;30(5):759-768.

27. Holcomb JB, McMullin NR, Pearse L, et al. Causes of death in U.S. Special Operations Forces in the global war on terrorism: 2001-2004. Ann Surg 2007;245(6):986-991.

28. Ramasamy A, Harrisson SE, Clasper JC, et al. Injuries from roadside improvised explosive devices. J Trauma 2008;65(4):910-914.

29. Heimbach DM, Afromowitz MA, Engrav LH, et al. Burn depth estimation—man or machine. J Trauma 1984;24(5):373-378.

30. Jaskille AD, Shupp JW, Jordan MH, et al. Critical review of burn depth assessment techniques: Part I. Historical review. J Burn Care Res 2009;30(6):937-947.

31. Wachtel TL, Berry CC, Wachtel EE, et al. The inter-rater reliability of estimating the size of burns from various burn area chart drawings. Burns 2000;26(2):156-170.

32. Frascone R, Kaye K, Dries D, et al. Successful placement of an adult sternal intraosseous line through burned skin. J Burn Care Rehabil 2003;24(5):306-308.

33. Alvarado R, Chung KK, Cancio LC, et al. Burn resuscitation. Burns 2009;35(1):4-14.

34. Chung KK, Wolf SE, Cancio LC, et al. Resuscitation of severely burned military casualties: fluid begets more fluid. J Trauma 2009;67(2):231-237; discussion 237.

35. Ennis JL, Chung KK, Renz EM, et al. Joint Theater Trauma System implementation of burn resuscitation guidelines improves outcomes in severely burned military casualties. J Trauma 2008;64(2 Suppl):S146-151; discussion S151-152.

36. Chung KK, Blackbourne LH, Wolf SE, et al. Evolution of burn resuscitation in operation Iraqi freedom. J Burn Care Res 2006;27(5):606-611.

37. Pruitt BA. Advances in fluid therapy and the early care of the burn patient. World J Surg 1978;2(2):139-150.

38. Graves TA, Cioffi WG, McManus WF, et al. Fluid resuscitation of infants and children with massive thermal injury. J Trauma 1988;28(12):1656-1659.

39. Pham TN, Cancio LC, Gibran NS, et al. American Burn Association practice guidelines: burn shock resuscitation. J Burn Care Res 2008;29(1):257-266.

40. Salinas J, Drew G, Gallagher J, et al. Closed-loop and decision-assist resuscitation of burn patients. J Trauma 2008;64(4 Suppl):S321-332.

41. Kuwa T, Jordan BS, Cancio LC. Use of power Doppler ultrasound to monitor renal perfusion during burn shock. Burns 2006;32(6):706-713.

42. Cancio LC, Kuwa T, Matsui K, et al. Intestinal and gastric tonometry during experimental burn shock. Burns 2007;33(7):879-884.

43. Pruitt BA Jr. Protection from excessive resuscitation: "pushing the pendulum back." J Trauma 2000;49(3):567-568.

44. Jaskille AD, Jeng JC, Sokolich JC, et al. Repetitive ischemia-reperfusion injury: a plausible mechanism for documented clinical burn-depth progression after thermal injury. J Burn Care Res 2007;28(1):13-20.

45. Cancio LC, Galvez E Jr, Turner CE, et al. Base deficit and alveolar-arterial gradient during resuscitation contribute independently but modestly to the prediction of mortality after burn injury. J Burn Care Res 2006;27(3):289-296.

46. Ivy ME, Atweh NA, Palmer J, et al. Intra-abdominal hypertension and abdominal compartment syndrome in burn patients. J Trauma 2000;49(3):387-391.

47. Greenhalgh DG, Warden GD. The importance of intra-abdominal pressure measurements in burned children. J Trauma 1994;36(5):685-690.

48. Tsoutsos D, Rodopoulou S, Keramidas E, et al. Early escharotomy as a measure to reduce intraabdominal hypertension in full-thickness burns of the thoracic and abdominal area. World J Surg 2003;27(12):1323-1328.

49. Latenser BA, Kowal-Vern A, Kimball D, et al. A pilot study comparing percutaneous decompression with decompressive laparotomy for acute abdominal compartment syndrome in thermal injury. J Burn Care Rehabil 2002;23(3):190-195.

50. Hobson KG, Young KM, Ciraulo A, et al. Release of abdominal compartment syndrome improves survival in patients with burn injury. J Trauma 2002;53(6):1129-1133.

51. O'Mara MS, Slater H, Goldfarb IW, et al. A prospective, randomized evaluation of intra-abdominal pressures with crystalloid and colloid resuscitation in burn patients. J Trauma 2005;58(5):1011-1018.

52. Saffle JI. The phenomenon of "fluid creep" in acute burn resuscitation. J Burn Care Res 2007;28(3): 382-395.

53. Oda J, Ueyama M, Yamashita K, et al. Hypertonic lactated saline resuscitation reduces the risk of abdominal compartment syndrome in severely burned patients. J Trauma 2006;60(1):64-71.

54. Bosch X, Poch E, Grau JM. Rhabdomyolysis and acute kidney injury. N Engl J Med 2009;361(1):62-72.

55. Ron D, Taitelman U, Michaelson M, et al. Prevention of acute renal failure in traumatic rhabdomyolysis. Arch Intern Med 1984;144(2):277-280.

56. Brown CV, Rhee P, Chan L, et al. Preventing renal failure in patients with rhabdomyolysis: do bicarbonate and mannitol make a difference? J Trauma 2004;56(6):1191-1196.

57. Homsi E, Barreiro MF, Orlando JM, et al. Prophylaxis of acute renal failure in patients with rhabdomyolysis. Ren Fail 1997;19(2):283-288.

58. Huerta-Alardín AL, Varon J, Marik PE. Bench-to-bedside review: rhabdomyolysis—an overview for clinicians. Crit Care 2005;9(2):158-169.

59. Conger JD. Interventions in clinical acute renal failure: what are the data? Am J Kidney Dis 1995;26(4):565-576.

60. Harrison HN, Moncrief JA, Ducket JW Jr, et al. The relationship between energy metabolism and water loss from vaporization in severely burned patients. Surgery 1964;56:203-211.

61. Shirani KZ, Vaughan GM, Robertson GL, et al. Inappropriate vasopressin secretion (SIADH) in burned patients. J Trauma 1983;23(3):217-224.

62. Kang SK, Kim W, Oh MS. Pathogenesis and treatment of hypernatremia. Nephron 2002;92(Suppl 1):14-17.

63. Fried LF, Palevsky PM. Hyponatremia and hypernatremia. Med Clin North Am 1997;81(3):585-609.

64. Lindner G, Schwarz C, Kneidinger N, et al. Can we really predict the change in serum sodium levels? An analysis of currently proposed formulae in hypernatraemic patients. Nephrol Dial Transplant 2008;23(11):3501-3508.

65. Lovén L, Nordström H, Lennquist S. Changes in calcium and phosphate and their regulating hormones in patients with severe burn injuries. Scand J Plast Reconstr Surg 1984;18(1):49-53.

66. Pruitt BA Jr, Dowling JA, Moncrief JA. Escharotomy in early burn care. Arch Surg 1968;96(4):502-507.

67. Brown RL, Greenhalgh DG, Kagan RJ, et al. The adequacy of limb escharotomies-fasciotomies after referral to a major burn center. J Trauma 1994;37(6):916-920.

68. Dulhunty JM, Boots RJ, Rudd MJ, et al. Increased fluid resuscitation can lead to adverse outcomes in major-burn injured patients, but low mortality is achievable. Burns 2008;34(8):1090-1097.

69. Ouellette EA, Kelly R. Compartment syndromes of the hand. J Bone Joint Surg Am 1996;78(10):1515-1522.

70. Salisbury RE, McKeel DW, Mason AD Jr. Ischemic necrosis of the intrinsic muscles of the hand after thermal injuries. J Bone Joint Surg Am 1974;56(8):1701-1707.

71. Murray CK, Hsu JR, Solomkin JS, et al. Prevention and management of infections associated with combat-related extremity injuries. J Trauma 2008;64(3 Suppl):S239-251.

72. Saffle JR, Schnelby A, Hofmann A, et al. The management of fractures in thermally injured patients. J Trauma 1983;23(10):902-910.

73. US Department of Defense (US DoD). Burns. In: Emergency War Surgery, Third United States Revision. Washington, DC: Department of the Army, Office of the Surgeon General, Borden Institute; 2004. p. 28.1-28.15.

74. Chu CS, McManus AT, Pruitt BA Jr, et al. Therapeutic effects of silver nylon dressings with weak direct current on *Pseudomonas aeruginosa*-infected burn wounds. J Trauma 1988;28(10):1488-1492.

75. Fong J, Wood F, Fowler B. A silver coated dressing reduces the incidence of early burn wound cellulitis and associated costs of inpatient treatment: comparative patient care audits. Burns 2005;31(5):562-567.

76. Tredget EE, Shankowsky HA, Groeneveld A, et al. A matched-pair, randomized study evaluating the efficacy and safety of Acticoat silver-coated dressing for the treatment of burn wounds. J Burn Care Rehabil 1998;19(6):531-537.

77. Gore DC, Beaston J. Infusion of hot crystalloid during operative burn wound debridement. J Trauma 1997;42(6):1112-1125.

78. Owens VF, Palmieri TL, Comroe CM, et al. Ketamine: a safe and effective agent for painful procedures in the pediatric burn patient. J Burn Care Res 2006;27(2):211-216; discussion 217.

79. Kotwal RS, O'Connor KC, Johnson TR, et al. A novel pain management strategy for combat casualty care. Ann Emerg Med 2004;44(2):121-127.

80. Wolfe RA, Roi LD, Flora JD, et al. Mortality differences and speed of wound closure among specialized burn care facilities. JAMA 1983;250(6):763-766.

81. Herndon DN, Barrow RE, Rutan RL, et al. A comparison of conservative versus early excision. Therapies in severely burned patients. Ann Surg 1989;209(5):547-552; discussion 552-553.

82. Thompson JT, Marks MW. Negative pressure wound therapy. Clin Plast Surg 2007;34(4):673-684.

83. Shuck JM, Pruitt BA Jr, Moncrief JA. Homograft skin for wound coverage. A study of versatility. Arch Surg 1969;98(4):472-479.

84. Goodwin CW, Maguire MS, McManus WF, et al. Prospective study of burn wound excision of the hands. J Trauma 1983;23(6):510-517.

85. Waymack JP, Pruitt BA Jr. Burn wound care. Adv Surg 1990;23:261-289.

86. Jones T, McDonald S, Deitch EA. Effect of graft bed on long-term functional results of extremity skin grafts. J Burn Care Rehabil. 1988;9(1):72-74.

87. Foster K, Greenhalgh D, Gamelli RL, et al. Efficacy and safety of a fibrin sealant for adherence of autologous skin grafts to burn wounds: results of a phase 3 clinical study. J Burn Care Res 2008;29(2):293-303.

88. Greenhalgh DG, Gamelli RL, Collins J, et al. Recombinant thrombin: safety and immunogenicity in burn wound excision and grafting. J Burn Care Res 2009;30(3):371-379.

89. Robertson RD, Bond P, Wallace B, et al. The tumescent technique to significantly reduce blood loss during burn surgery. Burns 2001;27(8):835-838.

90. Muller M, Gahankari D, Herndon DN. Operative wound management. In: Herndon DN, editor. Total burn care. 3rd ed. London: Saunders Elsevier; 2007. p. 177-195.

91. Herndon DN, ed. Total burn care. Philadelphia: Saunders Elsevier, 2007.

92. Sheridan RL, Behringer GE, Ryan CM, et al. Effective postoperative protection for grafted posterior surfaces: the quilted dressing. J Burn Care Rehabil 1995;16(6):607-609.

93. Teh BT. Why do skin grafts fail? Plast Reconstr Surg 1979;63(3):323-332.

94. Cancio LC, Howard PA, McManus AT, et al. Burn wound infections. In: Holzheimer RG, Mannic JA, editors. Surgical treatment—evidence-based and problem-oriented. New York: W. Zuckschwerdt Verlag GmbH; 2001. p. 671-683.

95. McManus AT, Mason AD Jr, McManus WF, et al. A decade of reduced gram-negative infections and mortality associated with improved isolation of burned patients. Arch Surg 1994;129(12):1306-1309.

96. Mozingo DW, McManus AT, Kim SH, et al. Incidence of bacteremia after burn wound manipulation in the early postburn period. J Trauma 1997;42(6):1006-1010.

97. Pruitt BA Jr, McManus AT, Kim SH, et al. Burn wound infections: current status. World J Surg 1998;22(2):135-145.

98. Brown TP, Cancio LC, McManus AT, et al. Survival benefit conferred by topical antimicrobial preparations in burn patients: a historical perspective. J Trauma 2004;56(4):863-866.

99. Wilhelmi BJ, Calianos TA II, Appelt EA, et al. Modified Dakin's solution for cutaneous vibrio infections. Ann Plast Surg 1999;43(4):386-389.

100. Wilmore DW, Long JM, Mason AD Jr, et al. Catecholamines: mediator of the hypermetabolic response to thermal injury. Ann Surg 1974;180(4):653-669.

101. Kelemen JJ III, Cioffi WG Jr, Mason AD Jr, et al. Effect of ambient temperature on metabolic rate after thermal injury. Ann Surg 1996;223(4):406-412.

102. Wilmore DW, Aulick LH, Mason AD, et al. Influence of the burn wound on local and systemic responses to injury. Ann Surg 1977;186(4):444-458.

103. Childs C. Fever in burned children. Burns Incl Therm Inj 1988;14(1):1-6.

104. Cancio LC, Pruitt BA Jr. Thermal injury. In: Tsokos GC, Atkins JL, editors. Combat medicine: basic and clinical research in military, trauma, and emergency medicine. Totowa, NJ: Humana Press; 2003. p. 291-324.

105. Czaja AJ, McAlhany JC, Pruitt BA Jr. Acute gastroduodenal disease after thermal injury. An endoscopic evaluation of incidence and natural history. N Engl J Med 1974;291(18):925-929.

106. Fadaak HA. Gastrointestinal haemorrhage in burn patients: the experience of a burn unit in Saudi Arabia. Ann Burns Fire Disasters 2000;13(2):81-83.

107. MacLaren R. A review of stress ulcer prophylaxis. J Pharm Pract 2002;15(2):147-157.

108. Moscona R, Kaufman T, Jacobs R, et al. Prevention of gastrointestinal bleeding in burns: the effects of cimetidine or antacids combined with early enteral feeding. Burns Incl Therm Inj 1985;12(1):65-67.

109. American Burn Association (ABA). Burn Center Referral Criteria. ABA Web site. Available at http://www.ameriburn.org/BurnUnitReferral.pdf. Accessed May 12, 2010.

110. Cancio LC, Pruitt BA Jr. Management of mass casualty burn disasters. Int J Disast Med 2004;2(4):114-129.

111. Beninati W, Meyer MT, Carter TE. The critical care air transport program. Crit Care Med 2008;36(7 Suppl):S370-376.

112. Bridges E, Evers K. Wartime critical care air transport. Mil Med 2009;174(4):370-375.

113. Rice DH, Kotti G, Beninati W. Clinical review: critical care transport and austere critical care. Crit Care 2008;12(2):207.

114. Barillo DJ, Dickerson EE, Cioffi WG, et al. Pressure-controlled ventilation for the long-range aeromedical transport of patients with burns. J Burn Care Rehabil 1997;18(3):200-205.

# CRITICAL CARE

*Chapter 13*

**Contributing Authors**
David Norton, MD, LTC, MC, US Air Force
Phillip Mason, MD, MAJ, US Air Force
Jay Johannigman, MD, COL, US Air Force Reserves

All figures and tables included in this chapter have been used with permission from Pelagique, LLC, the UCLA Center for International Medicine, and/or the authors, unless otherwise noted.

**Disclaimer**
The opinions and views expressed herein belong solely to those of the authors. They are not nor should they be implied as being endorsed by the United States Uniformed Services University of the Health Sciences, Department of the Army, Department of the Navy, Department of the Air Force, Department of Defense, or any other branch of the federal government.

# Table of Contents

# Introduction

The provision of critical care in the combat environment is never a passive process. There is always an opportunity to affect great change that can alter the course of a patient's recovery. A command of several core concepts is vital for those who practice in the combat intensive care unit (ICU). This chapter will review basic mechanical ventilation, pulmonary contusion management, acute respiratory distress syndrome management, endpoints of resuscitation, sepsis, several basic ICU care considerations for the combat casualty care (CCC) patient, and the critical care air transportation system. In a given day at a wartime trauma resuscitation hospital, a clinician will encounter every one of these issues. They are fundamental, common, and important to master.

# Mechanical Ventilation

The birth of the intensive care unit can be traced back to the application of invasive positive-pressure mechanical ventilation during the polio epidemic of 1952 in Denmark.[1] Prior to that time, positive-pressure ventilation (PPV) had been used only sparingly for a few decades by anesthesiologists in the operating room. Most of the mechanical ventilation provided to patients with neurologic disorders or respiratory failure prior to 1952 was done with negative-pressure ventilation (NPV) devices such as the cuirass respirator or the iron lung (tank respirator). While negative-pressure ventilation more accurately simulates normal physiologic breathing, positive-pressure ventilation is used almost exclusively in modern critical care, mainly due to improved access to the patient.

Mechanical ventilation has evolved as a discipline quite rapidly over the last few decades, and lessons learned are now paying substantial dividends with respect to morbidity and mortality. This section will focus primarily on the use of invasive mechanical ventilation to support the trauma patient encountered in the combat critical care setting. The use of noninvasive mechanical ventilation will be discussed in certain settings below where it may have a role, such as mild pulmonary contusion. The most important aspect of mechanical ventilation is defining the goals associated with its use in a given setting. A clear understanding of the clinical endpoint for this therapy will allow earlier liberation and improved outcomes.

## *Key Concepts*

Many trauma patients are placed on invasive mechanical ventilation primarily for airway protection early in a resuscitation or during perioperative periods. The method used to secure an airway depends upon the nature of the injury and the expected clinical course. Options include endotracheal intubation, nasotracheal intubation, cricothyroidotomy, and formal operative tracheotomy. Ensuring a stable, secure airway is always the first priority of any resuscitation. As vital as this step is, it is only the beginning. Mechanical ventilation is primarily a supportive therapy that buys time for an injury to heal, but it also has the ability to cause great harm if not used appropriately. A basic understanding of pulmonary system compliance, gas exchange, and ventilator-induced lung injury (VILI) is vital for its rational use.

> A clear understanding of the goals and clinical endpoint of mechanical ventilation will allow for earlier weaning and improved outcomes.

Compliance is defined as a change in volume divided by a change in pressure. In a given system, it may describe the change in volume expected if a given pressure is applied or vice versa. A system is said to be highly compliant when a large change in volume is associated with a small change in pressure.

With respect to invasive mechanical ventilation, pulmonary system compliance is assessed by the machine at bedside. This measurement is made at some distance from the patient, and its significance depends upon the clinical setting. Pulmonary system compliance is a combination of the pulmonary compliance and that of the chest wall. The lungs have a tendency to pull the chest wall centrally while the chest wall is inclined to pull the lungs outward. The balance of these two forces defines the pulmonary system compliance in a given patient. A lung that is stiff due to pulmonary edema surrounded by a normal chest wall may generate a similarly decreased pulmonary system compliance as a normal lung enclosed within a chest whose motion is restricted by a circumferential burn eschar. While esophageal manometry can be used to distinguish chest wall versus pulmonary contributions to the overall system compliance, bedside clinical assessment will need to be relied upon during CCC.

When a compliance abnormality is identified, it is helpful to classify it as a static or dynamic defect. If using a conventional volume-control mode, as described later in this chapter, a compliance defect will result in an elevated peak pressure. The peak pressure is the highest pressure generated as the machine pushes a given volume of gas into a patient's lungs. Once the initial portion of the breath is introduced, a more stable plateau pressure is reached until the end of inhalation.

A static compliance abnormality is one in which there is an elevated peak pressure as well as a similarly elevated plateau pressure. No matter how long the inspiration period lasts, an elevated pressure will continue to be noted that is similar to the peak pressure. Conditions causing stiff lungs such as pulmonary edema or a stiff chest wall will result in a static compliance abnormality. A dynamic compliance abnormality is characterized by an elevated peak pressure that is significantly higher than the plateau pressure, the breath has difficulty getting into the lungs initially, but then is able to overcome the obstruction. A common example of this is mucus or other secretions in the airways that is significant enough to hamper, but does not completely obstruct airflow.

Gas exchange in the lungs is accomplished at the level of the alveolar capillary interface. Ideally, flow of air into an alveolus and flow of blood into a surrounding capillary vessel bed should be matched. Areas of ventilation (V) should generally correspond to areas of perfusion (Q); V/Q = 1. When ventilation is present in the absence of blood flow (V/Q = infinity), this is known as dead-space ventilation.[2] The dead-space fraction is the ratio of dead-space (Vd) to tidal volume (Vt). The dead-space fraction is the portion of each breath that is unavailable for gas exchange. A normal person has a dead-space fraction of approximately 30 percent at rest that decreases to 18 percent at maximal exercise.[3] A higher dead-space fraction results in difficulty eliminating carbon dioxide.

Perfusion in the absence of ventilation makes it impossible for oxygen to diffuse from the airways into the blood and bind hemoglobin. Areas with preserved blood flow but an absence of ventilation (V/Q = 0) cause a right-to-left shunt.[2] The proportion of blood that passes from the right side of the heart to the left without being exposed to adequately ventilated alveoli is called the shunt fraction.

In the normal lung, there are three physiologically distinct zones with respect to gas exchange as described by West.[4] From the top to the bottom of the lungs, there is an increase in alveolar ventilation as well as an even greater relative increase in blood flow. The uppermost portions of the lung are characterized by West Zone 1 physiology and are defined by an alveolar pressure (Palv) that is greater than the pulmonary artery systolic (PAs) and pulmonary artery diastolic (PAd) pressures. In West Zone 1 conditions, dead-space ventilation always exists since V/Q is by definition infinite. In West Zone 2 sections, PAs pressure is greater than Palv, which is greater than PAd pressure. Finally, in West Zone 3 sections, PAs pressure is greater than PAd pressure, which is greater than Palv. The majority of gas exchange happens in West Zone 3 conditions in the spontaneously breathing adult in the mid and basilar portions of the lungs.[4]

Positive-pressure invasive mechanical ventilation is often used to support patients who have inadequate oxygenation (respiration). Options available to improve respiration include increasing the fraction of inspired oxygen ($FiO_2$) or increasing the mean airway pressure. There are several ways to increase the mean airway pressure including inverse ratio ventilation, application of positive end-expiratory pressure (PEEP), and purposefully allowing the development of intrinsic PEEP. Treatment of hypoxemic respiratory failure will be covered in more detail later in this chapter when pulmonary contusion and acute respiratory distress syndrome are addressed.

> Augmentation of oxygenation and elimination of carbon dioxide may be achieved though invasive mechanical ventilation.

Augmentation of carbon dioxide elimination (ventilation) is often facilitated with invasive mechanical ventilation. Each breath that is provided for the patient (Vt) can be thought of as a combination of a portion used for gas exchange (effective alveolar ventilation [Va]) and that lost to dead-space ventilation (Vd). Thus, Vt = Va + Vd. If one considers these components over the course of a minute (by multiplying each by the respiratory rate per minute), minute ventilation (Ve) = Va + Vd. Rearranging the equation for effective alveolar ventilation (Va) yields: Va = Ve − Vd = Ve (1 − Vd/Vt).

The actual partial pressure of carbon dioxide in arterial blood ($PaCO_2$) is a function of how much $CO_2$ is generated by the body ($VCO_2$) and how much is eliminated (largely dependent upon Va):

$$PaCO_2 = k(VCO_2)/Va = k(VCO_2)/Ve(1 − Vd/Vt).$$

The $CO_2$ production is generally proportional to the basal metabolic rate, and increases in times of physiologic stress and with temperature elevation. The respiratory quotient ($R_Q = VCO_2/VO_2$) of enteral and parenteral feeds may also impact $CO_2$ production in some critical care patients. Other than manipulating the $R_Q$ of feeds or controlling temperature, effective control of the $PaCO_2$ is largely a function of mechanical ventilation and the ability to control the minute ventilation (Ve), which is equal to the respiratory rate ($f$) multiplied times tidal volume (Ve = $f$ x Vt). It should be noted that overdistension of alveoli with excessive ventilator pressures or intravascular volume depletion can both lead to an increase in West Zone 1 conditions by increasing the dead-space fraction. This can happen in an unpredictable manner at times, but should be considered when carbon dioxide elimination is proving difficult with positive-pressure ventilation.

## Ventilator-Induced Lung Injury

One of the unfortunate lessons of critical care has been the realization that positive-pressure mechanical ventilation has the capacity to cause significant harm. Injury caused to the lung as a direct result of the use of a ventilator is called ventilator-induced lung injury (VILI). The pathophysiology of VILI is complex, but includes the effects of extrapulmonic air trapping (see barotrauma below) as well as the development of diffuse alveolar damage that is indistinguishable from that seen in acute respiratory distress syndrome (ARDS). As our understanding of VILI increases, so does the nosology to classify it. At present, it is helpful to think of four distinct subsets: barotrauma, volutrauma, atelectotrauma, and biotrauma.

> Morbidity associated with positive-pressure mechanical ventilation is termed ventilator-induced lung injury (VILI). It may be broadly classified into barotrauma, volutrauma, atelectotrauma, and biotrauma.

### Barotrauma

Barotrauma describes the most commonly appreciated adverse effects, such as the development of air collections outside of the lung, due to the use of inappropriately high pressure levels for a given clinical condition. While it is possible for a pneumothorax to develop directly at the periphery of the lung as a direct result of pressure changes, it is more frequently observed that air ruptures into the bronchovascular bundles first and dissects proximally resulting in a pneumomediastinum. Since the pleural space and the mediastinal space are separated by a pleural reflection on each side, a pneumothorax may or may not develop. Any subsequent pneumothorax will not necessarily form on the side of the initial airway defect. Finally, air may dissect in a cephalad or caudal direction, resulting in palpable air collections in the skin of the face, neck and chest, or intestinal wall (pneumatosis intestinalis) (Fig. 1).

### Volutrauma

Volutrauma describes a physical overdistension of alveolar lung units that leads to pulmonary inflammation and can trigger the development of diffuse alveolar damage. It may occur in association with barotrauma, especially when excessive ventilatory pressures are used. Volutrauma is most likely to be a problem in conditions characterized by uneven ventilation such as pulmonary contusion or ARDS. Air becomes preferentially diverted to alveolar units with preserved compliance, leading to their overdistension. Animal models demonstrate that alveolar overdistention is likely a larger contributor to the development of VILI than elevated intraalveolar pressures.[5] From a pressure standpoint, it is the transalveolar pressure that is most dangerous, rather than the absolute pressure applied by the ventilator. The transalveolar pressure is directly correlated with the subsequent volume of expansion and therefore the potential development of volutrauma.

### Atelectotrauma

Atelectotrauma refers to the repetitive opening and closing of alveolar lung units, which can lead to the development of local inflammation and diffuse alveolar damage. This occurs because opening and closing of alveoli that are adjacent to alveoli that are incapable of opening contribute to a shearing stress at their interface. Cytokines are released that perpetuate the local inflammatory response and may serve as a catalyst for injury in other parts of the body. This is one hypothesized mechanism for the development of multiple organ dysfunction syndrome and is more likely to be a major player in VILI associated with asymmetric lung injury.[5]

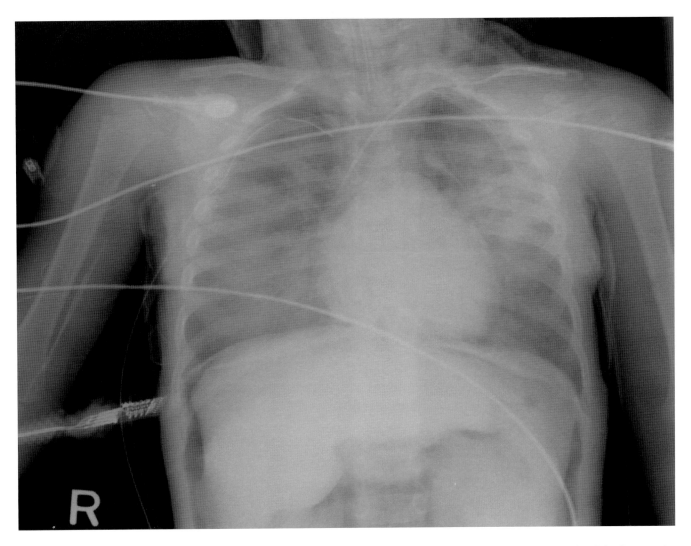

Figure 1. *Four-year-old child with severe ARDS at a Level III facility. Very high mean airway pressure requirements to maintain minimal oxygenation resulted in severe barotrauma.*

## Biotrauma

An emerging concept that links the three aforementioned mechanisms of VILI is that of biotrauma. Biotrauma describes the impact on the lungs and body of biologically active molecules such as inflammatory mediators that are released as a direct result of positive-pressure ventilation. Alveolar volume, pressure, and cyclical opening have all been associated with the development of biotrauma.[6,7] It is likely that biotrauma is a final common pathway resulting in lung injury for many otherwise seemingly disparate mechanisms. Use of antiinflammatory agents to prevent or mitigate the impact of VILI has thus far been unsuccessful, further underlining the importance of prevention.[8]

> Oxygen toxicity primarily leads to the development of pulmonary fibrosis. Efforts to limit the $FiO_2$ should be made whenever possible ($FiO_2$ less than 50 percent) to minimize this complication.

Oxygen toxicity should also be considered a local form of biotrauma. There is no "safe" level of oxygen supplementation since its presence in any concentration will be associated with some degree of oxidation and damage to tissues. Animal models have convincingly demonstrated that higher levels of oxygen supplementation lead to the development of a form of VILI that is independent of the effects of pressure, volume, and cyclical changes.[9] Oxygen toxicity leads primarily to the development of pulmonary fibrosis and efforts to limit the $FiO_2$ should be made whenever possible. While no completely safe threshold has been demonstrated convincingly in clinical trials, most advocate decreasing the $FiO_2$ to less than 50 percent as soon as possible.[10]

## *Basic Modes of Positive-Pressure Ventilation*

### Overview

The provision of positive-pressure ventilation can be accomplished in an ever-increasing variety of ways. The increasing complexity of computer-driven algorithms can be confusing, but focusing on the fundamentals can help the clinician choose an appropriate mode for a given clinical situation. This section reviews some basic concepts applicable to all methods of providing positive-pressure ventilation and how they apply to more common modes of ventilation in clinical use. At the heart of understanding the different modes of ventilation is appreciating the impact of compliance and how the ventilator and patient communicate with each other. As discussed previously, compliance is the change in volume over the change in pressure. At any given point in time, the pulmonary system has a given overall compliance that will dictate the pressure change expected if a volume is provided by the ventilator. Conversely, if a pressure is provided by the ventilator, the compliance will determine the volume that is generated. Generally, a positive-pressure breath provides a volume or a pressure as an independent variable to the patient, and the compliance of the pulmonary system determines the value of the dependent variable.

Communication between the ventilator and the patient is what defines the actual mode of ventilation. When a given mode of ventilation is chosen, a set of rules for communication between the patient and ventilator is established. At a basic level, the defining questions are as follows: (1) how does the machine know when to start a breath?; (2) how does the machine provide the breath?; and (3) how does the machine know when to stop giving the breath? The combination of answers to these three questions defines the basic rules of communication and, therefore, the ventilator mode.

The trigger is the signal to the ventilator that it is time to provide a positive-pressure breath. For the common modes of ventilation, the trigger for a given breath is time (a breath is delivered at a set rate regardless of patient effort) or patient-driven. A patient-triggered breath is provided when the patient initiates a predetermined negative inspiratory pressure or a change in flow in the ventilator circuitry. This is interpreted by the machine as a desire on behalf of the patient to receive a breath. Some modes have both time and patient triggers (assist-control), as will be discussed later.

Provision of a breath to the patient depends on whether the machine or the patient initiated the breath. When the breath is given to the patient in accordance with a predetermined rate, it is said to be a control breath. A breath that is given by the machine in response to initiation by the patient is said to be an assist breath. Occasionally, the patient may initiate a breath that is in close proximity to when a control breath was going to be given by the machine. Most current ventilators recognize this and provide the planned control breath rather than an assist one in order to maintain minimum minute ventilation and avoid patient-ventilator synchrony problems.

Modes of ventilation are generally referred to as volume-control or pressure-control modes. Volume control is unfortunately a misnomer. A volume-control breath delivers a set volume to the patient; however, flow is actually the controlled variable. A specific flow is given by the machine until a predetermined volume is achieved. It is more accurate to think of volume control as volume set and flow control. A pressure-control mode of ventilation does deliver a set pressure using a pressure control and is therefore an accurate description. The cycle defines how the machine knows to stop giving a breath to the patient and allow exhalation to begin. Available cycle mechanisms commonly used include time, volume, pressure, and flow. Time cycles are often used in both pressure- and volume-control modes where a set inspiratory to expiratory (I:E) ratio is important to maintain. Flow cycles are frequently applied to pressure-supported assist breaths in modes such as pressure-support ventilation, as will be described below.

With this brief background, it is now time to consider how trigger, control, and assist breath delivery and cycle define the modes that are commonly used for positive-pressure ventilation. A few less conventional modes will also be described that may be of use in the combat casualty critical care setting today or in the near future.

## Assist-Control (A/C)

*Trigger:*      Time (controlled breaths), Patient (assisted breaths)

*Breath Delivery:* Control (volume set and flow controlled)

           Assist (volume set and flow controlled)

*Cycle:*      Time or Volume

In A/C mode, a respiratory rate, tidal volume, and inspiratory flow rate are set by the operator. The combination of these three variables will define the I:E ratio. The patient can trigger an assist breath that is recognized by the machine as either a negative pressure or change in flow in a closed circuit. The assist breath given has an identical tidal volume to the control breaths. Cycling depends on the ventilator manufacturer. In the past, a volume cycle was used for both the controlled and assisted breaths, and an operator set flow rate would determine the I:E ratio. Most current ventilators provide a mechanism for setting an I:E ratio, and the machine will automatically determine a time cycle based on the average number of total breaths the patient is breathing per minute. To achieve the desired I:E ratio, the machine may vary the flow and/or have a built-in inspiratory hold after the set volume is applied in order to achieve the desired I:E ratio.

## Synchronized Intermittent Mandatory Ventilation (SIMV)

*Trigger:*      Time (controlled breaths), Patient (assisted breaths)

*Breath Delivery:* Control (volume set and flow controlled)

           Assist – none (SIMV) versus pressure-support (SIMV/PSV)

*Cycle:*      Time or Volume (controlled breaths), Flow (assisted breaths)

With SIMV mode ventilation, the operator determines a set respiratory rate and tidal volume, and cycling of controlled breaths is identical to that described in the A/C section. In fact, in a patient who takes no spontaneous breaths, SIMV mode is identical to A/C mode. Assisted breaths that are initiated by the patient have a trigger that can be either a change in flow or the generation of a predefined negative inspiratory pressure. When SIMV is used alone, there is no support given by the ventilator during an assist breath. The machine recognizes that a spontaneous breath has been initiated and responds by opening a valve that allows the patient to take as deep a breath without support as the patient can. Frequently, SIMV is combined with pressure-support ventilation (PSV). The combined SIMV/PSV mode allows an operator determined pressure-support to be applied by the ventilator through the inspiratory phase of an assist breath. The resulting tidal volume will be determined by the pulmonary system compliance at the time the breath is delivered and may or may not be similar to the set tidal volume delivered on controlled breaths. A flow cycle is used to terminate assist breaths in both SIMV and SIMV/PSV. The machine determines the maximal inspiratory flow at breath initiation and cycles the breath off when the inspiratory flow generated by the patient declines to a predetermined point, such as 20 to 25 percent of the maximal value.

> Although SIMV is frequently used in critical care units today, it cannot be recommended as a weaning mode of ventilation. The rationale for its use as a maintenance mode of ventilation, above other modes, has little support in the literature.

Synchronized intermittent mandatory ventilation was initially designed as a weaning mode where an operator could transition a patient to a completely spontaneous mode of ventilation from a completely controlled mode simply by decreasing respiratory rate over time. Unfortunately, SIMV performed inferiorly to PSV and T-piece trials in two major prospective, randomized weaning studies and delayed overall extubation time.[11,12] Several hypotheses have been proposed to explain these findings, many relating to the way in which SIMV was applied. Of note, research indicates that as the set respiratory rate declines as a percentage of the overall respiratory rate, the work of breathing goes up substantially.[13] Assisted breaths in the SIMV mode can be quite variable and may not be adequate. Proponents of SIMV argue that combining SIMV with PSV allows assist breaths that have less variability relative to the control breaths and therefore decreased work of breathing. Others argue that titrating PSV to achieve assist breaths that are similar to control breaths in SIMV/PSV is no different from what can more easily be accomplished with A/C. Although SIMV is frequently used in critical care units today, it cannot be recommended as a weaning mode, and the rationale for its use as a maintenance mode of ventilation above other modes has little support in the literature.[11,12,14]

## Pressure-Control Ventilation (PCV)

*Trigger:*     Time (controlled breaths), Patient (assisted breaths)

*Breath Delivery:* Control (pressure controlled)

               Assist (pressure controlled)

*Cycle:*       Time or Pressure

Pressure-control-ventilation mode is identical to A/C mode with the exception that the breath delivered in the control or assist setting is a pressure breath set by the operator. This mode is frequently utilized in disease states where pulmonary system compliance is limited, and it is perceived by the clinician that using a predefined pressure control will decrease the likelihood of barotrauma. It is also used in situations where manipulation of the I:E ratio to greater than or equal to 1:1 (inverse ratio ventilation) is felt to be advantageous. When volume control A/C is set appropriately, there is little advantage to the use of PCV even in disease states where both such concerns manifest, such as ARDS. Pressure-control ventilation and volume-control A/C are in actuality very similar modes of ventilation, and either can be used in most cases, the choice being largely related to operator comfort.

Pressure-control ventilation mode is frequently utilized in disease states where pulmonary system compliance is limited and where pressure control will decrease the likelihood of barotrauma.

Understanding the concept of compliance is key. A given volume can be given that will generate a certain pressure. Conversely, a pressure can be given that will generate a certain volume. The relationship between the volume and pressure is defined by the system compliance, and whether the breath is given as a volume or a pressure is largely irrelevant in most circumstances. When pressure-controlled breaths are used in conditions characterized by reduced pulmonary system compliance, inadequate tidal volumes are possible and should be watched for closely. Occult air trapping with significant intrinsic PEEP that is unrecognized will also result in a lower than expected tidal volume when using pressure-controlled breath delivery.

## Pressure-Support Ventilation (PSV)

*Trigger:* Patient
*Breath Delivery:* Pressure support
*Cycle:* Flow

Pressure-support ventilation is a mode of ventilation that is strictly an assist mode. The patient triggers the ventilator by generating a change in flow or a negative inspiratory pressure that is recognized by the ventilator. The machine then provides an operator defined pressure support throughout the inhalation portion of the breath until a flow cycle is reached. The breath cycles off typically when inspiratory flow drops below 20 to 25 percent of the maximal inspiratory flow. One concern related to PSV is the potential for its application in patients who have an inadequate respiratory drive or respiratory muscle strength. In either case, an inadequate minute ventilation may result. Most modern ventilators that have PSV as an option also allow a predefined backup control mode such as A/C that is automatically initiated when the minute ventilation is below a certain threshold. Some proprietary programs will only augment the number of breaths needed at a given time to achieve the minimum minute ventilation and will continue to allow the patient to otherwise remain in PSV. Pressure-support ventilation is commonly used as a weaning mode in the ICU, although with enough pressure support this mode can also be used quite effectively as a fully supportive mode, as long as the patient is able to generate an adequate respiratory effort.

Pressure-support ventilation is an assist mode commonly used to wean patients in the ICU.

Patients with significant air trapping may become dysynchronous with PSV. Prolonged exhalation times due to increased airway resistance (inflammation, secretions, etc.,) or increased compliance (emphysema) may result in incomplete alveolar emptying and the development of air trapping. Patients who have significant air trapping will be noted at end-exhalation to have a pressure within the lungs that is above atmospheric pressure (Patm). This is referred to as intrinsic positive-end expiratory pressure (iPEEP) or autoPEEP. The pressure difference between the intrinsic PEEP and atmospheric pressure can establish a significant expiratory flow between the gas exchanging units and the mouth, even when the patient considers the breath complete. This flow can be recognized by the ventilator and complicate the ability of the machine to accurately determine the proper time to end the inhalation portion of a breath that is flow cycled as in PSV. The machine may terminate the breath at a different time than the patient would prefer, creating the potential for significant dysynchrony. While use of PSV in patients with the potential for air trapping is not absolutely contraindicated, close attention should be paid to patient ventilator interaction.

The basic modes of ventilation, as presented here, represent the most commonly utilized methods of delivering positive-pressure breaths today. They are, however, very rudimentary modes with respect to their ability to accommodate the underlying neuromuscular processes involved in producing a patient breath. Several newer modes of ventilation are currently being evaluated and can be expected to be seen shortly in modern critical care units. Three of these modes are discussed below as they are used from time to time in the current combat casualty critical care environment.

## Advanced Modes of Positive-Pressure Ventilation

### Airway Pressure Release Ventilation (APRV)

Airway pressure release ventilation (APRV) is a time-triggered, pressure-controlled, time-cycled mode used in conditions where limiting airway pressure and manipulating the I:E ratio are both desirable, such as ARDS. High PEEP (PEEPh) and low PEEP (PEEPl) levels are set, as are the amount of time to be spent at the high PEEP level (Th) and the time to be spent at the low PEEP level (Tl). The patient spends at least 60 percent of the respiratory cycle at PEEPh, typically closer to 80 to 90 percent. If the patient attempts to take a spontaneous breath, the trigger can be either flow or a negative inspiratory pressure. Generally, spontaneous breaths in APRV are unassisted when taken while at PEEPh. They may be assisted by preset pressure support when taken during PEEPl; however, often they are not when the Tl is of a very short duration. When pressure support is used to assist a spontaneous breath taken at PEEPl, it is often set to be equal to the difference between PEEPh and PEEPl.

> Airway pressure release ventilation (APRV) is a time-triggered, pressure-controlled, and time-cycled mode used in conditions where limiting airway pressure and manipulating the I:E ratio are both desirable (e.g., ARDS).

The advantage of APRV is the ability to control mean airway pressure by varying the I:E ratio without having to force the patient to complete an entire respiratory cycle with each spontaneous breath. For instance, if a patient were undergoing inverse ratio ventilation using either A/C or PCV, each spontaneous breath would force an entire iteration of the breathing cycle. This can be extremely uncomfortable to a patient and frequently mandates very high levels of sedation or even chemical paralysis. With APRV, a spontaneous breath does not change where the patient is in the time-triggered, pressure-controlled, time-cycled breath. If a breath is taken, the patient takes what he can and returns immediately to the PEEPh or PEEPl plateau that he was previously on. This is more comfortable for the patient, in spite of the maintenance of a significantly inversed I:E ratio. As the lung injury improves, the Th and Tl can be manipulated to a more normal I:E ratio over time, allowing an easy transition to more traditional modes of ventilation, particularly PSV.

### Pressure-Regulated Volume Control (PRVC)

Pressure-regulated volume control (PRVC) is a time- and patient-triggered, volume set/pressure-supported, time-cycled (set inspiratory time, Ti) mode of ventilation that adjusts the pressure support over the course of several breaths to achieve a preset tidal volume. This ensures adequate minute ventilation while augmenting patient efforts to the minimal extent necessary. PRVC use can be difficult in patients with significant variability in spontaneous respiratory breath generation. The ventilator looks at the tidal volume achieved with a given pressure support during the set inspiratory time over the last several breaths and compares the average tidal volume achieved to the desired tidal volume. By calculating a compliance using the average tidal volume and the difference between the pressure support and the PEEP, the ventilator determines what increase in pressure support is necessary to achieve a target tidal volume. Unfortunately, variable pressure swings on a breath to breath basis can cause the ventilator to over or underestimate the optimal pressure support. Cough, significant patient movement, or tachypnea may all render PRVC a difficult mode to use and result in extreme patient work of breathing variability.

High-Frequency Ventilation (HFV)
High-frequency ventilation (HFV) has several variants that are all based on the idea of providing very low tidal volumes at very high respiratory rates. The most commonly studied of the HFV modes are high-frequency jet ventilation (HFJV) and high-frequency oscillatory ventilation (HFOV). High-frequency jet ventilation uses pulses of gas to generate very small tidal volumes at frequencies of one to 10 hertz (Hz). The mode was used initially for thoracic surgery involving the major airways, but today is generally limited to the pediatric critical care population. High-frequency oscillatory ventilation uses even higher frequencies of five to 50 Hz along with exceptionally small tidal volumes to maintain a predefined mean airway pressure in lung conditions with extremely limited pulmonary system compliance such as ARDS. Because of the extremely small tidal volumes being used, the method of gas exchange is fundamentally different when HFV is used relative to more conventional modes of ventilation. Chan et al. provided an excellent review of HFOV in the treatment of ARDS.[15] The use of HFOV in ARDS will be discussed in further detail below.

## Basic Ventilator Settings When Lungs Are Normal

When mechanical ventilation is used for patients with normal lungs, it is being done for airway protection during the initial resuscitative period (Fig. 2). When employing mechanical ventilation, careproviders must avoid VILI. Finally, some lung conditions not appreciated initially may evolve or develop over time, such as pulmonary contusions, tracheal injury, or acute lung injury. The initial ventilator settings considered here assume normal pulmonary system compliance and an absence of identifiable lung injury.[16,17,18]

It is recommended that most be placed on traditional A/C ventilation as follows: $FiO_2$ = 100 percent, $f$ = 16 to 20, Vt = 5 to 8 milliliters (ml) per kilogram (predicted body weight), PEEP = 5 centimeters (cm) $H_2O$ and flow = 60 liters per minute.[19]

The $FiO_2$ can be turned down quickly after intubation to the lowest amount necessary to keep pulse oximeter oxygen saturation ($SpO_2$) greater than 92 to 94 percent (a higher $SpO_2$ may be desired when shock states are present). In cases of hypoperfusion where the $SpO_2$ cannot be measured accurately, serial arterial blood gas assessments may need to be obtained to appropriately titrate the $FiO_2$.

> The $FiO_2$ should be titrated downward after intubation to the lowest amount necessary to keep $SpO_2$ greater than 92 to 94 percent.

The minute ventilation (Ve = $f$ x Vt) adequacy is determined primarily by the pH. Whatever minute ventilation is necessary to achieve an adequate pH is the goal of mechanical ventilation. Efforts to achieve a normal partial pressure of carbon dioxide in arterial blood ($PaCO_2$) are not generally productive. Partial

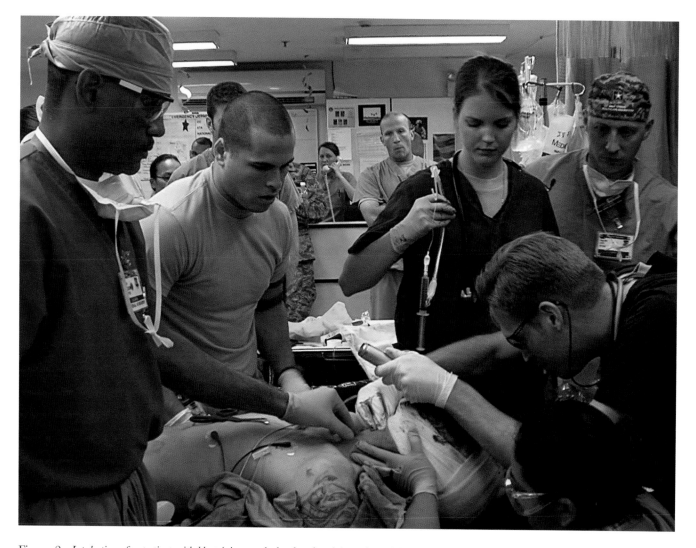

Figure 2. *Intubation of a patient with blast injury to the head and neck is performed during primary trauma survey to protect his airway.*

pressure of carbon dioxide in arterial blood manipulation should be more appropriately considered as a way of achieving a desired pH. In most patients, a pH above 7.25 is adequate, although 7.35 to 7.40 is ideal in most settings. In some conditions, such as those associated with significant cerebral edema, low pH should be rigorously avoided.[20,21] The tidal volume described here of 5 to 8 ml per kilogram is lower than the 8 to 12 ml per kilogram classically described for initial settings in a patient with normal lungs and more closely resembles recommendations for ventilation of ARDS patients. This is because a significant body of data is beginning to emerge that VILI also develops in normal lungs at volumes that were previously considered safe.[22,23] It is important to note that the weight used in these formulas is the predicted (ideal) body weight (PBW) as used in the ARDSnet trials (see section on ARDS):

PBW in kilograms (male) = 50 + 2.3 x (height in inches – 60)
PBW in kilograms (female) = 45.5 + 2.3 x (height in inches – 60)

To compensate for the lower tidal volume recommended here, a higher respiratory rate will also be necessary. Adjustments in the respiratory rate should be made as necessary to achieve the pH goals outlined previously, as long as the patient's spontaneous rate does not already exceed the machine set rate. If the spontaneous rate does already exceed the set rate, the set rate should be established as approximately 80 percent of the total rate, and further changes in the pH can be achieved with tidal volume manipulation. As the patient rate decreases, a decrease can be made in the set rate while attempting to keep the ratio of machine breaths to total breaths constant at about 80 percent. If the total rate does not exceed the set rate, then the set rate can be manipulated as necessary to achieve the pH goals described.

In the absence of any lung injury, PEEP greater than 5 cm $H_2O$ is generally not initially necessary. As the amount of time spent on the ventilator increases, dependent atelectasis frequently develops and can create a very significant shunt leading to hypoxemia. Increased levels of PEEP may need to be applied in order to combat the development of atelectasis or to counteract the effects of lung injury in evolution. The manipulation of PEEP will be discussed in more detail below as it pertains to pulmonary contusion and ARDS.

> In the absence of lung injury, PEEP greater than 5 cm $H_2O$ is generally not initially necessary. Increased levels of PEEP may be needed in order to prevent the development of atelectasis or to counteract the effects of lung injury in evolution.

There is rarely a significant benefit to the manipulation of flow. In patients with prolonged exhalation times, such as asthma and chronic obstructive pulmonary disease (COPD), flow is frequently increased in an attempt to decrease the I:E ratio and allow more time for exhalation. However, at a standard flow of 60 liters per minute, a tidal volume of 500 ml is supplied in 0.5 seconds (60 liters per minute = 1000 ml per second). Therefore, doubling the flow rate to 120 liters per minute will decrease the inspiratory time to 0.25 seconds, extending the exhalation time by only 0.25 seconds. Simply decreasing the respiratory rate from 20 to 12 will increase the expiratory time by two seconds without having to manipulate the flow at all.

# Pulmonary Contusion

### Basic Concepts
Pulmonary contusion represents a heterogeneous, generally asymmetric, lung injury that is associated with blunt trauma or blast injury (Fig. 3).[24,25] It frequently evolves over hours to days and can result in significant right-to-left shunt as well as impaired ventilation. Associated injuries may include injury to the pulmonary vasculature and the airways. If a major airway injury occurs in association with blunt trauma, it frequently will appear within 2.5 cm of the carina and may not be appreciated during the initial resuscitation.[26] Blast injury to the lungs can result from primary blast effects, penetrating trauma (projectiles), or blunt trauma that results in pulmonary contusion. The blunt trauma that is applied to the chest in the case of blast injury may be either from physical contact (being thrown against an object) or from air pressure waves. The development of pulmonary contusion in the setting of blast injury was said to be unlikely in the absence of tympanic membrane perforation.[27] Recent reports dispute the reliability of tympanic membrane rupture as a sensitive screening tool for primary blast injury detection.[28,29]

Blast injury to the lungs can result from primary blast effects, penetrating trauma (projectiles), or blunt trauma that results in pulmonary contusion. The blunt trauma that is applied to the chest in the case of blast injury may be either from physical contact (being thrown against an object) or from air pressure waves.

Contusion in the pulmonary parenchyma is characterized by collections of blood and exudative fluid in alveoli in response to destruction of the alveolar capillary interface by transmitted pressure. As the pressure waves propagate through the lung tissue, they transmit less energy per unit of lung tissue so the destruction is greatest closer to the point of impact. This is the primary reason for the asymmetric nature of the injury. Lobar collapse and focal atelectasis may also occur due to the collection of blood, blood clots, reactive airway secretions, mucus plugging, and occasionally aspirated secretions or foreign bodies such as teeth or food particles. All of these factors create significant regions of lung that have minimal ventilation but relatively preserved blood flow, resulting in right-to-left shunt development. The resulting hypoxemia may present fairly abruptly many hours after the initial injury.

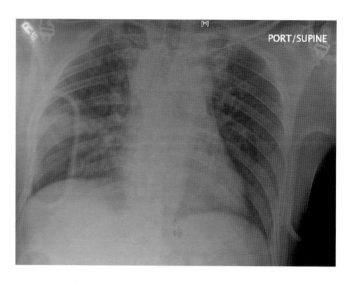

Figure 3. *Pulmonary contusion represents a heterogeneous, generally asymmetric, lung injury that is associated with blunt trauma or blast injury.*

Pulmonary system compliance decreases significantly with blunt trauma that is substantial enough to result in pulmonary contusion. Fractured ribs may limit the efficiency of rib cage movement, as may resultant pain. The particular condition of flail chest is characterized by the presence of two or more adjacent ribs that each have at least two sites of fracture (Fig. 4). Inspiration in the spontaneously breathing patient normally results from chest wall expansion and diaphragm contraction that generates a negative intrathoracic pressure relative to atmospheric pressure. This serves to draw the flail segment inward during inspiration and contributes to respiratory compromise. It also may not be recognized when a person is on positive-pressure mechanical ventilation because there is no mechanism for the flail chest to develop. The presence of significant chest wall injury of any kind can be expected to decrease the chest wall compliance.

The alveolar injury pattern described previously creates a decrease in lung compliance. The compliance is further decreased by any postobstructive atelectasis associated with airway occlusion by blood or other secretions. Inability to take deep breaths due to pain will contribute to the development of dependent atelectasis as well as make postobstructive atelectasis more likely. Decreased chest wall compliance and lung compliance both contribute to a limited total pulmonary system compliance. The limited compliance decreases the tidal volume that a patient is able to generate. In addition, given that a normal pair of lungs has a given amount of dead-space, a decreased tidal volume by necessity implies a greater dead-space fraction. A larger dead-space fraction means that there will be increased difficulty getting rid of carbon dioxide, so the body must compensate by increasing the minute ventilation ($Ve = f \times Vt$). Since tidal volume is limited, patients with significant pulmonary contusions are often noted to breath shallowly

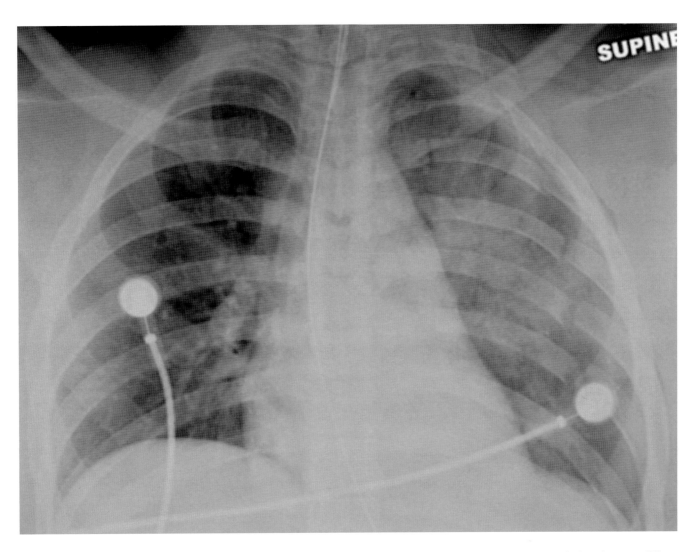

Figure 4. *Flail chest is described as the paradoxical movement of a segment of chest wall due to fractures of two or more ribs in at least two different sites. Here, multiple left-sided posterior rib fractures are noted.*

and rapidly as they try to increase respiratory rate. However, once tidal volume becomes sufficiently shallow and dead-space fraction significantly large, the patient is at great risk for the development of hypercarbic respiratory failure.

## Management

### Airway Protection and Pulmonary Toilet

Airway protection and ventilator support are extremely important facets of pulmonary contusion management. Upper airway control with endotracheal intubation or tracheostomy is generally accomplished early in the resuscitation of severely injured patients. Due to the progressive nature of pulmonary contusion symptomatology, careproviders should obtain early airway control and provide ventilator support for all moderate to severely symptomatic pulmonary contusion patients. Mildly symptomatic cases may be managed with supplemental oxygen, serial observation, and pulse oximetry.[30] Occasionally, patients may benefit from the use of noninvasive positive-pressure ventilation (NIPPV) if they are alert.[31]

Due to the progressive nature of pulmonary contusion symptomatology, early airway control and ventilator support should be provided to all moderate to severely symptomatic patients. Mildly symptomatic cases may be managed with supplemental oxygen, serial observation, and pulse oximetry.

The concept of airway protection in the case of pulmonary contusion also extends to airways that can be reached by flexible fiberoptic bronchoscopy easily, such as those serving the major pulmonary segments (Fig. 5). Bronchoscopy allows removal of clots and secretions, thereby decreasing the percentage of lung that may have been prone to postobstructive atelectasis.[32] A survey can be performed with flexible fiberoptic bronchoscopy to rule out any evidence of major airway injury and localize any major bleeding that may be present from vessel injury. Serial flexible fiberoptic bronchoscopy as the contusion progresses may be necessary to maintain adequate pulmonary toilet by clearing mucus plugging or inspissated secretions that may contribute to the late development of atelectasis. It should be noted that flexible fiberoptic bronchoscopy does not have the ability to clear blood or exudative secretions at the level of the alveoli.

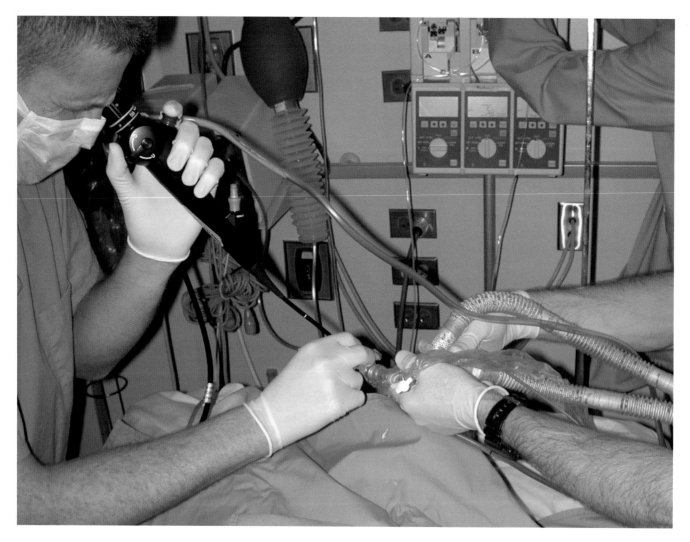

Figure 5. *Flexible fiberoptic bronchoscopy allows removal of blood clots and secretions, thereby decreasing the likelihood of postobstructive atelectasis.*

## Positive-Pressure Ventilation

Positive-pressure ventilation has a key role in the care of pulmonary contusions by supporting adequate gas exchange.[24] The application of a positive-pressure breath can augment the tidal volume enough to allow an adequate minute ventilation. The minute ventilation necessary may also be decreased by the use of positive-pressure ventilation since a more effective tidal volume will lead to a decreased dead-space fraction. Remembering that the $PaCO_2$ is inversely related to Ve $(1-Vd/Vt)$, it is easy to see that an augmented tidal volume will significantly improve ventilation in the setting of pulmonary compliance limitations.

As discussed earlier, positive-pressure ventilation can augment respiration (oxygenation) in two ways: increasing the $FiO_2$ and increasing the mean airway pressure. Increasing the mean airway pressure can be accomplished in several ways, but is easiest to do in the setting of pulmonary contusion by increasing the PEEP. Positive end-expiratory pressure results in an increased functional residual capacity (FRC), which is the volume of the lung at end-tidal exhalation. The increased functional residual capacity helps to maintain the patency of alveoli and counteract the tendency towards atelectasis and shunt development. The application of PEEP may also open some previously closed alveoli, further improving the shunt fraction.

> Positive-pressure ventilation is instrumental in the care of pulmonary contusions by supporting adequate gas exchange.

One potential complication of excessive PEEP application results from the asymmetric nature of the lung injury.[24] Any pressure applied by the ventilator will preferentially go first to portions of the lung with relatively normal compliance such as those that are not affected by the contusion. Serial increases in PEEP may paradoxically result in decreasing oxygenation if overdistension of normal lung becomes severe enough to decrease blood flow by the creation of West Zone 1 conditions. West Zone 1 conditions comprise alveolar pressures greater than pulmonary artery systolic pressures greater than pulmonary artery diastolic pressures. Blood will then preferentially flow to the contused lung units where ventilation is poor, increasing the shunt fraction and worsening hypoxemia. Increasing areas of West Zone 1 conditions by definition imply larger areas of dead-space ventilation, and the dead-space fraction is therefore increased leading to less effective ventilation. It is difficult to know in a given patient what level of PEEP may prove to be too much, but progressively worsening hypoxemia and hypercapnea in the setting of increasing levels of PEEP may imply that the level of PEEP being applied is excessive.

It is important to remember that positive pressure can be applied noninvasively (NIPPV). This is an excellent option for patients with mild pulmonary contusions, who otherwise are not in need of invasive mechanical ventilatory support. The appropriate use of NIPPV can be expected to result in decreased ventilator-associated pneumonia.[31] However, as contusions may heal slowly and may progress over several days, the decision to use NIPPV should be accompanied by aggressive serial clinical evaluations. Use of NIPPV also makes the use of flexible fiberoptic bronchoscopy for airway survey and serial pulmonary toilet difficult.

## Adjunctive Strategies

For patients with isolated pulmonary contusion, intravascular volume should be minimized to that necessary to ensure adequate systemic perfusion.[31] This will minimize the adverse effects on pulmonary physiology. When pulmonary contusion is encountered in the multisystem trauma patient, it may not be the dominant or most life-threatening injury. In such cases, intravascular volume should be maintained as dictated by the overall injury pattern, but fluid minimization should be accomplished when possible. Even in the setting of isolated pulmonary contusion, forced diuresis does not have a role except in patients who are otherwise intravascularly volume overloaded, as in the case of a congestive heart failure patient who may have sustained blunt thoracic trauma.[31]

In patients with isolated pulmonary contusion, intravascular volume administration should be kept to the minimum amount necessary to maintain adequate systemic perfusion.

Pain control is vital, as is stabilization of the chest wall. In the case of rib fractures, the application of positive-pressure ventilation may be all that is necessary for chest wall stabilization.[33] Direct fixation of rib fractures may be necessary in some cases, particularly when large areas of flail chest are involved.[33] Adequate pain control may be aided greatly by the use of epidural anesthesia and paravertebral blocks.[34] Such techniques may be especially effective in the marginal, unintubated patient. Most deployed medical facilities that have anesthesia support should be facile in these methods of achieving pain control.

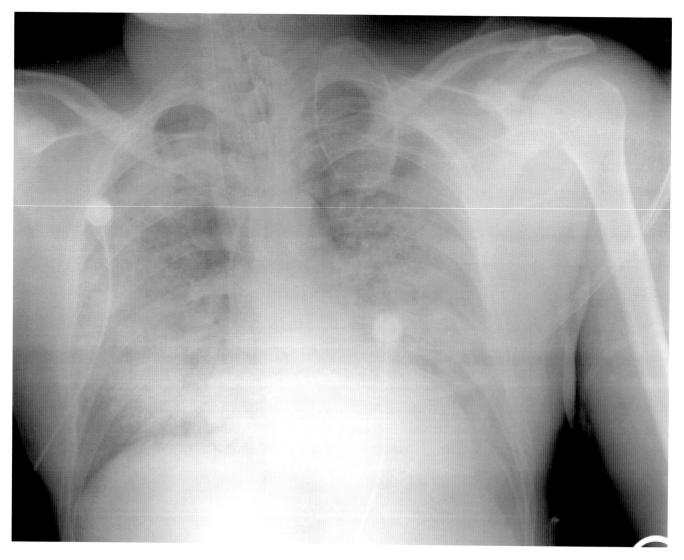

Figure 6. *Patient with severe ARDS following trauma. ARDS is a clinical syndrome characterized by noncardiogenic pulmonary edema in response to lung injury.*

Control of cough is debatable, and it is difficult to offer guidance that applies to all cases.[35] Cough is beneficial in that it may allow improved pulmonary toilet by dislodging clot and secretions in the airway, thereby decreasing postobstructive atelectasis. On the other hand, cough that is associated with significant chest wall pain may prolong the period where patients feel incapable of taking adequate deep breaths. This may contribute to hypercarbic respiratory failure as well as the development of more atelectasis. Cough in general should probably be encouraged, but any associated pain should be treated aggressively. Cough should only be suppressed when the pulmonary contusion is accompanied by active, uncontrolled pulmonary hemorrhage and intractable pain.

> Cough should only be suppressed when a pulmonary contusion is accompanied by active, uncontrolled pulmonary hemorrhage, or intractable pain. Otherwise, coughing should probably be encouraged, and any associated pain should be treated aggressively.

Chest physical therapy is often prescribed for patients in the ICU, but there is almost no literature supporting its use in any setting outside of that associated with bronchiectasis.[36,37] Some describe benefits in cases where postobstructive focal atelectasis is present, such as that associated with a maturing pulmonary contusion. If chest physical therapy is used for a pulmonary contusion patient, pain control is vital for the same reasons as outlined above with respect to cough.

The significant shunt associated with pulmonary contusion is due to a heterogenous, largely asymmetric process.[24,31] The injury process and resultant shunting associated with acute lung injury and the acute respiratory distress syndrome are also heterogenous but more likely to be symmetric (Fig. 6). There are significant differences in the management of these conditions as will be outlined in the next section.

# Acute Respiratory Distress Syndrome (ARDS)

## *Basic Concepts*
Acute lung injury (ALI) and ARDS both describe a common clinical syndrome characterized by the development of noncardiogenic pulmonary edema in response to a direct or indirect lung injury.[38] Both processes have an identical pathophysiologic origin and management is the same.[39] The difference between ALI and ARDS is one of severity with respect to the partial pressure of oxygen in arterial blood ($PaO_2$)/$FiO_2$ ratio and is therefore somewhat arbitrary. For this reason, ARDS will be used exclusively in this review to describe any patient with a clinical syndrome compatible with either ALI or ARDS. The American-European Consensus Criteria for ALI and ARDS both include the following characteristics: acute onset (less than seven days), diffuse bilateral patchy infiltrates seen on standard chest radiography, and an absence of left atrial hypertension clinically (or with a pulmonary capillary wedge pressure [PCWP] less than 18 mm Hg if a pulmonary artery catheter is already in place). As noted previously, ALI and ARDS differ only in the $PaO_2$/$FiO_2$ used for their definition. Acute respiratory distress syndrome is notable for a $PaO_2$/$FiO_2$ less than 200, while that of ALI is between 200 and 300.[39]

Acute respiratory distress syndrome can be caused by both direct and indirect injuries.[40] Direct causes include aspiration, pneumonia, blunt trauma to the chest, and other pulmonary processes that may trigger a significant inflammatory response. Indirect injury may cause ARDS by triggering systemic inflammation through the release of cytokines. Examples of indirect injury relevant to the critical care

ICU environment include multisystem trauma, shock, blood product transfusion, and sepsis. The common pathway for both direct and indirect causes is inflammation. When ARDS presents clinically, it usually develops several hours to days after the initial precipitating injury.[40,41]

> Acute lung injury and ARDS both describe a common clinical syndrome characterized by the development of noncardiogenic pulmonary edema in response to a direct or indirect lung injury.

The likelihood of ARDS development secondary to an underlying insult rises with the age of the patient. The mortality attributable to ARDS is approximately 40 percent but increases with the number of concomitant organ system failures.[40] The development of renal failure in the setting of ARDS denotes a particularly poor prognosis. A recent study demonstrated that the likelihood of eventual death due to ARDS is related to dead-space fraction on presentation.[42] Those with a higher dead-space fraction had a higher mortality. The mortality due to ARDS is improving with aggressive supportive therapy and an increasing appreciation of the role that mechanical ventilation can play in both recovery and injury propagation.[10]

The pathology associated with ARDS is that of diffuse alveolar damage, regardless of the inciting injury, which may represent a stereotypic lung injury and healing response.[40] There are two distinct clinical phases in the evolution of the lung injury: an exudative phase that predominates in the first five to seven days, followed by a proliferative phase after this point.[40] Cytokines and other inflammatory mediators initiate changes that lead to disruption of the normal alveolar-capillary interface and the introduction of exudative fluid into the alveolus. This causes two major changes: the first is inactivation of surfactant, and the second is sloughing of the alveolar and bronchial epithelial cells. Loss of surfactant function makes alveolar collapse more likely, and the loss of epithelial cells leads to hyaline membrane formation on the denuded basement membrane. The injury leads to attraction of neutrophils as well as stimulation of alveolar macrophages. These cells release several cytokines, proinflammatory agents as well as some antiinflammatory mediators. On balance, there is a net effect to perpetuate the inflammatory process and to recruit other neutrophils. It is not clear to what extent local release of these agents impacts other organ systems.

The late phase of ARDS evolution, the proliferative phase, is notable for the development of fibrotic changes in the interstitium and alveolar spaces.[40] There may be significant architectural distortion, and it is common to see an increase in dead-space fraction that may manifest as an increased $PaCO_2$ or a suddenly increased spontaneous minute ventilation. While it is convenient to think of ARDS pathophysiology as having two distinct phases, there is evidence of abnormal fibroproliferation early in the syndrome, and fibroblast mitogenic activity on bronchoalveolar lavage specimens has been correlated with mortality.[43] Most patients who die as a direct result of ARDS will do so during the exudative phase of the syndrome, but there is still a significant mortality risk for those in the fibroproliferative stage who require prolonged ventilation.[40] Their mortality is increasingly likely to be related to nosocomial complications as well as failure of other organ systems.

In a clinical sense, there are three distinct lung zones created in patients with ARDS. There are significant portions of the lung that are dominated by shunt physiology secondary to alveolar filling and atelectasis, associated both with the loss of surfactant and dependent collapse. Most of these areas will either heal or they will not irrespective of interventions. Vigorous efforts to open involved alveoli are unlikely to be of benefit and may be harmful to more compliant areas of the lungs. A second important lung zone is characterized by significant atelectasis or alveolar-capillary barrier damage that may be reversible. Some areas in this region may even open with the introduction of a positive-pressure breath but close as the breath is allowed to exit the lung. The cycle then repeats with each subsequent breath. This area is the battleground for ARDS supportive management. The goal is to utilize this region for gas exchange as much as possible while simultaneously protecting it from further injury evolution. The third lung zone is a relatively normal one. It is likely that there are significant inflammatory changes taking place in these regions as well, but from a gross macroscopic standpoint, this zone appears to behave in a normal physiologic manner. As described for the second region, one of the fundamental goals of ARDS care is to protect this normal lung zone from injury. Gattinoni et al. have used the term "baby lungs" when thinking about mechanical ventilation of ARDS patients, since a smaller than normal lung volume is actually available to perform the necessary physiologic function normally accomplished by the uninjured pulmonary system.[44]

The edema and atelectasis create a significant amount of physiologic right-to-left shunt that generally leads to progressive, severe hypoxemia. These changes also cause a significant reduction in lung compliance. Efforts to provide "normal" tidal volume breaths using a traditional volume-control mode will result in the development of very high peak and plateau pressures.[40,45] Use of a pressure-control mode with the intent of limiting these high pressures will often lead to very low tidal volumes.[46,47] Strategies for addressing both the shunt and compliance abnormalities will be discussed in further detail below.

Ventilator-induced lung injury is one of the significant dangers associated with the care of the ARDS patient.[7] Volutrauma in ARDS has been noted with excessive tidal volumes in both retrospective and prospective human trials and demonstrated convincingly in animal studies.[10] Volutrauma is felt to be one of the primary mediators of VILI in ARDS patients and has been the impetus for the low-tidal-volume strategies described below. Barotrauma was seen frequently in the past when overaggressive positive-pressure ventilation was applied to ARDS patients with severely limited lung compliance, resulting in very high transalveolar pressures. Atelectotrauma due to cyclic opening and closing of alveoli is of greatest concern at the edges of portions of the lung that are densely consolidated. Alveoli that open and close adjacent to those that are incapable of opening create a shearing force with each cycle. This shearing force may disrupt the alveolar-capillary interface and perpetuate the lung injury. Finally, biotrauma associated with mechanical ventilation use will exacerbate the underlying inflammatory milieu already present in the ARDS patient and may serve to encourage further lung injury. With this as a background, attention now turns to the complex task of ARDS management. Goals for management of ARDS include: (1) eliminate the source of the ARDS; (2) provide aggressive supportive care to allow time for healing to take place; and (3) do not cause further harm with iatrogenic interventions.

> Goals for management of ARDS include: (1) eliminate the source of the ARDS; (2) provide aggressive supportive care to allow time for healing to take place; and (3) do not cause further harm with iatrogenic interventions.

## *Mechanical Ventilation*

### Tidal Volume

Volutrauma has long been noted in animal models to both perpetuate existing ARDS and to cause a lung injury de novo with pathology consistent with diffuse alveolar damage. It was therefore hypothesized that using a lower tidal volume with mechanical ventilation may result in improved outcomes. Four randomized controlled trials conducted using so-called lung protective strategies were published in the late 1990's.[48,49,50,51] Only one of the four was able to demonstrate a statistically significant improvement in mortality.[48] A consortium of institutions known as the Acute Respiratory Distress Syndrome Clinical Trials Network (ARDSnet) led by the National Heart Lung and Blood Institute was formed in the mid 1990's to coordinate ARDS research efforts. They conducted a large phase III randomized controlled trial comparing a low tidal volume (4 to 6 ml per kilogram) versus high (conventional) tidal volume (12 ml per kilogram) that was published in 2000.[52] The low-tidal-volume intervention resulted in statistically significant improvements in mortality, ventilator-free days and organ-failure-free days. It should be noted that the weight used for the tidal volume calculation is the predicted body weight. This same low-tidal-volume strategy was used in subsequent ARDSnet studies described later that addressed issues such as optimal PEEP settings, fluid strategy and corticosteroid use in ARDS. A reproduction of the ARDSnet low-tidal-volume strategy is included in the Appendix.

An early criticism of the low-tidal-volume ARDSnet trial was that it is unclear from the design of the study that a low tidal volume of 4 to 6 ml per kilogram is optimal. Another explanation of the study findings perhaps is that a tidal volume of 12 ml per kilogram may be excessive and did not represent the common standard of care at the time the study was done.[53] The criticism has been countered by survey data from the mid 1990s demonstrating that average tidal volumes in use at the time of the study design were in fact similar to those produced in the ARDSnet study control group. At this point in time, the ARDSnet low-tidal-volume strategy is considered the standard of care for initial ventilator management of ARDS, and deviations from this basic protocol should only be made when it has failed in a given clinical setting.

> Low-tidal-volume strategy is considered the standard of care for initial ventilator management of ARDS.

Based on the ARDSnet study findings, initial ventilator settings for a patient with ARDS are illustrated below.[52] For patients who were previously receiving invasive mechanical ventilation prior to the diagnosis of ARDS, adjust the $FiO_2$ and PEEP as indicated in the Appendix. For patients who were intubated at the same time that the initial diagnosis of ARDS was made, begin with an $FiO_2$ of 100 percent, a PEEP of 10 cm $H_2O$ and titrate both according to the Appendix.

> 1. Assist-Control (A/C) Mode (volume set/flow controlled for assist and control breaths)
> 2. Initial Vt = 8 ml per kilogram (PBW)
>    PBW in kg (male) = 50 + 2.3 x (height in inches – 60)
>    PBW in kg (female) = 45.5 + 2.3 x (height in inches – 60)
> 3. Reduce Vt by 1 ml per kilogram until Vt = 6 ml per kilogram
> 4. Adjust $f$ (up to 35) and Vt (4 to 6 ml per kilogram) to achieve peak plateau pressure (Pplat) less than 30 cm $H_2O$ and pH 7.3 to 7.45
> 5. Bicarbonate can be added if pH is less than 7.3 and if $f$ is maximal at 35.
> 6. Initial $FiO_2$ and PEEP levels were not predefined in the ARDSnet low-tidal-volume study.

An important concern related to the use of low tidal volumes to limit plateau pressures in ARDS patients is the development of clinically significant respiratory acidosis. Previous research has demonstrated that moderate degrees of respiratory acidosis are well tolerated in most instances and therefore represent a small price to pay relative to the benefits of decreasing volutrauma and barotrauma.[54] This trade-off of ventilation for lung function preservation became known as permissive hypercapnia. The ARDSnet protocol allowed for the use of bicarbonate to help counteract the effects of hypercapnia and normalize the pH.[52] There was little difference in pH between intervention and control groups after the initial 72 hours. Other options in clinical practice include the use of proton scavengers such as tromethamine and less commonly limiting $CO_2$ production by manipulating the respiratory quotient of feeds, decreasing body temperature, or minimizing metabolic rate through deep sedation or paralysis. The use of permissive hypercapnia in the setting of a severe elevation in intracranial pressure should be avoided due to associated worsening elevations in intracranial pressure.[20,21,55,56]

> The use of low tidal volumes to limit plateau pressures in ARDS patients can lead to clinically significant respiratory acidosis. When permissive hypercapnia is practiced, the resultant acidemia can be mitigated by use of bicarbonate or other interventions.

## Positive End-Expiratory Pressure (PEEP)

The optimal PEEP to be used for mechanical ventilation of the ARDS patient is an area of great interest and few definite answers.[57] The maintenance of pressure in the airways at end-exhalation should help to prevent collapse of alveoli and preserve the current functional residual capacity, which is the volume in the lungs at the end of tidal exhalation. In ARDS, progressive atelectasis is a problem due to progression of the injury itself, as well as the effects of compression by a heavy, edematous lung on more dependent portions. The use of PEEP can counteract this trend.

An intuitive approach to the application of PEEP would involve the examination of a static pressure-volume curve as represented in Figure 7. Pressure is applied initially to the lung in an effort to cause inflation. The initial portion of the curve is characterized by little change in volume in spite of pressure application, which represents alveoli that are closed and will not open without a significant amount of energy. Once a critical opening pressure is reached, the compliance of the system improves markedly, and the lung opens quickly with relatively little subsequent pressure application. This critical opening pressure is referred to as the lower inflection point. At some point, the lung cannot expand further and compliance again drops drastically yielding no significant gain in volume regardless of the further application of pressure. This point of sudden decrease in compliance is called the upper inflection point.

Many experts have argued that the optimal PEEP should be one that is just above the lower inflection point, since the fundamental goal of PEEP is to prevent collapse of alveoli and loss of functional residual capacity. Others argue that it is more effective to use a higher level of PEEP just below the upper inflection point in order to maximize the ability to keep the lungs open. A third opinion relates to the fact that a static pressure-volume curve in ARDS often demonstrates a degree of hysteresis. The sigmoidal shape curve seen as air is pushed into the lungs is not identical to that seen when air is allowed to passively leave on exhalation. The exhalation curve is typically shifted slightly to the left, implying a higher lung volume at any given transpulmonary pressure relative to that seen on inhalation. Some advocate using the exhalation curve to determine the optimal PEEP rather than any point on the inhalation curve, since the goal is to help alveoli remain open as air leaves the lungs.

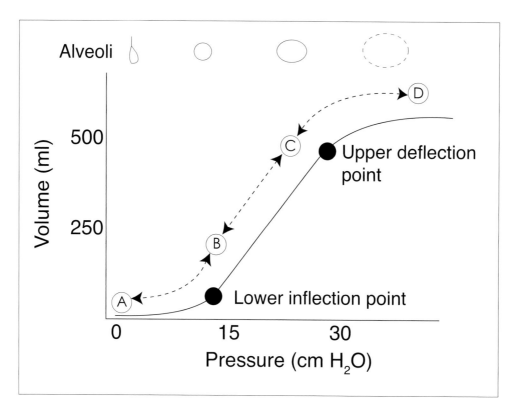

Figure 7. *An ARDS static compliance curve. Once a critical opening pressure is reached (B), the compliance of the system improves markedly and the lung opens quickly with relatively little subsequent pressure application.*

Several ventilator packages have sophisticated software algorithms available that can project a pressure-volume curve. However, measurement of a true static pressure-volume curve involves paralyzing the patient and serially measuring pressures after different volumes are introduced into the patient. In the day-to-day clinical management of an ARDS patient, this process is time consuming, risky for the patient, and not practical to consider several times a day when compliance may be expected to change rapidly.

Attempts to define the optimal use of PEEP have resulted in the evolution of two schools of thought, one advocating more moderate levels of PEEP and one favoring a high level of PEEP.[58,59]

Potential problems may be envisioned with both approaches. If a low-PEEP strategy is used, it may not be adequate enough to maximally prevent alveolar collapse. Additionally, worsening compliance due to evolution of the lung injury may lead to the emergence of an inadequate level of PEEP within hours or days that may have been adequate at the time it was set. If a low-PEEP strategy is used, close attention must be paid to the development of worsening compliance and shunt. The use of very high levels of PEEP may result in overdistension of relatively normal lung tissue. Excessive alveolar distending pressures may cause diversion of blood to less ventilated sections of the lung. This creates increased dead-space in the more compliant areas of lung and increased shunt in the more consolidated areas. Other complications to consider in the scenario would be atelectotrauma exacerbation at the interfaces between more and less compliant areas of lung, as well as volutrauma and possibly barotrauma in the overdistended lung regions. All of these effects would perpetuate biotrauma and add the effects of VILI to those already ongoing due to the ARDS.

In 2004, the ARDSnet published the results of a multicenter randomized controlled trial comparing a low-PEEP/high FiO$_2$ strategy to a high-PEEP/low FiO$_2$ strategy known as the Assessment of Low Tidal Volume and Elevated End-Expiratory Lung Volume to Obviate Lung Injury (ALVEOLI) trial.[59] The study enrolled 549 patients to completion and did not show a significant difference in terms of hospital mortality or ventilator-free days. The average PEEP in the low-PEEP group was 8.3 cm H$_2$O compared to 13.2 cm H$_2$O in the high-PEEP group. A subgroup analysis of the ALVEOLI trial compared the effects of recruitment maneuvers in ARDS patients who were ventilated in the high-PEEP group. Recruitment maneuvers were performed by transitioning the patient from A/C to continuous positive airway pressure (CPAP) with a pressure of 35 cm H$_2$O and maintaining this pressure for 30 seconds before transitioning back to A/C. There were some transient improvements in SpO$_2$ in some patients, but no sustained improvements after an hour were noted. Some patients experienced desaturation and hypotension as complications. A recent study compared the use of a moderate level of PEEP (5 to 9 cm H$_2$O; the minimal distension group) to an increased recruitment approach (increasing the PEEP to reach a plateau pressure of 28 to 30 cm H$_2$O).[60] All patients received a low-tidal-volume (6 ml per kilogram) strategy with volume set/flow controlled, A/C as the mode of mechanical ventilation. There was no significant difference in mortality, but the increased recruitment strategy led to a statistically significant improvement in the number of ventilator-free days and organ failure-free days. It should also be noted that adjunctive therapies such as prone positioning and inhaled nitric oxide were used more frequently in the minimal distension group. Meade et al. compared an "open-lung" strategy of ventilation versus the now standard ARDSnet low-tidal-volume algorithm in a multicenter randomized controlled trial published in 2008 involving 983 patients with ARDS.[61] The intervention group received a plateau pressure limit of 40 cm H$_2$O, pressure-control ventilation, and a significantly higher PEEP than that seen in the 2000 ARDSnet low-tidal-volume trial. There was no difference in mortality, but there was a statistically significant decrease in refractory hypoxemia and the use of rescue therapy (inhaled nitric oxide, prone positioning, high frequency oscillatory ventilation and extracorporeal membrane oxygenation) in the intervention group.

> In most cases of ARDS, the optimal PEEP is likely at least 10 to 12 cm H$_2$O. Higher levels should be attempted in patients with more severe ARDS manifestations, while close attention is paid to the development of iatrogenic complications.

Conclusions regarding PEEP remain a source of great debate. The data appears to favor a higher PEEP with respect to oxygenation, but there does not appear to be a mortality benefit to this approach.[59,61] Concern exists that excessively high levels of PEEP may perpetuate VILI, exacerbate hypoxemia and hypercapnia, and may cause hypotension.[62] The optimal PEEP is likely at least 10 to 12 cm H$_2$O in most cases, and higher levels should probably be attempted in patients with more severe ARDS manifestations while close attention is paid to the development of iatrogenic complications.[59,61]

Airway Pressure Release Ventilation (APRV)

Airway pressure release ventilation (APRV) has been used as an alternative mode of mechanical ventilation in the ARDS patient.[63,64] As discussed earlier, it involves controlling the mean airway pressure by cycling between two different levels of PEEP. The ability to generate a high mean airway pressure augments oxygenation, while the upper PEEP level serves to limit the plateau pressure generated by driving air into a noncompliant lung. The ability to limit the plateau pressure is an attractive feature of this mode of ventilation in ARDS, as is such a precise ability to control the mean airway pressure. The fact that the ventilator does not have to change its controlled pressure release cycle based upon patient effort is also very helpful and allows the use of very aggressive inverse ratio ventilation with less patient discomfort.[63] This allows a decreased requirement for sedation and chemical paralysis.[65]

One drawback of APRV mode is that the tidal volume generated by the controlled breaths is determined by the difference between the high PEEP and low PEEP levels. Most who use APRV tend to use relatively aggressive PEEPh levels but PEEPl levels of 0 to 5 cm $H_2O$. This large difference creates the potential for excessive tidal volume generation greater than 6 ml per kilogram and therefore may perpetuate VILI. The development of intrinsic PEEP may mitigate this concern somewhat since the time spent at the PEEPl is frequently very short. The time at the PEEPl is often set so that the expiratory flow versus time curve is only 80 to 90 percent of the way back to a baseline of zero flow when the machine cycles back to the PEEPh level. Significant intrinsic PEEP will cause the tidal volume to be proportional to the difference between the PEEPh and intrinsic PEEP rather than the larger difference between PEEPh and PEEPl.

> There is no data to support the use of APRV over other modes of ventilation in the setting of ARDS. It should be thought of as a potentially useful salvage therapy in the critical care setting for patients who have failed a traditional ARDSnet low-tidal-volume strategy.

At this time, there are no data to support a benefit of this mode of ventilation versus any other mode in the setting of ARDS. There are studies that describe the successful application of APRV for ARDS patients, and some major medical centers have a great deal of experience with the mode.[66] A randomized, open labeled, parallel assignment study comparing APRV to the ARDSnet low-tidal-volume standard of care for ALI/ARDS is currently enrolling patients.[67] At this time, APRV should be thought of as a potentially useful salvage therapy in the CCC setting for patients who have failed the traditional ARDSnet low-tidal-volume strategy.

## Adjunctive Strategies

Inhaled nitric oxide (iNO) has been used to cause selective pulmonary artery vasodilation in several conditions, including primary pulmonary hypertension, pulmonary reperfusion lung injury after pulmonary thromboendarterectomy, and ARDS in both adults in infants.[68,69,70] Inhaled nitric oxide is very short-acting and does not enter the systemic circulation to an appreciable extent. Its effects are therefore locally confined to well-ventilated alveoli, serving to improve ventilation-perfusion matching. Importantly, perfusion is diverted away from poorly ventilated regions, which has the effect of decreasing the shunt fraction and therefore improving hypoxemia. Several clinical trials have evaluated the use of iNO in ARDS with variable designs and outcomes. A recent meta-analysis concluded that there is a small but significant improvement in $PaO_2/FiO_2$ at 24 hours but no improvement in mortality and potential harm (renal dysfunction). Thus it cannot routinely recommended at this time.[69]

> Although there is a small but significant improvement in $PaO_2/FiO_2$ at 24 hours, inhaled nitric oxide fails to improve mortality, and cannot be routinely recommended for treatment of ARDS.

High-frequency oscillatory ventilation is the intellectually extreme manifestation of the low-tidal-volume approach. The majority of clinical experience with this mode of ventilation and its application in ARDS is confined to a few major academic medical centers. A study published by Derdak et al. in 2002 compared the use of HFOV versus a more conventional mode of ventilation.[71] There was no mortality benefit noted in that study, although there was a trend towards improved survival noted as many as 90 days after randomization (p = 0.1, 148 patients enrolled in the study). The average tidal volume in the conventional ventilation group was 10 ml per kilogram. There has not been a prospective randomized controlled trial comparing HFOV to the ARDSnet low-tidal-volume strategy. High-frequency oscillatory ventilation should be thought of as a rescue therapy only in centers with significant experience in its use. It may find wider application in the future as further prospective studies are conducted.

Extracorporeal membrane oxygenation (ECMO) has been used in neonatal intensive care for ARDS for several decades with success.[72] The therapy involves diverting blood through a filter outside of the body to allow gas exchange and then reintroducing the treated blood into the vasculature. A large prospective study evaluating the use of ECMO in adults with severe acute respiratory failure during the 1970's failed to show a significant benefit to the therapy.[73] Extracorporeal membrane oxygenation is used as therapy for ARDS in a few large medical centers today with relatively stringent criteria used for selection of patients believed to derive benefit. A portable extracorporeal carbon dioxide removal ($ECCO_2R$) device called the NovaLung® has been used in the ICU as rescue therapy for United States (US) service members wounded in Iraq with severe ARDS and for their critical care air transport out-of-theater. Rationale for this approach stems from allowing the use of very low minute ventilation in an effort to minimize ventilator induced lung injury.[74] Experience is limited, but anecdotal success has been encouraging.[75] Randomized controlled trials further evaluating ECMO and $ECCO_2R$ technology relative to ARDSnet low-tidal-volume standards are needed.

## Fluid Management

A recent study compared a conservative versus liberal fluid management strategy in ARDS.[76] The study also compared the use of a central venous catheter in the internal jugular or subclavian position versus a pulmonary artery catheter to guide assessment of intravascular volume status. The conservative fluid strategy limited fluid infusion and encouraged early diuresis. There was a profound difference in cumulative fluid balance between the liberal and conservative fluid groups by day seven after randomization. Of note, the cumulative fluid balance curves for the initial ARDSnet low-tidal-volume and ALVEOLI studies were almost identical to the liberal fluid curve in the Wiedeman et al. study.[52,59,76] With respect to fluid balance approaches, there was no significant difference in mortality; however, an improvement was noted in both ventilator-free days and ICU-free days in the conservative fluid group. There was no difference in any major outcome when comparing the use of a standard central venous catheter versus a pulmonary artery catheter. It is recommended that outside of the initial resuscitation for hypovolemic shock, intravascular volume be minimized to the extent possible. There does not appear to be a significant role for the routine use of a pulmonary artery catheter for the management of ARDS.

> Apart from the initial resuscitation for hypovolemic shock, intravascular fluid administration should be minimized during management of ARDS.

## Role of Corticosteroid Therapy

Corticosteroids have been evaluated in both the early and late phases of ARDS in several well-designed randomized controlled trials over the last fifteen years. An ARDSnet trial published in 2006 evaluating the efficacy and safety of corticosteroid use for persistent ARDS did not demonstrate a mortality benefit to their use.[77] In fact, corticosteroids started more that two weeks after onset of ARDS were associated with an increased mortality. There was a statistically significant improvement in ventilator-free days in the treatment group through 28 days after randomization. Two meta-analyses published recently arrived at conflicting conclusions.[78,79] Agarwal et al. were unable to find any benefit in mortality with the use of corticosteroids for ARDS in either the early or late phase.[78] Meduri et al. found a statistically significant improvement with the use of corticosteroids with respect to ventilator-free days as well as mortality.[79]

> The routine use of corticosteroids in either the early or late phase of ARDS is not recommended at this time.

Currently evidence suggests there may be some physiologic improvement with the use of corticosteroids for ARDS, particularly when started before the development of a significant amount of fibrosis.[80] There does not appear to be a consensus that mortality is improved with the therapy, and the potential for complications directly related to the therapy is significant. The routine use of corticosteroids in either the early or late phase of ARDS is not recommended at this time.

## Role of Prone Positioning

Prone positioning has been advocated as an adjunctive therapy for ARDS to improve oxygenation and has been studied prospectively in several trials.[81,82,83,84,85,86] The physiologic basis for improvements in oxygenation is not entirely clear, but is hypothesized to involve improved ventilation perfusion matching, regional changes in ventilation, and decreased compression of the dependent portions of the left lower lobe by the heart. Proning a patient with ARDS can be a difficult undertaking and requires a special bed that can assist in the position change and several personnel. In the CCC environment, a frame made by the Stryker company is available that can be used in the ICU and during critical care air transportation (Fig. 8). The potential for dislodgement of endotracheal tubes and lines is significant and may be life threatening for a patient with marginal oxygenation at baseline.

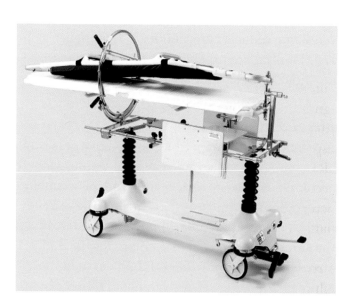

Figure 8. *A Stryker frame allows a patient to be turned to the prone position as a single unit without individually moving parts of the body.*

Gattinoni et al. were unable to demonstrate a mortality benefit to prone positioning for 304 ARDS patients enrolled in a randomized controlled trial, but a significant improvement in $PaO_2$ was noted in 70 percent of patients in the experimental group.[83] A post-hoc analysis was able to demonstrate an improvement in mortality in the quartile of patients with the lowest $PaO_2/FiO_2$ on enrollment as well as in the quartile of patients with the highest simplified acute physiology score (SAPS) II at enrollment. One criticism of the study was the relatively short duration of prone positioning. Of note, there was no difference in the number of endotracheal tubes that were dislodged between the experimental and control groups.

A 2002 review of the literature for the use of prone positioning with ARDS concluded that improvement in oxygenation can be expected in 70 to 80 percent of early ARDS patients undergoing prone positioning, but the effects of this improvement are not seen after seven days.[82] There does not appear to be a substantial mortality benefit and significant care must be taken during patient position changes. Finally, the incidence of pressure sores was increased in patients who were proned and related directly to the duration of time in the prone position. A recent prospective randomized trial evaluated the use of prone positioning for periods of at least 20 hours at a time for the treatment of moderate and severe ARDS.[86] The primary endpoint of all-cause mortality at 28 days was equivalent for both the supine and prone patient groups, as was a secondary endpoint of mortality at six months. In the severe ARDS patient group, there was a slight trend towards benefit with respect to mortality at both time points, but the difference did not reach statistical significance.[86]

| Prone positioning is not recommended for routine therapy of ARDS patients at this time. |
| --- |

Prone positioning is not recommended for routine therapy of ARDS patients at this time. It is recommended as an adjunctive therapy in patients with severe hypoxemia. Care should be taken to closely coordinate the efforts of those involved in proning the patient, and dislodgement of the endotracheal tube should be prevented at all costs.

## *Nutritional Goals*

Nutrition in the ICU is increasingly being appreciated as an active therapy with the potential for a significant impact on patient outcomes.[87] The patient with ARDS has an injury that is driven to a great extent by inflammatory mediators. Using any therapy, including nutrition, to help modulate the pathologic response is desirable. Several small studies suggest a possible benefit to the use of omega-3 fatty acids in ARDS as a mechanism for reducing inflammation.[88,89,90] The balance of fat versus carbohydrate in enteral feeds also significantly impacts the respiratory quotient and therefore the carbon dioxide production. An increased $CO_2$ production may complicate efforts to use permissive hypercapnia as a strategy in the management of ARDS.

A recent study evaluated the effect of a specific enteral feed on patients with sepsis and respiratory failure.[90] The experimental group was given a feed with significant amounts of omega-3 fatty acids (replacing omega-6 fatty acids which are metabolized to inflammatory mediators) as well as borage oil. They noted a statistically significant improvement in mortality and $PaO_2/FiO_2$ (at days four and seven) as well as an increase in ICU-free days and ventilator-free days. A major prospective randomized controlled trial that will address nutrition specifically in ARDS patients is currently underway in the ARDSnet consortium of research centers.

| While definitive data supporting the use of specific enteral feeds in ARDS are still lacking, the preponderance of available data at this time supports the use of feeds high in omega-3 fatty acids. |
| --- |

## *Summary*

Acute respiratory distress syndrome (ARDS) is a diffuse, heterogenous disorder resulting in significant shunt physiology and pulmonary compliance limitations that are seen commonly in the CCC ICU. The use of a low-tidal-volume, open-lung strategy can improve mortality by limiting the propagation of the lung injury and possibly decreasing the incidence of multisystem organ failure.

# Endpoints of Resuscitation

## *Basic Concepts*

At the most basic level, shock is defined as a state where there is inadequate oxygen available relative to the metabolic needs of the intracellular processes.[91] This may be a result of decreased oxygen delivery, increased oxygen requirement in the setting of fixed delivery, or an inability to utilize oxygen at the cellular level. It is important for the clinician to have a solid appreciation of oxygen delivery ($DO_2$), aerobic metabolic demand, oxygen uptake ($VO_2$), the oxygen extraction ratio (ER), and their interrelationships. In the normal healthy state, the oxygen uptake correlates directly with aerobic metabolic demand. As will be discussed shortly, conditions that affect the mitochondrial electron transport chain will influence the relationship between aerobic metabolic demand and oxygen uptake. Failure of appropriate aerobic metabolism defines the presence of shock, and resultant adverse outcomes are related both to the severity of the failure as well as its duration.[92]

> Ensuring adequate resuscitation and early recognition of hypoperfusion is critical in the treatment of shock.

Oxygen delivery is directly proportional to the oxygen content of the blood as well as the volume of blood transmitted to the body per-unit-time. The most important components of oxygen delivery are therefore hemoglobin (Hgb), oxygen saturation of hemoglobin ($SaO_2$), and the cardiac output (Q). The amount of oxygen dissolved in the blood is very small relative to that bound to hemoglobin. While the $PaO_2$ is included in the definition of oxygen delivery, it is physiologically of little importance.

Q = Stroke Volume x Heart Rate
$DO_2$ = Q x [1.39 x Hgb x $SaO_2$ + 0.0031 x $PaO_2$]

The interrelationship of oxygen uptake and oxygen delivery in the normal state is affected greatly by the integrity of the mitochondrial electron transport chain. Generally, there is an abundance of oxygen delivery relative to oxygen uptake. Efforts to increase oxygen delivery will not result in increased oxygen uptake. Below a critical oxygen delivery, the oxygen uptake is said to be supply dependent as the reduction-oxidation (redox) state of the mitochondrial electron transport chain changes towards a more reduced state in response to the oxygen delivery. The amount of oxygen utilized will mirror that which is provided, and the relationship is defined by the oxygen extraction ratio (ER = $VO_2/DO_2$). In a non-supply-dependent state where there is an abundance of oxygen delivery relative to oxygen uptake, the redox state of the electron transport chain adjusts towards increased oxidation to yield a progressively lower oxygen extraction ratio as oxygen delivery increases. A normal oxygen extraction ratio in this setting is approximately 15 to 30 percent. When oxygen delivery is limited enough to become supply dependent, a maximum oxygen extraction ratio is established by a maximally reduced electron transport chain. A normal global oxygen extraction ratio in the supply dependent setting is in the range of 60 to 70 percent; however, it should be recognized that each tissue has its own oxygen extraction ratio that may play a large role in determining its risk of injury in a given low oxygen supply state.

In patients who have sustained prolonged or severe decreases in oxygen delivery, expected redox changes may fail, leading to inefficient activity of the electron transport chain. The result is a lower than expected oxygen extraction ratio and the development of an oxygen uptake that becomes supply dependent across all levels of oxygen delivery. The inability to move away from supply dependence, even with supranormal oxygen delivery, signifies a failure of the expected change towards oxidation of the electron transport chain. Decoupling of the electron transport chain redox state from the oxygen delivery can result in the production of free radical mediated damage as well as the generation of reactive oxygen species. This decoupling is a commonly described phenomenon in patients who eventually develop progressive organ dysfunction as the trauma resuscitation evolves. Inefficient oxygen utilization can be difficult to detect at bedside, but inadequate oxygen availability at the cellular level will lead to increased rates of anaerobic metabolism that can be detected in a variety of different ways. Most methods investigated to detect the presence of anaerobic metabolism rely on secondary acid-base physiology changes reflecting the increased production of lactate and the increased consumption of bicarbonate.

In the CCC setting, hypovolemic shock is seen most frequently initially, and many patients may go on to develop distributive shock secondary to the systemic inflammatory response syndrome. Rapid resolution of the etiology is the most critical aspect of the management of either, but aggressive supportive care directed at normalization of oxygen delivery is vital.

> Hypovolemic shock is seen in the immediate phase of resuscitation, but distributive shock may follow, secondary to the systemic inflammatory response syndrome.

Markers of global perfusion adequacy do not necessarily mean that regional perfusion is intact. Inadequate regional perfusion that is clinically unrecognized is common and may be seen in as many as 85 percent of patients with normal bedside hemodynamics early in a major trauma resuscitation.[93,94] Uncompensated shock is generally easy to diagnose at bedside, as it is heralded by decreased urine output, tachycardia, and hypotension. Compensated shock is a condition characterized by normal bedside markers of resuscitation with underlying evidence of regional oxygen delivery inadequacy such as a progressive metabolic acidosis. It is clear that traditional bedside parameters available to the clinician are inadequate to establish an effective resuscitation endpoint. Available options for defining such an endpoint follow.

> Clinical markers such as decreased urine output, tachycardia, and hypotension may herald uncompensated shock. Conversely, clinical markers may be normal in compensated shock, and additional biochemical markers may be necessary to establish an effective resuscitation endpoint.

## *Lactate*

The use of lactate to assess resuscitation adequacy follows logically from the recognition that anaerobic metabolism leads to increased production. Understanding its strengths and weaknesses in this regard follow from an appreciation of how it is formed and subsequently cleared. Glycolysis, whether anaerobic in the cytoplasm or aerobic in the mitochondria, results in the production of a small amount of adenosine triphosphate (ATP) and pyruvate. Any stress state will increase the rate of glycolysis and result in increased pyruvate production. In an anaerobic environment, pyruvate is converted almost exclusively to lactate. In an aerobic environment, the majority of pyruvate is consumed by the tricarboxylic acid (TCA) cycle resulting in efficient production of ATP. However, even in an aerobic environment, there is a fixed ratio of lactate to pyruvate (a normal lactate to pyruvate ratio [L:P] is 10:1). Any increase in pyruvate production will also result in increased lactate production regardless of the availability of oxygen, but the percentage of pyruvate used to create lactate increases in the anaerobic environment (L:P greater than 30:1). Lactate is cleared from the body by actions of the liver (60 percent), kidney (30 percent), and muscle (10 percent).

> Lactate should not be used as a sole marker for adequacy of resuscitation in the CCC environment.

Lactate is increased in trauma resuscitation patients who are nonsurvivors relative to those who survive.[95] Time to resolution of lactic acidosis appears to be predictive of survival in the setting of trauma resuscitation as well as postoperative surgical patients being cared for in the ICU.[96,97] Use of lactate as an endpoint for resuscitation is appealing given its ease of measurement. However, its use is complicated by the fact that its generation is not completely related to the presence of anaerobic conditions, and its clearance may be delayed when liver or kidney damage is present. As a real-time marker of perfusion, both of these are important considerations. An elevated lactate level can serve as a useful prognostic marker.

In summary, an elevated lactate level has prognostic value, but a normal level is not helpful. Lactate should not be used as a sole marker for adequacy of resuscitation in the CCC environment.

## *Base Deficit*

The base deficit is a theoretical construct designed to simplify acid-base interpretation and has no true physiologic basis. It is the amount of bicarbonate in millimoles (mmol) per liter required to titrate one liter of whole blood to achieve a pH of 7.4, assuming the $PaCO_2$ of the patient is 40 mm Hg. The base deficit does not have any relationship to the cause of the acidemia, and the amount of base predicted assumes a stable acid-base system at the time of measurement.

One of the few areas in the critical care literature where base deficits have been shown to be of clinical benefit is in the setting of early trauma resuscitation.[98,99,100] This is a reflection of the fact that most cases of acidemia seen in this setting result from hypovolemic shock leading to inadequate oxygen delivery and the subsequent development of lactic acidosis. A progressively worsening base deficit argues that the resuscitative efforts are not adequate and should prompt the clinician to ensure adequate hemostasis, intravascular volume repletion, and replacement of hemoglobin.

> Base deficit has been shown to be of clinical benefit in guiding the management of hypovolemic patients during early trauma resuscitation. The base deficit should not be used to guide therapy after the initial resuscitative period, as too many variables affecting acid-base physiology are likely to exist.

Scenarios that will complicate the use of base deficit as an endpoint of resuscitation include any condition that impacts the acid-base status other than lactic acidosis.[95,101] A non-anion gap metabolic acidosis is frequently seen after aggressive crystalloid resuscitation, particularly if saline is used. This will worsen the base deficit and may not reflect inadequate resuscitation at all. Respiratory acidosis will worsen a base deficit, and a respiratory alkalosis will improve it. Exogenous bicarbonate therapy or buffers used in total parenteral nutrition (TPN) may also complicate the use of the base deficit as a marker of resuscitation adequacy. A final problem with the base deficit is that it is a more appropriate marker of global resuscitation than regional resuscitation.

An increased base deficit in the trauma resuscitation period has been correlated with increased resuscitation requirements in terms of fluid and blood as well as increased mortality.[99,102,103] The progression of the base deficit during resuscitation has also been correlated with worsened outcomes.[104] Serum bicarbonate levels correlate well with base deficit in trauma patients, but the serum lactate level is not well-predicted by the base deficit.[95,105]

Base deficit has value in predicting prognosis and guiding resuscitation in the hypovolemic patient. It is easy to measure at the bedside in austere environments and can be calculated with reasonable accuracy during critical care air transport using portable handheld arterial blood gas analyzers based upon measured pH and $PaCO_2$ values. It is not recommended for use as a resuscitation endpoint in patients who have other sources of acid-base physiology derangement, such as those who have received a significant amount of crystalloid fluid therapy. The base deficit should not be used to guide therapy after the initial resuscitative period, as too many variables affecting acid-base physiology are likely to exist other than lactic acidosis related to inadequate intravascular volume. Finally, the base deficit may be insensitive to the existence of regional hypoperfusion, and a normal base deficit should be therefore greeted with guarded optimism.

## *Supraphysiologic Oxygen Delivery Attainment*

The development of supply dependence of oxygen uptake on oxygen delivery has long been recognized in shock resuscitation as a marker of suboptimal oxygen utilization at the cellular level. Patients demonstrating decoupling of the electron transport chain demonstrate supply dependence across all levels of oxygen delivery and a lower maximal oxygen extraction ratio. It has been hypothesized that: (1) patients who are unable to generate an adequate oxygen delivery to meet the basic oxygen uptake needs of the body will do poorly; (2) increased aerobic metabolic needs in a time of stress will necessitate the generation of a higher than normal oxygen delivery, particularly when supply dependent physiology is present; and (3) the presence of a lower than normal maximal oxygen extraction ratio will also necessitate the generation of a supraphysiologic oxygen delivery.

Groundbreaking work by Shoemaker and colleagues found that high-risk surgical patients who survived were able to generate significantly higher cardiac indices and oxygen delivery values than nonsurvivors.[106,107] Early efforts to incorporate supraphysiologic oxygen delivery as a goal of resuscitation resulted in improved outcomes.[108,109] Subsequent studies using cardiac index and oxygen delivery goals defined by the experience of Shoemaker et al. were not successful in improving outcomes.[110,111] A study comparing clinical resuscitation using an oxygen delivery goal of 500 ml/min/m² versus the value of 600 ml/min/m² found no significant difference in outcomes.[112] There is difficulty in interpreting these studies because of significant variations in study design and patient population. A recent meta-analysis failed to show an overall benefit to the use of supraphysiologic oxygen delivery in surgical patient resuscitation.[113] However, a subset analysis of patients who had the intervention initiated before the onset of organ dysfunction did show a significant benefit.

Supraphysiologic oxygen delivery achievement is not recommended as a resuscitation endpoint for trauma patients encountered in the combat environment. Measurement is difficult to perform, and the data does not support a specific oxygen delivery goal that is absolutely better than any other in all patient populations. While it is true that severely ill patients are more likely to need a supraphysiologic oxygen delivery to meet oxygen uptake goals, the necessary oxygen delivery should be determined by targeting other endpoints of resuscitation.

## Mixed Venous Oxygen Saturation / Central Venous Oxygen Saturation

In a stressed patient with an intact ability to appropriately adjust the redox state of the mitochondrial electron transport chain toward reduction, supply dependence will develop below a critical oxygen delivery, and a maximal global oxygen extraction ratio of 65 to 70 percent can be expected. Measurement of the mixed venous oxygen saturation ($SvO_2$) in this case will yield a value of 30 to 35 percent, if one assumes that the $SaO_2$ is 100 percent. In the nonstressed state, the redox state of the electron transport chain favors oxidation, and the global oxygen extraction ratio is much lower than in the stressed state (typically less than 30 percent). Measurement of the mixed venous oxygen saturation in this setting, again assuming a $SaO_2$ of 100 percent, will be greater than 70 percent.

Measurement of mixed venous oxygen saturation has been hypothesized to be a useful endpoint of resuscitation because changes in its value theoretically reflect the balance between oxygen utilization and oxygen demand. A lower value, particularly less than 60 to 70 percent, indicates a relative inadequacy of oxygen delivery and a trend towards increased electron transport chain reduction in order to maintain adequate oxygen uptake relative to intracellular oxygen demand. A problem with this concept is commonly seen in the resuscitation of septic patients where decoupling is commonly seen, and oxygen uptake demonstrates supply dependence across a very broad range of oxygen delivery values, and a lower maximal oxygen extraction ratio is also seen. This reflects a significant inefficiency in oxygen utilization at the cellular level; however, the lower than expected oxygen extraction ratio may mask the inefficiency. A very low oxygen extraction ratio will result in a normalization of the mixed venous oxygen saturation that does not draw attention to the dysfunctional oxygen utilization at the cellular level. This scenario may also be observed in severely injured trauma patients who develop the systemic inflammatory response syndrome.

The measurement of mixed venous oxygen saturation is made using blood drawn from the distal tip of a pulmonary artery catheter. Efforts have been made to correlate the value of mixed venous oxygen saturation and the central venous oxygen saturation ($ScvO_2$) obtained from the distal tip of a central venous catheter positioned in the superior vena cava. It is normally expected that the two values will be slightly different owing to the contribution of blood from the coronary sinus as well as variable extraction of blood returning to the heart from the inferior vena cava relative to the superior vena cava. Several studies have noted a tight correlation between mixed venous oxygen saturation and central venous oxygen saturation, even if the actual values varied by a few percentage points.[114,115,116]

The mixed venous oxygen saturation was used as one of three goals for resuscitation in a prospective study of critically ill patients.[117] Patients were either resuscitated to a normal cardiac index, a supranormal cardiac index, or a mixed venous oxygen saturation of 70 percent. There were no differences in mortality or the development of multiple organ dysfunction syndrome.[117] Rivers et al. used a central venous oxygen saturation of 70 percent as one endpoint in their groundbreaking study of early goal-directed therapy in the treatment of severe sepsis and septic shock and demonstrated improved mortality.[118]

> Central venous oxygen saturation is recommended as one easily measured endpoint for resuscitation in the combat care environment. Central venous oxygen saturation less than 60 to 65 percent signifies inadequate resuscitation.

Central venous oxygen saturation is recommended as one easily measured endpoint for resuscitation in the combat care environment. A frankly low central venous oxygen saturation that is less than 60 to 65 percent should be taken as a marker of inadequate resuscitation.[119] Efforts should be made to ensure hemostasis, adequate intravascular volume, optimization of hemoglobin concentration, and oxygen saturation. Inotropic therapy can be considered if these parameters are all adequate but the central venous oxygen saturation remains low. There is no benefit to be gained from the placement of a pulmonary artery catheter specifically to measure the mixed venous oxygen saturation.

A normal central venous oxygen saturation should not be interpreted as confirming adequate resuscitation. Poor oxygen utilization at the cellular level may lead to a normalized central venous oxygen saturation while significant intracellular hypoxia continues. Efforts to confirm adequacy of regional oxygenation should continue if the central venous oxygen saturation is normal.

## Gastric Intramucosal pH (pHi)

Blood flow is not uniform across the tissues of the body, and decreased systemic perfusion pressures cause redistribution away from tissues that are not immediately necessary for survival. In hypovolemic shock, blood flow redistributes away from the gut mucosa early on and does not return until relatively late in the recovery process. Gut mucosa is one of the regions that is most sensitive to decreased perfusion pressure and therefore represents an excellent location to assess the adequacy of regional oxygen delivery.

Anaerobic metabolism in the gut mucosa leads to the increased production of tissue pressure of carbon dioxide ($PCO_2$), which rapidly equilibrates with the gastric secretions and lowers the gastric intramucosal pH (pHi). The gastric intramucosal pH can be measured using a gastric tonometry balloon or a continuous monitoring $CO_2$ electrode. A normal gastric intramucosal pH suggests adequate regional oxygen delivery, while an abnormally low gastric intramucosal pH suggests inadequate resuscitation in spite of possibly normal vital signs or markers of global oxygenation.

> If available, gastric intramucosal pH is recommended for the assessment of the adequacy of regional oxygen delivery in trauma patients in the combat care environment.

Several studies have noted a statistically significant correlation between a low gastric intramucosal pH and mortality.[120,121,122,123] When used as a prospective endpoint for a protocol driven resuscitation, a delay in achieving the gastric intramucosal pH goal was associated with increased mortality and the development of organ system failure.[124,125]

Gastric intramucosal pH is recommended for the assessment of the adequacy of regional oxygen delivery in trauma patients in the combat care environment if available. Gastric tonometry performed using saline filled probes with semipermeable membranes is unlikely to be widely used in most wartime critical care units, but continuous gastric $CO_2$ monitoring capability may be available in the near future as validation of increasingly portable technology continues. Such a capability would also be extremely useful in the critical care air transport setting.

## Sublingual PCO₂ (PslCO₂)

The measurement of sublingual $PCO_2$ ($PslCO_2$) concentrations is easy to do at the bedside and correlates well with gastric intramucosal pH.[126,127] A handheld monitor is used in much the same way as an oral temperature probe. The implications of an elevated sublingual $PCO_2$ are identical to those of a low gastric intramucosal pH, and a normal value is felt to represent normal regional oxygen delivery.

> The measurement of sublingual $PCO_2$ concentrations may be useful in assessing adequacy of resuscitation of trauma patients.

The use of sublingual $PCO_2$ as a noninvasive surrogate marker of gut mucosa perfusion has been described in two studies.[129,128] The sublingual $PCO_2$ has also been used in a prospective fashion to identify hemorrhage in penetrating trauma patients.[129] The degree of sublingual $PCO_2$ elevation correlated with the volume of blood loss.

The technology surrounding sublingual $PCO_2$ may be a very useful adjunct to the care of the combat trauma patient and represents a cheap, easily transportable method of assessing adequacy of resuscitation in austere environments. It is likely to offer the same benefits as gastric intramucosal pH assessment but will be much easier to perform.

## Tissue Carbon Dioxide and Oxygen Assessment

Transcutaneous oxygen content ($PO_2$) is expected to decrease when oxygen delivery is inadequate to meet demand. The development of anaerobic metabolism leads to the elevation of tissue $PCO_2$ in a fashion that is analogous to that described in the gut mucosa. Electrodes have been used to assess transcutaneous $PO_2$ and $PCO_2$ in critically ill trauma patients. Lower $PO_2$ values and higher $PCO_2$ values were associated with increased mortality.[130] One problem with older methods of assessing transcutaneous $PO_2$ and $PCO_2$ is that they were invasive. Near infrared spectroscopy (NIRS) offers a noninvasive method of assessing skeletal muscle oxyhemoglobin levels, which have been hypothesized to correlate with adequate regional oxygenation. Oxygen saturation of hemoglobin in tissue ($StO_2$) is the percentage of oxygenated hemoglobin relative to total hemoglobin. The oxygen saturation of hemoglobin in tissue was studied during the resuscitation of trauma patients and found to correlate well with oxygen delivery, lactate, and base deficit and less so with gastric intramucosal pH.[131] A prospective randomized observational study found that oxygen saturation of hemoglobin in tissue using NIRS technology was able to reliably identify severe shock but may not be able to reliably identify mild shock states.[132]

Tissue assessment of oxygenation may be useful as a resuscitation endpoint for trauma patients in the future, and NIRS technology may ensure ease of its application in the combat setting. At this time, it cannot be recommended as an endpoint of resuscitation due to its lack of demonstrated ability to identify early shock.

## Summary

Several of the commonly used endpoints of resuscitation such as mixed venous oxygen saturation, lactate concentration, and base deficit are useful in identifying global deficiencies in oxygen delivery. Increased sensitivity is required to identify patients with regional oxygen delivery abnormalities, and this capability is becoming available in the form of gastric intramucosal pH monitoring, sublingual $PCO_2$ assessment, and oxygen saturation of hemoglobin in tissue analysis. Markers of regional perfusion adequacy will likely largely replace global perfusion assessment in the future. Technological advancements will allow these more sensitive endpoints to be assessed in austere combat environments and during critical care air transport. A future frontier will involve the sensitive detection of oxygen utilization abnormalities at the cellular level. However, this capability will only be useful if therapies can be developed in the future that can act upon the information in a beneficial manner.

# Sepsis

## Definition of Sepsis

Sepsis is a clinical syndrome that is extremely common in the multisystem trauma patient and associated with great morbidity, mortality, and cost of care.[133,134] The presence of sepsis can be a challenge to identify in the combat casualty population since there are frequently numerous reasons for the presence of a systemic inflammatory state. However, early recognition and aggressive management of sepsis are necessary to maximize the chance of patient survival. Severe organ dysfunction associated with untreated infection has been recognized for over a millennium. Attempts to define the syndrome of sepsis did not become formalized in a largely agreed upon manner until 1991.[135] This consensus definition described the systemic inflammatory response syndrome (SIRS) as a condition that may result from either an infectious or noninfectious etiology. Sepsis was defined as the presence of SIRS most likely due to infection.

The traditional SIRS criteria are as follows:
- Temperature greater than 38°C or less than 36°C
- Heart rate greater than 90 beats per minute
- Respiratory rate greater than 20 breaths per minute or $PaCO_2$ less than 32 mm Hg
- White blood cells (WBCs) greater than 12,000 cells per cubic millimeter; less than 4,000 cells per cubic millimeter; or with greater than 10 percent band forms

| SIRS AND SEPSIS DEFINITION | |
|---|---|
| SIRS (Systemic Inflammatory Response Syndrome) | Two or more of the following criteria: <br> • Temperature > 38°C or <36°C <br> • Heart rate > 90 beats per minute <br> • Respiratory rate > 20 breaths per minute or $PaCO_2$ < 32 mm Hg <br> • WBCs > 12,000 cells per cubic millimeter or < 4,000 cells per cubic millimeter or > 10 percent immature (band) forms |
| Sepsis | Documented infection together with two or more SIRS criteria |
| Severe Sepsis | Sepsis associated with organ dysfunction, including, but not limited to, lactic acidosis, oliguria, hypoxemia, coagulation disorders, or an acute alteration in mental status |
| Septic Shock | Sepsis with hypotension, despite adequate fluid resuscitation, along with the presense of perfusion abnormalities. Patients who are on inotropic or vasopressor agents may not be hypotensive at the time when perfusion abnormalities are detected. |

Table 1. *Definition of SIRS and sepsis syndromes.*

Severe sepsis was defined as sepsis associated with evidence of organ dysfunction, hypoperfusion, or hypotension. Septic shock was defined as the persistence of organ dysfunction, hypoperfusion, or hypotension in spite of adequate fluid resuscitation. The diagnostic criteria for sepsis were revised in 2001 in an effort to incorporate new biomarkers of inflammation and offer an improved system for staging sepsis.[136] The PIRO staging system takes into account predisposition toward sepsis, the infectious insult likely to have caused the condition, the response of the body (SIRS), and evidence of organ dysfunction (Table 1). From a clinical standpoint, the initial consensus definitions offered in 1991 are most useful and worth committing to memory for every physician in the combat environment. The revised guidelines from 2001 are most useful for research protocol development, but the definitions of organ dysfunction can serve to remind the trauma critical care clinician of relevant physiologic variables to trend.

## Pathophysiology

Sepsis is characterized by four basic clinical defects: vasodilation, leaky endothelial membranes, disseminated intravascular coagulation, and cellular oxygen utilization inefficiency.[137] In a given patient, some of these defects may be more relevant than others. A distributive shock pattern with relative intravascular volume depletion is frequently seen, leading to organ hypoperfusion. Disseminated intravascular coagulation contributes significantly to ineffective end-organ oxygen delivery and can induce a systemic hypocoagulable state. The inefficient utilization of oxygen at the cellular level is a result of decoupling at the level of the mitochondrial electron transport chain as described in the previous section on endpoints of resuscitation. Mitigating the adverse impact of each of the aforementioned defects defines the goals of sepsis management.

## Prognosis

Severe sepsis and septic shock are associated with mortality rates of 30 to 60 percent.[133,134,138,139] In spite of improvements in critical care and the development of several broad-spectrum, highly active antibiotics, the mortality associated with sepsis has not improved greatly in the last several decades.[133,134] This is likely due to several factors, among them being a larger number of immunosuppressed patients, a higher proportion of elderly patients, and the emergence of several virulent pathogens with challenging patterns of antimicrobial drug resistance.

The expected mortality associated with infection is directly related to the development of severe sepsis or septic shock.[140] Multiple organ dysfunction syndrome as a result of inadequate oxygen delivery and ineffective oxygen utilization at the cellular level is a poor prognostic marker, and the mortality is related to the number of organ system failures present.[141] In the setting of sepsis some specific organ system dysfunctions are associated with higher odds of subsequent death, with hematologic and neurologic failure both being particularly concerning.[142]

## Management

Critical care is a process rather than the definition of a form of medicine that happens only in an ICU. Over the last two decades, the importance of an institutional approach to several complex care issues has been demonstrated. The management of sepsis involves the coordinated efforts of numerous healthcare providers and the synthesis of a large body of clinical data. It is vital that each institution adopt an aggressive, protocolized approach to the resuscitation of the septic patient.

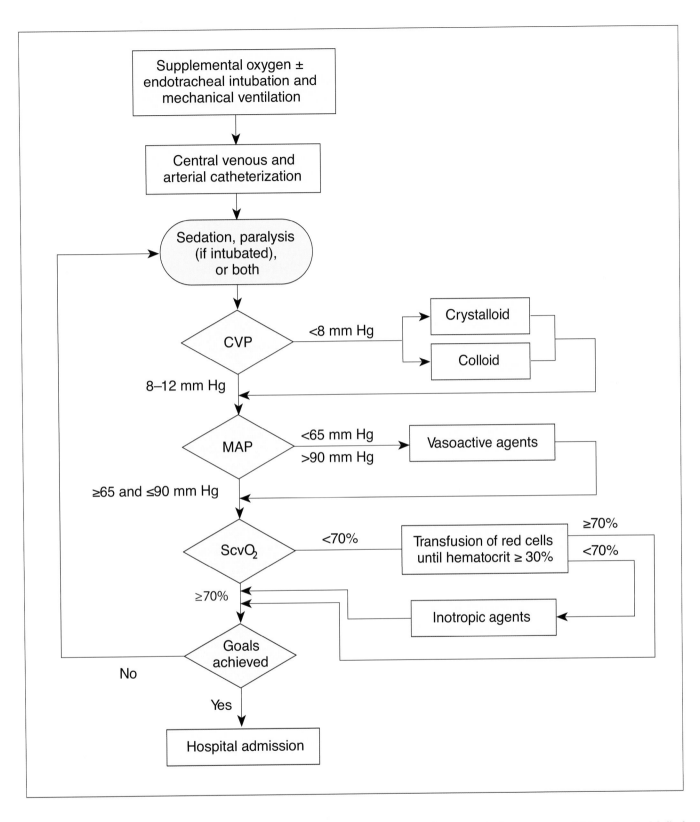

Figure 9. *Early goal-directed therapy protocol used by Rivers et al. in the management of severe sepsis. Image courtesy of Massachusetts Medical Society.*[118]

> The use of an early goal-directed therapy protocol for the management of severe sepsis has been shown to significantly improve mortality.

The use of an early goal-directed therapy protocol for the management of severe sepsis has been shown to significantly improve mortality (Fig. 9).[118] One of the most important aspects of this study was that resuscitations were initiated early in the emergency room setting and continued in the ICU.[118] Waiting for transfer to the ICU to begin aggressive resuscitation should never be considered an appropriate strategy. Several subsequent studies have described morbidity, mortality, and economic benefits associated with a protocolized, institutional approach to sepsis resuscitation.[143,144,145,146] Rivers et al. published an excellent review of one approach to implementation of an institutional commitment to sepsis resuscitation.[147]

## Infection Source Control

Perhaps the most important aspect of the management of the septic patient involves identification of the etiology of infection and ensuring adequate infection source control. While this seems intuitive, it is often forgotten as a fundamental priority during the initial activity surrounding other aspects of the resuscitation. Source identification and efforts to control the infection should be considered part of the initial resuscitation.[147,148,149] Timing of transport for radiologic studies or operative intervention will need to be individualized based on patient stability.

> The most important aspect of the management of the septic patient involves identification of the source of infection and achieving infection source control.

When drawing blood cultures, two or more cultures should be obtained.[150,151,152] Patients with indwelling catheters that have been in place for greater than 48 hours should have blood drawn through each lumen of each catheter.[148] The vascular device is more likely to be the source of the infection if cultures drawn through the line become positive more than two hours prior to cultures simultaneously drawn peripherally.[153,154] In the CCC setting, the use of empiric antibiotics is necessary while attempting to achieve successful source control. This involves the early identification of the etiology of infection as well as an understanding of the most likely associated microorganisms and any common antimicrobial resistance patterns. A recent series of articles regarding combat related infections and the experience in Operation Enduring Freedom (OEF) and Operation Iraqi Freedom (OIF) is helpful for physicians taking care of patients in these settings.[155,156]

## Resuscitation Goals

> The Surviving Sepsis Campaign 2008 guidelines recommend the following initial resuscitation goals:[148]
> 1. Central venous pressure (CVP) 8 to 12 mm Hg
>    8 mm Hg for unintubated patients
>    12 mm Hg for intubated patients
> 2. Mean arterial pressure (MAP) greater than or equal to 65 mm Hg
> 3. Urine output greater than 0.5 ml per kilogram per hour
> 4. Central venous oxygen saturation (ScvO$_2$) greater than or equal to 70 percent or mixed venous oxygen saturation (SvO$_2$) greater than or equal to 65 percent.

The resuscitation goals offered here are similar to those used in the early goal-directed therapy study by Rivers et al.[118] They do not offer a mechanism for evaluating regional oxygen delivery adequacy and should be supplemented at a given institution with intramucosal gastric pH, sublingual $PCO_2$, or oxygen saturation of hemoglobin in tissue assessment if available. In the typical CCC scenario, however, the resuscitation goals above are likely to be the best available.

## Intravascular Volume

Relative intravascular volume depletion is seen in sepsis as a result of vasodilation and endothelial leak. Hemorrhage in the trauma patient may also be a complicating factor. Maintaining an adequate intravascular volume is necessary to ensure adequate cardiac preload and therefore cardiac output. Decreased cardiac output will, by necessity, lead to a decrease in oxygen delivery which can be particularly important in sepsis where oxygen consumption may be supply-dependent.

Static measures are most often used in the ICU setting to estimate intravascular volume. The CVP is most often used at the bedside due to its ease of measurement, and there is no advantage to obtaining a pulmonary capillary wedge pressure over the CVP. Unfortunately, CVP is a very poor predictor of the intravascular volume status in the septic patient.[157] As an example, a CVP less than 5 mm Hg in sepsis has only a 47 percent positive predictive value for the presence of intravascular volume depletion.[158] Changes in intrathoracic pressure due to any cause may cause CVP to be an inaccurate representation of intravascular volume status. In the trauma ICU, mechanical ventilation and abdominal compartment syndrome are common complicating factors.[159,160]

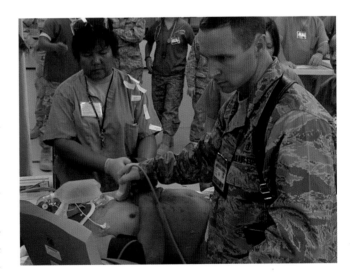

Dynamic measures such as pulse pressure variation are better predictors of intravascular volume status in sepsis than CVP.[161,162] As technology evolves, it is likely pulse pressure variation measurement capability will be available in the CCC setting. Transthoracic and transesophageal echocardiography have both been shown to be excellent markers of intravascular volume status as well.[163] Small portable ultrasound machines are commonly available at Level III facilities and may be useful when CVP and the clinical exam do not correlate (Fig. 10).

Figure 10. *Portable ultrasound machines, available at Level III facilities, may be used for hemodynamic assessment.*

Bedside ultrasonography available in Level III facilities has been shown to be an excellent marker of intravascular volume status.

The type of fluid used for resuscitation may depend on associated injuries, such as traumatic brain injury accompanied by intracranial pressure elevation, where hypertonic saline may be a preferred resuscitation fluid.[164,165] A recent large trial failed to show a benefit to the use of albumin or normal saline during the resuscitation of patients in the ICU.[166] However, the same outcomes were obtained using smaller resuscitation volumes in the colloid group. Two reviews of the topic also failed to show a significant outcome benefit using one or the other approach.[167]

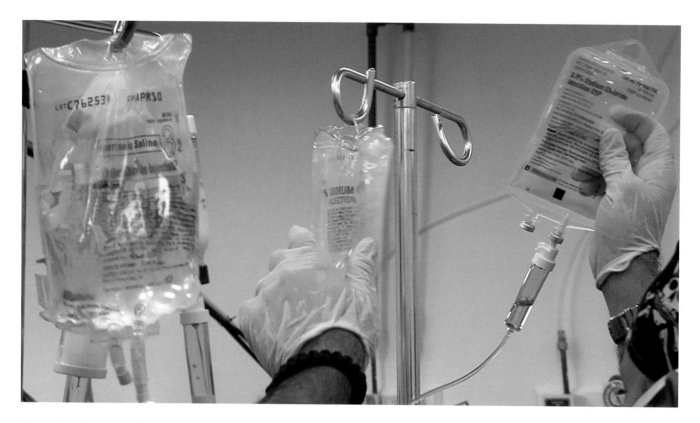

Figure 11. *Intravenous fluid administration should be performed aggressively during sepsis resuscitation.*

Fluid should be given in an aggressive manner early in sepsis resuscitation using boluses of greater than 1,000 ml crystalloid or greater than 300 to 500 ml colloid at a time until adequate cardiac filling pressures are obtained (Fig. 11).[148] After this point, intravascular volume supplementation should be eliminated until evidence of intravascular hypovolemia is once again demonstrated. Fluid balance is directly proportional to mortality. To some extent, this may reflect the severity of the underlying disease, but even when this is controlled for, there appears to be a benefit to minimizing intravascular volume overload after the initial resuscitation period.[168]

## Role of Vasopressors

The use of a vasopressor may be beneficial in the management of sepsis and should be thought of as a temporizing measure that is only used as long and as much as necessary.[148,169] A mean arterial pressure goal of 65 mm Hg is sufficient for most, but higher goals may be necessary as a way of preserving cerebral perfusion pressure in those with an elevated intracranial pressure. The human body tightly autoregulates blood flow to a given organ or tissue. This means that over a large range of blood pressure variation, the actual blood flow is controlled fairly precisely. In very low-pressure states, the blood pressure may fall below the pressure necessary for autoregulation, and the blood flow becomes linearly related to the pressure. In this setting, immediate improvement of the blood pressure will improve blood flow and oxygen delivery.[170,171] Patients with a history of essential hypertension may benefit from a higher mean arterial pressure due to a rightward shift in their normal autoregulatory range. Myocardial perfusion is a function of the difference between the diastolic blood pressure and the ventricular end-diastolic pressure. While the end-diastolic pressure is typically low early in the resuscitation of severe sepsis, it will normalize with resuscitation. Ensuring an adequate diastolic blood pressure can prevent myocardial ischemia or infarction.

The optimal vasopressor in sepsis depends upon the individual patient scenario.[169] The Surviving Sepsis Campaign 2008 guidelines suggest that either norepinephrine or dopamine be used as a first-line agent.[148] Patients who fail to respond should have epinephrine added to the vasopressor regimen. Vasopressin or phenylephrine can be considered for patients who are still hypotensive in spite of the above measures and who have been adequately volume resuscitated. Some studies have suggested that norepinephrine is a better first line choice of vasopressor in severe sepsis than dopamine. These studies evaluated the hemodynamic effects of norepinephrine versus dopamine in septic patients and demonstrated improved clinical outcomes and improved splanchnic circulation in patients treated with norepinephrine.[172,173,174] Recent studies analyzing the use of norepinephrine in septic shock have come to opposite conclusions, linking the use of norepinephrine to worse or equivalent outcomes relative to alternative vasoactive agents.[175] Epinephrine is an alternative vasopressor. It has been associated with elevation of lactic acid levels in the serum independent of oxygenation or blood flow. This is likely secondary to increased glycolysis and production of higher amounts of pyruvate with a normal L:P ratio of 10:1.[176]

Vasopressin levels are decreased in patients with severe sepsis and those who die from sepsis, when compared to those with mild sepsis and those who survive.[177] Two clinical studies have demonstrated a hemodynamic and vasopressor sparing benefit to the addition of a low-dose vasopressin infusion in patients with septic shock.[178,179] No mortality benefit was identified in either study. The recently completed Vasopressin and Septic Shock Trial (VASST) trial did not demonstrate a mortality benefit by adding vasopressin to a patient already being managed with norepinephrine.[180]

Dopamine is not recommended specifically for the prevention or management of acute renal failure in the septic patient. Several trials have failed to demonstrate benefit, while noting a decrease in splanchnic perfusion, associated with the use of dopamine (versus norepinephrine) in patients with severe sepsis.[181,182,183,184] Consensus opinion currently is that there is potential harm that may be expected when low-dose dopamine is used for renal failure prevention or management in the critically ill patient.[148,185]

> Vasopressors may be of benefit in the management of sepsis, but they should be viewed as a temporizing measure.

## Role of Corticosteroids

Corticosteroids should be added in total daily dose equivalents of hydrocortisone less than or equal to 300 milligrams (mg) intravenously daily in patients with hypotension associated with septic shock that is unresponsive to vasopressors or is of prolonged duration.[148,186] If a steroid is used with less mineralocorticoid activity than hydrocortisone, fludrocortisone can be added in a dose of 50 mcg per day. Three randomized controlled studies have shown clinical benefit to the use of corticosteroids in the setting of septic shock.[187,188,189] The first of these three studies was able to demonstrate a mortality reduction for patients who failed to increase their cortisol level more than 9 mcg per deciliter after an adrenocorticotropic hormone (ACTH) stimulation test.[187] The recently completed Corticosteroid Therapy of Septic Shock (CORTICUS) trial failed to show a mortality benefit to the use of corticosteroids in the setting of septic shock but did demonstrate faster resolution of shock in patients who were given steroids.[190] The response to an ACTH stimulation test did not predict those who responded to steroid therapy and those who did not. It is not clear from the study why improved resolution of the shock state with corticosteroids did not translate into a meaningful outcome advantage.

> The use of steroids in the management of refractory septic shock should be limited to patients who have failed at least two vasopressor agents.

The shock state associated with sepsis is frequently complicated by absolute or relative adrenal insufficiency. Unfortunately, the data supporting a benefit to the use of corticosteroids is minimal. Corticosteroids should be used in those with a previous condition requiring replacement and should be considered early in those who are likely to have secondary adrenal insufficiency due to chronic steroid therapy prior to the sepsis interval. The use of steroids strictly for the management of refractory septic shock should be limited to patients who have failed vasopressor therapy with at least two agents.

## Assessing Adequacy of Oxygen Delivery

An assessment of the adequacy of oxygen delivery with central venous oxygen saturation was part of the Rivers et al. early-goal directed therapy strategy for severe sepsis management and is recommended by the most recent Surviving Sepsis Campaign 2008 guidelines.[118,148] The goals are a central venous oxygen saturation greater than or equal to 70 percent or a mixed venous oxygen saturation greater than or equal to 65 percent depending on which is being followed in a given patient.

The topic of assessing adequacy of resuscitation was discussed in more detail previously, but a few concepts should be emphasized for the patient with severe sepsis. First, both central venous oxygen saturation and mixed venous oxygen saturation are markers of global oxygen delivery and may not be sensitive to regional inadequacy.[191] Where possible, technology to assess regional perfusion should be employed to supplement the data gained from the central venous oxygen saturation or mixed venous oxygen saturation. Just as a normal blood pressure does not mean that a patient is necessarily adequately resuscitated, neither does a normal central venous oxygen saturation.

A second important point regarding mixed venous oxygen saturation assessment is that a high value is commonly seen in very advanced septic shock. Because patients with septic shock frequently have decoupling of the mitochondrial electron transport chain, their oxygen consumption is supply dependent across most values of oxygen delivery, and the maximal oxygen extraction ratio may be profoundly decreased. A normal mixed venous oxygen value may be measured in spite of significant intracellular hypoxemia.[191] This perpetuates a shock state that may lead to death through the development of progressive multiple organ dysfunction.

The central venous oxygen saturation or mixed venous oxygen saturation is useful in identifying those with a need for further resuscitation when the values are low, but they are of little use when normal.[191] When low, the defective component of oxygen delivery must be identified, remembering that oxygen delivery is a function of cardiac output and oxygen content of the blood. If the central venous oxygen saturation or mixed venous oxygen saturation is low, efforts to ensure adequate hemoglobin oxygen saturation should be made first. Second, transfusion to a hemoglobin value of at least 10 g per deciliter should be considered.[148] Finally, if the mixed venous saturation remains low, an inotrope can be added with the intent of increasing cardiac output. The necessity of maintaining adequate intravascular volume during this process should be emphasized since an inadequate cardiac output can result from inadequate preload, direct myocardial suppression by cytokines in sepsis, or from myocardial infarction.

Central venous oxygen saturation or mixed venous oxygen saturation is useful in identifying patients needing further resuscitation when the values are low, but are of little use when normal.

## Blood Product Transfusion

The transfusion of blood products carries the potential for great benefit but also great harm to the patient and cost to society. In the CCC setting, it may be a very limited resource that must be used judiciously. Massive transfusion during a trauma resuscitation or transfusion goals associated with inadequately controlled hemorrhage are separate topics than the use of blood products strictly for the management of sepsis. Sepsis frequently develops during the course of care of the trauma patient rather than being present during the initial patient resuscitation. For the management of sepsis, component therapy is recommended rather than the use of whole blood.[148] Component therapy allows correction of identifiable defects (Fig. 12). Specific goals for the transfusion should be defined and effects of the therapy subsequently assessed.[192]

The most likely component to be considered for transfusion is packed red blood cells. The Transfusion Requirements in Critical Care (TRICC) trial demonstrated the adequacy of a conservative transfusion strategy in critically ill patients.[193] In spite of the linear relationship between oxygen uptake and oxygen delivery over a

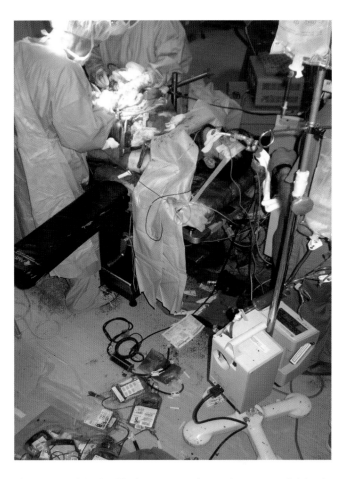

Figure 12. *Selective blood component therapy is recommended in the setting of sepsis complicated by coagulopathic bleeding.*

broad range of oxygen delivery, ineffective oxygen utilization precludes a significant oxygen uptake benefit from very aggressive red blood cell (RBC) transfusion in the setting of severe sepsis.[194] It is recommended that packed red blood cell therapy only be used when hemoglobin concentrations are less than 7 g per deciliter unless evidence of ongoing oxygen delivery inadequacy (e.g., low central venous oxygen saturation, myocardial ischemia, cerebral hypoperfusion) exists or active hemorrhage is present.[148] In that case, a hemoglobin goal of at least 10 g per deciliter is prudent, although overaggressive transfusion may be potentially harmful in the multisystem trauma patient, and these competing goals must be balanced carefully.[195] Once adequate oxygen delivery is felt to be present based upon available assessment tools, efforts to minimize red blood cell transfusion should be made.

It is recommended that packed red blood cell therapy only be used when the hemoglobin value is less than 7 g per deciliter, unless evidence of ongoing oxygen delivery inadequacy exists, or active hemorrhage is present.

Erythropoietin should not be used to improve hemoglobin or prevent future potential blood transfusions in the setting of sepsis. Two prospective clinical trials failed to demonstrate a significant benefit to the use of erythropoietin supplementation in critically ill patients.[196,197] Both of these studies show erythropoietin results in increased hemoglobin concentrations and decreased need for blood transfusion, but there is no data showing improved survival or clinical outcomes. Thus, it is not recommended in surviving sepsis guidelines.[148]

Correction of coagulopathy due to factor depletion or thrombocytopenia is not recommended strictly for the management of sepsis.[148,198] There may be settings where correction is desirable, as in the case of early trauma resuscitation, uncontrolled intracranial hemorrhage, or spinal surgery. Strict goals for resuscitation that are well-validated remain elusive and largely a matter of opinion. In the setting of sepsis, a platelet count of less than 5,000 per cubic millimeter should prompt transfusion, as should values of 5,000 per cubic millimeter to 30,000 per cubic millimeter when active bleeding is present.[148] Some procedures may require higher transfusion goals. There is no absolute international normalized ratio (INR) that should prompt transfusion of fresh frozen plasma in the absence of active bleeding or an anticipated procedure, but the risk of spontaneous intracranial hemorrhage correlates directly with anticoagulation intensity.[199,200]

Disseminated intravascular coagulation (DIC) results from an abnormal balance of procoagulant and anticoagulant factors in the blood that ultimately results in excessive accumulation of fibrin in the microvasculature. This contributes to organ dysfunction and may eventually lead to a generalized inability to form clot due to excessive consumption of coagulation factors. In the setting of active bleeding due to DIC, fresh frozen plasma may be considered in an attempt to improve the overall coagulopathy, platelet transfusion may be of benefit, and cryoprecipitate can be used to correct the fibrinogen deficiency. It is important to emphasize that all of these therapies are likely to be ineffective unless the source of the DIC is corrected. Specific goals for the supportive management of DIC will depend upon a bedside clinical assessment of any resulting hemorrhage.

## Role of Inotropic Therapy

The necessity of inotropic therapy may be suggested by the presence of a decreased central venous oxygen saturation in the setting of adequate intravascular volume repletion, hemoglobin oxygen saturation, and hemoglobin content.[170] If a pulmonary artery catheter is in place, a decreased cardiac output in the setting of normal or high cardiac filling pressures suggests a role for inotropic therapy. A pulmonary artery catheter is not necessary for the identification of the need for inotropic therapy or the utilization of an inotrope but may allow more accurate dose titration.

Dobutamine is the inotrope of choice in septic patients.[148,170,201] Dobutamine increases oxygen utilization, and care must therefore be exercised in states where cardiac oxygen delivery is marginal. When started, it is started at 5 micrograms (mcg) per kilogram per minute and titrated to a maximum dose of 20 mcg per kilogram per minute. If using a central venous catheter with the tip in the superior vena cava, the central venous oxygen saturation can be used to guide therapy. The dose is increased until the central venous oxygen saturation normalizes or the maximum dose is reached. Arrhythmias may complicate the ability to titrate dobutamine. If a pulmonary artery catheter is in place, the cardiac index can be trended, as can the mixed venous oxygen saturation.

A large part of the blood pressure improvement seen when dopamine is used as a vasopressor at moderate doses may be due to increased stroke volume; therefore, it can be considered an inotrope as well.[169] Norepinephrine has some inotropic properties, but its major mode of improving blood pressure is through peripheral vasoconstriction.[169]

## Role of Recombinant Human Activated Protein C (rhAPC)

The Recombinant Human Activated Protein C Worldwide Evaluation in Severe Sepsis (PROWESS) trial was the first to demonstrate a mortality benefit with the use of an agent (recombinant human activated protein C [rhAPC]) designed to prevent abnormal clotting in severe sepsis.[202] Subset analysis of the PROWESS trial found the greatest benefit in patients with more severe manifestations of sepsis. The process by which the PROWESS study was conducted and its conclusions (i.e., based on subgroup analysis) have generated controversy.[203] The limitations of rhAPC were delineated by the Administration of Drotrecogin Alfa (activated) in Early Stage Severe Sepsis (ADDRESS) trial, which was designed to evaluate the use of rhAPC in patients with severe sepsis but a low risk of death.[204] It was stopped early due to futility, and a subset analysis of patients with recent surgery and only a single-organ dysfunction had a significantly higher 28-day mortality if they received rhAPC. The study concluded that rhAPC (drotrecogin alfa or Xigris®) "should not be used in patients with severe sepsis who are at low risk for death, such as those with single-organ failure or an APACHE II score less than 25."

Recombinant human activated protein C has been recommended by some for patients with severe sepsis and either multiple organ failures or an APACHE II score greater than 25.[148] Use of rhAPC, specifically in the combat trauma population, needs to be tempered by a higher risk of bleeding noted in national surveys relative to that reported in the initial PROWESS trial.[205,206] Risks and benefits must be carefully assessed, and adequate hemostasis must be ensured. When used, it is best to initiate therapy with rhAPC as soon as the need is identified, since outcomes appear to be best when the therapy is introduced early.[207,208,209] The cost-effectiveness of administering rhAPC in all severe sepsis patients has been questioned, and calls for more selective use in this subset of high-risk patients have been made.[203]

## Management of Hyperglycemia

The publication in 2001 of a significant mortality benefit in critical care patients treated with an intensive insulin therapy protocol with resultant glucose values of 80 to 120 mg per deciliter was met with great enthusiasm.[210] Because this initial experience was primarily with surgical ICU patients, a subsequent study by the same author was conducted in the medical ICU population.[211] The medical ICU study was able to demonstrate a mortality benefit only in those patients with a length of stay greater than three days, which cannot be predicted when patients are admitted. It is important to note as well that the rate of significant hypoglycemia was 18 percent, relative to the 6.2 percent seen in the 2001 surgical ICU study. Both of these studies were performed at a single institution. While tight glucose control was adopted quickly by several major clinical organizations, the results of other studies have failed to demonstrate similar outcomes, and in fact, not only show no benefit, but provide evidence of harm.[212,213]

The recently completed Normoglycemia in Intensive Care Evaluation – Survival Using Glucose Algorithm Regulation (NICE-SUGAR) study randomized 6,104 critical care patients into intensive glucose control (81 to 108 mg per deciliter) versus conventional glucose control (180 mg per deciliter or less) groups and followed a number of variables over 90 days from enrollment.[214] The results are striking in their demonstration of a 2.6 percent mortality increase at 90 days in those treated with an intensive approach, although there was no significant difference in mortality at 28 days. Subgroup analysis in the NICE-SUGAR study noted a trend toward improved outcomes with conventional control in patients with severe sepsis, as well as those with an APACHE II score greater than 25 on admission.

> Moderate glucose control (less than 150 mg per deciliter) should be achieved using insulin infusion protocols in patients with sepsis.

Of particular relevance to the trauma critical care population was a trend toward improved outcomes in trauma patients with intensive insulin control. Excitement over this result should be tempered by the wide confidence intervals (0.50 to 1.18) and the fact that there was a statistically significant improvement in operative admission patients who were treated with conventional control. Hyperglycemia has been associated with worsened outcomes following traumatic brain injury and sepsis. At this time, it is recommended that moderate glucose control (less than 150 mg per deciliter) be achieved using insulin infusion protocols in patients with sepsis.[148] Future studies are needed to help clarify what degree of glucose control is most beneficial for the critically ill patient.

## Role of Bicarbonate Therapy

Bicarbonate therapy has been used in clinical practice for years in an attempt to mitigate the effects of acidemia caused by numerous metabolic and respiratory challenges. In the setting of sepsis-induced lactic acidosis, there does not appear to be any benefit to the routine use of bicarbonate therapy.[215,216]

It is hypothesized that conformational changes at the level of the sympathetic receptor occur at very low pH values that may lead to unresponsiveness to vasopressor therapy. There is no firm clinical data supporting an absolute pH where such an effect may occur. In the aforementioned studies, the number of patients enrolled with pH less than 7.15 was small.[215,216] The use of bicarbonate is associated with volume overload that may complicate other goals of sepsis therapy, particularly after the initial resuscitation phase. It is recommended in the Surviving Sepsis Campaign 2008 guidelines that bicarbonate not be used for the sole purpose of raising pH greater than 7.15 in an effort to improve hemodynamics.[148]

> In the setting of sepsis-induced lactic acidosis, there does not appear to be any benefit to the routine use of bicarbonate therapy.

For patients with profound acidemia, raising the pH may be an immediate lifesaving maneuver.[217] Manipulation of mechanical ventilation may allow a sufficient respiratory alkalosis to improve the overall pH adequately, or bicarbonate therapy may be utilized. In a theoretical sense, bicarbonate combines with hydrogen ions and eventually creates water and carbon dioxide via the action of carbonic anhydrase. Carbon dioxide readily crosses cell membranes and may therefore contribute to intracellular pH reduction in spite of improved pH in the blood. This might be more significant when sepsis is associated with ARDS or other conditions where ventilation is limited and carbon dioxide elimination is suboptimal. The potential for poor outcomes due to intracellular pH decrease associated with bicarbonate therapy has not been demonstrated conclusively in a prospective clinical fashion.

Other options for raising the pH include the use of tromethamine, which is a proton scavenger that is eliminated renally.[218] The tromethamine solution is hypertonic and has a pH of 8.6. The hypertonic nature of the solution can induce a mild osmotic diuresis and will result in improved urine output, but it should not be used as an agent to prevent or treat acute renal failure. For those with established renal failure, tromethamine is not appropriate given the necessity of renal clearance. Bicarbonate therapy is associated with a significant sodium load and increased generation of carbon dioxide; therefore, tromethamine may be preferred in patients with hypernatremia or a limited minute ventilation.[218] There is no evidence that outcomes are better with tromethamine versus bicarbonate therapy versus no therapy at all in the setting of lactic acidosis associated with severe sepsis.

Unfortunately, there is no clear guidance than can be offered for pH values less than 7.15. Until better data emerges, the decision to correct the pH and the best way to accomplish this goal are both up to the bedside clinician.

## Nutritional Goals

The literature regarding optimal nutrition for the septic patient continues to evolve, but few firm recommendations can be made at this time. It appears that septic patients have a higher basal energy expenditure than nonstressed patients.[219,220] Glutamine and arginine supplementation may be of benefit.[221,222] The method by which critical care patients are fed has generally received as much attention as what is fed (Fig. 13). Enteral nutrition is preferred over total parenteral nutrition when possible.[223,224] Enteral feeding is cheaper, preserves the integrity of the gut mucosa (possibly decreasing the incidence of multiple organ dysfunction syndrome), and has a lower rate of secondary infection. The exact timing of feed initiation is unclear. It seems intuitive that earlier achievement of adequate caloric intake would be beneficial. This has been demonstrated in the hypercatabolic adult burn patient population.[225] However, in the sepsis population undergoing initial resuscitation, it is unclear whether the body is able to use the nutrients provided to it. Decreased gut perfusion may also make the use of enteral nutrition risky, and total parenteral nutrition may be favored earlier if feeds are started during the periresuscitation period.

It is probably best to achieve adequate caloric intake as early as possible after the initial resuscitation period with enteral nutrition being favored over total parenteral nutrition unless there are significant contraindications (severe ileus, recent gastrointestinal surgery, etc.). The choice of feeds remains an unsettled matter with many favoring antioxidant formulas, although there is little outcome data at this point to argue for or against such recommendations.

> Enteral nutrition is preferred over total parenteral nutrition when possible and should be started as early as possible after the initial resuscitation period.

## Summary

The sepsis syndrome is characterized by vasodilation, leaky endothelial membranes, DIC, and ineffective oxygen utilization at the cellular level. It is associated with a high mortality. Early syndrome recognition, infection source control, and a protocolized approach to resuscitation are key factors for ensuring patient survival. Components of supportive therapy include maintenance of adequate intravascular volume, vasopressor support, inotropic support, moderate glucose control, rhAPC in select patients with severe sepsis, and the rational use of blood products. There may be a role for the use of corticosteroids in some patients, and the optimal nutrition strategy continues to emerge.

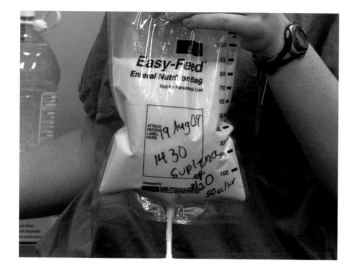

Figure 13. *Enteral nutrition is preferred over total parenteral nutrition.*

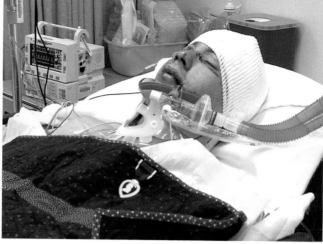

Figure 14. *Ventilator-associated pneumonia is defined as a pneumonia that arises after 48 to 72 hours of endotracheal intubation.*

# Basic Care Considerations in the Combat Casualty Care ICU

## *Combat-Associated Pneumonia Prevention*

Ventilator-associated pneumonia (VAP) is a frequent complication of prolonged mechanical ventilation that leads to increased duration of mechanical ventilation, prolongation of ICU care, and, most importantly, an increase in mortality.[226] Ventilator-associated pneumonia is defined as a pneumonia that arises after 48 to 72 hours of endotracheal intubation (Fig. 14).[227] Multidrug-resistant bacteria of nosocomial origin are more likely to be associated with ventilator-associated pneumonia after the first four to five days of hospitalization as the patient becomes colonized with organisms that live in an environment characterized by extraordinary antibiotic selection pressure. Organisms such as methicillin-resistant *Staphylococcus aureus* (MRSA) and multidrug-resistant gram-negative organisms such as *Pseudomonas aeruginosa* and *Acinetobacter baumanii* are commonly encountered.[227]

> Ventilator-associated pneumonia is a frequent complication of prolonged mechanical ventilation that leads to increased duration of mechanical ventilation, prolongation of ICU care, and increased mortality.

The flow of combat casualties out-of-theater in OEF and OIF for the vast majority of critically ill patients involves a handful of medical centers (Fig. 15). This is done to consolidate medical resources in a few locations and because patient flow via the air evacuation system uses aircraft of opportunity that are flying regularly established mission routes. Multidrug-resistant organisms are extremely common in these node locations, and patients who become colonized tend to carry such organisms to each successive node.[228] Of particular concern has been the emergence of extremely virulent multidrug-resistant acinetobacter and pseudomonas strains that have been associated with ventilator-associated pneumonia. The concept of "combat-associated pneumonia" as a variant of ventilator-associated pneumonia has emerged to accentuate the importance of these extremely difficult to treat, multidrug-resistant organisms as a cause of nosocomial pneumonia.[229] Combat-associated pneumonia also highlights the role that the nodal structure of patient flow plays in the emergence of multidrug-resistant organisms at each successive military treatment facility.[228]

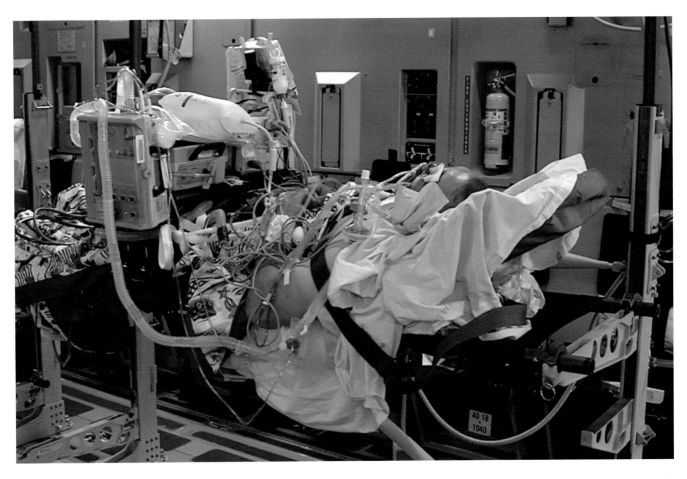

Figure 15. *Multidrug-resistant organisms are common in the evacuation chain, and patients who become colonized tend to carry such organisms to each successive facility.*

### COMBAT-ASSOCIATED PNEUMONIA PREVENTION BUNDLE

1. Keep head of bed elevated greater than 30 to 45 degrees at all times, unless contraindicated
2. Daily sedation interruption
3. Gastrointestinal bleeding prophylaxis
4. Deep venous thrombosis (DVT) prophylaxis
5. Heat and moisture exchanger (HME) use unless otherwise specified; no daily changes of HMEs
6. Oral care every two hours, with chlorhexidine every 12 hours
7. Consider vaccination with PNEUMOVAX® and influenza vaccine
8. Continuous subglottic suctioning endotracheal tube if duration of intubation expected to be greater than or equal to four days
9. No routine ventilator circuit changes

Table 2. *Combat-associated pneumonia prevention interventions.*

Prevention of combat-associated pneumonia in ventilated patients is vital since treatment is extremely difficult. The development of ventilator-associated pneumonia prevention bundles is now common practice in critical care units. A suggested combat-associated pneumonia bundle is depicted in Table 2. Posting these recommendations at bedside can serve as a helpful reminder for clinicians, nurses, and respiratory therapists. Such recommendations should also be included in standard ICU admission order sets. Critical care air transport teams can continue all of these recommendations during flight and should be encouraged to do so prior to each movement of an intubated patient.

In combat critical care units, consideration should be given to relatively liberal use of an invasive diagnostic strategy to confirm suspected cases of combat-associated pneumonia. Options include flexible fiberoptic bronchoscopy (with or without protected specimen brush) and blind bronchoalveolar lavage (BAL) using specially designed catheters. This will decrease the use of broad-spectrum antibiotics and hopefully decrease some of the selection pressure that exists in downrange ICUs.

## Deep Venous Thrombosis Prophylaxis

Multisystem trauma patients have numerous risk factors for the development of venous thromboembolic disease. In the combat environment, there is a higher likelihood of intravascular dehydration prior to injury that may contribute to an increased risk over that seen in the civilian trauma population in the US.[230] A more important distinction between the two populations is the periods of prolonged immobilization that will necessarily accompany air evacuation out of the combat theater.

Representatives from the American College of Chest Physicians recently reviewed the literature regarding a number of common patient populations encountered in the combat environment such as those with head and spine injuries, orthopedic injuries, and multisystem trauma.[231] Several insightful recommendations for each population are made and levels of evidence are reviewed.

> When possible, trauma patients should receive either graded compression stockings or intermittent pneumatic compression devices, given the higher than normal risk for venous thromboembolism in the combat environment.

Given the higher than normal risk for venous thromboembolism in the combat environment, it is recommended that each patient receive either graded compression stockings or intermittent pneumatic compression devices unless injury severity does not allow the placement of such devices on any extremity (Fig. 16). In addition, low-molecular-weight heparin dosed as 30 mg injected subcutaneously twice daily should be used unless contraindicated by active uncontrolled hemorrhage or recent intracranial bleeding.[231,232] An aggressive approach to venous thromboembolism prophylaxis in the combat trauma environment is wise since treatment with full-dose anticoagulation for DVT or pulmonary embolism (PE) may be problematic in patients with ongoing hemostasis inadequacy or who may need repeated trips to the operating room.

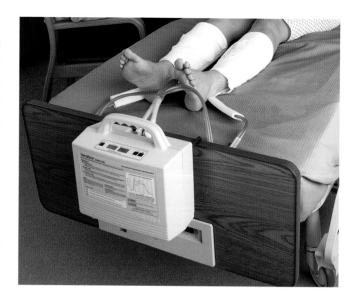

Figure 16. *Intermittent pneumatic compression devices are used for venous thromboembolism prophylaxis. Image courtesy of DJO, LLC.*

## Gastrointestinal Bleeding Prophylaxis

Stress gastritis is a common complication in critical care patients.[233] Significant risk factors for gastrointestinal bleeding due to stress gastritis include mechanical ventilation greater than 48 hours, coagulopathies, shock, sepsis, hepatic failure, renal failure, multiple trauma, greater than 35 percent total body surface area burn, head/spinal cord trauma, and a prior history of upper gastrointestinal hemorrhage.[234]

> All patients admitted to a combat ICU should be treated with an intravenous proton-pump inhibitor or $H_2$-receptor antagonist due to risk of stress gastritis.

All patients admitted to a combat ICU should be treated with an intravenous proton-pump inhibitor or $H_2$-receptor antagonist. This is generally continued even when the patient is tolerating enteral feeds, although some experts would consider discontinuation of prophylaxis at that point.[233]

## Preventive Care and Infection Control

Exposure keratopathy is common in the critical care setting when the eye is left exposed to dry air in patients who are not capable of spontaneously blinking (e.g., chemical sedation or central nervous system injury).[235] Efforts to protect the eyes with the regular application of lubrication is a basic necessity of care that can be overlooked during combat critical care with devastating consequences. Exposure keratopathy may lead to the development of infections that are extremely difficult to eradicate and frequently result in permanent loss of vision.[235]

Aggressive skin care is extremely important in the multisystem trauma patient due to the prolonged periods of immobility that often accompany convalescence.[236] Decubitus ulcers can develop quickly in dependent regions where weight is focused on a single point and allowed to compress the soft-tissue underneath. Common ulcer locations include the sacral region, heels, and portions of the body that are left pressed up against solid objects such as a bedrail. What appear at first to be small areas of redness can evolve over hours to days into large, poorly healing regions of necrotic soft-tissue that may require extensive debridement and occasional skin grafting.[237] There is also a risk for the development of osteomyelitis in exposed bone. Prevention involves frequent turning in an effort to continually redistribute pressure points as well as the use of foam blocks under the feet and legs.

> Aggressive skin care is extremely important in the multisystem trauma patient in order to prevent decubitus ulcers. Efforts to protect the eyes with regular application of lubrication are necessary to prevent exposure keratopathy.

Intensive care unit infection control measures are extremely important in the current mature theaters of combat in Afghanistan and Iraq. The spread of multidrug-resistant pathogens needs to be limited as much as possible in an effort to improve outcomes. The epidemiology, history, prevention, and treatment of combat-related infections were outlined in a recent series of articles.[155,228,238,239,240] Basic recommendations for preventing the spread of nosocomial multidrug-resistant pathogens include universal standard precautions, contact precautions with all direct patient care, consideration of cohorting patients who are likely to be in the ICU less than 72 hours, and antibiotic control. Antibiotic control recommendations include avoiding unnecessary use of broad-spectrum empiric antibiotics, establishment of a local antibiogram that can be used to guide initial therapy, and limiting antibiotic therapy duration as much as possible.[156]

## Structure of the Combat Casualty Care ICU

Critical care is a process that begins at the point of injury and continues until resolution of the physiologic insult. Care that is provided in the ICU is one piece of a larger systemic effort to provide care. The ICU is a complicated environment charged with the coordination of the efforts of many as a wealth of data is prioritized and acted upon. Traditionally, physicians have practiced in a relatively independent manner, and several different approaches to a given disease process may be expected at a given institution. Numerous studies in the last two decades have demonstrated that protocolized approaches to complex disease processes can result in better patient outcomes.[120,241,242,243] In many instances, the improved outcomes are as likely to be due to the development of an institutional approach to a given problem rather than the intervention per se. An institutional approach allows multiple services to prepare for involvement in a predictable fashion and improve efficiency. Additionally, a protocol allows more frequent adjustment of therapies in response to real-time data collection than is possible when decisions are deferred to once or twice daily physician rounds.

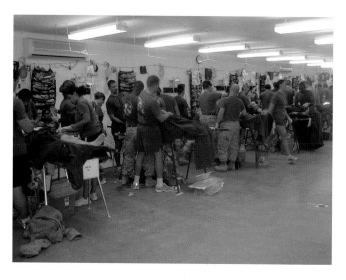

Figure 17. *The ability to adapt available resources to the needs of many will dictate the success or failure of a combat ICU. Image courtesy of Harold Bohman, MD, CAPT, MC, US Navy.*

The importance of multidisciplinary rounds cannot be overemphasized. While it has been demonstrated during the current OEF and OIF conflicts that an intensivist-directed ICU team improves outcomes in the combat theater, every member of the critical care team has a role to play and an expertise to bring to the bedside.[244] Simply adding a clinical pharmacist to daily rounds in the ICU improves mortality.[245] Multidisciplinary rounds offer both a chance to share ideas and impressions about a patient's care as well as a method of communicating a plan simultaneously to all of the care team members.

Telemedicine is in its infancy as a specialty but will be seen with increasing frequency in the combat environment in the next decade. The technology behind telemedicine is evolving rapidly and allows a limited resource to be in many places at once. It is a medicine force-multiplier that has the potential to help minimize the forward-positioned medical logistical footprint.

A final key concept regarding the structure of the combat casualty care ICU is the need for flexibility. The combat care environment is fluid and frequently unpredictable. Large numbers of patients may appear suddenly at anytime (Fig. 17). The ability to adapt the available, sometimes limited, resources to the needs of many will in large part dictate the success or failure of a combat ICU.[246] Deviations from optimum care are to be expected, but a firm understanding of the relevant medical concepts will help prioritize efforts and maximize the chances for a successful patient outcome.

# Critical Care Air Transport Team (CCATT)

## *Historical Background and System Basics*

All coalition patients with critical care requirements in the current conflicts in Afghanistan (OEF) and Iraq (OIF) are flown out-of-theater to Germany with the assistance of a Critical Care Air Transport Team (CCATT) (Fig. 18). A CCATT is composed of a physician with some critical care training, a critical care nurse, and a respiratory therapist. They are prepositioned in the area of operation to facilitate transport to Landstuhl Regional Medical Center (LRMC) in Germany, and more teams are prepositioned in Germany for transport back to the continental US.[247,248] Each team has a specified equipment allowance standard that is designed to support between three and six patients, with the number on a given mission being determined in part by the severity of illness. A CCATT represents an additional critical care capability that augments the capabilities of an air evacuation team. Air evacuation teams are composed of two to three nurses and four to seven technicians that provide care to non-critically injured patients and act as the liason between the CCATT and the aircraft crew members.[248,249]

> All coalition patients with critical care requirements in the current conflicts in Afghanistan (OEF) and Iraq (OIF) are flown out-of-theater to Germany with the assistance of a CCATT. Critical Care Air Transport Teams facilitate the rapid evacuation of severely ill patients, which translates both into better patient care as well as a significantly decreased forward medical footprint.

The birth of the CCATT asset can be traced back to 1988, when the program was first proposed by then Col PK Carlton, USAF, MC. Subsequent experiences in the Gulf War and Somalia highlighted a need for a coordinated approach to augmenting the in-flight critical care capability of standard air evacuation teams. A pilot program was formed in 1994 and the program was later formally adopted in 1996. The role of CCATT in patient movement has matured in the OEF and OIF areas of operation since 2001 and 2003, respectively.[250] Critical Care Air Transport Teams facilitate the rapid evacuation of severely ill patients, which translates both into better patient care as well as a significantly decreased forward medical footprint. The evolution of this unique capability has been one of the great success stories of military medicine during the current conflicts.

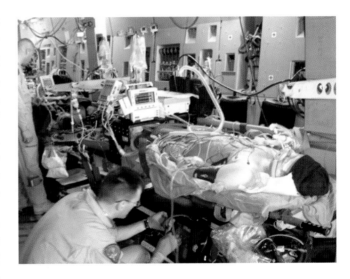

Figure 18. *A CCATT transports critically injured soldiers out-of-theater.*

The overall approach to care of the severely injured trauma patient has evolved in parallel with the CCATT system. The concept of damage control resuscitation emphasizes a first surgery to control immediately life-threatening hemorrhage while delaying more definitive surgical therapy until after a period of resuscitation that may take several hours to days.[251] In practice in OEF and OIF, patients will often have a first damage control surgery at a forward surgical location and are transported to a larger military trauma center in-theater by helicopter that is colocated with a CCATT. A second washout surgery may be performed at the trauma center and then the patient is flown with a CCATT to Germany.[252] During the five to nine hours in the air, the CCATT is able to continue an aggressive resuscitation and deliver a patient to Landstuhl that is better prepared for more definitive surgical therapy. The success of damage control resuscitation in civilian trauma settings and in other military conflicts has lent itself well to the CCATT concept, and the presence of this new capability allows damage control to be pursued without delaying patient transport.

The US Air Force used to have a fleet of dedicated air evacuation aircraft, the majority of which were C-9 aircraft based on the DC-9 airliner airframe (Fig. 19). A set fleet of aircraft was found to be expensive and inflexible since all of the aircraft had identical capabilities in terms of range and logistics footprint and were located in only a few locations worldwide. Today, the air evacuation system uses "aircraft of opportunity." Air evacuation and CCATT teams are designed to be modular and have been trained to use the unique capabilities of numerous aircraft to allow patient transport. Today, the majority of CCATT missions are flown on C-17 and C-130 aircraft. Refueling aircraft such as the KC-135 and KC-10 have been used, as has the largest aircraft in the US inventory, the C-5. CCATT missions in-theater are occasionally flown on HH-60 Black Hawk helicopters, and some missions in the continental US and Europe are conducted with the C-21, which is the military version of a standard Learjet.

When the critical care team downrange identifies the need for CCATT transport, an air evacuation liason officer is contacted. The air evacuation liaison officer notifies a local flight surgeon who can evaluate the patient and identify any special needs the patient may have in flight. The request is then forwarded to a Joint Patient Movement Requirement Center (JPMRC) in-theater. The request is cleared, and an effort is coordinated with the Tanker Airlift Control Center (TACC) to find an aircraft in the theater that can be made available for patient movement. The patient, an air evacuation team, and a CCATT are then assigned

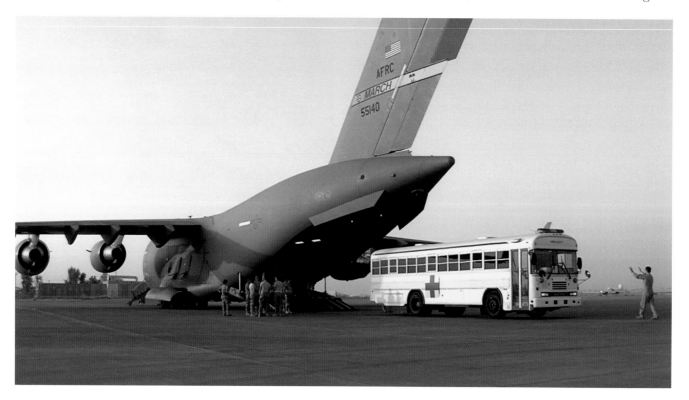

Figure 19. *C-17 aircraft is commonly used for CCATT missions.*

to that aircraft and preparations are made in the critical care unit for flight. While the system seems at first glance to be complex, it has become relatively efficient and results in much faster patient evacuation than in any prior conflict as well as a significantly decreased need for forward medical resources.[253]

## Challenges Associated with Critical Care in the Air

Critical care in the back of an aircraft can be challenging and represents a significant physiologic stressor for the patient. Older aircraft may have poor temperature control and are typically very cold in flight. While flying in-theater below a certain threshold altitude, aircraft are kept dark inside to minimize the chances of being shot down. Vibration and noise are common factors that make patient monitoring more difficult than on the ground. Aircraft cabins are typically pressurized to 6,000 to 8,000 feet leading to lower oxygen content in the air as well as a tendency for any gas contained within an enclosed space to expand. This can complicate the care of patients with closed eye injuries associated with air pockets in the vitreous or patients with unrecognized pneumothoraces. Finally, acceleration changes associated with steep combat takeoffs and landings may contribute to the development of increased intracranial pressures in patients with traumatic brain injury.[254,255]

> Physiologic stressors associated with cabin temperature, vibration and noise, air pressure, and steep combat takeoffs and landings may compound patient morbidity.

Perhaps the biggest challenge facing the CCATT when caring for a patient is the reality that there are limited options for assistance. The medical equipment that accompanies a CCATT is designed to support numerous interventions such as endotracheal intubation, central venous catheter insertion, arterial line placement, emergent tracheostomy, and chest tube thoracostomy. However, there are occasions when it is necessary to divert an aircraft to allow urgent transport of a patient to a ground based medical facility. Luckily, this has been a rare occurrence. A specialized Acute Lung Rescue Team (ALRT) is positioned at Landstuhl Regional Medical Center to assist in the evacuation of OEF/OIF patients with profound respiratory failure that may exceed basic CCATT capabilities.[76]

The relatively austere, resource-limited environment that a CCATT practices within demands that every effort be made prior to the flight to anticipate complications that may arise. With experience during a deployed rotation, the sending ICU teams and CCATTs become very adept at anticipating the needs of a patient. Those with marginal oxygenation on the ground should be intubated prior to flight.[256] Developing extremity compartment syndromes should be addressed with fasciotomies, and abdominal compartment syndromes should lead to laparotomy and the placement of an adjustable temporary abdominal closure.[250,257] Patients with suspected intracranial pressure elevations should be considered for early placement of intracranial pressure monitoring capability.[255] Blood products that may be needed for resuscitation and medications such as antibiotics and vasopressors should be identified prior to the mission.

> The biggest challenge facing the CCATT when caring for a patient is that there are limited options for assistance, and every effort must be made prior to the flight to anticipate complications that may arise.

The use of the air evacuation system with CCATT augmentation has resulted in excellent patient outcomes, increased speed of evacuation, and a decreased downrange medical footprint. Even in its relative infancy, the CCATT capability is demonstrating a new way to allocate medical resources in the combat care environment. The successful evolution of the system has created a new paradigm for how major industrialized countries involved in protracted wartime operations will address the care of their wounded warriors.

## Summary

Aggressive, attentive, evidence-based critical care is a key component of recovery for the multisystem trauma patient. The ability to adapt the lessons of the medical literature to the challenges of the combat environment often determines the difference between a successful or poor patient outcome. Those who have the privilege of caring for our nation's heroes will always look back on the experience as one of the defining moments of their lives. Even in the most austere settings, there is no limit to the good that can be done.

# References

1. Colice GL. Historical perspective on the development of mechanical ventilation. In: Tobin MJ, editor. Principles and practice of mechanical ventilation. 2nd ed. New York: McGraw-Hill, 2006. p. 1-36.

2. West JB. Ventilation. In: West JB. Pulmonary pathophysiology: The essentials. 7th ed. Baltimore: Lippincott Williams & Wilkins, 2008. p. 3-16.

3. Salzman SH. Cardiopulmonary exercise testing. In: ACCP pulmonary board review 2008: course syllabus. Northbrook: American College of Chest Physicians, 2008.

4. West JB. Gas exchange. In: West JB, editor. Pulmonary pathophysiology: the essentials. 7th ed. Baltimore: Lippincott Williams & Wilkins, 2008. p. 17-36.

5. Dreyfuss D, Soler P, Basset G, et al. High inflation pressure pulmonary edema. Respective effects of high airway pressure, high tidal volume, and positive end-expiratory pressure. Am Rev Respir Dis 1988;137(5):1159-1164.

6. Santos CC, Zhang H, Liu M, et al. Bench-to-bedside review: Biotrauma and modulation of the innate immune response. Crit Care 2005;9(3):280-286.

7. Dreyfuss D, Saumon G. Ventilator-induced lung injury: lessons from experimental studies. Am J Respir Crit Care Med 1998;157(1):294-323.

8. Halbertsma FJ, Vaneker M, Scheffer GJ, et al. Cytokines and biotrauma in ventilator-induced lung injury: a critical review of the literature. Neth J Med 2005;63(10):382-392.

9. Carvalho CR, de Paula Pinto Schettino G, Maranhao B, et al. Hyperoxia and lung disease. Curr Opin Pulm Med 1998;4(5):300-304.

10. Girard TD, Bernard GR. Mechanical ventilation in ARDS: a state-of-the-art review. Chest 2007;131(3):921-929.

11. Brochard L, Rauss A, Benito S, et al. Comparison of three methods of gradual withdrawal from ventilatory support during weaning from mechanical ventilation. Am J Respir Crit Care Med 1994;150(4):896-903.

12. Esteban A, Frutos F, Tobin MJ, et al. A comparison of four methods of weaning patients from mechanical ventilation. Spanish Lung Failure Collaborative Group. N Engl J Med 1995;332(6):345-350.

13. Marini JJ, Smith TC, Lamb VJ. External work output and force generation during synchronized intermittent mandatory ventilation – effect of machine assistance on breathing effort. Am Rev Respir Dis 1988;138(5):1169-1179.

14. Butler R, Keenan SP, Inman KJ, et al. Is there a preferred technique for weaning the difficult-to-wean patient? A systematic review of the literature. Crit Care Med 1999;27(11):2331-2336.

15. Chan KP, Stewart TE, Mehta S. High-frequency oscillatory ventilation for adult patients with ARDS. Chest 2007;131(6):1907-1916.

16. Schmidt GA, Hall JB. Management of the ventilated patient. In: Hall JB, Schmidt GA, Wood LDH, editors. Principles of critical care. 3rd ed. New York: McGraw-Hill, 2005. p. 517-536.

17. Sessler CN, Krieger BP. Mechanical ventilatory support. In: ACCP Pulmonary board review course syllabus 2008. Northbrook: American College of Chest Physicians, 2008.

18. Wilson WC, Minokadeh A, Ford R, et al. Mechanical ventilation. In: Wilson WC, Grande CM, Hoyt DB, editors. Trauma critical care, volume 2. New York: Informa Healthcare USA, Inc., 2007. p. 505-524.

19. Holets S, Hubmayr RD. Conventional methods of ventilatory support. In: Tobin MJ, editor. Principles and practice of mechanical ventilation. 2nd ed. New York: McGraw-Hill, 2006. p. 163-326.

20. Stocchetti N, Maas AI, Chieregato A, et al. Hyperventilation in head injury: a review. Chest 2005;127(5):1812-1827.

21. Marik PE, Varon J, Trask T. Management of head trauma. Chest 2002;122(2):699-711.

22. Gajic O, Dara SI, Mendez JL, et al. Ventilator-associated lung injury in patients without acute lung injury at the onset of mechanical ventilation. Crit Care Med 2004;32(9):1817-1824.

23. MacIntyre NR. Is there a best way to set tidal volume for mechanical ventilatory support? Clin Chest Med 2008;29(2):225-231.

24. Cohn SM. Pulmonary contusion: review of the clinical entity. J Trauma 1997;42(5):973-979.

25. Hwang JCF, Amador ER, Hanowell LH. Critical care considerations following chest trauma. In: Wilson WC, Grande CM, Hoyt DB, et al., editors. Trauma critical care, volume 2. New York: Informa Healthcare USA, Inc., 2007. p. 465-484.

26. Dries DJ. Trauma and thermal injury. In: American College of Chest Physicians, ed. ACCP Critical care board review course syllabus 2008. Northbrook: ACCP, 2008.

27. DePalma RG, Burris DG, Champion HR, et al. Blast injuries. N Engl J Med 2005;352(13):1335-1342.

28. Harrison, CD, Bebarta VS, Grant GA. Tympanic membrane perforation after combat blast exposure in Iraq: a poor biomarker of primary blast injury. J Trauma 2009;67(1):210-211.

29. Ritenour AE, Baskin TW. Primary blast injury: update on diagnosis and treatment. Crit Care Med 2008;36(7 Suppl): S311-317.

30. Wanek S, Mayberry JC. Blunt thoracic trauma: flail chest, pulmonary contusion and blast injury. Crit Care Clin 2004;20(1):71-81.

31. Simon B, Ebert J, Bokhari F, et al. Practice management guideline for "pulmonary contusion – flail chest." Eastern Association for the Surgery of Trauma (EAST) 2006 June [cited 2010 Jan 15]. Available from: URL: http://www.east.org/tpg/pulmcontflailchest.pdf.

32. Kreider ME, Lipson DA. Bronchoscopy for atelectasis in the ICU: a case report and review of the literature. Chest 2003;124(1):344-350.

33. Nirula R, Diaz JJ Jr, Trunkey DD, et al. Rib fracture repair: indications, technical issues, and future directions. World J Surg 2009;33(1):14-22.

34. Karmakar MK, Ho AM. Acute pain management of patients with multiple fractured ribs. J Trauma 2003;54(3):615-625.

35. Eccles R. Importance of placebo effect in cough clinical trials. Lung 2010;188(Suppl 1);S53-61.

36. Dodek P, Keenan S, Cook D, et al. Evidence-based clinical practice guideline for the prevention of ventilator-associated pneumonia. Ann Intern Med 2004;141(4):305-313.

37. Stiller K. Physiotherapy in intensive care: towards and evidence-based practice. Chest 2000;118(6):1801-1813.

38. Sessler CN. Hypoxemic respiratory failure. In: ACCP Pulmonary board review course syllabus 2008. Northbrook: American College of Chest Physicians, 2008.

39. Bernard GR, Artigas A, Brigham KL, et al. The American-European Consensus Conference on ARDS: definitions, mechanisms, relevant outcomes and clinical trial coordination. Am J Respir Crit Care Med 1994;149(3 Pt 1):818-824.

40. Ware LB, Matthay MA. The acute respiratory distress syndrome. N Engl J Med 2000;342(18):1334-1349.

41. Hudson LD, Milberg JA, Anardi D, et al. Clinical risks for development of acute respiratory distress syndrome. Am J Respir Crit Care Med 1995;151(2 Pt 1):293-301.

42. Nuckton TJ, Alonso JA, Kallet RH, et al. Pulmonary dead-space fraction as a risk factor for death in the acute respiratory distress syndrome. N Engl J Med 2002;346(17):1281-1286.

43. Marshall RP, Bellingan G, Webb S, et al. Fibroproliferation occurs early in the acute respiratory distress syndrome and impacts on outcome. Am J Respir Crit Care Med 2000;162(5):1783-1788.

44. Gattinoni L, Pesenti A. The concept of "baby lung." Intensive Car Med 2005;31(6):776-784.

45. Gattinoni L, Caironi P. Refining ventilatory treatment for acute lung injury and acute respiratory distress syndrome. JAMA 2008;299(6):691-693.

46. Marik PE, Krikorian J. Pressure-controlled ventilation in ARDS: a practical approach. Chest 1997;112(4):1102-1106.

47. Esteban A, Alia I, Gordo F, et al. Prospective randomized trial comparing pressure-controlled ventilation and volume-controlled ventilation in ARDS. For the Spanish Lung Failure Collaborative Group. Chest 2000;117(6):1690-1696.

48. Amato MB, Barbas CS, Medievos DM, et al. Effect of a protective-ventilation strategy on mortality in the acute respiratory distress syndrome. N Engl J Med 1998;338(6):347-354.

49. Brower RG, Shanholtz CB, Fessler HE, et al. Prospective, randomized controlled clinical trial comparing traditional versus reduced tidal volume ventilation in acute respiratory distress syndrome patients. Crit Care Med 1999;27(8):1492-1498.

50. Brochard L, Roudot-Thoraval F, Roupie E, et al. Tidal volume reduction for prevention of ventilator-induced lung injury in acute respiratory distress syndrome. The Multicenter Trial Group on Tidal Volume reduction in ARDS. Am J Respir Crit Care Med 1998;158(6):1831-1838.

51. Stewart TE, Meade MO, Cook DJ, et al. Evaluation of a ventilation strategy to prevent barotraumas in patients at high risk for acute respiratory distress syndrome. Pressure- and Volume-Limited Ventilation Strategy Group. N Engl J Med 1998;338(6):355-361.

52. NIH ARDS Network. Ventilation with lower tidal volumes as compared with traditional tidal volumes for acute lung injury and the acute respiratory distress syndrome. N Engl J Med 2000;342(18):1301-1308.

53. Eichacker PQ, Gerstenberger EP, Banks SM, et al. Meta-analysis of acute lung injury and acute respiratory distress syndrome trials testing low tidal volumes. Am J Respir Crit Care Med 2002;166(11):1510-1514.

54. Carvalho CR, Barbas CS, Medeiros DM, et al. Temporal hemodynamic effects of permissive hypercapnia associated with ideal PEEP in ARDS. Am J Respir Crit Care Med 1997;156(5):1458-1466.

55. Weber T, Tschernich H, Sitzwohl C, et al. Tromethamine buffer modifies the depressant effect of permissive hypercapnia on myocardial contractility in patients with acute respiratory distress syndrome. Am J Respir Crit Care Med 2000;162(4 Pt 1):1361-1365.

56. Kregenow DA, Swenson ER. The lung and carbon dioxide: implications for permissive and therapeutic hypercapnia. Eur Respir J 2002;20(1):6-11.

57. MacIntyre NR. Is there a best way to set positive expiratory-end pressure for mechanical ventilatory support in acute lung injury? Clin Chest Med 2008;29(2):233-239.

58. Levy MM. Optimal PEEP in ARDS. Changing concepts and current controversies. Crit Care Clin 2002;18(1):15-33.

59. Brower RG, Lanken PN, MacIntyre N, et al. National Heart, Lung and Blood Institute ARDS Clinical Trials Network. Higher versus lower positive end-expiratory pressures in patients with the acute respiratory distress syndrome. N Engl J Med 2004;351(4):327-336.

60. Mercat A, Richard JC, Vielle B, et al. Positive end-expiratory pressure setting in adults with acute lung injury and acute respiratory distress syndrome: a randomized controlled trial. JAMA 2008;299(6):646-655.

61. Meade MO, Cook DJ, Guyatt GH et al. Ventilation strategy using low tidal volumes, recruitment maneuvers, and high positive end-expiratory pressure for acute lung injury and acute respiratory distress syndrome: a randomized controlled trial. JAMA 2008;299(6):637-645.

62. Antonelli M, Azoulay E, Bonten M, et al. Year in review in Intensive Care Medicine, 2008: II. Experimental, acute respiratory failure and ARDS, mechanical ventilation and endotracheal intubation. Intensive Care Med 2009;35(2):215-231.

63. Putensen C, Wrigge H. Clinical review: biphasic positive pressure and airway pressure release ventilation. Crit Care 2004;8(6):492-497.

64. Kaplan LJ, Bailey H, Formosa V. Airway pressure release ventilation increases cardiac performance in patients with acute lung injury/acute respiratory distress syndrome. Crit Care 2001;5(4):221-226.

65. Putensen C, Zech S, Wrigge H, et al. Long-term effects of spontaneous breathing during ventilatory support in patients with acute lung injury. Am J Respir Crit Care Med 2001;164(1):43-49.

66. Putensen C, Hering R, Muders T, et al. Assisted breathing is better in acute respiratory failure. Curr Opin Crit Care 2005;11(1):63-68.

67. Tumlin JA, et al. Airway pressure release ventilation (APRV) is superior to ARDS net low tidal volume-cycled ventilation in ALI/ARDS patients. PRESSURE Trial. Clinicaltrials.gov (identifier NCT00793013).

68. Ballard RA, Truog WE, Cnaan A, et al. Inhaled nitric oxide in preterm infants undergoing mechanical ventilation. N Engl J Med 2006;355(4):343-353.

69. Adhikari NK, Nurns KE, Friedich JO, et al. Effect of nitric oxide on oxygenation and mortality in acute lung injury: systematic review and meta-analysis. BMJ 2007;334(7597):779.

70. Taylor RW, Zimmerman JL, Dellinger RP, et al. Low-dose inhaled nitric oxide in patients with acute

lung injury: a randomized controlled trial. JAMA 2004;291(13):1603-1609.

71. Derdak S, Mehta S, Stewart TE, et al. High-frequency oscillatory ventilation for acute respiratory distress syndrome in adults: a randomized, controlled trial. Am J Respir Crit Care Med 2002;166(6):801-808.

72. Mugford M, Elbourne D, Field D. Extracorporeal membrane oxygenation for severe respiratory failure in newborn infants. Cochrane Database Syst Rev 2008;(3):CD001340.

73. Zapol WM, Snider MT, Hill JD, et al. Extracorporeal membrane oxygenation in severe acute respiratory failure. A randomized prospective study. JAMA 1979;242(20):2193-2196.

74. Gattinoni L, Presenti A, Mascheroni D, et al. Low frequency positive-pressure ventilation with extracorporeal $CO_2$ removal in severe acute respiratory failure. JAMA 1986;256(7):881-886.

75. Dorlac GR, Fang R, Pruitt VM, et al. Air transport of patients with severe lung injury: development and utilization of the Acute Lung Rescue Team. J Trauma 2009;66(4 Suppl):S164-171.

76. National Heart, Lung and Blood Institute Acute Respiratory Distress Syndrome (ARDS) Clinical Trials Network. Wiedemann HP, Wheeler AP, Bernard GR, et al. Comparison of two fluid-management strategies in acute lung injury. N Engl J Med 2006;354(24):2564-2575.

77. Steinberg KP, Hudson LD, Goodman RB, et al. Efficacy and safety of corticosteroids for persistent acute respiratory distress syndrome. N Engl J Med 2006;354(16):1671-1684.

78. Agarwal R, Nath A, Aggarwal AN, et al. Do glucocorticoids decrease mortality in acute respiratory distress syndrome? A meta-analysis. Respirology 2007;12(4):585-590.

79. Meduri GU, Golden E, Freire AX, et al. Methylprednisolone infusion in early severe ARDS: results of a randomized controlled trial. Chest 2007;131(4):954-963.

80. Meduri GU, Marik PE, Chrousos GP, et al. Steroid treatment in ARDS: a critical appraisal of the ARDS network trial and the recent literature. Intensive Care Med 2008;34(1):61-69.

81. Ward N. Effects of prone position in ARDS. An evidence-based review of the literature. Crit Care Clin 2002;18(1):35-44.

82. Pelosi P, Brazzi L, Gattinoni L. Prone position in acute respiratory distress syndrome. Eur Respir J 2002;20(4):1017-1028.

83. Gattinoni L, Tognoni G, Pesenti A, et al. Effect of prone positioning on the survival of patients with acute respiratory failure. N Engl J Med 2001;345(8):568-573.

84. Guerin C, Gaillard S, Lemasson S, et al. Effects of systematic prone positioning in hypoxemic acute respiratory failure: a randomized controlled trial. JAMA 2004;292(19):2379-2387.

85. Mancebo J, Fernandez R, Blanch L, et al. A multicenter trial of prolonged prone ventilation in severe acute respiratory distress syndrome. Am J Respir Crit Care Med 2006;173(11):1233-1239.

86. Taccone P, Pesenti A, Latini R, et al. Prone positioning in patients with moderate and severe acute respiratory distress syndrome; a randomized controlled trial. JAMA 2009;302(18):1977-1984.

87. Montejo JC, Zarazaga A, Lopez-Martinez J, et al. Immunonutrition in the intensive care unit. A systematic review and consensus statement. Clin Nutr 2003;22(3):221-233.

88. Gadek JE, DeMichele SJ, Karlstad MD, et al. Effect of enteral feeding with eicosapentaenoic acid, gamma-linolenic acid, and antioxidants in patients with acute respiratory distress syndrome. Enteral Nutrition in ARDS Study Group. Crit Care Med 1999;27(8):1409-1420.

89. Murthy R, Murthy M. Omega-3 fatty acids as anti-inflammatory agents. A classical group of nutraceuticals. J Neutraceuticals Funct Med Foods 1999;2(1):53-72.

90. Pontes-Arruda A, Aragao AM, Albuquerque JD. Effects of enteral feeding with eicosapentaenoic acid, gama-linolenic acid, and antioxidants in mechanically ventilated patients with severe sepsis and septic shock. Crit Care Med 2006;34(9):2325-2333.

91. Cain JG, Cohen JB, Kistler B, et al. Shock. In: Wilson WC, Grande CM, Hoyt DB, editors. Trauma critical care, volume 2. New York: Informa Healthcare USA, Inc., 2007. p. 313-336.

92. Tisherman SA, Barie P, Bokhari F, et al. Clinical practice guideline: endpoints of resuscitation. J Trauma 2004;57(4):898-912.

93. Scalea TM, Maltz S, Yelon J, et al. Resuscitation of multiple trauma and head injury: role of crystalloid fluids and inotropes. Crit Care Med 1994;22(10):1610-1615.

94. Abou-Khalil B, Scalea TM, Trooskin SZ, et al. Hemodynamic responses to shock in young trauma patients: need for invasive monitoring. Crit Care Med 1994;22(4):633-639.

95. Mikulaschek A, Henry SM, Donovan R, et al. Serum lactate is not predicted by anion gap or base excess after trauma resuscitation. J Trauma 1996;40(2):218-222; discussion 222-224.

96. Abramson D, Scalea TM, Hitchcock R, et al. Lactate clearance and survival following injury. J Trauma 1993;35(4):584-588; discussion 588-589.

97. McNelis J, Marini CP, Jurkiewicz A, et al. Prolonged lactate clearance is associated with increased mortality in the surgical intensive care unit. Am J Surg 2001;182(5):481-485.

98. Kaplan LJ, Kellum JA. Initial pH, lactate, anion gap, strong ion difference, and strong anion gap predict outcome from major vascular injury. Crit Care Med 2004;32(5):1120-1124.

99. Davis JW, Shackford SR, MacKersie RC, et al. Base deficit as a guide to volume resuscitation. J

Trauma 1988;28(10):1464-1467.

100. Porter JM, Ivatury RR. In search of the optimal end points of resuscitation in trauma patients: a review. J Trauma 1998;44(5):908-914.

101. Brill SA, Stewart TR, Brundage SI, et al. Base deficit does not predict mortality when secondary to hyperchloremic acidosis. Shock 2002;17(6):459-462.

102. Rutherford EJ, Morris JA Jr, Reed GW, et al. Base deficit stratifies mortality and determines therapy. J Trauma 1992;33(3):417-423.

103. Krishna G, Sleigh JW, Rahman H. Physiological predictors of death in exsanguinating trauma patients undergoing conventional trauma surgery. Aust N Z J Surg 1998;68(12):826-829.

104. Siegel JH, Rivkind AI, Dalal S, et al. Early physiologic predictors of injury severity and death in blunt multiple trauma. Arch Surg 1990;125(4):498-508.

105. Eachempati SR, Reed RL 2nd, Barie PS. Serum bicarbonate concentration correlates with arterial base deficit in critically ill patients. Surg Infect (Larchmt) 2003;4(2):193-197.

106. Shoemaker WC, Montgomery ES, Kaplan E, et al. Physiologic patterns in surviving and nonsurviving shock patients. Use of sequential cardiorespiratory variables in defining criteria for therapeutic goals and early warning of death. Arch Surg 1973;106(5):630-636.

107. Shoemaker WC, Appel P, Bland R. Use of physiologic monitoring to predict outcome and to assist in clinical decisions in critically ill postoperative patients. Am J Surg 1983;146(1):43-50.

108. Fleming A, Bishop M, Shoemaker W, et al. Prospective trial of supranormal values as goals of resuscitation in severe trauma. Arch Surg 1992;127(10):1175-1181.

109. Bishop MH, Shoemaker WC, Appel PL, et al. Prospective, randomized trial of survivor values of cardiac index, oxygen delivery, and oxygen consumption as resuscitation endpoints in severe trauma. J Trauma 1995;38(5):780-787.

110. Durham RM, Neunaber K, Mazuski JE, et al. The use of oxygen consumption and delivery as endpoints for resuscitation in critically ill patients. J Trauma 1996;41(1):32-39; discussion 39-40.

111. Velmahos GC, Demetriades D, Shoemaker WC, et al. Endpoints of resuscitation of critically injured patients: normal or supranormal? A prospective randomized trial. Ann Surg 2000;232(3):409-418.

112. McKinley BA, Kozar RA, Cocanour CS, et al. Normal versus supranormal oxygen delivery goals in shock resuscitation: the response is the same. J Trauma 2002;53(5):825-832.

113. Kern JW, Shoemaker WC. Meta-analysis of hemodynamic optimization in high-risk patients. Crit Care Med 2002;30(8):1686-1692.

114. Ladakis C, Myrianthefs P, Karabinis A, et al. Central venous and mixed venous oxygen saturation in critically ill patients. Respiration 2001;68(3):279-285.

115. Edwards JD, Mayall RM. Importance of the sampling site for measurement of mixed venous oxygen saturation in shock. Crit Care Med 1998;26(8):1356-1360.

116. Reinhart K, Rudolph T, Bredle DL, et al. Comparison of central-venous to mixed-venous oxygen saturation during changes in oxygen supply/demand. Chest 1989;95(6):1216-1221.

117. Gattinoni L, Brazzi L, Pelosi P, et al. A trial of goal-oriented hemodynamic therapy in critically ill patients. SvO$_2$ Collaborative Group. N Engl J Med 1995;333(16):1025-1032.

118. Rivers E, Nguyen B, Havstad S, et al. Early goal-directed therapy in the treatment of severe sepsis and septic shock. N Engl J Med 2001;345(19):1368-1377.

119. Rivers EP, Ander DS, Powell D. Central venous oxygen saturation monitoring in the critically ill patient. Curr Opin Crit Care 2001;7(3):204-211.

120. Gys T, Hubens A, Neels H, et al. The prognostic value of gastric intramural pH in surgical intensive care patients. Crit Care Med 1988;16(12):1222-1224.

121. Gutierrez G, Bismar H, Dantzker DR, et al. Comparison of gastric intramucosal pH with measures of oxygen transport and consumption in critically ill patients. Crit Care Med 1992;20(4):451-457.

122. Roumen RM, Vreugde JP, Goris RJ. Gastric tonometry in multiple trauma patients. J Trauma 1994;36(3):313-316.

123. Chang MC, Cheatham ML, Nelson LD, et al. Gastric tonometry supplements information provided by systemic indicators of oxygen transport. J Trauma 1994;37(3):488-494.

124. Ivatury RR, Simon RJ, Havriliak D, et al. Gastric mucosal pH and oxygen delivery and oxygen consumption indices in the assessment of adequacy of resuscitation after trauma: a prospective, randomized study. J Trauma 1995;39(1):128-134.

125. Ivatury RR, Simon RJ, Islam S, et al. A prospective randomized study of end points of resuscitation after major trauma: global oxygen transport indices versus organ-specific gastric mucosal pH. J Am Coll Surg 1996;183(2):145-154.

126. Ristagno G, Tang W, Sun S, et al. Role of buccal PCO$_2$ in the management of fluid resuscitation during hemorrhagic shock. Crit Care Med 2006;34(12 Suppl):S442-446.

127. Marik PE. Sublingual capnography: a clinical validation study. Chest 2001;120(3):923-927.

128. Povoas HP, Weil MH, Tang W, et al. Comparisons between sublingual and gastric tonometry during hemorrhagic shock. Chest 2001;118(4):1127-1132.

129. Baron BJ, Sinert R, Zehtabchi S, et al. Diagnostic utility of sublingual $PCO_2$ for detecting hemorrhage in penetrating trauma patients. J Trauma 2004;57(1):69-74.

130. Tatevossian RG, Wo CC, Velmahos GC, et al. Transcutaneous oxygen and $CO_2$ as early warning of tissue hypoxia and hemodynamic shock in critically ill emergency patients. Crit Care Med 2000;28(7):2248-2253.

131. McKinley BA, Marvin RG, Cocanour CS, et al. Tissue hemoglobin $O_2$ saturation during resuscitation of traumatic shock monitored using near infrared spectrometry. J Trauma 2000;48(4):637-642.

132. Crookes BA, Cohn SM, Bloch S, et al. Can near-infrared spectroscopy identify the severity of shock in trauma patients? J Trauma 2005;58(4):806-813; discussion 813-816.

133. Angus DC, Linde-Zwirble WT, Lidicker J, et al. Epidemiology of severe sepsis in the United States: analysis of incidence, outcome, and associated costs of care. Crit Care Med 2001;29(7):1303-1310.

134. Dombrovskiy VY, Martin AA, Sunderram J, et al. Rapid increase in hospitalization and mortality rates for severe sepsis in the United States: a trend analysis from 1993 to 2003. Crit Care Med 2007;35(5):1244-1250.

135. Bone RC, Balk RA, Cerra FB, et al. Definitions for sepsis and organ failure and guidelines for the use of innovative therapies in sepsis. The ACCP/SCCM Consensus Conference Committee. American College of Chest Physicians/Society of Critical Care Medicine. Chest 1992;101(6):1644-1655.

136. Levy MM, Fink MP, Marshall JC, et al. 2001 SCCM/ESICM/ACCP/ATS/SIS International Sepsis Definitions Conference. Crit Care Med 2003;31(4):1250-1256.

137. Hotchkiss RS, Karl IE. The pathophysiology and treatment of sepsis. N Engl J Med 2003;348(2):138-150.

138. Annane D, Aegerter P, Jars-Guincestre MC, et al. Current epidemiology of septic shock: the CUB-Rea network. Am J Respir Crit Care Med 2003;168(2):165-172.

139. Ely EW, Goyette RE. Sepsis with acute organ dysfunction. In: Hall JB, Schmidt GA, Wood LDH, editors. Principles of critical care. New York: McGraw-Hill, 2005. p. 505-524.

140. Alberti C, Brun-Buisson C, Goodman SV, et al. Influence of systemic inflammatory response syndrome and sepsis on outcome of critically ill infected patients. Am J Respir Crit Care Med 2003;168(1):77-84.

141. Varpula M, Tallgren M, Saukkonen K, et al. Hemodynamic variables related to outcome in septic shock. Intensive Care Med 2005;31(8):1066-1071.

142. Vincent JL, de Mendonca A, Cantraine F, et al. Use of the SOFA score to assess the incidence of organ dysfunction/failure in intensive care units: results of a multicenter, prospective study. Working group on "sepsis-related problems" of the European Society of Intensive Care Medicine. Crit Care Med 1998;26(11):1793-1800.

143. Kortgen A, Niederprum P, Bauer M. Implementation of an evidence-based "standard operating procedure" and outcome in septic shock. Crit Care Med 2006;34(4):943-949.

144. Micek ST, Roubinian N, Heuring T, et al. Before-after study of a standardized hospital order set for the management of septic shock. Crit Care Med 2006;34(11):2707-2713.

145. Nguyen HB, Corbett SW, Steele R, et al. Implementation of a bundle of quality indicators for the early management of severe sepsis and septic shock is associated with decreased mortality. Crit Care Med 2007;35(4):1105-1112.

146. Shorr AF, Micek ST, Jackson WL Jr, et al. Economic implications of an evidence-based sepsis protocol: can we improve outcomes and lower costs? Crit Care Med 2007;35(5):1257-1262.

147. Rivers EP, Ahrens T. Improving outcomes for severe sepsis and septic shock: tools for early identification of at-risk patients and treatment protocol implementation. Crit Care Clin 2008;24(3 Suppl):S1-47.

148. Dellinger RP, Levy MM, Carlet JM, et al. Surviving sepsis campaign: international guidelines for management of severe sepsis and septic shock: 2008. Crit Care Med 2008;36(1):296-327.

149. Jimenez MF, Marshall JC. Source control in the management of sepsis. Intensive Care Med 2001;27 (Suppl 1):S49-62.

150. Bouza E, Sousa D, Rodriguez-Creixems M, et al. Is the volume of blood cultured still a significant factor in the diagnosis of bloodstream infections? J Clin Microbiol 2007;45(9):2765-2769.

151. Mermel, LA, Maki DG. Detection of bacteremia in adults: consequences of culturing an inadequate volume of blood. Ann Intern Med 1993;119(4):270-272.

152. Connell TG, Rele M, Cowley D, et al. How reliable is a negative blood culture result? Volume of blood submitted for culture in routine practice in a children's hospital. Pediatrics 2007;119(5):891-896.

153. Blot F, Schmidt E, Nitenberg G, et al. Earlier positivity of central-venous- versus peripheral-blood cultures is highly predictive of catheter-related sepsis. J Clin Microbiol 1998;36(1):105-109.

154. Mermel LA, Farr BM, Sherertz RJ, et al. Guidelines for the management of intravascular catheter-related infections. Clin Infect Dis 2001;32(9):1249-1272.

155. Murray CK, Hsu JR, Solomkin JS, et al. Prevention and management of infections associated with combat-related extremity injuries. J Trauma 2008;64(3 Suppl):S239-251.

156. Hospenthal DR, Murray CK, Andersen RC, et al. Guidelines for the prevention of infection after combat-related injuries. J Trauma 2008;64(3 Suppl):S211-220.

157. Magder S, Bafaqeeh F. The clinical role of central venous pressure measurements. J Intensive Care Med 2007;22(1):44-51.

158. Osman D, Ridel C, Ray P, et al. Cardiac filling pressures are not appropriate to predict hemodynamic response to volume challenge. Crit Care Med 2007;35(1):64-68.

159. Bendjelid K, Romand JA. Fluid responsiveness in mechanically ventilated patients: a review of indices used in intensive care. Intensive Care Med 2003;29(3):352-360.

160. Malbrain ML, Deeren D, De Potter TJ. Intra-abdominal hypertension in the critically ill: it is time to pay attention. Curr Opin Crit Care 2005;11(2):156-171.

161. Michard F, Boussat S, Chemla D, et al. Relation between respiratory changes in arterial pulse pressure and fluid responsiveness in septic patients with acute circulatory failure. Am J Respir Crit Care Med 2000;162(1):134-138.

162. De Backer D, Heenen S, Piagnerelli M, et al. Pulse pressure variations to predict fluid responsiveness: influence of tidal volume. Intensive Care Med 2005;31(4):517-523.

163. Charron C, Caille V, Jardin F, et al. Echocardiographic measurement of fluid responsiveness. Curr Opin Crit Care 2006;12(3):249-254.

164. Doyle JA, Davis DP, Hoyt DB. The use of hypertonic saline in the treatment of traumatic brain injury. J Trauma 2001;50(2):367-383.

165. White H, Cook D, Venkatesh B. The use of hypertonic saline for treating intracranial hypertension after traumatic brain injury. Anesth Analg 2006;102(6):1836-1846.

166. Finfer S, Bellomo R, Boyce N, et al. A comparison of albumin and saline for fluid resuscitation in the intensive care unit. N Engl J Med 2004;350(22):2247-2256.

167. Choi PT, Yip G, Quinonez LG, et al. Crystalloids vs. colloids in fluid resuscitation: a systematic review. Crit Care Med 1999;27(1):200-210.

168. Durairaj L, Schmidt GA. Fluid therapy in resuscitated sepsis: less is more. Chest 2008;133(1):252-263.

169. Hollenberg SM. Vasopressor support in septic shock. Chest 2007;132(5):1678-1687.

170. Hollenberg SM, Ahrens TS, Annane D, et al. Practice parameters for hemodynamic support of sepsis in adult patients: 2004 update. Crit Care Med 2004;32(9):1928-1948.

171. LeDoux D, Astiz ME, Carpati CM, et al. Effects of perfusion pressure on tissue perfusion in septic shock. Crit Care Med 2000;28(8):2729-2732.

172. Martin C, Papazian L, Perrin G, et al. Norepinephrine or dopamine for the treatment of hyperdynamic septic shock? Chest 1993;103(6):1826-1831.

173. Martin C, Viviand X, Leone M, et al. Effect of norepinephrine on the outcome of septic shock. Crit Care Med 2000;28(8):2758-2765.

174. De Backer D, Creteur J, Silva E, et al. Effects of dopamine, norepinephrine and epinephrine on the splanchnic circulation in septic shock: which is best? Crit Care Med 2003;31(6):1659-1667.

175. Leone M, Martin C. Vasopressor use in septic shock: an update. Curr Opin Anaesthesiol 2008;21(2):141-147.

176. Levy B, Bollaert PE, Charpentier C, et al. Comparison of norepinephrine and dobutamine to epinephrine for hemodynamics, lactate metabolism, and gastric tonometric variables in septic shock: a prospective, randomized study. Intensive Care Med 1997;23(3):282-287.

177. Landry DW, Levin HR, Gallant EM, et al. Vasopressin deficiency contributes to the vasodilation of septic shock. Circulation 1997;95(5):1122-1125.

178. Patel BM, Chittock DR, Russell JA, et al. Beneficial effects of short-term vasopressin infusion during severe septic shock. Anesthesiology 2002;96(3):576-582.

179. Dunser MW, Mayr AJ, Ulmer H, et al. Arginine vasopressin in advanced vasodilatory shock. Circulation 2003;107(18):2313-2319.

180. Russell JA, Walley KR, Singer J, et al. Vasopressin versus norepinephrine infusion in patients with septic shock. N Engl J Med 2008;358(9):877-887.

181. Bellomo R, Chapman M, Finfer S, et al. Low-dose dopamine in patients with early renal dysfunction: a placebo-controlled randomized trial. Australian and New Zealand Intensive Care Society (ANZICS) Clinical Trials Group. Lancet 2000;356(9248):2139-2143.

182. Marik PE, Iglesias J. Low-dose dopamine does not prevent acute renal failure in patients with septic shock and oliguria: NORASEPT II Study Investigators. Am J Med 1999;107(4):387-390.

183. Marik PE, Mohedin M. The contrasting effects of dopamine and norepinephrine on systemic and splanchnic oxygen utilization in hyperdynamic sepsis. JAMA 1994;272(17):1354-1357.

184. Neviere R, Mathieu D, Chagnon JL, et al. The contrasting effects of dobutamine and dopamine on gastric mucosal perfusion in septic patients. Am J Respir Crit Care Med 1996;154(6 Pt 1):1684-1688.

185. Holmes CL, Walley KR. Bad medicine: low-dose dopamine in the ICU. Chest 2003;123(4):1266-1275.

186. Annane D, Bellissant E, Bollaert PE, et al. Corticosteroids in the treatment of severe sepsis and septic shock in adults: a systematic review. JAMA 2009;301(22):2362-2375.

187. Annane D, Sebille V, Charpentier C, et al. Effect of treatment with low doses of hydrocortisone and

fludrocortisone on mortality in patients with septic shock. JAMA 2002;288(7):862-871.

188. Briegel J, Forst H, Haller M, et al. Stress doses of hydrocortisone reverse hyperdynamic septic shock: a prospective, randomized, double-blind, single-center study. Crit Care Med 1999;27(4):723-732.

189. Bollaert PE, Charpentier C, Levy B, et al. Reversal of late septic shock with supraphysiologic doses of hyrdrocortisone. Crit Care Med 1998;26(4):645-650.

190. Sprung CL, Annane D, Keh D, et al. Hydrocortisone therapy for patients with septic shock. N Engl J Med 2008;358(2):111-124.

191. Trzeciak S, Rivers EP. Clinical manifestations of disordered microcirculatory perfusion in severe sepsis. Crit Care 2005;9 (Suppl 4):S20-26.

192. Lorente JA, Landin L, De Pablo R, et al. Effects of blood transfusion on oxygen transport variables in severe sepsis. Crit Care Med 1993;21(9):1312-1318.

193. Hebert PC, Wells G, Blajchman MA, et al. A multicenter, randomized, controlled clinical trial of transfusion requirements in critical care. Transfusion Requirements in Critical Care Investigators, Canadian Critical Care Trials Group. N Engl J Med 1999;340(6):409-417.

194. Fernandes CJ Jr, Akamine N, De Marco FV, et al. Red blood cell transfusion does not increase oxygen consumption in critically ill septic patients. Crit Care 2001;5(6):362-367.

195. Sondeen J, Coppes VG, Gaddy CE, et al. Potential resuscitation strategies for treatment of hemorrhagic shock. Presented at the RTO HFM Symposium on "Combat casualty care in ground based tactical situation: trauma technology and emergency medical procedures," St Pete Beach, FL 16-18 August 2004. RTO-MP-HFM-109.

196. Corwin HL, Gettinger A, Rodriguez RM, et al. Efficacy of recombinant human erythropoietin in the critically ill patient: a randomized, double-blind, placebo-controlled trial. Crit Care Med 1999;27(11):2346-2350.

197. Corwin HL, Gettinger A, Pearl RG, et al. Efficacy of recombinant human erythropoietin in critically ill patients: a randomized controlled trial. JAMA 2002;288(22):2827-2835.

198. Dara SI, Rana R, Afessa B, et al. Fresh frozen plasma transfusion in critically ill medical patients with coagulopathy. Crit Care Med 2005;33(11):2667-2671.

199. Aguilar MI, Hart RG, Kase CS, et al. Treatment of warfarin-associated intracerebral hemorrhage: literature review and expert opinion. Mayo Clin Proc 2007;82(1):82-92.

200. Rosand J, Eckman MH, Knudsen KA, et al. The effect of warfarin and intensity of anticoagulation on outcome of intracerebral hemorrhage. Arch Intern Med 2004;164(8);880-884.

201. Beale RJ, Hollenberg SM, Vincent JL, et al. Vasopressor and inotropic support in septic shock: an evidence-based review. Crit Care Med 2004;32(11 Suppl):S455-465.

202. Bernard GR, Vincent JL, Laterre PF, et al. Efficacy and safety of recombinant human activated protein C for severe sepsis. N Engl J Med 2001;344(10):699-709.

203. Costa V, Brophy JM. Drotrecogin alfa (activated) in severe sepsis: a systematic review and new cost-effectiveness analysis. BMC Anesthesiol 2007; 7:5.

204. Abraham E, Laterre PF, Garg R, et al. Drotrecogin alfa (activated) for adults with severe sepsis and a low risk of death. N Engl J Med 2005;353(13):1332-1341.

205. Kanji S, Perreault MM, Chant C, et al. Evaluating the use of Drotrecogin alfa (activated) in adult severe sepsis: a Canadian multicenter observational study. Intensive Care Med 2007;33(3):517-523.

206. Bertolini G, Rossi C, Anghileri A, et al. Use of Drotrecogin alfa (activated) in Italian intensive care units: the results of a nationwide survey. Intensive Care Med 2007;33(3):426-434.

207. Ely EW, Laterre PF, Angus DC, et al. Drotrecogin alfa (activated) administration across clinically important subgroups of patients with severe sepsis. Crit Care Med 2003;31(1):12-19.

208. Fourrier F. Recombinant human activated protein C in the treatment of severe sepsis: an evidence-based review. Crit Care Med 2004;32(11 Suppl):S534-541.

209. Vincent JL, Bernard GR, Beale R, et al. Drotrecogin alfa (activated) treatment in severe sepsis from the global open-label trial ENHANCE: further evidence for survival and safety and implications for early treatment. Crit Care Med 2005;33(10):2266-2277.

210. Van den Berghe G, Wouters P, Weekers F, et al. Intensive insulin therapy in the critically ill patients. N Engl J Med 2001;345(19):1359-1367.

211. Van den Berghe G, Wilmer A, Hermans G, et al. Intensive insulin therapy in the medical ICU. N Engl J Med 2006;354(5):449-461.

212. Brunkhorst FM, Kuhnt E, Engel CE, et al. Intensive insulin therapy in patients with severe sepsis and septic shock is associated with an increased rate of hypoglycemia – results from a randomized multicenter study (VISEP). Infection 2005;33:19-20.

213. Brunkhorst FM, Engel C, Bloos F, et al. Intensive insulin therapy and pentastarch resuscitation in severe sepsis. N Engl J Med 2008;358(2):125-139.

214. NICE-SUGAR Study Investigators, Finfer S, Chittock DR, Su SY, et al. Intensive versus conventional glucose control in critically ill patients. N Engl J Med 2009;360(13):1283-1297.

215. Cooper DJ, Walley KR, Wiggs BR, et al. Bicarbonate does not improve hemodynamics in critically ill

patients who have lactic acidosis: a prospective, controlled clinical study. Ann Intern Med 1990;112(7):492-498.

216. Mathieu D, Neviere R, Billard V, et al. Effects of bicarbonate therapy on hemodynamics and tissue oxygenation in patients with lactic acidosis: a prospective, controlled clinical study. Crit Care Med 1991;19(11):1352-1356.

217. Sabatini S, Kurtzman NA. Bicarbonate therapy in severe metabolic acidosis. J Am Soc Nephrol 2008;20(4):692-695.

218. Hoste EA, Colpaert K, Vanholder RC, et al. Sodium bicarbonate versus THAM in ICU patients with mild metabolic acidosis. J Nephrol 2005;18(3):303-307.

219. Perez J, Dellinger RP; International Sepsis Forum. Other supportive therapies in sepsis. Intensive Care Med 2001;27 (Suppl 1):S116-127.

220. Uehara M, Plank LD, Hill GL. Components of energy expenditure in patients with severe sepsis and major trauma: a basis for clinical care. Crit Care Med 1999;27(7):1295-1302.

221. Novak F, Heyland DK, Avenell A, et al. Glutamine supplementation in serious illness: a systematic review of the evidence. Crit Care Med 2002;30(9):2022-2029.

222. Barbul A. Arginine: biochemistry, physiology, and therapeutic implications. JPEN J Parenter Enteral Nutr 1986;10(2):227-238.

223. Kreymann KG, Berger MM, Deutz NE, et al. ESPEN guidelines on Enteral Nutrition: Intensive care. Clin Nutr 2006;25(2):210-223.

224. Gramlich L, Kichian K, Pinilla J, et al. Does enteral nutrition compared to parenteral nutrition result in better outcomes in critically ill adult patients? A systematic review of the literature. Nutrition 2004;20(10):843-848.

225. Wasiak J, Cleland H, Jeffery R. Early versus late enteral nutritional support in adults with burn injury: a systematic review. J Hum Nutr Diet 2007;20(2):75-83.

226. Heyland DK, Cook DJ, Griffith L, et al. The attributable morbidity and mortality of ventilator-associated pneumonia in the critically ill patient. The Canadian Clinical Trials Group. Am J Respir Crit Care Med 1999;159(4 Pt 1):1249-1256.

227. American Thoracic Society, Infectious Disease Society of America. Guidelines for the management of adults with hospital-acquired, ventilator-associated, and healthcare-associated pneumonia. Am J Respir Crit Care Med 2005;171(4):388-416.

228. Murray CK. Epidemiology of infections associated with combat-related injuries in Iraq and Afghanistan. J Trauma 2008;64(3 Suppl):S232-238.

229. Conger NG, Landrum ML, Jenkins DH, et al. Prevention and management of infections associated with combat-related thoracic and abdominal cavity injuries. J Trauma 2008;64(3 Suppl):S257-264.

230. Isenbarger DW, Atwood JE, Scott PT, et al. Venous thromboembolism among United States soldiers deployed to Southwest Asia. Thromb Res 2006;117(4):379-383.

231. Hirsh J, Guyatt G, Albers GW, et al. Executive Summary: American College of Chest Physicians Evidence-Based Clinical Practice Guidelines. 8th ed. Chest 2008;133(6 Suppl):71S-109S.

232. Cordts PR, Brosch LA, Holcomb JB. Now and then: combat casualty care policies for Operation Iraqi Freedom and Operation Enduring Freedom compared with those of Vietnam. J Trauma 2008;64(2 Suppl):S14-20.

233. Ali T, Harty RF. Stress-induced ulcer bleeding in critically ill patients. Gastroenterol Clin North Am 2009;38(2):245-265.

234. Cook DJ, Fuller HD, Guyatt GH. Risk factors for gastrointestinal bleeding in the critically ill patient. Canadian Critical Care Trials Group. N Engl J Med 1994;330(6):377-381.

235. Rosenberg JB, Eisen LA. Eye care in the intensive care unit: narrative review and meta-analysis. Crit Care Med 2008;36(12):3151-3155.

236. Eachempati SR, Hydo LJ, Barie PS. Factors influencing the development of decubitus ulcers in critically ill surgical patients. Crit Care Med 2001;29(9):1678-1682.

237. Levi B, Rees R. Diagnosis and management of pressure ulcers. Clin Plastic Surg 2007;34(4):735-748.

238. D'Avignon LC, Saffle JR, Chung KK, et al. Prevention and management of infections associated with burns in the combat casualty. J Trauma 2008;64(3 Suppl):S277-286.

239. Wortmann GW, Valadka AB, Moores LE. Prevention and management of infections associated with combat-related central nervous system injuries. J Trauma 2008;64(3 Suppl):S252-S256.

240. Murray CK, Hinkle MK, Yun HC. History of infections associated with combat-related injuries. J Trauma 2008;64(3 Suppl):S221-S231.

241. Marelich GP, Murin S, Battistella F, et al. Protocol weaning of mechanical ventilation in medical and surgical patients by respiratory care practitioners and nurses: effect on weaning time and incidence of ventilator-associated pneumonia. Chest 2000;118(2):459-467.

242. Ely EW, Baker AM, Dunagan DP, et al. Effect on the duration of mechanical ventilation of identifying patients capable of breathing spontaneously. N Engl J Med 1996;335(25):1864-1869.

243. Ely EW, Bennett PA, Bowton DL, et al. Large scale implementation of a respiratory therapist-driven protocol for ventilator weaning. Am J Respir Crit Care Med 1999;159(2):439-446.

244. Lettieri CJ, Shah AA, Greenburg DL. An intensivist-directed intensive care unit improves clinical outcomes in a combat zone. Crit Care Med 2009;37(4):1256-1260.

245. MacLaren R, Bond CA, Martin SJ, et al. Clinical and economic outcomes of involving pharmacists in the direct care of critically ill patients with infections. Crit Care Med 2008;36(12):3184-3189.

246. Grathwohl KW, Venticinque SG. Organizational characteristics of the austere intensive care unit: the evolution of military trauma and critical care medicine; applications for civilian medical systems. Crit Care Med 2008;36(7 Suppl):S275-S283.

247. Johannigman JA. Critical care aeromedical teams (CCATT): then, now and what's next. J Trauma 2007;62(6 Suppl):S35.

248. Johannigman JA. Maintaining the continuum of en route care. Crit Care Med 2008;36(7 Suppl):S377-382.

249. Bridges E, Evers K. Wartime critical care air transport. Mil Med 2009;174(4):370-375.

250. Beninati W, Meyer MT, Carter TE. The critical care air transport program. Crit Care Med 2008;36(7 Suppl):S370-376.

251. Blackbourne LH. Combat damage control surgery. Crit Care Med 2008;36(7 Suppl):S304-310.

252. Fang R, Pruitt VM, Dorlac GR, et al. Critical care at Landstuhl Regional Medical Center. Crit Care Med 2008;36(7 Suppl):S383-387.

253. McNeil JD, Pratt JW. Combat casualty care in an air force theater hospital: perspectives of recently deployed cardiothoracic surgeons. Semin Thorac Cardiovasc Surg 2008;20(1):78-84.

254. Warren J, Fromm RE Jr, Orr RA, et al. Guidelines for the inter- and intrahospital transport of critically ill patients. Crit Care Med 2004;32(1):256-262.

255. Andersson N, Grip H, Lindvall P, et al. Air transport of patients with intracranial air: computer model of pressure effects. Aviat Space Environ Med 2003;74(2):138-144.

256. Parsons CJ, Bobechok WP. Aeromedical transport: its hidden problems. Can Med Assoc J 1982;126(3):237-243.

257. Rice DH, Kotti G, Beninati W. Clinical review: critical care transport and austere critical care. Crit Care 2008;12(2):207.

# Appendix

## SUMMARY OF VENTILATOR PROCEDURES*

| VARIABLE | GROUP RECEIVING TRADITIONAL TIDAL VOLUMES | GROUP RECEIVING LOWER TIDAL VOLUMES |
|---|---|---|
| Ventilator mode | Volume assist-control | Volume assist-control |
| Initial tidal volume (ml/kg of predicated body weight) [†] | 12 | 6 |
| Plateau pressure (cm of water) | ≤ 50 | ≤ 30 |
| Ventilator rate setting needed to achieve a pH goal of 7.3 to 7.45 (breaths/min) | 6-35 | 6-35 |
| Ratio of the duration of inspiration to the duration of expiration | 1:1 - 1:3 | 1:1 - 1:3 |
| Oxygenation goal | $PaO_2$, 55-80 mm Hg, or $SpO_2$, 88-95% | $PaO_2$, 55-80 mm Hg, or $SpO_2$, 88-95% |
| Allowable combinations of $FiO_2$ and PEEP (cm of water) [‡] | 0.3 and 5 | 0.3 and 5 |
| | 0.4 and 5 | 0.4 and 5 |
| | 0.4 and 8 | 0.4 and 8 |
| | 0.5 and 8 | 0.5 and 8 |
| | 0.5 and 10 | 0.5 and 10 |
| | 0.6 and 10 | 0.6 and 10 |
| | 0.7 and 10 | 0.7 and 10 |
| | 0.7 and 12 | 0.7 and 12 |
| | 0.7 and 14 | 0.7 and 14 |
| | 0.8 and 14 | 0.8 and 14 |
| | 0.9 and 16 | 0.9 and 16 |
| | 0.9 and 18 | 0.9 and 18 |
| | 1.0 and 18 | 1.0 and 18 |
| | 1.0 and 20 | 1.0 and 20 |
| | 1.0 and 22 | 1.0 and 22 |
| | 1.0 and 24 | 1.0 and 24 |
| Weaning | By pressure support; required by protocol when $FiO_2$ ≤ 0.4 | By pressure support; required by protocol when $FiO_2$ ≤ 0.4 |

* $PaO_2$ denotes partial pressure of arterial oxygen, $SpO_2$ oxyhemoglobin saturation measured by pulse oximetry, $FiO_2$ fraction of inspired oxygen, and PEEP positive end-expiratory pressure.

† Subsequent adjustments in tidal volumes were made to maintain a plateau pressure of 50 cm of water in the group receiving traditional tidal volumes and 30 cm of water in the group receiving lower tidal volumes.

‡ Further increases in PEEP, to 34 cm of water, were allowed but were not required.

*NIH ARDS Network. Ventilation with lower tidal volumes as compared with traditional tidal volumes for acute lung injury and the acute respiratory distress syndrome. N Engl J Med 2000;342:1301-1308. Copyright © 2000 Massachusetts Medical Society. All rights reserved.*

# Abbreviations and Acronyms

## A

AAN: American Academy of Neurology
ABA: American Burn Association
ABC: airway, breathing, and circulation
ABLS: Advanced Burn Life Support
A/C: assist-control
ACTH: adrenocorticotropic hormone
ADDRESS: Administration of Drotrecogin Alfa (activated) in Early Stage Severe Sepsis (trial)
AFSOC: Air Force Special Operations Command
AFTH: Air Force Theater Hospital
AIREVAC: air evacuation
AIS: Abbreviated Injury Scale
ALI: acute lung injury
ALRT: Acute Lung Rescue Team
ALVEOLI: Assessment of Low Tidal Volume and Elevated End-Expiratory Lung Volume to Obviate Lung Injury (trial)
AMEDD: US Army Medical Department
ANFO: ammonium nitrate/fuel oil
AOR: area of responsibility
AP: anteroposterior
APD: afferent papillary defect
aPLT: apheresis platelet
APRV: alternating pressure release ventilation
aPTT: activated partial thromboplastin time
ARDS: acute respiratory distress syndrome
ARDSnet: Acute Respiratory Distress Syndrome Clinical Trials Network
ATLS: Advanced Trauma and Life Support
ATP: adenosine triphosphate

## B

BAL: bronchoalveolar lavage
BAMC: Brooke Army Medical Center
BP: blood pressure
BSMC: Brigade Support Medical Company
BSS: balanced salt solution
BTBIS: Brief TBI Screen
BUMED: Bureau of Medicine and Surgery

## C

CASEVAC: casualty evacuation
CBF: cerebral blood flow
CCATT: Critical Care Air Transport Team/Critical Care Aeromedical Transport Team
CCC: combat casualty care
CDC: Centers for Disease Control and Prevention
CENTCOM: US Central Command
CHS: combat health support
cm: centimeter
CN: cranial nerve
COG: Clinical Operating Guidelines
CONUS: continental United States
COPD: chronic obstructive pulmonary disease
CORTICUS: Corticosteroid Therapy of Septic Shock (trial)
CPAP: continuous positive airway pressure
CPG: Clinical Practice Guidelines
CPK: creatinine phosphokinase

CPP: cerebral perfusion pressure
CPR: cardiopulmonary resuscitation
CRTS: Casualty Receiving and Treatment Ship
CS: compartment syndrome
CSH: Combat Support Hospital
CT: computed tomography
CTA: computed tomographic angiography
CVP: central venous pressure
CVR: cerebral vascular resistance

**D**
D10: 10% dextrose
D25: 25% dextrose
D5: 5% dextrose
D50: 50% dextrose
DCR: damage control resuscitation
DCS: damage control surgery
DECRA: Decompressive Craniectomy (trial)
DIC: disseminated intravascular coagulation
DIMOC: Defense Imagery Management Operations Center
$DO_2$: oxygen delivery
DOD: Department of Defense
DVT: deep venous thrombosis

**E**
$ECCO_2R$: extracorporeal carbon dioxide removal
ECMO: extracorporeal membrane oxygenation
ED: emergency department
EFP: explosively formed projectile
EMEDS: Expeditionary Medical Support
EMF: Expeditionary Medical Facility
EMS: emergency medical services
EMT: emergency medical technician; also Emergency & Military Tourniquet
EMT-B: emergency medical technician–basic
ENT: ear-nose-throat
EOD: explosive ordnance disposal
ER: oxygen extraction ratio
$EtCO_2/ETCO_2$: end-tidal carbon dioxide
ETT: endotracheal tube
exam: examination

**F**
FAST: Focused Assessment with Sonography for Trauma
FDA: Food and Drug Administration
FFP: fresh frozen plasma
$FiO_2$: fraction of inspired oxygen
Fr: French (gauge system used to measure catheter size)
FRC: functional residual capacity
FRSS: Forward Resuscitative Surgical System
FST: Forward Surgical Team
FTSG: full-thickness skin graft
FWB: fresh whole blood

**G**
g: gram
GCS: Glasgow Coma Scale
GSW: gunshot wound

## H

HEAT: high-explosive antitank
HFJV: high-frequency jet ventilation
HFOV: high-frequency oscillation ventilation
HFV: high-frequency ventilation
Hgb: hemoglobin
HIV: human immunodeficiency virus
HME: heat and moisture exchanger
HMMWV: High-Mobility Multipurpose Wheeled Vehicle ("Humvee")
HMX: cyclotetramethylene tetranitramine
HPMK: Hypothermia Prevention and Management Kit
HPPL: high-pressure pulsatile lavage
HR: heart rate
HSS: Health Services Support
HTS: hypertonic saline

## I

I:E: inspiratory to expiratory ratio
ICP: intracranial pressure
ICRC: International Committee for the Red Cross
ICU: intensive care unit
IED: improvised explosive device
I MEF: First Marine Expeditionary Force
in-lbs: inch-pounds
iNO: inhaled nitric oxide
INR: international normalized ratio
IO: intraosseous
IOFB: intraocular foreign body
IOP: intraocular pressure
IPEEP: intrinsic positive end-expiratory pressure
ISS: Injury Severity Score
IV: intravenous
IVC: inferior vena cava

## J

JP: Jackson Pratt
JPTA: Joint Patient Tracking Application
JTTR: Joint Theater Trauma Registry
JTTS: Joint Theater Trauma System

## K

KCl: potassium chloride
K.E.D.: Kendrick® Extrication Device
KIA: killed in action
K-wires: Kirschner wires

## L

labs: laboratory tests
LMA: laryngeal-mask airway
LOC: loss of consciousness
LOS: length of hospital stay
L:P: lactate to pyruvate ratio
LR: lactated Ringer's
LRMC: Landstuhl Regional Medical Center
LZ: landing zone

**M**

MACE: Military Acute Concussion Evaluation
MAP: mean arterial pressure
MASH: Mobile Army Surgical Hospital
mcg: microgram
MEDEVAC: medical evacuation
mEq: milliequivalent
METTAG: Medical Emergency Triage Tag
METT-TC: mission, equipment, terrain and weather, time, troops, and civilians
MFST: Mobile Field Surgical Team
mg: milligram
ml: milliliter
mm: millimeter
MODS: multiple organ dysfunction syndrome
mOsm: milliosmole
MRAP: mine-resistant ambush-protected (vehicles)
MRI: magnetic resonance imaging
MRSA: methicillin-resistant *Staphylococcus aureus*
m/sec: meters per second
MTF: Medical Treatment Facility

**N**

NASCIS: National Acute Spinal Cord Injury Study
NATO: North Atlantic Treaty Organization
NG: nasogastric
NICE-SUGAR: Normoglycemia in Intensive Care Evaluation-Survival Using Glucose Algorithm Regulation (study)
NIPPV: noninvasive positive-pressure ventilation
NIRS: near infrared spectroscopy
NOE: naso-orbito-ethmoid
NPO: nil per os (nothing by mouth)
NPV: negative-pressure ventilation
NS: normal saline
NSAID: nonsteroidal anti-inflammatory drug

**O**

OEF: Operation Enduring Freedom
OIF: Operation Iraqi Freedom
OR: operating room
OTFC: oral transmucosal fentanyl citrate

**P**

PA: posterior-anterior
PAd: pulmonary artery diastolic
PAI-1: plasminogen-activator inhibitor type 1
PALS: Pediatric Advanced Life Support
Palv: alveolar pressure
2-PAM: pralidoxime chloride
$PaO_2$: partial pressure of oxygen in arterial blood/arterial blood gas
PAs: pulmonary artery systolic
Patm: pressure above atmospheric pressure
PBW: predicted (ideal) body weight
$PCO_2$: partial pressure of carbon dioxide
PCR: patient care report
PCV: pressure-control ventilation
PCWP: pulmonary capillary wedge pressure
PE: pulmonary embolism
PEEP: positive end-expiratory pressure

PEEPh: high positive end-expiratory pressure
PEEPl: low positive end-expiratory pressure
PETN: pentaerythritol tetranitrate
pHi: gastric mucosal pH
PPE: personal protective equipment
Pplat: peak plateau pressure
PPV: positive-pressure ventilation
PRBCs: packed red blood cells
PROWESS: Recominant Human Activated Protein C Worldwide Evaluation in Severe Sepsis (trial)
PRVC: pressure-regulated volume control
PslCO$_2$: sublingual PCO$_2$
PSV: pressure-support ventilation
PT: prothrombin time
PTSD: posttraumatic stress disorder
PTTV: percutaneous transtracheal ventilation

## Q
Q: cardiac output; also areas of perfusion

## R
RBC: red blood cell
RDX: cyclotrimethylene trinitramine
REACH: Registry of Emergency Airways at Combat Hospital
RESCUEip: Randomized Evaluation of Surgery with Craniectomy for Uncontrollable Elevation of Intra-Cranial Pressure (trial)
RFVIIa: recombinant factor VIIa
RhAPC: recombinant human activated protein
RPG: rocket-propelled grenade
RR: respiratory rate
RSI: rapid sequence intubation
RTS: Revised Trauma Score

## S
SALT: Sort, Assess, Life-Saving, Triage/Treat/Transport
SaO$_2$: oxygen saturation of hemoglobin
SAPS: simplified acute physiology score
SBIR: Small Business Innovation Research
SBP: systolic blood pressure
SCIWORA: spinal cord injury without radiographic abnormality
ScvO$_2$: central venous oxygen saturation
SEAL: Sea-Air-Land (US Navy)
SIADH: syndrome of inappropriate antidiuretic hormone
SIMV: synchronized intermittent mandatory ventilation
SIRS: systemic inflammatory response syndrome
SOF: Special Operations Forces
SOMI: sternal occipital mandibular immobilizer
SPO$_2$: pulse oximeter oxygen saturation
SSTP: Surgical Shock Trauma Platoon
START®: Simple Triage And Rapid Treatment
StO$_2$: oxygen saturation of hemoglobin in tissue
STP: Shock Trauma Platoon
STSG: split-thickness skin graft
SvO$_2$: mixed venous oxygen saturation

## T
TACC: Tanker Airlift Control Center
TACEVAC: tactical evacuation
TATRC: Telemedicine and Advanced Technology and Research Center

TBI: traumatic brain injury
TBSA: total body surface area
TCA: tricarboxylic acid
TCCC: Tactical Combat Casualty Care
Th: high PEEP level
THAM: tromethamine
TIC: Troops in Contact
Tl: low PEEP level
TNT: 2,4,6-trinitrotoluene
TOC: Tactical Operations Center
TPN: total parenteral nutrition
TRICC: Tranfusion Requirements in Critical Care

**U**
US: United States
USAF: United States Air Force
USAISR: United States Army Institute of Surgical Research
USMC: United States Marine Corps
USN: United States Navy
USSOCOM: US Special Operations Command
UXO: unexploded ordnance

**V**
V: areas of ventilation
Va: alveolar ventilation
V.A.C.®: vacuum-assisted closure
VAP: ventilated-associated pneumonia
VASST: Vassopressin and Septic Shock Trial
VBIED: vehicle-borne improvised explosive device
$VCO_2$: carbon dioxide generated by the body
Vd: dead-space ventilation
VDR-4®: Volumetric Diffusive Respiration (ventilator)
Ve: minute ventilation
VEC: Vertebrace® Extrication Collar
VILI: ventilator-induced lung injury
$VO_2$: oxygen uptake
VS: vital signs; also Valsella Meccanotechnica SpA (producer of the VS-16 Italian antitank blast mine)
Vt: tidal volume
VTOL: Vertical Take-Off and Landing

**W**
WBB: walking blood bank
WBC: white blood cell
WDMET: Wound Data and Munitions Effectiveness Team
WRAMC: Walter Reed Army Medical Center
WWI: World War I
WWII: World War II

# Index